Crohn's Disease and Ulcerative Colitis: From Pathophysiology to Novel Therapeutic Approaches (2nd Edition)

Crohn's Disease and Ulcerative Colitis: From Pathophysiology to Novel Therapeutic Approaches (2nd Edition)

Guest Editor

Dingpei Long

MDPI

Basel • Beijing • Wuhan • Barcelona • Belgrade • Novi Sad • Cluj • Manchester

Guest Editor
Dingpei Long
Institute for Biomedical
Sciences
Georgia State University
Atlanta
USA

Editorial Office
MDPI AG
Grosspeteranlage 5
4052 Basel, Switzerland

This is a reprint of the Special Issue, published open access by the journal *Biomedicines* (ISSN 2227-9059), freely accessible at: https://www.mdpi.com/journal/biomedicines/special_issues/BDFO7J4Q6Q.

For citation purposes, cite each article independently as indicated on the article page online and as indicated below:

Lastname, A.A.; Lastname, B.B. Article Title. *Journal Name* **Year**, *Volume Number*, Page Range.

ISBN 978-3-7258-6394-5 (Hbk)
ISBN 978-3-7258-6395-2 (PDF)
https://doi.org/10.3390/books978-3-7258-6395-2

Contents

About the Editor

Dingpei Long

Dingpei Long received his BS, MS, and PhD degrees from Southwest University in Chongqing, China. He is a Specially Appointed Research Fellow and doctoral supervisor at the State Key Laboratory of Resource Insects, Southwest University. His research focuses on translational therapeutics for inflammatory bowel disease, integrating oral nanomedicines, microbiome-informed targeted delivery, and silk-based biomaterials to treat colonic inflammation and its complications, in line with this Reprint's emphasis on mechanism-guided, model-informed, patient-centered care. He completed postdoctoral and project-lead training at Georgia State University and conducted visiting research at Radboud University Nijmegen. He has led nearly twenty funded projects supported by the National Natural Science Foundation of China, Erasmus+, and the Crohn's and Colitis Foundation. His honors include National High-Level Youth Talent support, Chongqing Youth Talent awards, and a Young Investigator Award from the Crohn's and Colitis Congress. He has authored about sixty peer-reviewed papers, holds multiple patents, and serves on several journal editorial boards. As Guest Editor, he aims to bridge mucosal pathophysiology with microbiome-aware drug delivery and pragmatic clinical decision-making to accelerate precision therapy in inflammatory bowel disease.

Preface

This Reprint, Crohn's Disease and Ulcerative Colitis: From Pathophysiology to Novel Therapeutic Approaches, Second Edition, surveys contemporary science and care for inflammatory bowel disease. Its subject is the biology and management of Crohn's disease and ulcerative colitis. Its scope spans eighteen peer reviewed contributions, including basic and translational studies, clinical research, systematic reviews, and meta analyses. Our aim is to connect mechanisms with decisions at the bedside, to clarify where evidence is strong, and to highlight promising directions that merit careful testing.

The motivation for assembling this Reprint is twofold. First, rapid advances in mucosal immunology, genetics, and the microbiome are changing how we define targets and measure success. Second, the field now has tools to personalize therapy, from model informed dosing and route selection to pharmacogenetic markers of response, while keeping patient-centered outcomes and extraintestinal disease in view. The collection brings forward work on epithelial injury and pyroptosis, bile acid signaling, mucosa associated dysbiosis and oral pathobionts, comparative effectiveness of interleukin 12 and 23 blockade, and new links between IBD and related immune mediated diseases. Together, these studies outline a practical pathway toward precision care.

This Reprint is addressed to clinicians in gastroenterology and related specialties, to researchers in immunology, microbiology, pharmacology, and genetics, and to trainees who seek an integrated, current perspective. We hope it serves as a concise reference for daily practice and a catalyst for collaboration across disciplines.

Dingpei Long
Guest Editor

biomedicines

MDPI

Editorial

Mechanisms for Precision, Patient-Centered Therapy in Inflammatory Bowel Disease

Dingpei Long [1,2]

[1] State Key Laboratory of Resource Insects, Institute of Sericulture and Systems Biology, Southwest University, Chongqing 400715, China; dplong@swu.edu.cn
[2] Digestive Disease Research Group, Institute for Biomedical Sciences, Georgia State University, Atlanta, GA 30303, USA

1. Introduction

Inflammatory bowel disease (IBD), encompassing Crohn's disease (CD) and ulcerative colitis (UC), arises from genetic susceptibility, environmental triggers, dysbiotic microbiota, and mucosal immune dysregulation [1–4]. Aberrant innate and adaptive immune responses to commensals drive chronic injury, while bile acid signaling and epithelial barrier failure further modulate inflammation [5–7]. Dysbiosis extends across gut and oral niches. Mucosa-associated microbial shifts are linked to drug tolerance, and the detection of oral fungi and herpesviruses in IBD suggests a potential oral–gut axis [8–11]. Epidemiology shows a rising global burden with substantial complications and cancer risk, reinforcing treat-to-target care and multidisciplinary management of extraintestinal manifestations (EIMs) [3,12,13].

Diagnostic approaches are shifting from invasive endoscopy toward noninvasive biomarkers and histology: CRP and fecal calprotectin are widely used to monitor disease activity, while histologic healing correlates with outcomes and is increasingly pursued as a therapeutic goal [13–15]. Therapeutics have expanded beyond 5-ASA, steroids, and thiopurines to include biologics (anti-TNF, anti-integrin, anti-IL-12/23) and oral small molecules (JAK, S1P modulators), thereby improving remission rates and promoting mucosal healing. However, many patients still experience primary nonresponse, loss of response, or adverse events [7,8,16,17]. Real-world considerations include the possibility that co-therapy potentially attenuating vedolizumab effectiveness, as well as the use of pediatric combination strategies (e.g., methotrexate with infliximab) [18]. Lifestyle and dietary guidance merit individualized approaches; for instance, coffee is often neutral or beneficial rather than uniformly contraindicated [19]. Precision delivery and chemoprevention concepts are advancing via oral nano- and microtechnologies and biomaterials (including silk-based systems), with preclinical efficacy for colitis and colitis-associated neoplasia [20–22]. Moreover, comorbidities such as irritable bowel syndrome (IBS) overlap, fibromyalgia/chronic fatigue, and obesity with its proinflammatory effects further shape outcomes and care pathways [23]. Altogether, this Special Issue (Second Edition) comprises 18 articles that collectively traverse pathophysiology, diagnostics, and therapy, bridging laboratory insights with pragmatic clinical decision-making.

2. Cross-Cutting Themes: Toward Precise, Mechanism-Guided Care

Mechanistic convergence and tractable targets. A representative preclinical study demonstrates that inhibiting caspase-1-dependent pyroptosis via TLR4/NF-κB and inflammasome pathways attenuates colitis and repairs barrier function, positioning pyroptosis as a promising therapeutic axis in UC [24]. Complementing innate immune targets, a narrative synthesis highlights epithelial, immune, and microbial crosstalk as the foundation for both current and emerging therapies [25], while a state-of-the-art review details how bile acids operate as signaling metabolites with therapeutic leverage points across receptors and metabolic circuits [26].

Microbiome-aware management. Multiple studies illustrate that mucosa-associated dysbiosis and even extra-intestinal microbial niches may shape clinical phenotypes and treatment tolerance. A study in UC links 5-aminosalicylic acid intolerance with specific mucosal microbial signatures [27], whereas a study in CD describes how commonly used therapies (5-ASA, azathioprine, infliximab) are associated with shifts toward short-chain-fatty-acid producers [28]. Extending beyond the gut, a focused study catalogs emerging oral fungi and herpesviruses in IBD, underscoring an oral–gut axis relevant to opportunistic infection risk [29]. At the same time, a real-world analysis of dietary habits finds that coffee appears to be neutral or even beneficial for inflammation in many patients, supporting individualized counseling over blanket restriction [30]. Finally, a forward-looking review **distills microbiome targets and strategies** under development, from refined FMT to next-generation probiotics [31].

Model-informed therapeutics and precision selection. Pharmacologic contributions emphasize not only ***which*** drug to use, but ***how*** to use it. Physiologically based pharmacokinetic (PBPK) simulations raise route- and weight-specific considerations for infliximab, cautioning that flat subcutaneous dosing may under-expose heavier adults, while weight-band dosing is more appropriate in pediatric settings [32]. A formal external evaluation of vedolizumab population PK models underscores both current limitations and their utility for simulation-based dose planning [33]. A meta-analysis clarifies that subcutaneous and intravenous IL-12/23 blockades perform comparably for induction and maintenance in moderate-to-severe CD, enabling preference- and resource-sensitive route choice [34]. Beyond PK, whole-exome sequencing identifies variants enriched among vedolizumab non-responders (e.g., in classical IBD-immunity genes), foreshadowing pharmacogenetic triage for biologics [35]. A newly added genetics study identifies shared etiologies between IBD and several other immune-mediated diseases and reveals novel loci with functional annotations and mechanistic plausibility; these finding reinforce the importance of genotype-informed therapeutic stratification [36].

Patient-centered outcomes and systemic disease. Several reviews remind us that IBD is a systemic disorder: extraintestinal manifestations (EIMs) require multidisciplinary strategies [12], with ocular complications demanding coordinated gastro-ophthalmology care and awareness of therapy-related effects [37]. A population-based structural equation analysis shows that perceived health $\rightarrow$ control $\rightarrow$ acceptance is a reproducible pathway; in high-burden IMIDs such as IBD, acceptance exerts a particularly strong influence on lived experience, supporting the integration of psychosocial support into routine care [38].

3. Overview of the 18 Articles by Domain

3.1. Mechanisms and Preclinical Therapeutics

- **Pyroptosis inhibition in UC (original research)**. Inhibiting caspase-1-dependent pyroptosis through TLR4/NF-κB and inflammasome modulation reduces colitis and restores barrier integrity, highlighting pyroptosis as a promising druggable target [24].
- **Pathogenesis synthesis (review)**. This narrative review integrates epithelial, immune, microbial, and environmental cues to map IBD pathobiology and explores the resulting therapeutic implications [25].
- **Bile-acid signaling (review)**. Bile acids are reframed as signaling mediators with entry points for intervention at both the receptor and metabolic levels [26].

3.2. Microbiome, Diet, and Mucosal Healing

- **Mucosa-associated microbiota and drug intolerance (original research).** Patients with UC who have 5-ASA intolerance exhibit distinct mucosal microbiota compositions, suggesting that first-line treatment choices could be stratified based on microbiome profiles [27].
- **Drug–microbiome interplay in CD (original research).** Mesalazine, azathioprine, and infliximab use is associated with shifts toward short-chain fatty acid (SCFA)-producing taxa and greater microbial evenness relative to untreated disease [28].
- **Oral pathobionts in IBD (original research).** Fungal and viral colonization of the oral cavity is documented in IBD, highlighting a potential extraintestinal reservoir of dysbiosis [29].
- **Dietary perspective: coffee (original research).** In a real-world cohort, many patients continue coffee consumption and do not experience worsened symptoms. In UC, coffee users were observed to have lower fecal calprotectin levels, suggesting a benign or even beneficial effect [30].
- **Microbiome-targeted therapies (review).** This review provides an overview of fecal microbiota transplantation (FMT) refinement, live biotherapeutics, and engineered strategies aligned to host–microbe mechanisms [31].

3.3. Clinical Pharmacology and Comparative Effectiveness

- **Infliximab PBPK (original research).** Virtual adult and pediatric populations show route- and weight-dependent exposure differences; notably, flat subcutaneous (SC) dosing may underdose heavier adults, advocating for exposure-guided adjustments [32].
- **Vedolizumab population-PK models (original research).** An external evaluation suggests that existing models are imperfect for a priori individualization but are useful for simulation-guided regimen planning and, with therapeutic drug monitoring (TDM), for dose optimization [33].
- **IL-12/23 inhibitors: SC vs. IV (systematic review/meta-analysis).** Comparable efficacy and safety across routes support delivery aligned with patient preference in moderate-to-severe CD [34].
- **Pharmacogenetics of vedolizumab response (original research).** Whole-exome sequencing (WES) in a Middle Eastern cohort identifies rare variants enriched in non-responders across canonical IBD-inflammation genes, pointing to biomarker-guided biologic selection [35].

3.4. Clinical Management and Complications

- **Postoperative recurrence in CD (review/meta-analysis).** Risk stratification, endoscopic monitoring, and early biologic prophylaxis—often using an anti-TNF agent as first-line therapy—serve as the cornerstones of recurrence prevention and management [39].
- **Extraintestinal disease (review).** A comprehensive review of EIMs (extraintestinal manifestations) outlines the pathophysiology and treatment principles across joints, skin, eyes, and the hepatobiliary system, emphasizing the need for integrated care [12].
- **Ocular involvement (review).** Episcleritis tends to track with luminal disease activity, whereas uveitis often diverges. Notably, therapy can both treat ocular complications and, in rare cases, precipitate them—care pathways should anticipate both possibilities [37].

3.5. Genetics and Biomarkers

- **Shared genetic etiologies across IMIDs (original research—newly added).** Multi-trait genome-wide association studies (GWAS) and integrative analyses reveal significant genetic relationships between IBD and several other immune-mediated inflammatory diseases (e.g., axial spondyloarthritis, psoriasis, uveitis/iridocyclitis, psoriatic arthritis). These analyses also identify new loci with functional annotations. Together, these findings underscore a germline foundation for precision stratification [36].

- **Diagnostic/functional candidates in UC (original research).** SLC26A2 is downregulated in active UC and is linked to IL-17 signaling and epithelial barrier pathways, suggesting significant diagnostic and therapeutic relevance [40].

4. Looking Ahead

Priorities converge on mechanism-guided, model-informed, patient-centered precision care. First, mechanistic hypotheses (e.g., pyroptosis, epithelial transport, bile acid circuits) should be embedded in clinical trials and combination therapeutic strategies to move beyond the ceiling of monotherapy [6,7,41]. Second, precision dosing and route selection should be operationalized using PBPK and population-PK tools that support exposure-guided use of infliximab and vedolizumab. Subcutaneous vs. intravenous IL-12/23 blockade shows comparable efficacy, thereby enabling delivery based on patient preference [7,14,42,43]. Furthermore, pharmacogenetics data (for example, WES signals linked to vedolizumab nonresponse) should inform triage and sequencing. Third, treatment targets must broaden to include histologic remission, biomarker normalization, dysbiosis correction, and improved quality of life, aligning with treat-to-target frameworks and concurrent EIM management [12–15,43].

Microbiome-directed care is progressing from proof-of-concept to standardized platforms: multidonor FMT, defined consortia, and probiotic- and metabolite-based strategies tailored to host–microbe states [2,9,19]. Regenerative and interventional solutions—from mesenchymal cell therapies for fistulizing disease to advanced surgical-biologic hybrids—should be integrated with precision medicine pathways [41,43,44]. Real-world modifiers (e.g., concomitant proton pump inhibitor use), pediatric-to-adult transitions, and the immunometabolic impacts of obesity all warrant proactive management [18,45]. Adjacent innovations, oral nanomedicine and biomaterials for targeted delivery and chemoprevention, can reduce systemic exposure while sustaining mucosal control [20–22]. Finally, combination and sequencing algorithms—supported by decision frameworks and shared decision-making—aim to deliver durable, steroid-free remission with minimal complications for patients across diverse IBD phenotypes [13,17,41,43].

Funding: This work was supported by the Academician Foundation Program of Chongqing (cstb2023yszx-jcx0003), the Fundamental Research Funds for the Central Universities (SWU-KF25005), and the Venture and Innovation Support Program for Chongqing Overseas Returnees (cx2024003).

Acknowledgments: I am grateful to the authors of the published papers for their valuable contributions and to the reviewers for the rigorous evaluations. I also wish to express my gratitude to the editorial board of the journal for their support.

Conflicts of Interest: The author declares no conflict of interest.

References

1. Kaser, A.; Zeissig, S.; Blumberg, R.S. Inflammatory Bowel Disease. *Annu. Rev. Immunol.* **2010**, *28*, 573–621. [CrossRef]
2. Shan, Y.; Lee, M.; Chang, E.B. The Gut Microbiome and Inflammatory Bowel Diseases. *Annu. Rev. Med.* **2022**, *73*, 455–468. [CrossRef]
3. Zhang, Y.; Chu, X.; Wang, L.; Yang, H. Global patterns in the epidemiology, cancer risk, and surgical implications of inflammatory bowel disease. *Gastroenterol. Rep.* **2024**, *9*, 12. [CrossRef] [PubMed]
4. Solitano, V.; Bernstein, C.N.; Dotan, I.; Dignass, A.; Domislici, R.; Dubinsky, M.C.; Gearry, R.B.; Hart, A.; Kaplan, G.G.; Ma, C.; et al. Shaping the future of inflammatory bowel disease: A global research agenda for better management and public health response. *Nat. Rev. Gastro. Hepat.* **2025**, *22*, 438–452.

5. Peyrin-Biroulet, L.; Reinisch, W.; Colombel, J.; Mantzaris, G.J.; Kornbluth, A.; Diamond, R.; Rutgeerts, P.; Tang, L.K.; Cornillie, F.J.; Sandborn, W.J. Clinical disease activity, C-reactive protein normalization, and mucosal healing in Crohn's disease in the SONIC trial. *Gut* **2014**, *63*, 88–95. [CrossRef] [PubMed]
6. Neurath, M.F. Current and emerging therapeutic targets for IBD. *Nat. Rev. Gastroenterol. Hepatol.* **2017**, *14*, 269–278. [CrossRef]
7. Moschen, A.R.; Tilg, H.; Raine, T. IL-12, IL-23 and IL-17 in IBD: Immunobiology and therapeutic targeting. *Nat. Rev. Gastroenterol. Hepatol.* **2019**, *16*, 185–196. [CrossRef]
8. Raine, T.; Bonovas, S.; Burisch, J.; Kucharzik, T.; Adamina, M.; Annese, V.; Bachmann, O.; Bettenworth, D.; Chaparro, M.; Czuber-Dochan, W.; et al. ECCO Guidelines on Therapeutics in Ulcerative Colitis: Medical Treatment. *J. Crohn's Colitis* **2022**, *16*, 2–17. [CrossRef]
9. Xu, L.; Liu, B.; Huang, L.; Li, Z.; Cheng, Y.; Tian, Y.; Pan, G.; Li, H.; Xu, Y.; Wu, W.; et al. Probiotic Consortia and Their Metabolites Ameliorate the Symptoms of Inflammatory Bowel Diseases in a Colitis Mouse Model. *Microbiol. Spectr.* **2022**, *10*, e0065722. [CrossRef]
10. Sheng, K.; Xu, Y.; Kong, X.; Wang, J.; Zha, X.; Wang, Y. Probiotic Bacillus cereus Alleviates Dextran Sulfate Sodium-Induced Colitis in Mice through Improvement of the Intestinal Barrier Function, Anti-Inflammation, and Gut Microbiota Modulation. *J. Agric. Food Chem.* **2021**, *69*, 14810–14823. [CrossRef]
11. Jeong, J.J.; Kim, K.A.; Jang, S.E.; Woo, J.Y.; Han, M.J.; Kim, D.H. Orally Administrated Lactobacillus pentosus var. plantarum C29 Ameliorates Age-Dependent Colitis by Inhibiting the NF-κB Signaling Pathway via the Regulation of Lipopolysaccharide Production by Gut Microbiota. *PLoS ONE* **2015**, *10*, e0116533. [CrossRef]
12. Faggiani, I.; Fanizza, J.; D'Amico, F.; Allocca, M.; Zilli, A.; Parigi, T.L.; Barchi, A.; Danese, S.; Furfaro, F. Extraintestinal Manifestations in Inflammatory Bowel Disease: From Pathophysiology to Treatment. *Biomedicines* **2024**, *12*, 1839. [CrossRef]
13. Kelly, C.; Sartor, R.B.; Rawls, J.F. Early subclinical stages of the inflammatory bowel diseases: Insights from human and animal studies. *Am. J. Physiol-Gastrl.* **2025**, *328*, G17–G31. [CrossRef] [PubMed]
14. Sands, B.E. Biomarkers of Inflammation in Inflammatory Bowel Disease. *Gastroenterology* **2015**, *149*, 1275–1285.e2. [CrossRef] [PubMed]
15. Louis, E. Fecal calprotectin: Towards a standardized use for inflammatory bowel disease management in routine practice. *J. Crohn's Colitis* **2014**, *9*, 1–3. [CrossRef] [PubMed]
16. Feagan, B.G.; Rutgeerts, P.; Sands, B.E.; Hanauer, S.; Colombel, J.F.; Sandborn, W.J.; Assche, G.V.; Axler, J.; Kim, H.-J.; Danese, S. Vedolizumab as Induction and Maintenance Therapy for Ulcerative Colitis. *N. Engl. J. Med.* **2013**, *369*, 699–710. [CrossRef]
17. Jeong, D.Y.; Kim, S.; Son, M.J.; Son, C.Y.; Kim, J.Y.; Kronbichler, A.; Lee, K.H.; Shin, J.I. Induction and maintenance treatment of inflammatory bowel disease: A comprehensive review. *Autoimmun. Rev.* **2019**, *18*, 439–454. [CrossRef]
18. Szemes, K.; Farkas, N.; Sipos, Z.; Bor, R.; Fabian, A.; Szepes, Z.; Farkas, K.; Molnar, T.; Schafer, E.; Szamosi, T.; et al. Co-Administration of Proton Pump Inhibitors May Negatively Affect the Outcome in Inflammatory Bowel Disease Treated with Vedolizumab. *Biomedicines* **2024**, *12*, 158. [CrossRef]
19. Paramsothy, S.; Yang, Y.; Zhang, J.; Wang, R.; Cheng, B.; Kalambhe, D.; Wang, Y.; Gu, Z.; Chen, D.; Wang, B.; et al. Multidonor intensive fecal microbiota transplantation for active ulcerative colitis: A randomized placebo-controlled trial. *Lancet* **2017**, *389*, 1218–1228. [CrossRef]
20. Zhao, Y.; Yang, Y.; Zhang, J.; Wang, R.; Cheng, B.; Kalambhe, D.; Wang, Y.; Gu, Z.; Chen, D.; Wang, B.; et al. Lactoferrin-mediated macrophage targeting delivery and patchouli alcohol-based therapeutic strategy for inflammatory bowel diseases. *Acta Pharm. Sin. B* **2020**, *10*, 1966–1976. [CrossRef]
21. Long, D.; Merlin, D. Micro- and nanotechnological delivery platforms for treatment of dysbiosis-related inflammatory bowel disease. *Nanomedicine* **2021**, *16*, 1741–1745. [CrossRef]
22. Long, D.; Alghoul, Z.; Sung, J.; Yang, C.; Merlin, D. Oral administration of M13-loaded nanoliposomes is safe and effective to treat colitis-associated cancer in mice. *Expert Opin. Drug Deliv.* **2023**, *20*, 1443–1462. [CrossRef] [PubMed]
23. Black, C.J.; Ford, A.C. Irritable bowel syndrome: A spotlight on future research needs. *Lancet Gastroenterol.* **2021**, *6*, 419–422.
24. Li, J.; Wu, H.; Zhou, J.; Jiang, R.; Zhuo, Z.; Yang, Q.; Chen, H.; Sha, W. Ruscogenin Attenuates Ulcerative Colitis in Mice by Inhibiting Caspase-1-Dependent Pyroptosis via the TLR4/NF-κB Signaling Pathway. *Biomedicines* **2024**, *12*, 989.
25. Calvez, V.; Puca, P.; Di Vincenzo, F.; Del Gaudio, A.; Bartocci, B.; Murgiano, M.; Iaccarino, J.; Parand, E.; Napolitano, D.; Pugliese, D.; et al. Novel Insights into the Pathogenesis of Inflammatory Bowel Diseases. *Biomedicines* **2025**, *13*, 305. [CrossRef]
26. Bai, S.H.; Chandnani, A.; Cao, S. Bile Acids in Inflammatory Bowel Disease: From Pathophysiology to Treatment. *Biomedicines* **2024**, *12*, 2910. [CrossRef]
27. Matsumoto, H.; Sasahira, M.; Go, T.T.; Yo, S.; Ninomiya, T.; Osawa, M.; Handa, O.; Umegami, E.; Inoue, R.; Shiotani, A. Characteristics of Mucosa-Associated Microbiota in Ulcerative Colitis Patients with 5-Aminosalicylic Acid Intolerance. *Biomedicines* **2024**, *12*, 2125. [CrossRef]
28. Yang, X.; Zhang, Y.; Gao, C.; Pan, Y.; Du, S.; Xiao, S.; Zhou, Z. The Effect of Drugs on the Intestinal Microbiota in Crohn's Disease. *Biomedicines* **2024**, *12*, 2241. [CrossRef]

29. Oliveira, M.M.E.; Campos, L.B.; Brito, F.; de Carvalho, F.M.; Silva-Junior, G.O.; da Costa, G.L.; Pinto, T.N.; de Sousa, R.M.P.; Miranda, R.; Castro, R.; et al. Oral Microbiota and Inflammatory Bowel Diseases: Detection of Emerging Fungal Pathogens and Herpesvirus. *Biomedicines* **2025**, *13*, 480. [CrossRef]
30. Neamți, L.; Gheorghe, S.R.; Ventuneac, A.; Drugan, T.; Drugan, C.; Silaghi, C.N.; Ciobanu, L.; Crăciun, A.M. Impact of Coffee Consumption on Subjective Perception and Inflammatory Markers in Patients with Inflammatory Bowel Diseases. *Biomedicines* **2024**, *12*, 1733. [CrossRef]
31. Sivakumar, N.; Krishnamoorthy, A.; Ryali, H.; Arasaradnam, R.P. Gut Microbial Targets in Inflammatory Bowel Disease: Current Position and Future Developments. *Biomedicines* **2025**, *13*, 716. [CrossRef]
32. Petric, Z.; Gonçalves, J.; Paixão, P. Infliximab in Inflammatory Bowel Disease: Leveraging Physiologically Based Pharmacokinetic Modeling in the Clinical Context. *Biomedicines* **2024**, *12*, 1974. [CrossRef]
33. Jovanović, M.; Homšek, A.; Marković, S.; Kralj, Đ.; Svorcan, P.; Knežević Ivanovski, T.; Odanović, O.; Vučićević, K. Review and External Evaluation of Population Pharmacokinetic Models for Vedolizumab in Patients with Inflammatory Bowel Disease: Assessing Predictive Performance and Clinical Applicability. *Biomedicines* **2025**, *13*, 43. [CrossRef] [PubMed]
34. Alwisi, N.; Ismail, R.; Al-Kuwari, H.; Al-Ansari, K.H.; Al-Matwi, M.A.; Aweer, N.A.; Al-Marri, W.N.; Al-Kubaisi, Y.; Al-Mohannadi, M.; Hamran, S.; et al. Comparative Efficacy of Subcutaneous Versus Intravenous Interleukin 12/23 Inhibitors for the Remission of Moderate to Severe Crohn's Disease: A Systematic Review and Meta-Analysis. *Biomedicines* **2025**, *13*, 702. [CrossRef] [PubMed]
35. Aljohani, H.; Anbarserry, D.; Mosli, M.; Ujaimi, A.; Bakhshwin, D.; Elango, R. High-Throughput Whole-Exome Sequencing and Large-Scale Computational Analysis to Identify the Genetic Biomarkers to Predict the Vedolizumab Response Status in Inflammatory Bowel Disease Patients from Saudi Arabia. *Biomedicines* **2025**, *13*, 459. [CrossRef] [PubMed]
36. Liu, X.; Li, D.; Zhang, Y.; Liu, H.; Chen, P.; Zhao, Y.; Ruscitti, P.; Zhao, W.; Dong, G. Identifying Common Genetic Etiologies Between Inflammatory Bowel Disease and Related Immune-Mediated Diseases. *Biomedicines* **2024**, *12*, 2562. [CrossRef]
37. Richardson, H.; Yoon, G.; Moussa, G.; Kumar, A.; Harvey, P. Ocular Manifestations of IBD: Pathophysiology, Epidemiology, and Iatrogenic Associations of Emerging Treatment Strategies. *Biomedicines* **2024**, *12*, 2856. [CrossRef]
38. Folkertsma, T.S.; Bloem, S.; Vodegel, R.M.; Bos, R.; Tack, G.J. Disease Acceptance and Control from the Subjective Health Experience Model as Health Perception Predictors in Immune-Mediated Inflammatory Diseases. *Biomedicines* **2025**, *13*, 538. [CrossRef]
39. Olteanu, A.O.; Klimko, A.; Tieranu, E.N.; Bota, A.D.; Preda, C.M.; Tieranu, I.; Pavel, C.; Pahomeanu, M.R.; Toma, C.V.; Saftoiu, A.; et al. Managing Crohn's Disease Postoperative Recurrence Beyond Prophylaxis: A Comprehensive Review with Meta-Analysis. *Biomedicines* **2024**, *12*, 2434. [CrossRef]
40. Qian, L.; Hu, S.; Zhao, H.; Han, Y.; Dai, C.; Zan, X.; Zhi, Q.; Xu, C. The Diagnostic Significance of SLC26A2 and Its Potential Role in Ulcerative Colitis. *Biomedicines* **2025**, *13*, 461. [CrossRef]
41. Wang, K.; Zhu, Y.; Liu, K.; Zhu, H.; Ouyang, M. Adverse events of biologic or small molecule therapies in clinical trials for inflammatory bowel disease: A systematic review and meta-analysis. *Heliyon* **2024**, *10*, e25357. [CrossRef]
42. Hou, Q.; Huang, J.; Ayansola, H.; Masatoshi, H.; Zhang, B. Intestinal Stem Cells and Immune Cell Relationships: Potential Therapeutic Targets for Inflammatory Bowel Diseases. *Front. Immunol.* **2021**, *11*, 623691. [CrossRef]
43. Weizman, A.V.; Nguyen, G.C.; Seow, C.H.; Targownik, L.; Murthy, S.K.; Boland, K.; Afzal, N.M.; Khanna, R.; Jones, J.; Afif, W.; et al. Appropriateness of biologics in the management of Crohn's disease using RAND/UCLA appropriateness methodology. *Inflamm. Bowel Dis.* **2019**, *25*, 328–335. [CrossRef]
44. DeLeon, M.F.; Hull, T.L. Treatment Strategies in Crohn's-Associated Rectovaginal Fistula. *Clin. Colon Rectal Surg.* **2019**, *32*, 261–267. [CrossRef]
45. Versini, M.; Jeandel, P.Y.; Rosenthal, E.; Shoenfeld, Y. Obesity in autoimmune diseases: Not a passive bystander. *Autoimmun. Rev.* **2014**, *13*, 981–1000. [CrossRef]

biomedicines

MDPI

Article

Ruscogenin Attenuates Ulcerative Colitis in Mice by Inhibiting Caspase-1-Dependent Pyroptosis via the TLR4/NF-κB Signaling Pathway

Jingwei Li [1,†], Huihuan Wu [2,†], Jialiang Zhou [3], Rui Jiang [1], Zewei Zhuo [1], Qi Yang [1], Hao Chen [1,*] and Weihong Sha [1,*]

1 Department of Gastroenterology, Guangdong Provincial People's Hospital (Guangdong Academy of Medical Sciences), Southern Medical University, Guangzhou 510080, China; lijingwei@gdph.org.cn (J.L.); 202121050713@mail.scut.edu.cn (R.J.); zhuozewei@gdph.org.cn (Z.Z.); yangqi5056@163.com (Q.Y.)

2 Department of Gastroenterology, The Sixth Affiliated Hospital, School of Medicine, South China University of Technology, Foshan 528200, China; wuhuihuan@gdph.org.cn

3 Department of Neonatal Surgery, Guangdong Women and Children Hospital, Guangzhou 511400, China

* Correspondence: chenhao@gdph.org.cn (H.C.); shaweihong@gdph.org.cn (W.S.)

† These authors contributed equally to this work.

Abstract: Inflammatory bowel diseases (IBD) are chronic inflammatory disorders affecting the digestive tract, including ulcerative colitis and Crohn's disease. Ruscogenin, a prominent steroidal sapogenin present in radix ophiopogon japonicus, has shown a protective effect on attenuating the inflammatory response associated with inflammatory diseases, but the efficacy of ruscogenin in IBD remains unclear. The aim of this study is to explore the effect of ruscogenin on intestinal barrier dysfunction and inflammatory responses as well as the underlying mechanism in ulcerative colitis. A dextran sulfate sodium salt (DSS)-induced C57BL/6 mouse colitis model was employed for the in vivo studies, while in vitro experiments were performed in THP-1 cells and human intestinal epithelial cells involved in inducing inflammatory responses and pyroptosis using LPS/nigericin. The results indicated that ruscogenin treatment attenuated the symptoms of ulcerative colitis, reduced the release of inflammatory cytokines and the expression of pyroptosis-associated proteins, and restored the integrity of the intestinal epithelial barrier in colon tissue in mice. Moreover, ruscogenin inhibited LPS/nigericin-induced pyroptosis in THP-1 cells. Mechanically, ruscogenin inhibited NLRP3 inflammasome activation and canonical pyroptosis, at least in part, through the suppression of the TLR4/NF-κB signaling pathway. These findings might provide new insights and a solid foundation for further exploration into the therapeutic potential of ruscogenin in the treatment of IBD.

Keywords: ruscogenin; ulcerative colitis; pyroptosis; caspase-1; TLR4

1. Introduction

Inflammatory bowel diseases (IBD) are chronic inflammatory disorders affecting the gastrointestinal tract, with ulcerative colitis (UC) and Crohn's disease being the two primary subtypes [1,2]. These conditions are characterized by recurring episodes of inflammation in the intestines, leading to various debilitating symptoms and impaired quality of life for affected individuals. The incidence and prevalence of IBD in the newly industrialized countries in Asia, the Middle East, and South America have steadily increased over the past decade [3]. It is estimated that an ageing IBD population will bring new challenges and complexities to gastroenterology clinics in the world in 2025 [4]. The etiology of IBD remains complex and multifactorial, but researchers have recently confirmed that dysregulated immune responses, defects in the intestinal epithelial barrier, and altered cell death processes play vital roles in the pathogenesis of these diseases [5]. To date, the main drug for the treatment of IBD include 5-aminosalicylates, corticosteroids, immunosuppressive drugs, and biological drug targeting at cytokines. Nevertheless, the prohibitive cost of monoclonal antibodies and the potential side effects associated with corticosteroids and immunosuppressive drugs impose limitations on their long-term utilization [6]. The development of novel drugs and improvement of the treatment strategy by implementing personalized medicine are warranted to achieve optimal disease control. Therefore, the development of potential innovative strategies for IBD treatment is highly urgent.

Pyroptosis is a highly regulated form of programmed cell death, which is a physiological response to host defense against microbial infections and tissue injury [7]. Pyroptosis plays an vital role in the occurrence and progression of various inflammatory diseases such as IBD [8,9]. The activation of pyroptosis involves different caspases, the most significant of which is the canonical pyroptosis pathway dependent on caspase-1 [10]. In the canonical pyroptosis pathway, the activation of the NLRP3 inflammasome recruits ASC and caspase-1 precursors and leads to subsequent activation of caspase-1. On the one hand, activated caspase-1 cleaves GSDMD to produce the N terminus, which binds to the cell membrane to form a membrane pore, leading to cell rupture. At the same time, activated caspase-1 cleaves and activates the inflammatory cytokines IL-1β and IL-18, which are then released to the outside of the cell through the membrane pores to cause inflammation. Moderate pyroptosis eradicates pathogenic microorganisms and induces tissue repair and slowly subsides after the removal of foreign bodies or repair of tissue damage. The vicious circle of dysregulated cell death, intestinal barrier destruction, and consequent inflammation lies at the core of chronic inflammatory diseases [11]. Thus, the accurate regulation of pyroptosis is a potential therapeutic strategy for IBD.

The Toll-like receptors 4 (TLR4) pathway is a key player in pyroptosis [12]. When cells are exposed to exogenous or endogenous stimuli, the pattern recognition receptors (PRRs) on the cell membrane activates TLR4 by recognizing pathogen-associated molecular patterns (PAMPs) or damage-associated molecular patterns (DAMPs) released by body cells. TLR4 promotes the transfer of nuclear transcription factor NF-κB into the nucleus through the MyD88 pathway. Then, NF-κB can not only promote the expression of NLRP3 to participate in the regulation of inflammasomes but also promote the expression of various pro-inflammatory genes, including inflammatory cytokines and chemokines [13]. Therefore, TLR4/NF-κB signaling pathways play an important role in regulating inflammatory responses and pyroptosis [14].

Given the complexity and limited treatment options for IBD, researchers have turned their attention to herbal medicine as potential interventions [15]. Ruscogenin, a prominent steroidal sapogenin present in radix ophiopogon japonicus, has emerged as a promising candidate for attenuating the inflammatory response associated with inflammatory diseases and cardiovascular diseases [16]. Notably, a previous study uncovered that ruscogenin has a protective effect on lung epithelial injury induced by LPS, and the possible mechanism is related to the inhibition of the NF-κB signaling pathway [17]. Moreover, recent studies have shown that ruscogenin alleviates particulate acute lung injury in mice by protecting the pulmonary endothelial barrier and inhibiting the TLR4 signaling pathway [18,19]. Another study found that ruscogenin attenuates cerebral ischemia-induced blood–brain barrier dysfunction by inhibiting NLRP3 inflammasome activation [20]. However, to date, there is a dearth of literature documenting the utilization of ruscogenin as a therapeutic intervention for IBD. In addition, the efficacy and mechanism of ruscogenin in ameliorating dextran sulfate sodium salt (DSS)-induced colitis by mitigating the extent of pyroptosis through regulating TLR4/NF-κB signaling pathway remains unclear and deserves further investigation.

In summary, we hypothesize that the administration of ruscogenin can attenuate DSS-induced colitis by improving intestinal barrier function, reducing the inflammation response and regulating pyroptosis via TLR4/NF-κB signaling pathway. The main purpose of this study is to elucidate the specific mechanism of ruscogenin in treating DSS-induced colitis model. The results of this study will provide promising treatment options and theoretical basis for the treatment of IBD patients.

2. Materials and Methods

2.1. Animal Experiments

SPF male C57BL/6 mice aged 6–8 weeks (weight 18–25 g) were purchased from Guangdong Province Animal Experiment Center. The mice were acclimated in their cages for a week before the experiments were conducted. The animals were maintained in standard condition at 23 ± 2 °C and (50 ± 10) % humidity, with a 12/12 h light and dark cycle and free access to water and food. All animal care and experiments were carried out in accordance with institutional animal care and use committee guidelines, and the procedures were approved by the ethics committee of Guangdong Provincial People's Hospital, Guangzhou, China (approval number: KY-N-2022-084-02; approval date: 30 August 2022).

2.2. Chemicals and Reagents

Ruscogenin (Rus, purity 99%; chemical formula: C27H42O4; molecular weight: 430.62) was purchased from J&K Scientific Ltd. (San Jose, CA, USA). Dextran sulfate sodium salt (DSS, molecular weight: 36,000–50,000) was purchased from MP Biomedicals (Irvine, CA, USA). Dulbecco's modified eagle medium (DMEM), RPMI 1640 medium, and fetal bovine serum (FBS) were purchased from Gibco (Carlsbad, CA, USA). LPS was purchased from Sigma-Aldrich (St. Louis, MO, USA). Nigericin was purchased from Invitrogen (Carlsbad, CA, USA). Overexpression plasmids for Flag-tagged TLR4 (pLV3-CMV-TLR4(human)-3×Flag-EF1a-CopGFP-Puro) and control plasmid were purchased from Miaoling Biology (Wuhan, China). The primary antibodies using in Western blotting were purchased from Abcam (Cambridge, UK) and Cell Signaling Technology (Boston, MA, USA), and the HRP-conjugated anti-rabbit and anti-mouse IgG antibodies were purchased from Cell Signaling Technology (Boston, MA, USA). The primary antibodies and the appropriate fluorescence conjugated secondary antibodies used in immunofluorescence staining were purchased from Abcam (Cambridge, UK).

2.3. DSS-Induced Colitis Model and Animal Experiment Design

The SPF male C57BL/6 mice were randomly divided into five groups. The mice in the control group (Ctrl) were treated with drinking water. The mice in the DSS model group (DSS) were administered drinking water that contains 3.5% DSS for 7 days. The mice in the Rus 0.5 mg/kg group (Rus 0.5) were administered drinking water containing 3.5% DSS for 7 days, followed by 0.5 mg/kg ruscogenin treatment by gavage daily. The mice in the Rus 5 mg/kg group (Rus 1) were administered drinking water containing 3.5% DSS for 7 days, followed by 1.0 mg/kg ruscogenin treatment by gavage daily. The mice in the Rus 2 mg/kg group (Rus 2) were administered drinking water containing 3.5% DSS for 7 days, followed by 2.0 mg/kg Ruscogenin treatment by gavage daily. Animals were monitored daily by weight and disease activity index score. After 7 days, the drinking water was switched to normal water for 1 day, and all the mice were euthanized on day 8. The serum and colon tissues samples were collected for subsequent analysis. The colon was excised from the cecum to 2 cm above the anus. The length of the colon was measured, which indirectly specified the inflammatory index of the colon.

2.4. Assessment of Disease Activity Index

To evaluate the disease activity index (DAI) of the mice in each group, the body weight, feces shape, and gross rectal bleeding of the mice were recorded and scored, according to the previous study [21]. In short, (1) loss of weight: less than 1%, score 0; less than 5%, greater than 1%, score 1; less than 10%, greater than 5%, score 2; less than 20% but greater than 10%, score 3; more than 20%, score 4; (2) feces shape: normal shape, score 0; loose stools score 1; liquid stools, score 3; and diarrhea score 4; (3) gross rectal bleeding: normal, score 0; mild bleeding, score 2; obvious bleeding, score 4.

2.5. Histological Evaluation

After 8 days, the mice were euthanized, and the colon tissues of each group were collected. The colon tissues were fixed with 10% formalin and embedded in paraffin. Then, colon tissues were cut into slices and stained with hematoxylin and eosin (H&E). The histology score was determined by multiplying the percent involvement of each of the five histological subscores [22]. For each parameter (0, absent; 1, mild; 2, moderate; 3, severe): mononuclear cell infiltrate (0–3), epithelial injury/erosion (0–3), crypt hyperplasia (0–3), polymorphonuclear cell infiltrates (0–3), and transmural inflammation (0–4). Extent factor was derived according to percent area involvement: 0, 0%; 1, <10%; 2, 10–25%; 3, 25–50%; and 4, >50%.

2.6. Cell Culture

Human acute monocytic leukemia THP-1 was purchased from Cell Bank of the Chinese Academy of Sciences (Shanghai, China). THP-1 cells were cultured in RPMI 1640 medium, supplemented with 10% FBS and 0.05 mM β-mercaptoethanol. Human intestinal epithelial cells (HIEC) and HEK-293T cells were purchased from Cell Bank of the Chinese Academy of Sciences (Shanghai, China) and were maintained in DMEM with 10% FBS. Cells were cultured in a humidified environment with 5% CO_2 at 37 °C. Differentiation of THP-1 cells was induced by 0.5 mM phorbol 12-myristate 13-acetate (PMA, Sigma Aldrich, St. Louis, MO, USA) for 3 h. The differentiated cells were washed three times with PBS. In this study, cells were seeded in 6-well plates at a density of 5×10^6 cells per well overnight. THP-1 cells were stimulated with LPS and nigericin to activate NLRP3 inflammasomes to mimic inflammatory environment in vitro. First, the cells were pre-treated with DMSO or different concentrations of ruscogenin for 24 h (2.5 μmol/L, 5 μmol/L, and 10 μmol/L), then treated with 100 ng/mL LPS, or left untreated for 4 h in serum-free medium, followed by treatment with 1 μM nigericin (Invitrogen, Carlsbad, CA, USA) for 4 h, as previously described [23]. The experimental groups for this study were defined as follows: Ctrl: normal control group; LPS: 100 ng/mL LPS exposure for 4 h and followed by treatment with 1 μM nigericin for 4 h; Rus 2.5 μM: 2.5 μM ruscogenin pretreatment for 24 h prior to LPS exposure for 4 h, followed by treatment with 1 μM nigericin for 4 h; Rus 5 μM: 5 μM ruscogenin pretreatment for 24 h prior to LPS exposure for 4 h, followed by treatment with 1 μM nigericin for 4 h; Rus 10 μM: 10 μM ruscogenin pretreatment for 24 h prior to 100 ng/mL LPS exposure for 4 h, followed by treatment with 1 μM nigericin for 4 h. For TLR4 overexpression experiment, normal THP-1 cells were treated with LPS/nigericin or ruscogenin (10 μM). THP-1 cells transfected with TLR4-plasmid were treated with LPS/nigericin and ruscogenin (10 μM). In brief, DMSO or 10 μM ruscogenin pretreatment for 24 h prior to 100 ng/mL LPS exposure was followed by treatment with 1 μM nigericin for 4 h.

2.7. Cell Viability Assay

The effects of ruscogenin on THP-1 cells was measured by using the cell counting kit-8 (CCK-8) assay (Guangzhou Bin Peng Biotechnology, Guangzhou, China). In brief, THP-1 cells were seeded in 96-well plates at 5×10^4 per well overnight. Cells were treated with complete medium containing ruscogenin (0–320 μM) for 24 h, and then, 10 μL of CCK-8 reagent was added to each well and incubated for 2–3 h at 37 °C. The optical density (OD) value at 450 nm was detected using a microplate reader.

2.8. Cell Transfection

To further clarify the potential molecular mechanism of ruscogenin in inhibiting LPS/nigericin-primed pyroptosis, HEK-293T cells were transfected with Flag-TLR4 plasmid and control plasmid using Lipofectamine 2000 (Invitrogen, Carlsbad, CA, USA), and then, the culture medium was changed to normal complete medium after 4–6 h. THP-1 cells were cultured in 6-well plates. After 48 h and 72 h, viral fluids were obtained and used to infect THP-1 cells. After transfection, puromycin was used to select successfully transfected THP-1 cells.

2.9. ELISA

The levels of IL-6, TNF-α, MCP-1, and IL-18 in the colon tissue of the mice and the collected cell culture media were detected by ELISA kits (Proteintech, Wuhan, China; Cusabio, Beijing, China; Beyotime Biotechnology, Shanghai, China). The assay followed the instruction manual.

2.10. Quantitative Real-Time Polymerase Chain Reaction (qPCR)

Total RNA were extracted from colon tissues and cells using the Total RNA Isolation Kit (Vazyme, Nanjing, China). Reverse transcription was carried out using the Prime Script TM RT-PCR Kit (Takara, Otsu, Japan). Then, qPCR was performed with the Biorad CFX Connect (Biorad, Hercules, CA, USA) using the ChamQ Universal SYBR qPCR Master Mix (Vazyme, Nanjing, China), according to the manufacturer's instructions. The $2^{-\Delta\Delta Ct}$ method was used to calculate the relative expressions of mRNAs, and the levels of the target genes were normalized to that of the *GAPDH* gene. Primer sequences used in this study are listed in Table S1.

2.11. Western Blotting

The Western blotting was carried out exactly as previously described [24]. The total proteins were extracted from mice colon tissues and cells as well as supernatant with RIPA lysis buffer containing protease and phosphatase inhibitor (Beyotime Biotechnology, Shanghai, China). The protein concentrations were determined with an BCA protein assay kit (Leagene Biotechnology, Beijing, China). The samples were prepared in 4× sodium dodecyl sulfate–polyacrylamide gel electrophoresis (SDS-PAGE) sample loading buffer (Invitrogen, Carlsbad, CA, USA). Protein samples were subjected to SDS-PAGE and transferred to PVDF membranes. After incubation with 5% non-fat milk, the membranes were incubated with indicated primary antibodies at 4 °C overnight. Then, the membranes were washed with TBS containing 0.1% Tween-20 (TBST) three times and then incubated with the HRP-conjugated anti-rabbit or anti-mouse IgG antibodies for 2 h at room temperature. Finally, the membranes were washed three times with TBST, the protein bands were visualized using an ECL Western Blotting Substrate (Biosharp, Anhui, China), and the signals were recorded with the Image Quant LAS 500 System (Cytiva, Marlborough, MA, USA). The results were quantified using Image J 1.8.0 software (http://rsb.info.nih.gov/ij/, accessed on 1 February 2024) and normalized to GAPDH or Tubulin. The antibodies used in this study are listed in Table S2.

2.12. Immunofluorescence Staining

Cells were seeded in confocal dish at a density of 5 × 10^3 cells overnight. The cells were pre-treated with DMSO or ruscogenin (2.5 μM, 5 μM, and 10 μM) for 24 h, then treated with 100 ng/mL LPS, or left untreated for 4 h, followed by treatment with 1 μM nigericin for the indicated time. After removing the culture medium, cells were washed three times with PBS and fixed in 4% paraformaldehyde at room temperature for 30 min. The fixed cells were washed with PBS and blocked with 5% goat serum in PBS for 30 min at room temperature. The cells were then incubated with primary antibody overnight at 4 °C. After that, the cells were washed three times with PBS containing 0.1% Tween-20 (PBST), followed by secondary antibodies. Finally, antifade mounting medium with DAPI (Sigma-Aldrich, St Louis, MO, USA) was used to stain the cell nuclei at an indicated concentration. At least five fields per dish were randomly selected for observation, and the semiquantitative analysis of relative fluorescence intensity was analyzed by Image J 1.8.0 software (http://rsb.info.nih.gov/ij/, accessed on 1 February 2024). The antibodies used in this study are listed in Table S2.

2.13. Statistical Analysis

Statistical analysis was performed using IBM SPSS Statistics 22.0 (Chicago, IL, USA) and GraphPad Prism 9.0 (GraphPad Software, San Diego, CA, USA). The data of continuous variables fitting a normal distribution are presented as mean ± SD, and at least three independent experiments were performed in duplicate. The comparison of means of two independent samples was performed by two-tailed unpaired Student's *t*-test. The comparisons of means of multiple groups were analyzed by one-way or two-way ANOVA followed by post hoc multiple comparisons. Data of non-continuous variables are presented as median (Q1, Q3), and the comparison of the medians of multiple independent samples was performed using the Kruskal–Wallis test, followed by Dunn's multiple comparisons test. A $p < 0.05$ was considered as statistically significant.

3. Results

3.1. Ruscogenin Treatment Inhibits LPS/Nigericin-Induced Inflammatory Responses in THP-1 Cell and Improves the Intestinal Epithelial Barrier Function in Injured HIEC

Macrophages are the main natural immune cells that play a vital role in inflammatory response. To detect the effect of ruscogenin in vitro, in this study, an in vitro macrophage inflammation model was established using THP-1 cells, wherein inflammation was induced by using LPS and nigericin. Firstly, the potential cytotoxicity of ruscogenin was evaluated by the CCK-8 assay. THP-1 cells were incubated with different concentrations of ruscogenin for 24 h. As shown in Figure 1A, ruscogenin treatment at concentrations below 20 μM for 24 h did not result in a decrease in the viability of THP-1 cells compared to the untreated control group. However, when the concentration of ruscogenin reached 20 μM, the cell viability of THP-1 was 9.3% lower than that of the control group (100% vs. 90.7%, $p = 0.03$), which means that slight toxicity was observed. Moreover, the cell viability of THP-1 decreased from 82.0% to 42.8% as the concentration of ruscogenin increased from 40 μM to 320 μM, exhibiting a significant dose-dependent cytotoxicity. Consequently, 2.5 μM, 5 μM, and 10 μM ruscogenin were selected as the low-, medium-, and high-dose groups, respectively, for further studies.

Inflammatory mediators are key players in the progression of IBD, contributing significantly to the advancement of the disease. To investigate whether ruscogenin possessed anti-inflammatory effects on THP-1 macrophages, THP-1 cells were treated with 2.5 μM, 5 μM, and 10 μM ruscogenin for 24 h. Subsequently, the cells were primed with 100 ng/mL LPS for 3 h in a serum-free medium, and then, the NLRP3 inflammasome was activated using 1 μM nigericin for 4 h. The supernatant levels of TNF-α, IL-6, and MCP-1 in the culture medium were detected via ELISA assay. After LPS stimulation, the concentrations of TNF-α, IL-6, and MCP-1 in the THP-1 cell supernatant surged to (485.5 ± 19.5), (708.0 ± 17.5), and (267.4 ± 8.4) pg/mL, respectively, which were at least three times higher than those in the control group ($p < 0.001$). Interestingly, ruscogenin treatment led to a significant decrease in the concentrations of these cytokine. Particularly, in the 10 μM ruscogenin treatment group, these cytokine concentrations decreased to (246.0 ± 17.3), (274.6 ± 14.2), and (75.9 ± 3.7) pg/mL, respectively ($p < 0.001$). Then, the mRNA expression of these inflammatory factors was detected with qPCR. Compared with the control group, the mRNA levels of TNF-α, IL-6, and MCP-1 were markedly elevated in the LPS group (Figure 1B–E). Interestingly, treatment with ruscogenin significantly reduced the mRNA levels of TNF-α, IL-6, and MCP-1, especially treatment with 10 μM ruscogenin ($p < 0.001$). These findings suggest that ruscogenin therapy may effectively mitigate the production of pro-inflammatory cytokines, thereby attenuating the inflammatory response.

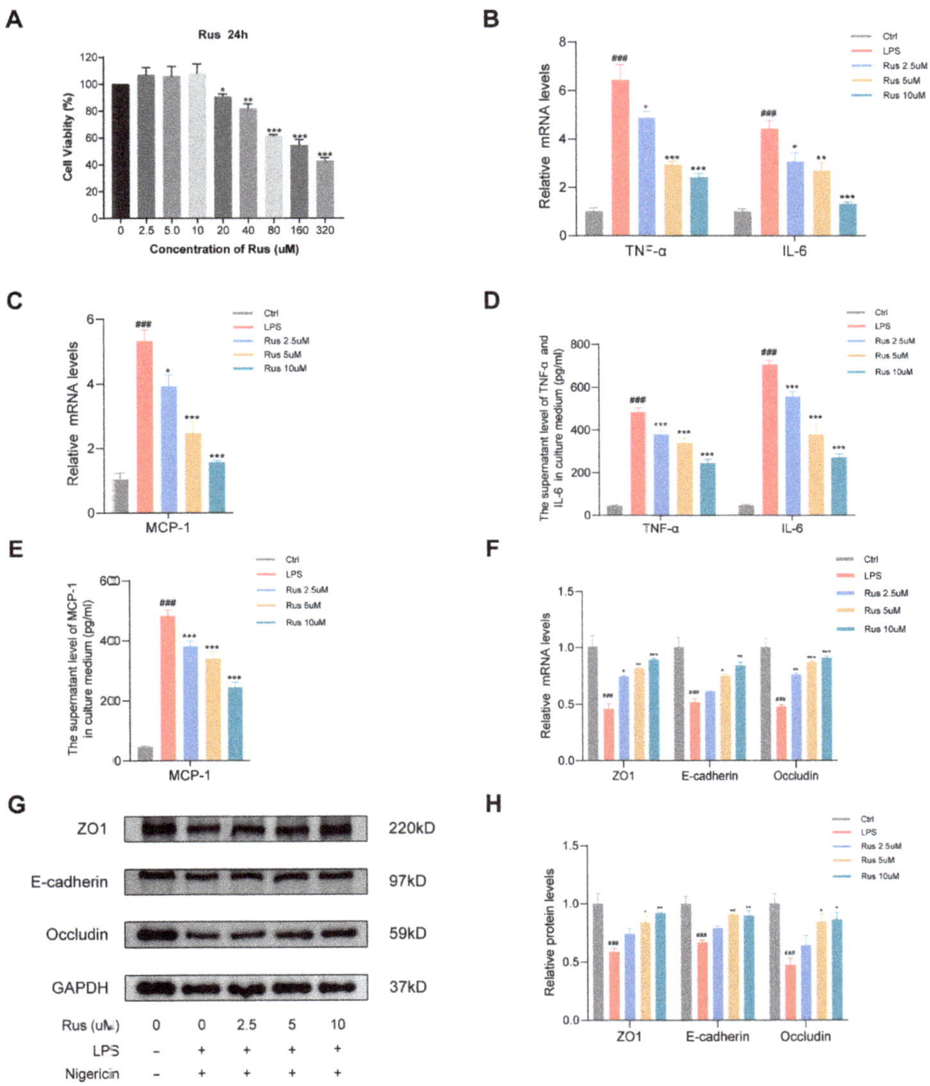

Figure 1. Ruscogenin treatment inhibited LPS-induced inflammatory responses in THP-1 cells and improves the intestinal epithelial barrier function in HIEC. (**A**) THP-1 cells were treated with DMSO or different concentrations of ruscogenin (2.5–320 μM) for 24 h, and the cell viability was determined by CCK-8 assay. (**B**,**C**) The mRNA expression of TNF-α, IL-6, and MCP-1 was detected with qPCR in THP-1 cells. (**D**,**E**) The supernatant levels of TNF-α, IL-6, and MCP-1 in the culture medium of THP-1 cells were detected via ELISA assay. (**F**) The mRNA expression of ZO1, E-cadherin, and occludin was detected with qPCR in HIEC. (**G**,**H**) The protein expression of ZO1, E-cadherin, and occludin in HIEC was analyzed by Western blotting and grayscale scanning analysis. Rus, ruscogenin; Ctrl, control group; LPS, LPS (100 ng/mL) exposure for 4 h group; Rus 2.5 μm, 2.5 μM ruscogenin pretreatment for 24 h prior to LPS exposure for 4 h, followed by treatment with 1 μM nigericin for 4 h group; Rus 5 μm, 5 μM ruscogenin pretreatment for 24 h prior to LPS exposure for 4 h, followed by treatment with 1 μM nigericin for 4 h group; Rus 10 μM, 10 μM ruscogenin pretreatment for 24 h prior to LPS exposure for 4 h, followed by treatment with 1 μM nigericin for 4 h group. Data are presented as the mean ± SD. ### $p < 0.001$ versus the control group; * $p < 0.05$, ** $p < 0.01$, and *** $p < 0.001$ versus the LPS group.

To assess whether ruscogenin treatment could improve the intestinal epithelial barrier function, we conducted Western blotting analysis and qPCR to detect the expression of tight junction proteins in HIEC, including ZO1, E-cadherin, and occludin. HIEC were treated with 2.5 μM, 5 μM, and 10 μM ruscogenin for 24 h, followed by 100 ng/mL LPS for 3 h in serum-free medium and 1 μM nigericin for 4 h. As shown in Figure 1F–H, both the mRNA and protein levels of ZO1, E-cadherin, and occludin were significantly reduced after LPS/nigericin administration compared to the control group. When compared with the LPS/nigericin group, ruscogenin treatment effectively increased the expression levels of ZO1, E-cadherin, and occludin, thereby preserving the integrity of the intestinal barrier against the damage caused by LPS/nigericin treatment. Thus, these findings suggest that ruscogenin treatment inhibited LPS/nigericin-induced inflammatory responses in THP-1 cell and improved the intestinal epithelial barrier in injured HIEC.

3.2. Ruscogenin Suppresses the LPS/Nigericin-Induced Caspase-1-Dependent Pyroptosis in Macrophages

Next, we explored whether ruscogenin exerts its anti-inflammatory effect by suppressing the inflammasome activation and whether ruscogenin could suppress pyroptosis in LPS/nigericin-primed macrophages in vitro. Mature IL-1β and IL-18 are produced by cleavage of IL-1β precursor and IL-18 precursor by cleaved caspase-1 [13]. The human macrophage THP-1 cells were pretreated with ruscogenin, followed by LPS priming and nigericin induction, as described above. As shown in Figure 2A,B, compared with the control group, the Western blotting results showed that the expression of IL-1β was significantly elevated in the LPS/nigericin-induced group. Interestingly, pretreatment with ruscogenin significantly suppressed the expression of mature IL-1β. The same results were verified by qPCR (Figure 2C). The supernatants of the culture medium were collected, and the levels of mature IL-18 were analyzed by ELISA assay. Consistently, ruscogenin decreased the production of IL-18 ($p < 0.01$), while high concentrations of ruscogenin treatment had the biggest effects (Figure 2D,E). These results together indicate that ruscogenin treatment significantly inhibited LPS/nigericin-induced IL-1β and IL-18 release.

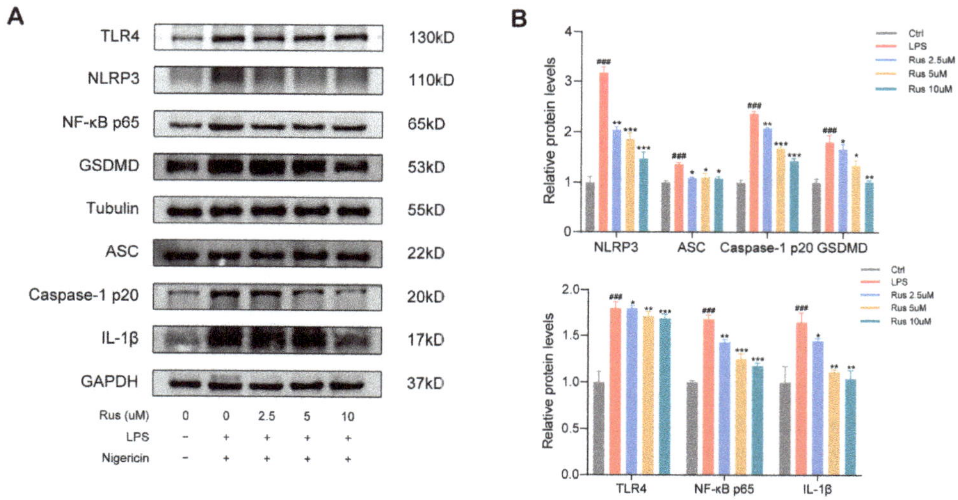

Figure 2. *Cont.*

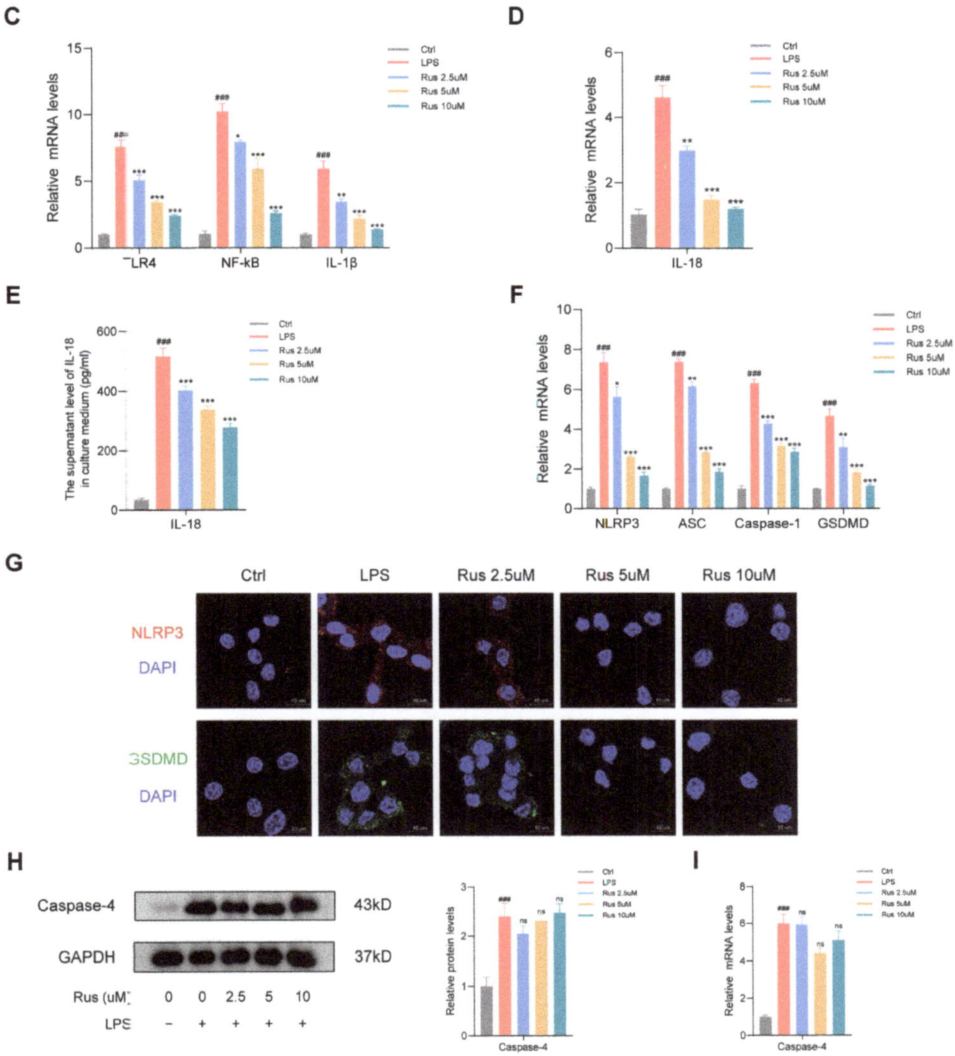

Figure 2. Ruscogenin suppresses the LPS/nigericin-induced caspase-1-dependent pyroptosis in macrophages. (**A**,**B**) The protein expressions of TLR4, NF-κB p65, NLRP3, ASC, caspase-1 p20, GSDMD, and IL-1β in THP-1 cells were analyzed by Western blotting and grayscale scanning analysis. (**C**) The mRNA expression levels of TLR4, NF-κB, and IL-1β in THP-1 cells were analyzed by qPCR. (**D**) The mRNA expression level of IL-18 was analyzed by qPCR. (**E**) The supernatant level of IL-18 in the culture medium of THP-1 cells was detected via ELISA assay. (**F**) The mRNA expressions levels of NLRP3, ASC, Caspase-1 p20, and GSDMD in THP-1 cells were analyzed by qPCR. (**G**) Immunofluorescence of NLRP3 and GSDMD in THP-1 cells. Scale bar: 10 μm. (**H**) After THP-1 cells were induced non-canonical pyroptosis using LPS, the protein expressions level of caspase-4 was analyzed by Western blotting. (**I**) After THP-1 cells were induced to non-canonical pyroptosis using LPS, the mRNA expressions level of caspase-4 was analyzed by qPCR. Rus, ruscogenin. Ctrl, control group; LPS, 100 ng/mL LPS; Rus 2.5 μm, 100 ng/mL LPS + 2.5 μM Rus; Rus 5 μm, 100 ng/mL LPS + 5 μM Rus; Rus 10 μm, 100 ng/mL LPS + 10 μM Rus. Data are presented as the mean ± SD. ns, not significant. ### $p < 0.001$ versus the control group; * $p < 0.05$, ** $p < 0.01$, and *** $p < 0.001$ versus the LPS group.

The NLRP3 inflammasome is an essential multiple protein complex comprised of NLRP3, ASC, and pro-caspase-1 that plays a crucial role in the development of canonical pyroptosis. The cleavage and activation of caspase-1 relies on the activation of NLRP3 inflammasome, and activated caspase-1 mediates the cleavage and activation of GSDMD, which is the executor of pyroptosis. We wondered whether ruscogenin might suppress the production of NLRP3, ASC, or caspase-1, so we detected the proteins extracted from the human macrophages THP-1 cells treated with ruscogenin. The results showed that the protein expression levels of NLRP3, ASC, caspase-1 p20, and GSDMD were upregulated in the LPS/nigericin-primed THP-1 cells but were significantly decreased after ruscogenin treatment, and 10 μM ruscogenin was more effective (Figure 2A,B). Additionally, the mRNA expression levels of NLRP3, ASC, caspase-1, and GSDMD were significantly higher in the LPS/nigericin-induced group than in the untreated control group by at least 300% ($p < 0.001$), whereas pretreatment with ruscogenin notably inhibited the expression of these genes (Figure 2C,F). The immunofluorescence staining showed that NLRP3 was elevated by LPS/nigericin stimulation, but the effect could be reversed by ruscogenin treatment (Figure 2G). Moreover, the results of immunofluorescence staining of GSDMD also indicated the suppressive functions of ruscogenin on LPS/nigericin-induced canonical pyroptosis (Figure 2G).

Furthermore, to investigate whether ruscogenin affects the non-canonical inflammasome pathway, we stimulated THP-1 with LPS to activate caspase-4 to mimic pyroptosis triggered by the non-canonical inflammasome pathway, according to the previous studies [25,26]. As shown in Figure 2H, the protein levels of caspase-4 were considerably increased after LPS treatment in comparison to the control group ($p < 0.001$). Nonetheless, ruscogenin treatment did not suppress the mRNA levels of caspase-4. In addition, the qPCR results indicated that ruscogenin treatment failed to rescue the increased mRNA levels of caspase-4 induced by LPS treatment (Figure 2I). This suggests that ruscogenin had little effect on the non-canonical pyroptosis pathway. Taken together, all these results indicated that ruscogenin could inhibit NLRP3 inflammasome activation and caspase-1-dependent pyroptosis in THP-1 cells.

3.3. Ruscogenin Ameliorates LPS/Nigericin-Induced Pyroptosis via Downregulating the Activation of NLRP3 Inflammasome and through TLR4/NF-κB Axis in Macrophages

To explore the specific molecular mechanisms underlying the protective effects of ruscogenin on macrophages against inflammation and pyroptosis, we examined mRNA expression and protein levels of the upstream signaling molecules of TLR4–NF-κB signaling pathway. Western blotting and qPCR results showed that LPS/nigericin stimulation triggered the activation of TLR4 and NF-κB. Ruscogenin administration inhibited the expression of TLR4 and NF-κB, and the higher dose was more effective (Figure 2A,B). To confirm the effects of ruscogenin on LPS/nigericin-induced inflammation and pyroptosis in macrophages and to determine whether it plays a role through the TLR4/NF-κB signaling pathway, we established a THP-1 cell line overexpressing TLR4 using Flag-TLR4 plasmid and control plasmid. With a successful transfection (Figure 3A), we stimulated the transfected THP-1 cells with LPS and nigericin. The pyroptosis pathway-related protein expression was determined by Western blotting. As shown in Figure 3B–E, the results showed that compared with the control group, LPS/nigericin stimulation significantly elevated the protein and mRNA expression levels of TLR4, NF-κB p65, NLRP3, caspase-1, GSDMD, and IL-1β in THP-1 cells transfected control plasmid. Furthermore,10 μM ruscogenin treatment reduced the protein and mRNA level of TLR4, NF-κB p65, NLRP3, caspase-1, GSDMD, and IL-1β, but the expression levels of these pyroptosis pathway-related proteins and genes were markedly increased in TLR4-overexpressed THP-1 cells, even though they were treated with 10 μM ruscogenin. The results of NLRP3 immunofluorescence staining were identical to those of qPCR and Western blotting (Figure 3F). Collectively, these results indicating that ruscogenin ameliorated LPS/nigericin-induced inflammatory response and pyroptosis in macrophages, at least in part, through the TLR4/NF-κB signaling pathway.

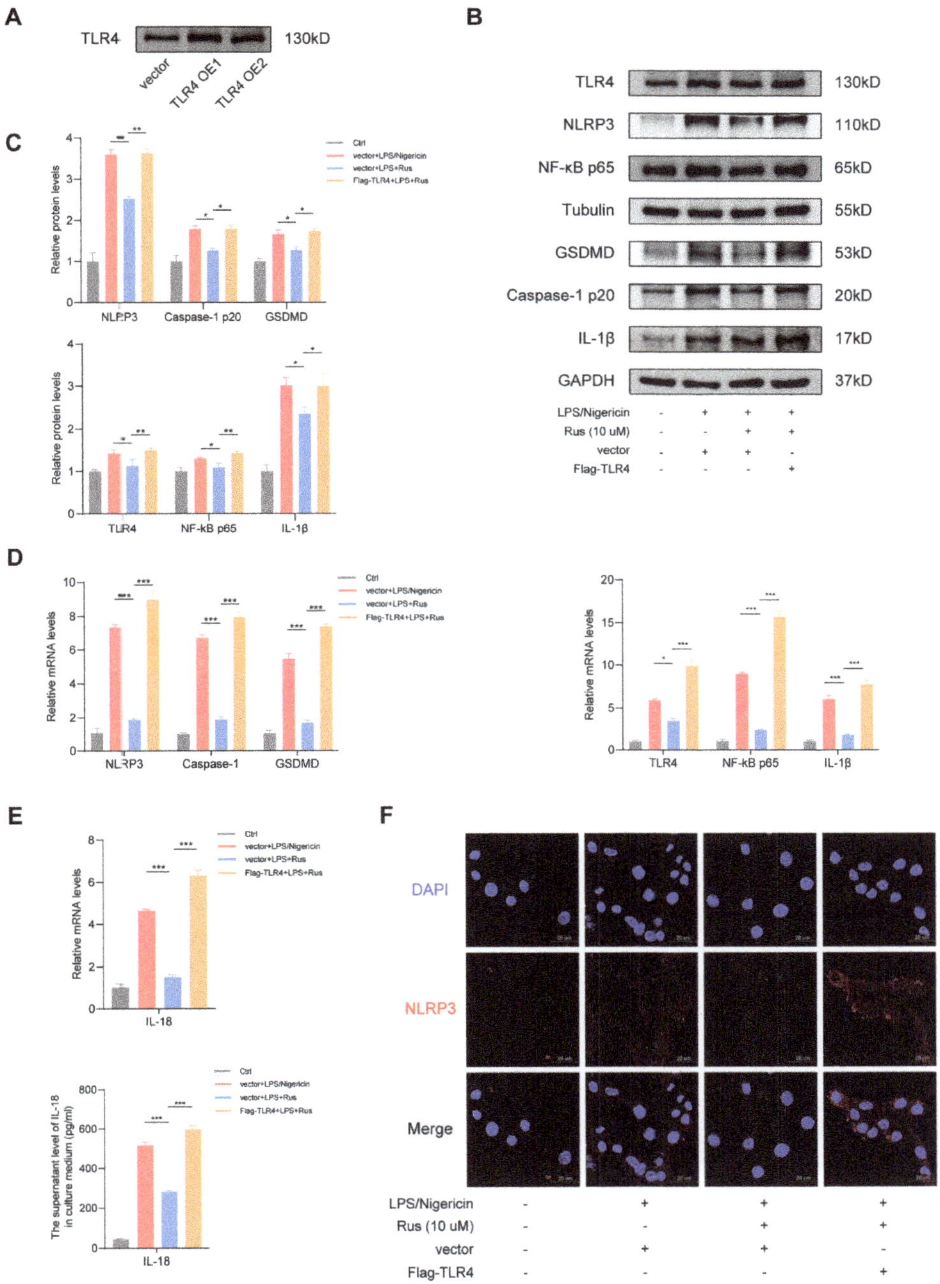

Figure 3. Ruscogenin ameliorates LPS/nigericin-induced pyroptosis via downregulating the activation of NLRP3 inflammasome and through TLR4/NF-κB axis in macrophages. (**A**) A overexpressed TLR4 THP-1 cell line were established using Flag-TLR4 plasmid and control plasmid. The expression level of TLR4 was detected by Western blotting. (**B**) The protein expressions of NLRP3 and IL-1β in THP-1 cells with overexpressed TLR4 were analyzed by western blotting and grayscale scanning analysis. (**C**) The protein expressions of TLR4, NF-κB, GSDMD, and caspase-1 p20 in THP-1 cells with overexpressed TLR4 were analyzed by Western blotting. (**D**) The mRNA expressions level of

NLRP3, IL-18, and IL-1β were analyzed by qPCR. (**E**) The mRNA expressions level of TLR4, NF-κB, GSDMD, and caspase-1 p20 were analyzed by qPCR. (**F**) Immunofluorescence of NLRP3 in THP-1 cells with overexpressed TLR4. Scale bar: 20 μm. Rus, ruscogenin; Ctrl, normal THP-1 cells treated with DMSO; vector + LPS/nigericin, THP-1 cells transfected with control plasmid were treated with LPS/nigericin for 4 h; vector + LPS + Rus, THP-1 cells transfected with control plasmid were treated with 10 μM ruscogenin for 24 h, followed by LPS/nigericin 4 h; Flag-TLR4 + LPS + Rus, THP-1 cells transfected with TLR4-plasmid were treated with 10 μM ruscogenin for 24 h and then LPS/nigericin for 4 h. Data are presented as the mean ± SD. * $p < 0.05$, ** $p < 0.01$, and *** $p < 0.001$.

3.4. Ruscogenin Treatment Attenuates DSS-Induced Colitis in Mice

Next, we used 3.5% DSS to induce colitis in mice and evaluated the treatment effects of ruscogenin in vivo. The design of the experiment is shown in Figure 4A. In brief, the mice were treated with drinking water containing 3.5% DSS and with different doses of ruscogenin (0.5 mg/kg, 1 mg/kg, and 2 mg/kg) for 7 days. We evaluated colitis by closely monitoring the clinical symptoms of IBD, which include diarrhea, bloody feces, body weight loss, and colon shortening. As shown in Figure 4B, the results of two-way ANOVA showed that administration time, dose, and their interaction all had effects on the body weight of mice. We wanted to explore the difference in body weight among the groups of mice after 7 days of continuous administration. On day 8, the body weight of mice in the DSS group was significantly reduced compared with that in the control group (17.4 ± 0.9 g vs. 24.3 ± 0.2 g, $p < 0.001$), while 1 mg/kg ruscogenin treatment markedly attenuated the induced loss of body weight by 3.5% DSS (19.1 ± 1.1 g vs. 17.4 ± 0.9 g, $p = 0.02$), and high-dose ruscogenin (2 mg/kg) had a greater treatment effect on body weight loss (20.2 ± 0.7 g vs. 17.4 ± 0.9 g, $p < 0.001$). The median DAI score of the mice in the DSS group was higher than that of the control group on day 8 ($p < 0.001$). Interestingly, compared with DSS group, 0.5 mg/kg ruscogenin treatment decreased the median DAI score of mice (5.0 (4.0, 5.0) vs. 9.0 (8.5, 9.5), $p < 0.001$), while 2 mg/kg ruscogenin administration was more effective (3.0 (3.0, 3.75) vs. 9.0 (8.5, 9.5), $p < 0.001$) (Figure 4C). All the mice were euthanized on day 8, and the colon tissues and serum were collected for further analysis. The DSS-treated mice exhibited shorter and erythematous colons, both of which are characteristic indicators of colitis (4.7 ± 0.2 cm vs. 6.8 ± 0.3 cm, $p < 0.001$). However, these colonic abnormalities were effectively rescued by ruscogenin (Figure 4D,E). In addition, H&E staining of colon tissue sections is shown in Figure 4G. Compared with the control group, the H&E staining of the colon tissue in the DSS model group showed incomplete colonic mucosa, destruction and irregular arrangement of glandular structure, disappearance of crypt structure, and a large number of inflammatory cells having infiltrated the mucosa and submucosa, accompanied by edema. However, the administration of ruscogenin dramatically ameliorated the histopathological manifestations of colitis. The intestinal crypt and glandular structure of the mice treated with ruscogenin was more obvious than that of the DSS model group, and less inflammatory cell infiltration was observed in the mucosa, which was similar to that of the untreated mice. Thus, the median histological scores were also substantially lower in the ruscogenin treatment groups than in the DSS group, and high-dose ruscogenin showed greater efficacy (Figure 4F). All these results suggest that ruscogenin treatment significantly alleviated DSS-induced colitis in mice, effectively attenuating the clinical symptoms of colitis.

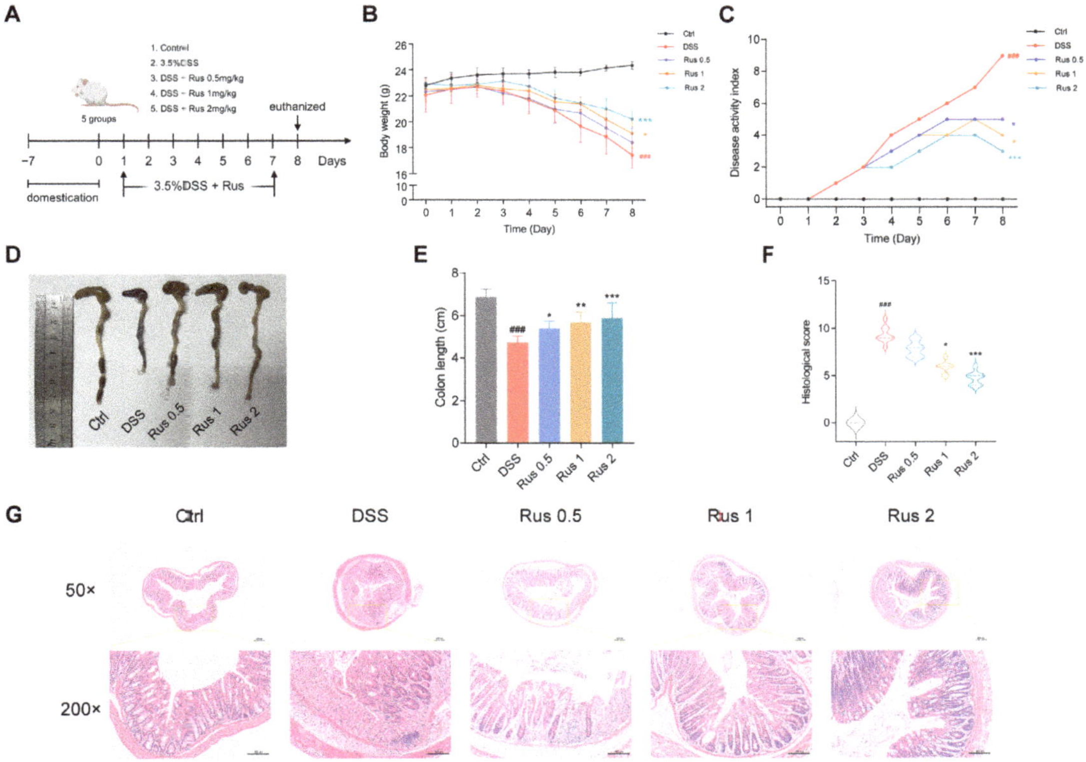

Figure 4. Ruscogenin attenuated the severity of DSS-induced colitis in mice. (A) Overview of the experimental protocol. C57BL/6 mice (n = 5–7 mice/group) were fed with distilled water or water containing 3.5% DSS and were intragastric injected with DMSO or ruscogenin (0.5/1/2 mg/kg) daily. Seven days later, all the water was changed to distilled water, and on the 8th day, the mice were euthanized, and their colon tissues were collected. (B) The body weight of each group. (C) The disease activity index of each group. (D,E) Colon tissues of mice were evaluated at the time of necropsy with representative macroscopic images. (F) Histological scores. At the center of each violin picture is a thick line that represents the median of the data. The upper and lower lines represent the first quartile and the third quartile. (G) Representative images of H&E staining of colon sections (magnification, 50× and 200×). The scale bars are 200 μm and 100 μm, respectively. DSS, Dextran sulfate sodium salt; Rus, ruscogenin; Ctrl, control group. DSS, 3.5% DSS group; Rus 0.5, 3.5% DSS + Rus 0.5 mg/kg group; Rus 1, 3.5% DSS + Rus 1 mg/kg group; Rus 2, 3.5% DSS + Rus 2 mg/kg group. Data in B and E are presented as the mean ± SD. Data in C are presented as the median. Data in F are presented as the median (Q1, Q3). ### $p < 0.001$ versus the control group; * $p < 0.05$, ** $p < 0.01$, and *** $p < 0.001$ versus the DSS group.

3.5. Ruscogenin Reduces the Inflammatory Response and Improves the Intestinal Barrier Function

To further evaluate the anti-inflammatory effects of ruscogenin, the expression of inflammatory cytokines IL-6, TNF-α, and MCP-1 were detected by qPCR (Figure 5A). Furthermore, the concentrations of IL-6, TNF-α, and MCP-1 in colon tissues were evaluated by ELISA (Figure 5B). All these results showed that the levels of these inflammatory cytokines were increased in the DSS group compared to that of in the control group, while ruscogenin treatment significantly reduced the levels of these inflammatory cytokines, especially in the Rus 2 group. Previous studies have demonstrated that epithelial barrier disruption is one of the main characteristics of IBD. Western blotting analysis, qPCR, and immunofluorescence staining were used to further determine whether ruscogenin could improve the intestinal mucosal barrier function in DSS-induced colitis. The mRNA expression levels of ZO1, E-cadherin, and occludin were significantly decreased in colon tissue in the DSS-administered mice compared to the control groups, but these changes were restored by ruscogenin treatment in a dose-dependent manner (Figure 5C). Moreover, Western blotting and immunofluorescence staining results were consistent with qPCR results and showed that DSS administration reduced the expression of E-cadherin, occludin, and ZO1, while ruscogenin treatment increased the level of these tight junction proteins in colon tissues from DSS-induced colitis mice, indicating that ruscogenin can improve intestinal barrier integrity in mice with colitis (Figure 5D–G). In short, the above results indicate that ruscogenin attenuates inflammatory response in DSS-induced colitis mice, and ruscogenin prevents the DSS-induced colitis by regulating tight junction proteins and improving the intestinal barrier function.

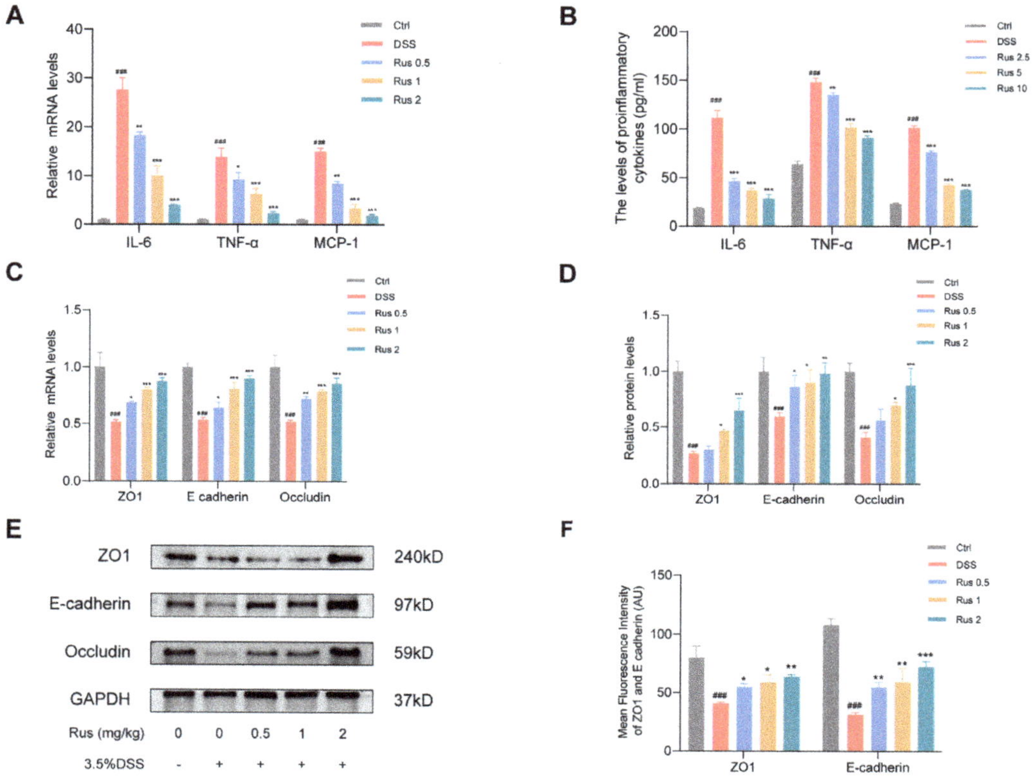

Figure 5. *Cont.*

G

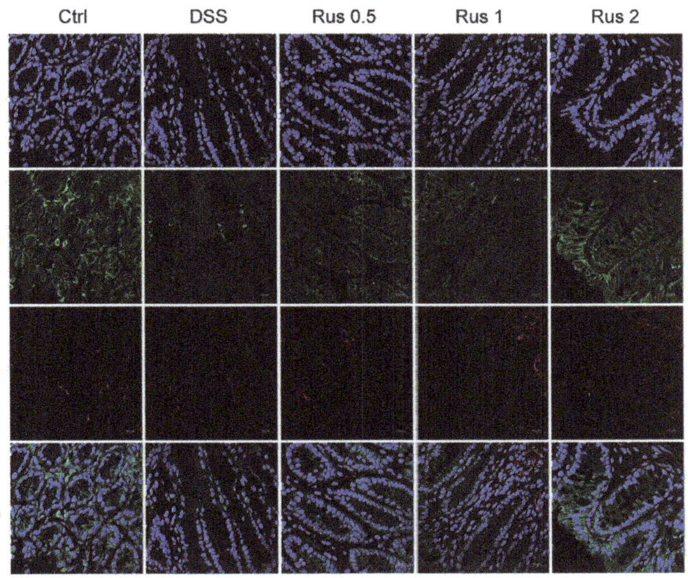

Figure 5. Effect of ruscogenin treatment on inflammatory cytokines and intestinal tight junction protein in DSS-induced mice colitis. (**A**) qPCR analysis of the mRNA expression level of inflammatory cytokines IL-6, TNF-α, and MCP-1 in colon tissues. (**B**) The levels of IL-6, TNF-α, and MCP-1 in colon tissues were detected by ELISA. (**C**) The mRNA expression levels of ZO1, E-cadherin, and occludin were analyzed by qPCR. (**D**,**E**) The protein expressions of ZO1, E-cadherin, and occludin in colon tissues were analyzed by Western blotting and grayscale scanning analysis. (**F**,**G**) The expressions of ZO1 and E-cadherin in colon tissue were analyzed by immunofluorescence staining. DAPI, blue; ZO1, red; E-cadherin, green. Scale bar: 20 μm. Rus, ruscogenin; Ctrl, control group; DSS, 3.5% DSS group; Rus 0.5, 3.5% DSS + Rus 0.5 mg/kg group; Rus 1, 3.5% DSS + Rus 1 mg/kg group; Rus 2, 3.5% DSS + Rus 2 mg/kg group. Data are presented as the mean ± SD. ### $p < 0.001$ versus the control group; * $p < 0.05$, ** $p < 0.01$, and *** $p < 0.001$ versus the DSS group.

3.6. Ruscogenin Alleviates DSS-Induced Colitis in Mice by Inhibiting NLRP3 Inflammasome Activation and Caspase-1-Dependent Pyroptosis

Previous reports have demonstrated a significant correlation between the activity of NLRP3 inflammasomes and the development as well as the pathogenesis of IBD. They have also found that IBD patients exhibit high expression of pyroptosis-related factors both at the mRNA level and protein level [12]. Based on the findings from in vitro experiments indicating that ruscogenin exhibited the ability to inhibit inflammation and pyroptosis, we proceeded to explore whether ruscogenin could alleviate DSS-induced colitis by inhibiting the NLRP3 inflammasome and pyroptosis via the TLR4–NF-κB signaling pathway. We conducted qPCR, ELISA, Western blotting, and immunofluorescence staining to measure the expression of pyroptosis-related molecular levels. As shown in Figure 6A–D, the mRNA expression levels of NLRP3, caspase-1, GSDMD, IL-18, and IL-1β of the mice in the DSS group were upregulated after DSS administration, but these indicators were significantly decreased after the mice were treated with ruscogenin, and 2 mg/kg ruscogenin administration was more obvious ($p < 0.001$). All these results were consistent with the results of Western blotting, showing that the protein expression levels of NLRP3, caspase-1, GSDMD, and IL-1β in colon tissues of the mice were markedly reduced in both the Rus 1 group and Rus 2 group compared with the DSS model group (Figure 6E–G). Consistent with the in vitro results, ruscogenin treatment inhibited the expression of TLR4 and NF-κB, and the higher dose was more effective (Figure 6E–G). Taken together, these results highlight that the protective effect of ruscogenin on DSS-induced colitis was associated with the attenuation of NLRP3 inflammasome activation and caspase-1-dependent pyroptosis by inhibiting the TLR4/NF-κB pathway.

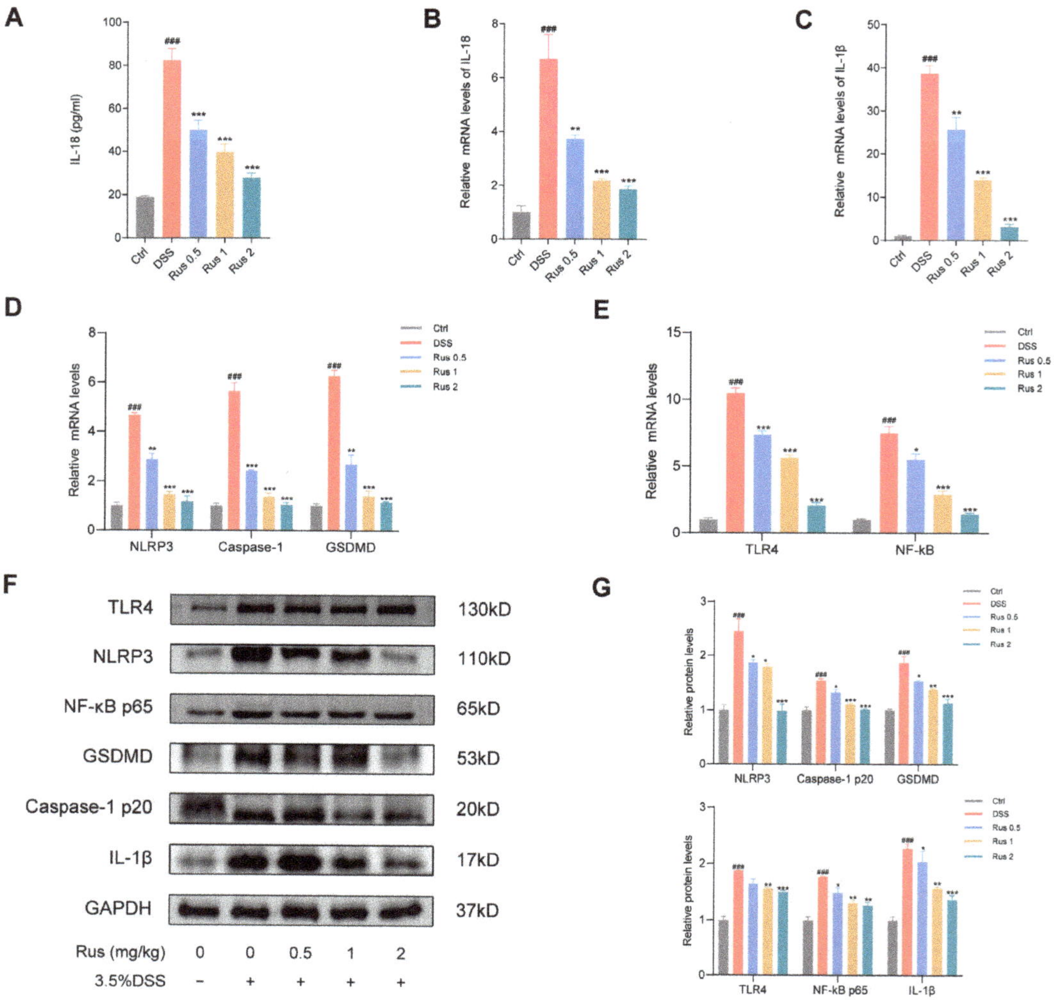

Figure 6. Ruscogenin treatment inhibits the activation of NLRP3 inflammasome and caspase-1-dependent pyroptosis in DSS-induced mice colitis. (**A**) The levels of IL-18 in colon tissues were detected by ELISA. (**B**) The mRNA expressions level of IL-18 was analyzed by qPCR. (**C**) The mRNA expressions level of IL-1β was detected by qPCR. (**D**,**E**) The mRNA expression levels of NLRP3, caspase-1 p20, GSDMD, TLR4, and NF-κB were analyzed by qPCR. (**F**,**G**) The protein expression levels of NLRP3, caspase-1 p20, GSDMD, TLR4, NF-κB p65, and IL-1β in colon tissues were analyzed by Western blotting and grayscale scanning analysis. Rus, ruscogenin; Ctrl, control group; DSS, 3.5% DSS group; Rus 0.5, 3.5% DSS + ruscogenin 0.5 mg/kg group; Rus 1, 3.5% DSS + ruscogenin 1 mg/kg group; Rus 2, 3.5% DSS + ruscogenin 2 mg/kg group. Data are presented as the mean ± SD. ### $p < 0.001$ versus the control group; * $p < 0.05$, ** $p < 0.01$, and *** $p < 0.001$ versus the DSS group.

4. Discussion

In this study, we used a DSS-induced mice colitis model and LPS/nigericin-induced THP-1 macrophages to illustrate ruscogenin's capacity to inhibit the inflammatory response and pyroptosis. Ruscogenin significantly inhibited LPS/nigericin-induced canonical pyroptosis in human monocytic leukemia cell THP-1 but had minimal impact on LPS-induced non-canonical pyroptosis in THP-1 cells. Moreover, it displayed a mitigating effect on DSS-induced colitis in vivo. In terms of the underlying mechanism, the TLR4/NF-κB pathway plays a vital role in the activation of NLRP3 inflammasome and caspase-1-dependent canonical pyroptosis instead of caspase-1-independent non-canonical pyroptosis [27]. By using a TLR4 overexpression plasmid, we found that ruscogenin treatment potentially alleviates DSS-induced colitis in mice by inhibiting NLRP3 inflammasome activation and canonical pyroptosis, and the protective effect may be related to the suppression of the TLR4/NF-κB signaling pathway. Through a combination of in vitro and in vivo experiments, we successfully demonstrated the therapeutic effects and potential mechanism of ruscogenin.

The doses of ruscogenin used for animal experiments in our study were 0.5, 1, and 2 mg/kg, based on the previous study [18,19]. The DSS-induced mice colitis model is a well-established and widely used model for studying the pathogenesis and drug efficacy of human UC [28]. The therapeutic efficacy of ruscogenin is manifested in the significant reduction of UC symptoms like diarrhea and rectal bleeding in mice treated with DSS. Additionally, ruscogenin administration led to the reversal of weight loss and a decrease in DAI scores. Colonic shortening, a common symptom induced by DSS, was notably alleviated with ruscogenin treatment. Histopathological evaluations revealed that the mice in the DSS group exhibited irregularities in the submucosa and crypt structures, but these abnormalities were significantly improved in the groups treated with ruscogenin. These findings indicate that ruscogenin may be a good candidate drug for the treatment of UC.

Recent research has indicated a strong correlation between the expression of proinflammatory molecules and intestinal epithelial barrier disruption and the occurrence and progression of UC, contributing to intestinal immune system disorders [29]. Intestinal epithelial cells typically serve as the first line of defense against intestinal diseases. The physical function of the intestinal barrier is damaged due to the accumulation of pyroptosis in intestinal epithelial cells and the dysfunction of tight junction proteins, which consequently leads to an increase in intestinal permeability [30]. Colonic inflammation can occur due to the presence of intestinal pathogens invasion as well as the breakdown of tight junctions caused by a continuous cycle of releasing both pro-inflammatory and anti-inflammatory factors [31]. This process triggers the adaptive immune system, leading to the activation of antigen-presenting cells and the transformation of naive T cells into effector T cells like Th1, Th2, Th17, and natural killer T cells [32]. These cells generate a variety of proinflammatory cytokines, including IL-1β, which activate macrophages to release a large number of cytokines, such as TNF-α, IL-6, and MCP-1, causing tissue damage. TNF-α, an early endogenous mediator in major inflammatory diseases, can disrupt the function of the intestinal barrier. IL-1β and MCP-1 also play a vital role in regulating inflammation, particularly in the early stages, leading to colonic inflammation. Recent studies have shown that advanced therapies targeting specific inflammatory pathways can treat moderate-to-severe UC [29,33]. In this study, our findings showed a significant increase in the levels of TNF-α, IL-6, and MCP-1 after the administration of DSS or LPS/nigericin. Interestingly, ruscogenin treatment reduced the levels of these proinflammatory cytokines in both colon tissues and culture medium supernatant as well as the expression of their corresponding mRNAs. Moreover, we confirmed the disruption of tight junction proteins in DSS-treated mice, while administration of ruscogenin significantly improved the intestinal barrier function by increasing ZO1, occludin, and E-cadherin expressions during epithelial damage. Therefore, these data demonstrate that ruscogenin treatment alleviates DSS-induced colitis by decreasing the secretion of inflammatory factors and repairing the expression of tight junctions and their associated proteins.

Pyroptosis serves as an immune defense mechanism against invading pathogens, characterized by cell membrane disruption and the secretion of inflammatory cytokines. However, when pyroptosis becomes uncontrolled due to overactive inflammasomes, it can lead to significant cell membrane damage and an excessive release of inflammatory factors, disrupting homeostasis and potentially leading to the development of various diseases. Recent studies have shown that pyroptosis is involved in the pathogenesis of UC [11,34]. Thus, the control of inflammatory response and pyroptosis of macrophage prevents extensive tissue damage in UC. Regarding LPS/nigericin-induced inflammatory and canonical pyroptosis, it is well known that TLR4 initiates the immune response by recognizing LPS. The most important pathway for LPS activation is the MyD88-dependent pathway [35]. First, after LPS stimulation, the intracellular Toll/IL-1 receptor structural domain of TLR4 binds to MyD88, which then induces NF-κB signaling, causing elevated expression of NLRP3, pro-IL-18, and pro-IL-1β. Then, nigericin indirectly activates NLRP3, leading to NLRP3 inflammatory complex assembly and caspase-1 activation. As a downstream mediator of the TLR4 signaling pathway, NF-κB is a transcription factor involved in various pathophysiological processes, including inflammation, pyroptosis, and immune processes [14,36]. Ruscogenin showed prominently anti-inflammatory activity in animal experimental models of cerebral ischemic injury, acute lung injury, and hepatic injury [17,18,20,37]. A previous study indicated that the possible molecular mechanism by which ruscogenin inhibits the inflammatory response is mainly related to the inhibition of the NF-κB signaling pathway [17]. Wu et al. found that ruscogenin ameliorated LPS-induced apoptosis of pulmonary endothelial cells mainly by targeting TLR4 [19]. Interestingly, another study conducted by Wang et al. also suggested that ruscogenin effectively alleviates particulate matter-induced acute lung injury probably by inhibiting TLR4/MyD88 signaling pathway. TLR4 might be vital for particulate matter to initiate pulmonary lesions and for ruscogenin to exert treatment effect on lung injury [18]. A newly published study reported that ruscogenin attenuates SARS-CoV-2 E protein-induced pyroptosis by inhibiting NLRP3 inflammasome activation [38]. Consistently, in this study, our novel data showed that ruscogenin effectively inhibited caspase-1-dependent pyroptosis via inhibiting the activation of NLRP3 inflammasome. Moreover, to exclude that ruscogenin affects pyroptosis through the caspase-4-dependent non-canonical inflammasome pathway, we analyzed the effect of ruscogenin on the non-canonical inflammasome pathway by stimulating HIEC with LPS alone. The results demonstrated that ruscogenin had little effect on the caspase-4-dependent non-canonical inflammasome pathway. Further results found that ruscogenin failed to ameliorate LPS/nigericin-induced pyroptosis and NLRP3 inflammasome activation when overexpressing TLR4, indicating that TLR4 is a potential target of ruscogenin, which is consistent with the findings of other studies mentioned above. Thus, our findings confirmed that this protective effect of ruscogenin may be related to TLR4/NF-κB pathway inhibition. It might provide a promising strategy for the treatment of UC patients. In short, we successfully demonstrated the therapeutic effects and potential mechanism of ruscogenin in the treatment of UC.

Aside from these findings, several potential limitations of this present study exist. For instance, the results of this study showed that ruscogenin inhibited the TLR4/NF-κB pathway, but the mediator involved is still unclear and needs to be explored. Furthermore, although we confirmed the finding that ruscogenin inhibits pyroptosis and thereby alleviates colitis through the TLR4/NF-κB pathway, transgenic mouse experiments are necessary to verify this pathway before using ruscogenin in IBD patients. Finally, ruscogenin restored the intestinal barrier in UC by reducing inflammatory responses and inhibiting pyroptosis. However, ruscogenin may also improve intestinal barrier function and inflammation through other means, and whether ruscogenin could protect the intestinal barrier disruption through other related signaling pathways remains unclear and deserves further research.

5. Conclusions

In summary, this study elucidated the efficient protective role of ruscogenin against DSS-induced colitis and demonstrated that ruscogenin alleviates DSS-induced colitis in mice by inhibiting NLRP3 inflammasome activation and caspase-1-dependent canonical pyroptosis, probably due to the suppression of the TLR4/NF-κB signaling pathway. These findings might provide new insights and a solid foundation for further exploration into the therapeutic potential of ruscogenin in the treatment of IBD.

Supplementary Materials: The following supporting information can be downloaded at: https://www.mdpi.com/article/10.3390/biomedicines12050989/s1, Table S1. Primers used in qPCR; Table S2. Antibodies.

Author Contributions: J.L., H.W., H.C. and W.S. performed study concept and design; J.L., H.W., J.Z., R.J., Z.Z., Q.Y., H.C. and W.S. provided acquisition, analysis, and interpretation of data and statistical analysis; R.J., Z.Z. and Q.Y. provided technical and material support; J.L. and H.W. wrote the original draft; J.L. and J.Z. revised the manuscript; H.C. and W.S. developed the methodology and undertook review revision of the paper. All authors have read and agreed to the published version of the manuscript.

Funding: The National Natural Science Foundation of China (U23A20408, 82171698, 82170561, 81741067, 81300279), the Natural Science Foundation for Distinguished Young Scholars of Guangdong Province (2021B1515020003), the Climbing Program of Introduced Talents and High-level Hospital Construction Project of Guangdong Provincial People's Hospital (DFJH201803, KJ012019099, KJ012021143, KY012021183), and the Guangdong Basic and Applied Basic Research Foundation (2022A1515012081).

Institutional Review Board Statement: The study was conducted in accordance with the Declaration of Helsinki, and approved by the Ethics Committee of Guangdong Provincial People's Hospital, Guangzhou, China (approval number: KY-N-2022-084-02; approval date: 30 August 2022).

Informed Consent Statement: Not applicable.

Data Availability Statement: The original contributions presented in the study are included in the article/Supplementary Material. Further inquiries can be directed to the corresponding author.

Acknowledgments: The authors would like to sincerely thank Zhong and the staff of the Central Laboratory of Guangdong Provincial People's Hospital for their assistance in technical support.

Conflicts of Interest: The authors declare that they have no competing interests.

Abbreviations

IBD, inflammatory bowel disease; UC, ulcerative colitis; Rus, ruscogenin; NLRP3, NOD-like receptor pyrin domain-containing protein 3; ZO1, Zonula occludens 1; TLR4, Toll-like receptors 4; PRR, pattern recognition receptor; PAMP, pathogen-related molecular pattern; DAMP, damage-related molecular pattern; IL-1β, interleukin-1β; GSDMD, gasdermin D; LPS, lipopolysaccharide; H&E, hematoxylin and eosin; DAI, disease activity index; CCK-8, cell counting kit-8; qPCR, quantitative real-time polymerase chain reaction.

References

1. Kobayashi, T.; Siegmund, B.; Le Berre, C.; Wei, S.C.; Ferrante, M.; Shen, B.; Bernstein, C.N.; Danese, S.; Peyrin-Biroulet, L.; Hibi, T. Ulcerative colitis. *Nat. Rev. Dis. Primers* **2020**, *6*, 74. [CrossRef]
2. Roda, G.; Chien Ng, S.; Kotze, P.G.; Argollo, M.; Panaccione, R.; Spinelli, A.; Kaser, A.; Peyrin-Biroulet, L.; Danese, S. Crohn's disease. *Nat. Rev. Dis. Primers* **2020**, *6*, 22. [CrossRef]
3. Ng, S.C.; Shi, H.Y.; Hamidi, N.; Underwood, F.E.; Tang, W.; Benchimol, E.I.; Panaccione, R.; Ghosh, S.; Wu, J.C.Y.; Chan, F.K.L.; et al. Worldwide incidence and prevalence of inflammatory bowel disease in the 21st century: A systematic review of population-based studies. *Lancet* **2017**, *390*, 2769–2778. [CrossRef]
4. Kaplan, G.G. The global burden of IBD: From 2015 to 2025. *Nat. Rev. Gastroenterol. Hepatol.* **2015**, *12*, 720–727. [CrossRef]
5. Chang, J.T. Pathophysiology of Inflammatory Bowel Diseases. *N. Engl. J. Med.* **2020**, *383*, 2652–2664. [CrossRef] [PubMed]

6. Jeong, D.Y.; Kim, S.; Son, M.J.; Son, C.Y.; Kim, J.Y.; Kronbichler, A.; Lee, K.H.; Shin, J.I. Induction and maintenance treatment of inflammatory bowel disease: A comprehensive review. *Autoimmun. Rev.* **2019**, *18*, 439–454. [CrossRef] [PubMed]
7. Man, S.M.; Karki, R.; Kanneganti, T.D. Molecular mechanisms and functions of pyroptosis, inflammatory caspases and inflammasomes in infectious diseases. *Immunol. Rev.* **2017**, *277*, 61–75. [CrossRef]
8. Chen, G.Y.; Nunez, G. Inflammasomes in intestinal inflammation and cancer. *Gastroenterology* **2011**, *141*, 1986–1999. [CrossRef] [PubMed]
9. Zhou, C.B.; Fang, J.Y. The role of pyroptosis in gastrointestinal cancer and immune responses to intestinal microbial infection. *Biochim. Biophys Acta Rev. Cancer* **2019**, *1872*, 1–10. [CrossRef]
10. Kesavardhana, S.; Malireddi, R.K.S.; Kanneganti, T.D. Caspases in Cell Death, Inflammation, and Pyroptosis. *Annu. Rev. Immunol.* **2020**, *38*, 567–595. [CrossRef]
11. Patankar, J.V.; Becker, C. Cell death in the gut epithelium and implications for chronic inflammation. *Nat. Rev. Gastroenterol. Hepatol.* **2020**, *17*, 543–556. [CrossRef] [PubMed]
12. Chen, X.; Liu, G.; Yuan, Y.; Wu, G.; Wang, S.; Yuan, L. NEK7 interacts with NLRP3 to modulate the pyroptosis in inflammatory bowel disease via NF-κB signaling. *Cell Death Dis.* **2019**, *10*, 906. [CrossRef]
13. Shi, J.; Gao, W.; Shao, F. Pyroptosis: Gasdermin-Mediated Programmed Necrotic Cell Death. *Trends Biochem. Sci.* **2017**, *42*, 245–254. [CrossRef]
14. Kondylis, V.; Kumari, S.; Vlantis, K.; Pasparakis, M. The interplay of IKK, NF-κB and RIPK1 signaling in the regulation of cell death, tissue homeostasis and inflammation. *Immunol. Rev.* **2017**, *277*, 113–127. [CrossRef] [PubMed]
15. Guo, B.J.; Bian, Z.X.; Qiu, H.C.; Wang, Y.T.; Wang, Y. Biological and clinical implications of herbal medicine and natural products for the treatment of inflammatory bowel disease. *Ann. N. Y. Acad. Sci.* **2017**, *1401*, 37–48. [CrossRef] [PubMed]
16. Chen, M.H.; Chen, X.J.; Wang, M.; Lin, L.G.; Wang, Y.T. Ophiopogon japonicus--A phytochemical, ethnomedicinal and pharmacological review. *J. Ethnopharmacol.* **2016**, *181*, 193–213. [CrossRef]
17. Sun, Q.; Chen, L.; Gao, M.; Jiang, W.; Shao, F.; Li, J.; Wang, J.; Kou, J.; Yu, B. Ruscogenin inhibits lipopolysaccharide-induced acute lung injury in mice: Involvement of tissue factor, inducible NO synthase and nuclear factor (NF)-κB. *Int. Immunopharmacol.* **2012**, *12*, 88–93. [CrossRef]
18. Wang, Y.-w.; Wu, Y.-h.; Zhang, J.-z.; Tang, J.-h.; Fan, R.-p.; Li, F.; Yu, B.-y.; Kou, J.-p.; Zhang, Y.-y. Ruscogenin attenuates particulate matter-induced acute lung injury in mice via protecting pulmonary endothelial barrier and inhibiting TLR4 signaling pathway. *Acta Pharmacol. Sin.* **2020**, *42*, 726–734. [CrossRef]
19. Wu, Y.; Yu, X.; Wang, Y.; Huang, Y.; Tang, J.; Gong, S.; Jiang, S.; Xia, Y.; Li, F.; Yu, B.; et al. Ruscogenin alleviates LPS-triggered pulmonary endothelial barrier dysfunction through targeting NMMHC IIA to modulate TLR4 signaling. *Acta Pharm. Sin. B* **2022**, *12*, 1198–1212. [CrossRef]
20. Cao, G.; Jiang, N.; Hu, Y.; Zhang, Y.; Wang, G.; Yin, M.; Ma, X.; Zhou, K.; Qi, J.; Yu, B.; et al. Ruscogenin Attenuates Cerebral Ischemia-Induced Blood-Brain Barrier Dysfunction by Suppressing TXNIP/NLRP3 Inflammasome Activation and the MAPK Pathway. *Int. J. Mol. Sci.* **2016**, *17*, 1418. [CrossRef]
21. Egger, B.; Bajaj-Elliott, M.; MacDonald, T.T.; Inglin, R.; Eysselein, V.E.; Büchler, M.W. Characterisation of acute murine dextran sodium sulphate colitis: Cytokine profile and dose dependency. *Digestion* **2000**, *62*, 240–248. [CrossRef] [PubMed]
22. Adolph, T.E.; Tomczak, M.F.; Niederreiter, L.; Ko, H.J.; Bock, J.; Martinez-Naves, E.; Glickman, J.N.; Tschurtschenthaler, M.; Hartwig, J.; Hosomi, S.; et al. Paneth cells as a site of origin for intestinal inflammation. *Nature* **2013**, *503*, 272–276. [CrossRef] [PubMed]
23. Wu, H.; Tu, S.; Zhuo, Z.; Jiang, R.; Zeng, R.; Yang, Q.; Lian, Q.; Sha, W.; Chen, H. Investigating the Mechanisms of Bisdemethoxycurcumin in Ulcerative Colitis: Network Pharmacology and Experimental Verification. *Molecules* **2022**, *28*, 68. [CrossRef] [PubMed]
24. Chen, H.; Zhang, H.; Zheng, Y.; Min, X.; Luo, Y.; Zhou, W.; Ma, F.; Li, J.; Lu, Q.; Zhang, C.; et al. Prolyl hydroxylase 2 silencing enhances the paracrine effects of mesenchymal stem cells on necrotizing enterocolitis in an NF-kappaB-dependent mechanism. *Cell Death Dis.* **2020**, *11*, 188. [CrossRef] [PubMed]
25. Kayagaki, N.; Wong, M.T.; Stowe, I.B.; Ramani, S.R.; Gonzalez, L.C.; Akashi-Takamura, S.; Miyake, K.; Zhang, J.; Lee, W.P.; Muszyński, A.; et al. Noncanonical inflammasome activation by intracellular LPS independent of TLR4. *Science* **2013**, *341*, 1246–1249. [CrossRef] [PubMed]
26. Yang, J.; Zhao, Y.; Shao, F. Non-canonical activation of inflammatory caspases by cytosolic LPS in innate immunity. *Curr. Opin. Immunol.* **2015**, *32*, 78–83. [CrossRef]
27. Broz, P.; Dixit, V.M. Inflammasomes: Mechanism of assembly, regulation and signalling. *Nat. Rev. Immunol.* **2016**, *16*, 407–420. [CrossRef] [PubMed]
28. Okayasu, I.; Hatakeyama, S.; Yamada, M.; Ohkusa, T.; Inagaki, Y.; Nakaya, R. A novel method in the induction of reliable experimental acute and chronic ulcerative colitis in mice. *Gastroenterology* **1990**, *98*, 694–702. [CrossRef]
29. Gros, B.; Kaplan, G.G. Ulcerative Colitis in Adults: A Review. *JAMA* **2023**, *330*, 951–965. [CrossRef]
30. Dai, Z.; Liu, W.C.; Chen, X.Y.; Wang, X.; Li, J.L.; Zhang, X. Gasdermin D-mediated pyroptosis: Mechanisms, diseases, and inhibitors. *Front. Immunol.* **2023**, *14*, 1178662. [CrossRef]
31. Shawki, A.; McCole, D.F. Mechanisms of Intestinal Epithelial Barrier Dysfunction by Adherent-Invasive Escherichia coli. *Cell Mol. Gastroenterol. Hepatol.* **2017**, *3*, 41–50. [CrossRef] [PubMed]

32. Akuzum, B.; Lee, J Y. Context-Dependent Regulation of Type17 Immunity by Microbiota at the Intestinal Barrier. *Immune. Netw* **2022**, *22*, e46. [CrossRef]
33. McLean, M.H.; Neurath, M.F.; Durum, S.K. Targeting interleukins for the treatment of inflammatory bowel disease-what lies beyond anti-TNF therapy? *Inflamm. Bowel. Dis.* **2014**, *20*, 389–397. [CrossRef]
34. Zhen, Y.; Zhang, H. NLRP3 Inflammasome and Inflammatory Bowel Disease. *Front. Immunol.* **2019**, *10*, 276. [CrossRef] [PubMed]
35. Rahimifard, M.; Maqbool, F.; Moeini-Nodeh, S.; Niaz, K.; Abdollahi, M.; Braidy, N.; Nabavi, S.M.; Nabavi, S.F. Targeting the TLR4 signaling pathway by polyphenols: A novel therapeutic strategy for neuroinflammation. *Ageing Res. Rev.* **2017**, *36*, 11–19. [CrossRef]
36. Zhang, Q.; Lenardo, M.J.; Baltimore, D. 30 Years of NF-κB: A Blossoming of Relevance to Human Pathobiology. *Cell* **2017**, *168*, 37–57. [CrossRef] [PubMed]
37. Elsawy, H.; Rajendran, P.; Sedky, A.M.; Alfwuaires, M. Ruscogenin Protects Against Deoxynivalenol-Induced Hepatic Injury by Inhibiting Oxidative Stress, Inflammation, and Apoptosis Through the Nrf2 Signaling Pathway: An In vitro Study. *Saudi. J. Med. Med. Sci.* **2022**, *10*, 207–215.
38. Huang, H.; Li, X.; Zha, D.; Lin, H.; Yang, L.; Wang, Y.; Xu, L.; Wang, L.; Lei, T.; Zhou, Z.; et al. SARS-CoV-2 E protein-induced THP-1 pyroptosis is reversed by Ruscogenin. *Biochem. Cell Biol.* **2023**, *101*, 303–312. [CrossRef]

biomedicines

MDPI

Review

Novel Insights into the Pathogenesis of Inflammatory Bowel Diseases

Valentin Calvez [1,2,†], Pierluigi Puca [1,2,†], Federica Di Vincenzo [2], Angelo Del Gaudio [2], Bianca Bartocci [2], Marco Murgiano [2], Jacopo Iaccarino [2], Erfan Parand [2], Daniele Napolitano [1], Daniela Pugliese [1,2], Antonio Gasbarrini [2] and Franco Scaldaferri [1,2,*]

1 IBD Unit, UOC CEMAD Medicina Interna e Gastroenterologia, Centro Malattie dell'Apparato Digerente, Dipartimento di Scienze Mediche e Chirurgiche Addominali ed Endocrino Metaboliche, Fondazione Policlinico Universitario Agostino Gemelli IRCCS, 00168 Rome, Italy; valentino.calvez@gmail.com (V.C.); pierluigi.puca@unicatt.it (P.P.); danielenapolitano1977@gmail.com (D.N.); daniela.pugliese@policlinicogemelli.it (D.P.)

2 Dipartimento di Medicina e Chirurgia Traslazionale, Università Cattolica del Sacro Cuore, 00168 Rome, Italy; federica.divincenzo30@gmail.com (F.D.V.); delgaudioangelo@gmail.com (A.D.G.); biancab97@hotmail.it (B.B.); marcomurgiano1@gmail.com (M.M.); ja.iaccarino@gmail.com (J.I.); erfanparand1380@gmail.com (E.P.); antonio.gasbarrini@unicatt.it (A.G.)

* Correspondence: franco.scaldaferri@policlinicogemelli.it

† These authors contributed equally to this work.

Abstract: Inflammatory bowel diseases (IBDs), encompassing Crohn's disease and ulcerative colitis, are complex chronic disorders characterized by an intricate interplay between genetic predisposition, immune dysregulation, gut microbiota alterations, and environmental exposures. This review aims to synthesize recent advances in IBD pathogenesis, exploring key mechanisms and potential avenues for prevention and personalized therapy. A comprehensive literature search was conducted across major bibliographic databases, selecting the most recent and impactful studies on IBD pathogenesis. The review integrates findings from multi-omics analyses, single-cell transcriptomics, and longitudinal cohort studies, focusing on immune regulation, gut microbiota dynamics, and environmental factors influencing disease onset and progression. Immune dysregulation, including macrophage polarization (M1 vs. M2) and Th17 activation, emerges as a cornerstone of IBD pathogenesis. Dysbiosis, as a result of reduced alpha and beta diversity and overgrowth of harmful taxa, is one of the main contributing factors in causing inflammation in IBD. Environmental factors, including air and water pollutants, maternal smoking, and antibiotic exposure during pregnancy and infancy, significantly modulate IBD risk through epigenetic and microbiota-mediated mechanisms. While recent advances have supported the development of new therapeutic strategies, deeply understanding the complex dynamics of IBD pathogenesis remains challenging. Future efforts should aim to reduce the burden of disease with precise, personalized treatments and lower the incidence of IBD through early-life prevention and targeted interventions addressing modifiable risk factors.

Keywords: inflammatory bowel disease; pathogenesis; immune system; gut microbiota; exposome; genetics; air pollution; water pollution

1. Introduction

Inflammatory bowel disease (IBD), encompassing Crohn's disease (CD) and ulcerative colitis (UC), is a complex condition characterized by chronic inflammation of the gastrointestinal tract. The pathogenesis of IBD is multifactorial and still not completely clarified.

Interactions among genetic predispositions, environmental influences, immune system dysfunctions, and alterations in the gut microbiota are involved. Gaining insight into such topics is of paramount importance for unraveling the mechanisms underlying IBD and developing effective therapeutic strategies and potentially for implementing effective prevention strategies [1].

The mainstay of IBD pathogenesis lies in a dysregulated immune response to gut microbiota. In healthy individuals, the immune system maintains a delicate balance that allows for tolerance to commensal microbes while mounting an appropriate response to pathogenic organisms. However, in genetically susceptible individuals, this balance is disrupted. Environmental factors such as diet, infections, and stress can exacerbate this dysregulation, leading to an inappropriate inflammatory response. This inflammatory milieu is primarily driven by T-helper (Th) cell responses. Th1 and Th17 cells are particularly implicated in Crohn's disease and ulcerative colitis, respectively. The activation of these cells results in the production of pro-inflammatory cytokines that perpetuate tissue damage and inflammation [2].

Genetic factors also play a significant role in IBD susceptibility. Numerous susceptibility loci have been identified through genome-wide association studies, indicating that specific genetic variations can influence an individual's immune response and microbiome composition. For instance, genes associated with autophagy and immune regulation are critical in maintaining intestinal homeostasis. However, genetic predisposition alone does not account for the entirety of disease variance; environmental triggers are essential in modulating these genetic risks [3].

The gut microbiota further complicates the pathogenesis of IBD. Dysbiosis, or an imbalance in microbial communities within the gut, has been consistently observed in IBD patients. This dysbiosis is characterized by reduced microbial diversity and an increase in pathogenic bacteria, which can breach the intestinal barrier and activate immune responses. The interplay between dysbiosis and immune dysfunction creates a feedback loop that exacerbates inflammation and contributes to the chronic nature of IBD [4].

Finally, the exposome—encompassing all environmental exposures—intersects with the other mentioned factors to influence disease outcomes. Factors such as dietary habits, antibiotic use, and exposure to pollutants can significantly impact gut health [5].

The pathogenesis of IBD is a multifaceted interplay between genetic susceptibility, environmental triggers, immune system dysregulation, and gut microbiota alterations. Recent advances in research have shed light on these aspects, revealing new avenues also for therapeutic interventions. This review discusses recent studies, emerging fields of research and novel insights that continue to enhance our understanding of IBD pathogenesis. Gaining insight into these topics is crucial for developing effective therapeutic strategies and exploring preventive approaches. Furthermore, a deeper understanding of pathogenetic mechanisms could pave the way for novel tools to identify patients with severe prognoses or therapy resistance at an early stage. Last but not least, novel biomarkers for non-invasive disease monitoring could emerge [6].

Building on these recent advances, this review delves deeper into the multifaceted pathogenesis of IBD, examining the interplay between the immune system, gut microbiota alterations, genetic predispositions, and environmental factors. Each section integrates established knowledge with the latest discoveries, offering novel perspectives that could inform therapeutic strategies, diagnostic tools, or preventive approaches.

2. The Innate and Adaptive Immune System

An aberrant immune response against epithelial elements and the intestinal microflora is the point of convergence of all the pathogenetic mechanisms of IBD [7].

The immune system includes two main compartments: innate and adaptive responses. The advent of single cell transcriptomics has revolutionized the investigation of the immune system, particularly T-cell populations. Recent studies indicate that, in the context of IBD, while the epithelial and stromal compartments undergo significant transcriptional shifts, the immune system exhibits profound alterations in both cell composition and abundance [8].

2.1. Innate Immune System

The epithelial layer, encompassing enterocytes and goblet cells, is the first gate of innate immunity. It plays a protective role thanks to its barrier function against pathogens [9]. Furthermore, the depletion or destruction of the mucus layer has been associated with the development of UC [10]. Previous studies have already highlighted that intestinal goblet cells play a role in the onset of Th17-based colitis, by delivering soluble antigens to $CD103^+$ dendritic cells. Recent evidence shows that the mucus reduction observed in UC is associated with a reduction in both the number and size of goblet cells. Furthermore, reduced glycosylation of the mucin 2 (MUC2) protein amplifies the inflammatory response to *E. coli*, driven by NF-kB signaling [11]. Evidence from single-cell RNA sequencing suggests that mucosal barrier malfunctioning may stem from the production of ectopic mucin. Specifically, transcripts of mucin 1 (MUC1), a mucin typically produced in the stomach, have been identified in the colonic mucosa of patients with CD [8]. Remarkably, recent studies based on single-cell transcriptomics show that ileal epithelial cells from pediatric patients with treatment-naïve CD have an overexpression of S100A9, a calprotectin subunit. This finding underscores the direct involvement of the epithelial barrier to the immune process underlying IBD [12].

Among the cellular populations involved in innate immunity, innate lymphoid cells (ILCs) are coming to the spotlight. ILCs are circulant and resident lymphocytes with a role in regulating tissue homeostasis and immune responses [13]. Various subtypes of ILCs have been identified, including ILC1s, which are primarily expressed in the upper gastrointestinal tract, and ILC3s, predominantly found in the ileum and colon [14]. Within this cellular subset, the enigmatic and controversial role of ILC3s is being investigated. ILC3s produce IL-17 and IL-22 and express receptors for IL-1 and IL-23 [15]. On one side, an imbalance in the activity of ILC3s is associated with reduced gut barrier integrity and increased susceptibility to inflammation. For example, Bao and colleagues recently demonstrated that, in a dextran sodium sulfate (DSS) mouse model of colitis, the exposure to bacterial sphingolipids leads to a reduced IL-22 secretion from ILC3s with consequent worsening of colitis [16]. On the contrary, in other models of colitis (such as anti-CD40 antibody-induced acute colitis), the inflammation is driven by the IL-22 produced by ILC3s [17]. Furthermore, specific subsets of ILC3s, such as $NKp44^+$, have a protective effect against CD and UC [18].

Macrophages, key players in innate immunity, mainly arise from monocytes and can be classified into M1 (inflammatory) and M2 (anti-inflammatory) types. M1 macrophages, activated by cytokines like IFN-γ and TNF-α, release cytokines (IL-12, IL-23) and reactive species that drive inflammation and pathogen clearance. In the gut, they disrupt tight junctions and induce epithelial cell apoptosis, worsening inflammation. M2 macrophages, marked by IL-4, IL-10, and CD206, promote tissue repair and resolve inflammation [19,20]. In UC, especially during the active phase, most macrophages in the lamina propria exhibit the M1 phenotype, which contributes to mucosal damage by disrupting tight junction proteins, compromising the epithelial barrier, and inducing apoptosis in epithelial cells. This results in heightened inflammation and further exacerbation of the disease [21]. On the contrary, increasing the proportion of M2 macrophages can alleviate symptoms of colitis in murine models, suggesting their protective role in IBD [22,23]. Novel insights on the role of macrophage polarization derive from single-cell and spatial transcriptomics. Garrido-Trigo and colleagues, upon identifying M0 macrophages within the colonic mucosa, highlighted significant variability in the transcriptional profiles of M1 macrophages in patients with IBD. Three major categories of M1 macrophages were identified: M1 ACOD1 (aconitate decarboxylase 1), M1 CXCL5 (CXC ligand 5), and the IDA (inflammation-dependent alternative) macrophage cluster. Notably, M1 macrophages in patients with UC (but not CD) exhibited elevated expression of neuregulin 1, a gene belonging to the epidermal growth factor family [24].

Myeloid cells, mainly neutrophils and macrophages, are also responsible for S100A9 calprotectin subunit. The role of calprotectin as an IBD biomarker has been known for some time [25]. However, recent evidence on the role of S100A9 in contributing to IBD pathogenesis is coming to the spotlight. In fact, S100A9 acts as an alarmin, a type of signaling molecule that is released during cellular stress or injury. It can activate immune responses by binding to Toll-like receptor 4 (TLR4) and other receptors, leading to the production of pro-inflammatory cytokines such as IL-1β, IL-6, and TNF-α. Furthermore, it also contributes to further neutrophils' recruitment. Notably, S100A9 may also interact with the gut microbiota, promoting dysbiosis. These features suggest that S100A9 could represent a new actor in the pathogenesis of IBD [26,27].

Natural killer (NK) cells, involved in both innate and adaptive immunity, recognize stress-induced and virus-infected cells. Found in the gut epithelium and stroma, they interact with various cell types and encounter antigens from microorganisms and the microbiota. In a healthy state, NK cells support immune responses by producing IFN-γ, enhancing anti-bacterial defenses [28]. In IBD patients, peripheral NK cells are dysregulated and produce high levels of pro-inflammatory cytokines, such as IL-17A and TNF-α, but exhibit diminished killing abilities. Additionally, these NK cells show reduced mitochondrial mass and impaired oxidative phosphorylation, indicating compromised cellular metabolism. The activity of mTORC1 (mammalian target of rapamycin complex 1), a key metabolic regulator, is also limited in both resting and cytokine-stimulated NK cells, contributing to their dysfunctional state in IBD. In CD, mucosal NK cells expressing NKp44 and NKp46 produce pro-inflammatory cytokines like IFNγ upon activation by intestinal macrophages, contributing to local inflammation. Conversely, in UC, NK cells appear to regulate the Th1/Th2 balance, with NKG2D$^+$ NK cells playing a potential regulatory role in modulating Th2-mediated responses [29]. The mechanisms of the innate immune system implicated in IBD pathogenesis are summarized in Figure 1.

2.2. *Adaptive Immune System*

Unlike the innate immune response, which acts as the first line of defense, the adaptive immune system is characterized by its ability to recognize specific antigens and mount a tailored response. In IBD, this response often becomes dysregulated, leading to chronic inflammation. The pathogenesis of IBD is thought to involve an inappropriate immune reaction against the gut microbiota and dietary antigens in genetically susceptible individuals. Key players in the adaptive immune response include various T-cell subsets, such as T helper cells (Th1, Th2, Th17), cytolytic CD8$^+$ cells, and regulatory T cells (Tregs). An imbalance between pro-inflammatory and anti-inflammatory Tregs is the mainstay of IBD pathogenesis [30,31].

Th1 polarization remains a mainstay of immune activation in IBD. Recent evidence obtained with single-cell transcriptomics confirms the presence of IFNG$^+$ TNF$^+$ T cells in mucosal and blood samples of patients with IBD, especially CD [32]. However, over the last years, increasing attention has been given to the role of Th17. In inflamed biopsies from patients with IBD, Medina and colleagues found a predominance of Th17 polarized lymphocytes overexpressing STAT3 (signal transducer and activator of transcription 3) and IL23R. Interestingly, according to single-cell transcriptional analysis, several lymphocytes showed a hybrid Th1/Th17 transcriptional profile, expressing genes such as CCL20 (C-C motif chemokine ligand 20), GZMA (granzyme A), GZMK (granzyme K), ITGA1 (integrin subunit alpha 1), CXCR3 (C-X-C motif chemokine receptor 3), GYG1 (glycogenin-1), CXCR6, LGALS3 (Galectin-3), and CCL5. Such cellular subpopulation was more abundant in inflamed tissues rather than non-inflamed areas and biopsies from healthy controls [33]. New transcriptional factors associated with the stimulation or inhibition of Th17 differentiation are being investigated. For example, the transcription factor ELF4 can both suppress inflammatory Th17 cell activity and induce macrophage M2 polarization [34].

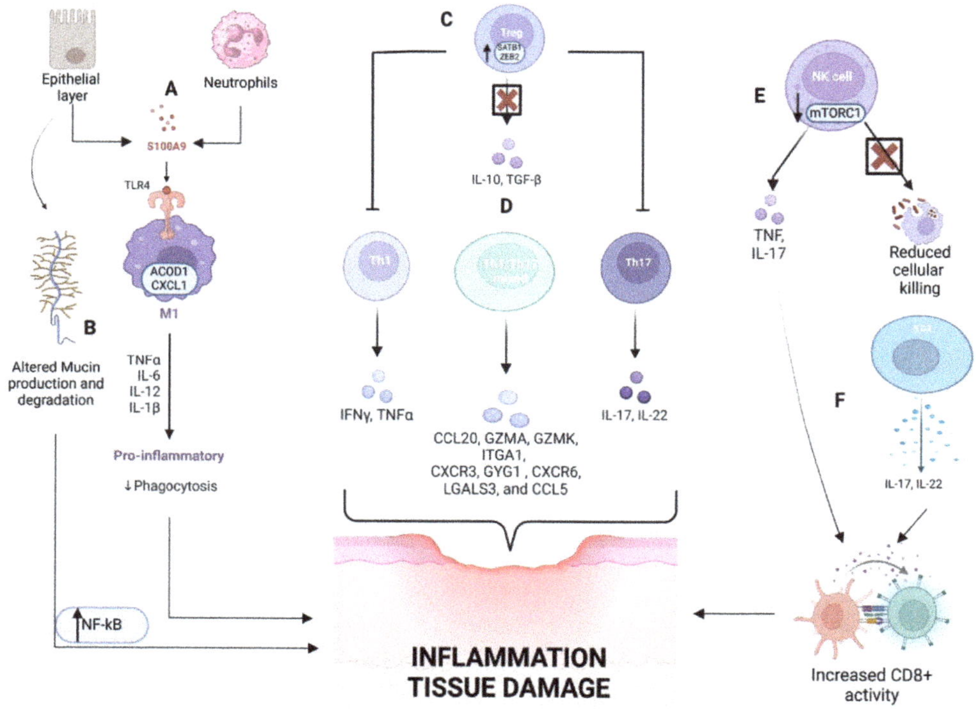

Figure 1. Dysregulated immune responses contributing to inflammation and tissue damage in IBD pathogenesis. Epithelial barrier disruption and neutrophil recruitment trigger the release of S100A9, which activates Toll-like receptor 4 (TLR4) signaling in M1 macrophages. These macrophages produce pro-inflammatory cytokines (TNFα, IL-6, IL-12, IL-1β), promoting inflammation and reducing phagocytosis (**A**). Altered production and glycosylation of mucin molecules contribute to amplify inflammation via NFkB (**B**). Dysregulated T-cell responses include reduced regulatory T cell (Treg) activity (**C**) and increased Th1, Th17, and mixed Th1/Th17 responses, producing IFNγ, TNFα, IL-17, and IL-22. These cytokines induce recruitment of inflammatory cells and expression of chemokines (CCL20, GZMA, ITGA1, etc.), amplifying tissue damage (**D**). NK cells with impaired mTORC1 signaling show reduced cytotoxicity, further aggravating inflammation (**E**). Innate lymphoid cells (ILC3) produce IL-17 and IL-22, enhancing $CD8^+$ T cell activation and exacerbating tissue injury (**F**).

It must be mentioned that a recent study by Tanemoto and colleagues proved the existence of a cellular subpopulation presenting mixed CD4/CD8 transcriptional activity. Such cells are closer to the $CD4^+$ population in terms of transcriptional analysis but also express CD8-related transcripts such as perforins or granzymes [35]. Activated cytotoxic $CD8^+$ T cells contribute to the initiation and progression of IBD. Several subtypes of $CD8^+$

are known, including conventional cytotoxic (or cytolytic) T lymphocytes (CTLs) and $CD8^+$ regulatory T cells [36]. Extensive insight into the role of $CD8^+$ in UC is provided by Corridoni et al. thanks to single-cell transcriptomics. On one side, $CD8^+$ lymphocytes are implicated in tissue damage through the production of TNF-α and other pro-inflammatory cytokines; on the other hand, some post-effector $CD8^+$ T cells exhibit regulatory characteristics that may help mitigate excessive inflammation. Furthermore, the study also identifies terminally differentiated dysfunctional $CD8^+$ T cells that express IL-26, a cytokine shown to attenuate acute colitis severity in a humanized mouse model [37]. $CD8^+$ cells have been found to be related to disease activity, especially in CD. In fact, both in blood and intestinal samples of patients with active CD, CD39-expressing $CD8^+$ T cells often showed signs of exhaustion, meaning they were less effective at responding to infections or inflammation [38].

Finally, an imbalance in the number and functionality of T regulatory lymphocytes is associated with the onset of IBD. $Foxp3^+$ Treg cells are essential for suppressing inflammation, primarily through the production of IL-10 in response to TGFβ1 (transforming growth factor beta 1) stimulation [39]. Interestingly, it has been recently postulated that diets with high amounts of fatty acids can induce ferroptosis of such cellular subtype, leading to colitis worsening [40]. Surprisingly, single-cell transcriptional analysis in mucosal samples of patients with UC shows that Tregs are numerically increased in comparison to healthy controls. This could be related to the need for dampening inflammation. Conversely, transcriptional profiles of this cellular lineage are altered in UC, with the overexpression of transcripts (including SATB1, special AT-rich sequence-binding protein-1, and ZEB2, Zinc finger E-box-binding homeobox 2) that should be instead be suppressed for normal Treg functioning. It has to be remarked that, according to new evidence, tissue and circulating Tregs are not the only to be considered: in fact, mesenteric lymph nodes represent a critical site of effect of Tregs [41,42]. The key mechanisms of the adaptive immune system contributing to IBD pathogenesis are illustrated in Figure 1.

Given the critical role of the immune system in the pathogenesis of IBD, innovative therapeutic strategies are being explored to modulate immune responses and promote healing, one of which involves the application of mesenchymal stem cells (MSCs). MSCs possess unique properties, including immunomodulation, anti-inflammatory effects, and tissue regeneration, which make them suitable for addressing the complex pathogenesis of IBD. In Crohn's disease, MSC therapy has received Food and Drug Administration approval for use in refractory cases, especially for complications such as fistulas and sphincter insufficiency. The mechanism of action of MSCs involves the secretion of bioactive factors that modulate the immune response, reduce inflammation, and promote healing of damaged intestinal tissue. They achieve this by downregulating pro-inflammatory cytokines and enhancing anti-inflammatory pathways, thereby restoring intestinal homeostasis. Moreover, MSCs exhibit low immunogenicity, allowing them to evade immune detection and reducing the risk of adverse reactions [43–45].

3. Gut Microbiota

Nowadays, the dissemination of integrated multi-omic analysis allows us to define disease-specific signatures. Common and recognizable profiles that characterize and distinguish IBDs are defined. For example, a recent study provides a multi-omic-based definition of gut microbiota, mycobiota, and metabolic signature in UC [46].

From an early age, the composition of microbiota is influenced and modified by several factors, including exposure to antibiotics. A systematic review has evaluated the impact of antibiotics on the infant gut microbiome composition and resistome in infants in low- to middle-income countries settings. Antibiotics disrupt microbiome diversity and taxonomy, with effects likely mediated by antibiotic class, duration of administration, and follow-up time [47]. The association between antibiotic exposure and an increased risk of developing IBD has been confirmed by a recent meta-analysis involving 99,104 IBD patients and 2,273,336 controls, reporting an odds ratio (OR) of 1.66 (95% CI, 1.28–2.16) [48]. Notably, exposure to cephalosporins was strongly associated with new-onset IBD (OR, 1.62; 95% CI, 1.26–2.08), as was exposure to penicillins (OR, 1.50; 95% CI, 1.14–1.98) and macrolides (OR, 1.50; 95% CI, 1.14–1.98). Similarly, quinolones (OR, 1.49; 95% CI, 1.45–1.54), tetracyclines (OR, 1.49; 95% CI, 1.44–1.54), and metronidazole/tinidazole (OR, 1.34; 95% CI, 1.30–1.38) were significantly linked to an increased IBD risk [47]. In children, the cumulative frequency of antibiotic use plays a critical role in the risk of developing IBD. While a single dispensation within the year preceding diagnosis was not significantly associated with IBD risk, cumulative exposure—defined as two or more dispensations within the same timeframe—was linked to a significantly higher risk. Prolonged antibiotic exposure further increases the risk of developing IBD, with an odds ratio (OR) of 1.49 (95% CI, 1.12–1.98) for exposure over three years and 1.46 (95% CI, 1.37–1.55) for exposure over two years [48]. Data from Sweden and Norway further underscore the importance of early antibiotic use. Among 103,046 children, 395 developed IBD, with a higher risk observed in those exposed to antibiotics during the first year of life (HR = 1.33; 95% CI, 1.01–1.76) compared to those without exposure. In contrast, the frequency of infections did not show a significant association with IBD risk [49].

The composition of microbiota in IBD patients significantly differs compared to healthy individuals. Beta-diversity, defined as the difference in types of microbes between multiple samples, and alpha-diversity, defined as the difference within an ecosystem or a sample, are both reduced in microbiota of IBD patients compared to healthy individuals, particularly if looking at the stability of the microbiome of patients over time [50]. As confirmed by recent meta-analysis, which has included 13 studies, reduced alpha-diversity is a consistent feature of both CD and UC but was more pronounced in CD (OR of 3.20, 95% CI: 2.09–4.88, $p < 0.001$) [51]. More in depth, key alterations include a decrease in beneficial *Firmicutes* and *Bacteroidetes*, alongside an increase in pathogenic *Proteobacteria*. Recent studies have confirmed such trend reporting that, specifically, the abundance of *Faecalibacterium prausnitzii* and *Roseburia intestinalis*, both known for their anti-inflammatory properties, is markedly reduced in IBD patients, while *Escherichia coli* and other members of the *Proteobacteria* phylum show increased prevalence, correlating with disease severity and inflammation levels [52,53].

Gut microbiota contributes to determining intestinal inflammation mainly through its interaction with the immune system (Figure 2). For example, germ-free mice colonized by gut microbiota from IBD patients show an elevation of Th17 and Th2 cells, with concomitant reduction of RORγt$^+$ Treg cells [54]. Interestingly, recent evidence shows that adherent-invasive *Escherichia coli* (AIEC) has the ability to attach to and penetrate epithelial cells, stimulating the secretion of interleukin-1 beta (IL-1β) from macrophages, which stimulates the differentiation of Th17 cells; in the same way, *Klebsiella pneumoniae* and *Klebsiella aerogenes* enhance the release of pro-inflammatory cytokines (particularly IL-1β and IL-18) from dendritic cells and macrophages, promoting the differentiation of Th1 and Th17 cells. Moreover, mucolytic bacteria like *Ruminococcus gnavus* are able to produce polysaccharides that stimulate tumor necrosis factor (TNF) secretion from dendritic cells [55]. Similarly, mice administered with DSS show more elevated IL-6 and IL-1β serum concentrations and monocyte-chemoattractant protein (MCP)-1 when receiving oral gavage of *C. difficile* after the DSS [56].

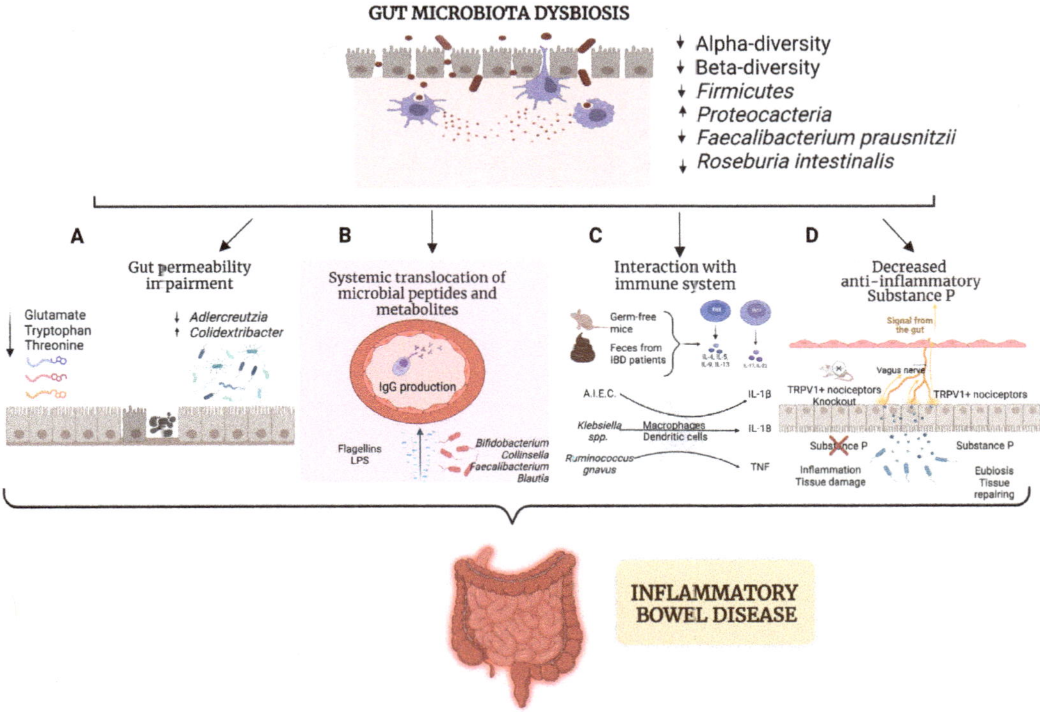

Figure 2. The impact of gut microbiota dysregulation on IBD pathogenesis. Reduced microbial diversity, depletion of beneficial taxa such as *Faecalibacterium prausnitzii* and *Roseburia intestinalis*, and enrichment of pathogenic taxa like *Proteobacteria* are the core features of gut dysbioisis. This disruption impairs gut permeability by reducing key amino acids and altering microbial composition, allowing microbial components to penetrate the intestinal barrier (**A**). Translocated microbial peptides and metabolites, such as flagellins and LPS, enter systemic circulation, triggering IgG production and amplifying inflammation (**B**). Immune system activation involves increased inflammatory cytokine production following exposure to microbial products, as observed in germ-free mice receiving fecal transplants from IBD patients. Pathogenic bacteria, including *Klebsiella* spp. and *Ruminococcus gnavus*, further stimulate macrophages and dendritic cells to release pro-inflammatory cytokines like IL-1β, IL-18, and TNF (**C**). Additionally, dysbiosis disrupts TRPV1^{+} nociceptor signaling, reducing levels of the anti-inflammatory mediator Substance P. This impairment compromises vagus nerve-mediated tissue repair, enhances inflammation, and deranges pain perception (**D**).

As mentioned, the intestinal mucus layer plays a central role in maintaining gut homeostasis. Understanding how gut microbiota interacts with mucus layer could represent a key factor in elucidating IBD pathogenesis. To such a purpose, a recent study demonstrated that mice deficient in the MUC2 protein also exhibit specific microbiota features impacting colitis severity [57]. Furthermore, the administration of *Lactobacillus reuteri* leads to a mitigation of colitis symptoms in DSS-induced colitis mice. This effect is mediated by the synthesis of indole-3-acetic acid (IAA), a tryptophan derivate, and to the thickening of the colonic mucus layer [58]. The mucus layer is not the only constituent of intestinal permeability. The association between gut microbiome composition and impaired barrier function is a mainstay of the IBD pathogenesis. Recent evidence suggests that decreased prevalence of *Adlercreutzia* (with anti-inflammatory properties), coupled with increased abundance of *Colidextribacter* (with a role in cellular oxidative stress), are related to impaired intestinal permeability. Moreover, the depletion of microbial pathways associated with the biosynthesis of the amino acids glutamate, tryptophan, and threonine suggests the role of microbiota-metabolites in driving altered gut permeability [59].

Gut microbiota could induce damage even outside of the gut. In fact, translocation of pathogens from mucosal surfaces into peripheral tissues can directly stimulate immune cells to produce many proinflammatory cytokines, increasing intestinal inflammation [60] (Figure 2). A cross-sectional study focused on characterizing the adaptive immunoglobulin response to human-derived microbiota flagellins in CD and UC. In particular, patients with CD, but not patients with UC, show increased serum IgG antibody responses to human ileal-localized *Lachnospiraceae flagellins*, with a subset of patients that also show increased CD4 cells against such antigens [61]. More recently, a correlation between a subset of commensal gut microbiota constituents that translocate across the gut barrier and systemic immunoglobulin G (IgG) responses has been described in mice and humans. In particular, the systemic IgG ranges were detectable against translocating gut bacteria and taxa that can be proinflammatory, such as *Bifidobacterium*, *Collinsella*, *Faecalibacterium*, and *Blautia* genera. In addition, patients with CD exhibited greater IgG targeting of gut commensals than UC patients [62].

The taxonomical impairment in gut microbiota results in a shift in the metabolomic profile of IBD patients. Functional modifications also play an important role in developing IBD [63]. The most relevant modifications are represented by higher levels of organic acids and amino acids such as tryptophan, glutamine, arginine, 5-hydroxytryptophan, and histidine, along with a decrease in short-chain fatty acids (SCFA) [64]. However, the role of these metabolites in IBD is still unsolved. The latest evidence reveals that a mixture of SCFA-producing bacterial strains attenuates UC in DSS-mice models by inducing M2 macrophage polarization and inhibiting JAK/STAT3/FOXO3 axis activation [65].

In recent years, focus has been given to the so-called "neglected microbiome" (fungi, protozoa, and viruses), which have also shown a great relevance in the IBD pathogenesis. Regarding the gut virome, *Siphoviridae* and *Myoviridae* (which belong to the order of *Caudovirales*) are significantly enriched in IBD patients, while *Quimbyviridae* are decreased [66]. Specific changes have also been highlighted between CD and UC patients in terms of virome. Patients with CD exhibit greater prevalence of the *Hepeviridae* family and a reduction of the *Virgaviridae* family; conversely, UC patients show an abundance of transcripts encoded by *Orthoepadnaviridae* [67]. The alterations in the virome significantly contribute to the pathogenesis of IBD through different pathways, such as altering the integrity of the intestinal mucosa; stimulating the immune response by influencing the host bacteria; releasing bacterial components after lysis or transcytosis; and inducing IFN type-I response in immune cells, which can worsen intestinal inflammation and increase the severity of the disease [68]. A recent study demonstrates how bacteriophage can influence the bacteria microbiota. Monocolonized germ-free mice with *Bacteroides fragilis* NCTC 9343 in the presence of Barc2635, a lytic double-stranded DNA bacteriophage belonging to the *Caudoviricete*, show a switch of the polysaccharide A (PSA) promoter of *B. fragilis* in the "OFF" state causing reduced a decrease in Tregs with a consequent reduction in inflammation [69]. Fecal virome transplantation (FVT) experiments using human fecal virus-like particles (VLPs) in a mouse model confirmed the roles of IBD viral signatures in disease progression. The expression levels of E-cadherin, β-catenin, and occludins were upregulated in the HF-FVT (Healthy Donor Fecal Virome Transplantation) group and downregulated in the IBD-FVT group, indicating worsened gut permeability in the IBD-FVT group. Additionally, the IBD-FVT group exhibited significantly greater levels of inflammatory cytokines, including TNF-α, IL-6, IFN-γ, and IL-1β. These findings indicate that the colonization of viruses from healthy donors has a mitigating effect on colitis in a mouse model, whereas that of viruses from IBD patients exacerbates colitis with a substantial expansion of IBD-enriched viral operational taxonomic units (vOTUs) within the mouse gut microbiota [66]. The rise of high-throughput sequencing also allowed a better understanding about fungal dysbiosis and the implication in the pathogenesis of IBD. *Didymellaceae*, *Saccharomycetales*, *Malassezia*, *Wickerhamomyces*, *Cutaneotrichosporon*, *Saccharomyces*, *Clavispora*, *Alternaria*, and *Candida* are major fungal markers in UC [46]. In 2,4,6-trinitrobenzenesulfonic acid (TNBS)-derived colitis mice models, fungi depletion protects against the progression of the disease. The mechanisms through which fungi promote pro-inflammatory response in IBD relies on CD4$^+$ T cells, which are stimulated to produce IFN-γ, IL-17A, and TNF-α [70]. The loss of integrity of IECs through the disruption of tight junction (TJ) Occludin and ZO-1 lead to the penetration of pathogens like fungi and bacteria into the mucosal barrier and consequently activate TLRs, Dectin-1, and caspase-recruitment domain 9 (CARD9), inducing a more severe inflammatory phenotype [71].

Finally, gut microbiota could play a role in determining IBD susceptibility, even through the interaction with the peripheral nervous system (PNS) (Figure 2). For example, a recent study analyzed the role of TRPV1$^+$ nociceptors in regulating the composition of the intestinal microbiota through substance P, which limits inflammation and promotes intestinal tissue protection, restoring intestinal homeostasis. In particular, in the absence of TRPV1$^-$ nociceptors, vancomycin-sensitive Gram-positive bacterial communities lead to enhanced susceptibility to DSS-induced colitis in mice. Moreover, mono-colonization of a consortium of Gram-positive bacteria *Clostridium* spp. in germ-free mice with disrupted nociception was able to exacerbate intestinal inflammation. In contrast, mono-colonization of nociceptor-sufficient germ-free mice with *Clostridium* spp. was tissue protective. Mechanistically, disruption of nociception resulted in decreased levels of substance P, and the therapeutic delivery of substance P promoted tissue-protective effects exerted by TRPV1$^+$ nociceptors in a microbiota-dependent manner [72].

Building on the growing understanding of the gut microbiota's role in inflammation and disease, fecal microbiota transplantation (FMT) has gained attention as a therapeutic strategy to restore microbial balance by transferring fecal microbiota from healthy donors to recipients. FMT has demonstrated its effectiveness in *Clostridioides difficile* infection [73]. Starting from this, FMT has been tested as a new promising therapeutic strategy in IBD. As evidence of the role of the gut microbiota as a trigger of inflammation, studies have been performed on FMT in patients with mild-to-moderate UC, demonstrating effectiveness in inducing clinical remission, despite the heterogeneity in design protocols, regarding routes of FMT administration, inclusion criteria, and follow-up periods. These results confirmed the possible use of FMT as a therapeutic option in UC patients. Nevertheless, the insufficient data about long-term effects and the variability in study designs currently do not allow FMT to be recommended as a standard treatment in clinical practice [73,74]. The efficacy of FMT in CD remains unclear. Some studies suggest a potential role in the induction and maintenance of clinical response and remission. However, the lack of randomized clinical trials and robust data currently does not support the application of FMT in CD patients [75].

4. Genetics

Genetics has long been recognized as a predisposing factor in the development of IBD, but its role has evolved over the years. While the focus on genetic factors may not be as prominent as it once was, recent studies continue to reveal intriguing insights into how genetic variations contribute to IBD susceptibility.

4.1. Polygenic Contributions to IBD

Several genes have been historically linked to an increased risk of IBD. Nucleotide Binding Oligomerization Domain Containing 2 (NOD2) was the first gene identified as a susceptibility factor for CD. It is involved in recognizing bacterial components and initiating immune responses. Variants in this gene impair autophagy, affecting bacterial clearance and immune regulation [76]. Among the genes associated with IBD, IL23R is notable for its protective alleles. The R381Q polymorphism reduces the risk of Crohn's disease by approximately threefold, and additional rare protective variants, such as G149R and V362I, further support the gene's protective role. These findings underscore the importance of IL23R in the IL23/Th17 signaling pathway, which plays a critical role in regulating $CD4^{+}$ Th17 cell differentiation. These insights underscore the therapeutic potential of targeting this pathway in IBD. Mutations in autophagy-related genes, such as ATG16L1 (Autophagy-Related 16 Like 1) and IRGM (Immunity-Related GTPase M), have been linked to immune response dysregulation. Additionally, genes involved in interleukin signaling pathways, including STAT3, TYK2, and JAK2, as well as PTPN2 (Tyrosine-protein phosphatase non-receptor type 2), which is associated with other autoimmune diseases, have been shown to contribute to the development of IBD [77].

An interesting genetic locus possibly involved in the predisposition to IBD is OCTN1/Slc22a4. OCTN1 (organic cation transporter, novel, type 1) is an organic cation transporter expressed in various tissues throughout the body. It is particularly abundant in intestinal epithelial cells, especially in the small intestine and colon, where it plays a crucial role in the absorption of specific molecules. Additionally, OCTN1 was also found in the proximal tubules of the kidney, liver, skeletal muscle, and placenta. In the gut, OCTN1 could be involved in the traffic of bacterial molecules, contributing to IBD pathogenesis. Polymorphisms in OCTN1 had been previously associated with predisposition of IBD (UC in particular) and occurrence of GI cancer in young individuals. Furthermore, OCTN1 facilitates the absorption of ergothioneine, a key antioxidant that protects intestinal cells from oxidative stress. When OCTN1 is dysfunctional, antioxidant protection is reduced, making the gut more vulnerable to inflammation. Recent evidence has shed new light on the role of this genetic locus. According to Del Chierico and colleagues, OCTN1 deficient mice ($OCTN1^{-/-}$) show reduced DSS-induced colitis severity and a higher baseline percentage of Treg, T memory, Th2, and Th17 cells [78–81].

CARD9 has recently emerged as a potential predisposing factor for IBD. This enigmatic protein interacts with Toll-like receptors (TLRs) to activate innate immunity via mitogen-activated protein kinases (MAPK) and nuclear factor kappa-light-chain-enhancer of activated B cells (NF-kB). The majority of CARD9 variants (such as rs10870077, rs4077515, and rs10781499) have a proinflammatory effect and represent predisposing variants to IBD. In contrast, uncommon variants such as rs141992399 and rs200735402 have an anti-inflammatory effect and act as protective from IBD [82]. It has been recently demonstrated that CARD9 also drives cellular apoptosis. In particular, CARD9-deficient mice show increased neutrophil apoptosis and are more susceptible to intestinal inflammation [83]. Finally, CARD9 is involved in the recovery from colitis through the production of IL-22 and other antimicrobial peptides [84]. Several other functions have been proposed for CARD9, including other immunomodulatory activities and control of tumorigenesis [82].

Polymorphisms and genetic variants of genes encoding for inflammatory cytokines have acquired recent relevance in the field of IBD susceptibility. TNF superfamily member 15 (TNFSF15) is the gene that encodes tumor necrosis factor-like cytokine 1A (TLA1), a member of the TNF cytokines superfamily. It interacts with its receptor DR3, encoded by the TNFRSF25 gene. Several roles are being investigated for TNFSF15 variants, including IBD susceptibility and fibrosis development [85]. More in depth, the binding of TNFSF 15 to DR3 results in increased bacterial uptake via PDK1 by phagocytic cells. Furthermore, the TNFSF 15-DR3 interaction leads to increased production of reactive oxygen species and reactive nitrogen species, as well as the activation of autophagy pathways. Taken all together, these modifications lead to increased intracellular bacterial clearance [86]. A Genome-Wide Association Study (GWAS) and a Transcriptome-Wide Association Study (TWAS), conducted on a Japanese population, identified a significant association between TNFSF15 expression in whole blood and the development of CD [87]. This association has been confirmed by a meta-analysis including eight studies and a total of 2682 patients. rs6478109 polymorphisms were significantly associated with the onset of CD (not UC), independent from disease phenotype [88].

4.2. Monogenic IBD

Monogenic forms of IBD, although rare, are typically severe and resistant to conventional therapies [89]. Unlike polygenic or idiopathic IBD, monogenic forms follow Mendelian inheritance patterns and are associated with specific genetic mutations [90]. Advances in next-generation sequencing have led to the identification of over 80 causal genes, IL10RA/IL10RB (interleukin 10 receptor alpha/beta), XIAP (X-linked inhibitor of apoptosis protein), CYBB (cytochrome b-245 beta chain), LRBA (lipopolysaccharide-responsive and beige-like anchor protein), and TTC7A (tetratricopeptide repeat domain 7A), which provide valuable insights into distinct disease mechanisms [91]. These mutations often disrupt key immune processes, underscoring the importance of precise genetic diagnosis. Mutations in genes regulating phagocyte functions—such as bacterial killing, cell migration, or inflammatory pathways—can drive monogenic IBD. For instance, antimicrobial activity is notably impaired in chronic granulomatous disease (CGD), which is linked to NADPH oxidase complex mutations. Nearly half of CGD patients develop intestinal inflammation, illustrating how genetic disruptions in microbial clearance can directly contribute to IBD pathogenesis [92]. Furthermore, recent discoveries, such as mutations in CYBC1 and Protein Kinase C Delta (PRKCD), have highlighted additional failures in microbial killing mechanisms that exacerbate disease severity [93,94]. Endothelial cell dysfunction also plays a critical role in some forms of monogenic IBD. Mutations in CD55, for example, enhance complement activation, which damages cells and amplifies inflammation [95]. Similarly, mutations in solute carrier organic anion transporter family member 2A1 (SLCO2A1) impair prostaglandin clearance, leading to chronic intestinal bleeding and further complicating disease management [93]. Together, these genetic abnormalities demonstrate the complex cellular disruptions underlying monogenic IBD.

Monogenic IBD is often characterized by early onset, atypical family history, unusual endoscopic findings, and extra-intestinal manifestations. These clinical features can help distinguish it from polygenic forms, enabling earlier and more targeted interventions. While emerging therapies such as hematopoietic stem cell transplantation and gene therapy using lentiviral vectors have shown promise, significant challenges remain in translating these advances into routine clinical practice [96]. Concerns about long-term safety and scalability highlight the need for continued research and validation of these novel approaches.

4.3. Genetics–Microbiota Interactions

Recent research has brought increasing attention to the dynamic interplay between host genetics and the gut microbiota in the pathogenesis of IBD. This relationship is bidirectional, with host genetic variations influencing microbial communities, while microbial proteins, in turn, modulate host gene expression. Understanding this complex interaction is key to uncovering novel pathways in IBD development and progression. Host genetic variations play a significant role in shaping the composition and functionality of the gut microbiota. For example, variants in genes such as IL17REL (interleukin 17 receptor E-like), MYRF (myelin regulatory factor), SEC16A (SEC16 homolog A, endoplasmic reticulum export factor), and WDR78 (WD repeat domain 78) have been linked to changes in microbiota diversity. In particular, MYRF variations are associated with reduced production of short-chain fatty acids (SCFAs), which are essential for maintaining gut health and mitigating inflammation [79]. These findings suggest that genetic predispositions can directly impact the microbial environment, creating conditions conducive to IBD. Conversely, microbial proteins can influence host gene expression, further complicating the immune response. For example, a study by Sudhakar and colleagues (2022) demonstrated how specific microbial proteins interact with host genes to modulate immune responses and inflammatory pathways in Crohn's disease [97]. These interactions underscore the intricate feedback loop between the microbiome and host genetics, wherein dysbiosis not only results from but also exacerbates genetic vulnerabilities.

This evolving understanding of genetics–microbiota interactions has significant implications for IBD treatment. It highlights the potential for integrated therapeutic approaches that target both genetic and microbial contributors to disease. By combining genetic profiling with microbiota analysis, clinicians may be able to develop personalized treatment strategies that address the root causes of IBD.

5. The Exposome

Several modifiable environmental factors, collectively referred to as the "exposome", have been investigated for their association with IBD risk [98]. While smoking remains the only well-established risk factor [99], evidence for other modifiable factors influencing disease susceptibility is steadily emerging, though preventive strategies have yet to be fully developed. We have comprehensively gathered all available evidence on environmental modifiable risk factors for CD and UC, categorizing them by life period—childhood or adulthood—in which they exert influence.

5.1. Childhood Exposures

Several prenatal and birth-related factors have been suggested to influence the development of CD or UC in various studies. Growing evidence suggests that in utero environmental exposures can influence epigenetic programming in the fetus, potentially shaping lifelong health risks, including susceptibility to inflammatory conditions [100–102]. These epigenetic modifications may also be inherited by future generations, representing transgenerational epigenetic inheritance [103,104]. For instance, studies have identified that an excessive intake of certain micronutrients, such as folate, vitamin B12, or methionine, in the maternal diet could increase the risk of colitis in offspring [105]. Additionally, maternal infections during pregnancy might trigger IL-6 production, leading to epigenetic changes in fetal intestinal epithelial stem cells and predisposing the child to inflammatory diseases [106]. These early-life exposures are part of the broader childhood exposome, as highlighted in a 2020 study by van der Sloot et al., which investigated 36 factors and identified prenatal smoking as a significant risk factor for CD (OR 1.89; 95% CI 1.38–2.59) and a nominally significant risk factor for UC (OR 1.61; 95% CI 1.16–2.23), even after accounting for smoking in later life [107]. Mechanistically, maternal smoking has been associated with persistent alterations in DNA methylation, miRNA dysregulation, and gut microbiome alterations in the exposed offspring [108–110].

In contrast, breastfeeding has been shown to exert a protective effect against CD (OR 0.71; 95% CI 0.59–0.85), UC (OR 0.78; 95% CI 0.67–0.91), and overall IBD (OR 0.74; 95% CI 0.66–0.83), with longer breastfeeding durations linked to lower disease risk [111,112]. Notably, this protective effect is stronger in Asian populations for CD (OR 0.31; 95% CI 0.20–0.48) compared to Caucasians, and in studies conducted before 2000, where IBD risk was reduced more significantly (OR 0.58 versus 0.82) [111]. Similarly, van der Sloot et al. identified a modest protective effect of breastfeeding on CD (OR 0.56; 95% CI 0.37–0.87) [107], while Gordon et al. (2022) reported that any form of breastfeeding, including mixed feeding, reduced UC onset risk (OR 0.48; 95% CI 0.25–0.93, $p = 0.03$), although no significant effect was observed for CD in twin pairs with IBD [113]. Breastfeeding's protective effect is hypothesized to stem from its role in establishing a healthy gut microbiota and supporting innate mucosal immunity development [114,115]. Conversely, the absence of breastfeeding has been linked to increased *Clostridium difficile* colonization and other immune-mediated diseases, including IBD.

Similarly, other early-life factors, such as mode of delivery, have been investigated for their potential influence on IBD risk. The impact of cesarean delivery, however, has shown inconsistent findings, with some studies linking cesarean births to an increased risk of CD (OR 1.38; 95% CI 1.12–1.70), but not UC or overall IBD [116–118]. Other research has found no significant differences in the incidence of CD or UC between cesarean and vaginal deliveries [112]. In the same vein, factors such as preterm birth, birthweight, and birth length have not been consistently associated with IBD risk [107].

On the other hand, as previously discussed in the gut microbiota section, the use of antibiotics during pregnancy or early life has been implicated as a potential risk factor for IBD. Antibiotics may disrupt the gut microbiota, reducing its diversity and taxonomic richness while altering its metabolic function [119–121]. For example, antibiotics have been associated with an increased risk of CD (OR 1.74; 95% CI 1.35–2.23) and IBD overall (OR 1.57; 95% CI 1.27–1.94), with a dose–response effect observed in pediatric CD (OR 2.75; 95% CI 1.72–4.38) [122]. This impact is especially pronounced in CD, where antibiotics exacerbate dysbiosis, a characteristic feature of the disease [123,124].

The "hygiene hypothesis" has also been proposed to explain IBD pathogenesis, suggesting that reduced exposure to environmental microorganisms disrupts immune system balance, increasing susceptibility to autoimmune conditions. A meta-analysis found that living near farm animals (OR 0.46; 95% CI 0.20–0.72), having pets (OR 0.77; 95% CI 0.59–0.94), sharing a home (OR 0.49; 95% CI 0.25–0.75), bed-sharing (OR 0.54; 95% CI 0.43–0.65), and having two or more siblings (OR 0.93; 95% CI 0.88–0.98) were protective against CD [125]. Similarly, these factors, except having siblings, along with access to hot water (OR 0.76; 95% CI 0.57–0.95) and a personal toilet (OR 0.73; 95% CI 0.59–0.88), conferred protection against UC [126]. Conversely, urban living has been associated with a higher incidence of CD (IRR 1.42; 95% CI 1.26–1.60) and IBD overall (OR 1.35; 95% CI 1.15–1.58) [127]. However, more recent studies have not confirmed the association between sibling presence and IBD risk, although other hygiene-related markers still point to a protective pattern. Notably, pet ownership during early life was shown to exert a protective effect, particularly in the first year of life, against CD (OR 0.30; 95% CI 0.22 –0.40) and UC (OR 0.32; 95% CI 0.24–0.44), with significant effects persisting throughout childhood [107].

Infection with Helicobacter pylori appears to offer protection against IBD, with a stronger effect observed in children compared to adults (OR 0.24 vs. 0.46) [128–131]. This association is thought to be mediated by immune modulation, including Toll-like receptor

2 activation, interleukin-10 production, inhibition of type I interferon and interleukin-12 production, and regulatory T-cell accumulation [132–134]. Reduced exposure to infectious agents during childhood may limit microbiota diversity and promote a pro-inflammatory Th2 immune response, increasing IBD risk [119,135]. Additionally, maternal exposure to farm environments has been shown to increase both the number and function of cord-blood regulatory T cells [136].

Other factors associated with increased IBD risk include low fruit intake, low physical activity, appendectomy, frequent childhood gastroenteritis admission, previous exposure to antibiotics and certain vaccinations, and early dietary introduction of gluten and sugar [137,138]. Notably, Piovani et al., among seven vaccinations, found that only the poliomyelitis vaccine was associated with IBD in a small meta-analysis [139]. Similarly, Ungaro et al. reported a significant association between antibiotic exposure and an elevated risk CD (OR 1.74; 95% CI 1.35–2.23) and IBD overall (OR 1.57; 95% CI 1.27–1.94), but not UC. A dose–response relationship was identified, with a stronger effect observed in pediatric CD (OR 2.75; 95% CI 1.72–4.38). All antibiotic classes, except for narrow-spectrum penicillins, were linked to an increased risk of IBD [122]. The biological plausibility of these findings is supported by the known impact of antibiotics on the gut microbiota. Antibiotics reduce both the taxonomic richness and diversity of the microbiome [119,120], impairing its metabolic function [121]. This disruption appears more pronounced in CD compared to UC, as antibiotics have been shown to exacerbate the dysbiosis characteristic of CD [123,124]. Stressful life events, such as parental divorce or a family death, have also been implicated [140,141]. Chronic stress is a well-established risk factor for both IBD onset and exacerbation. Recent findings highlight the role of enterochromaffin cells (EC) in gut sensing mechanisms that influence anxiety-like behaviors, as well as the impact of chronic stress and elevated corticosteroid levels on inflammatory enteric glial cells, which in turn activate immune cells [142,143]. This cascade can lead to various physiological alterations in the intestine, including increased gastrointestinal secretion, increased intestinal permeability, reduced mucosal blood flow, and alterations of the gut microbiota composition, thereby increasing the risk of IBD [144–146]

5.2. Adulthood Exposures

Besides childhood, numerous environmental factors have been studied for IBD risk also in adulthood. One of the most common problems of the modern era is air pollution, and in recent years the interest in this topic has also grown in the field of IBD [144,147,148]. From a pathogenetic point of view, environmental pollutants can alter the redox balance at the level of the intestinal barrier, oxidizing the lipids of the intestinal epithelium [149,150]. Oxidative stress, moreover, can cause damage to the mucous layer of the gastrointestinal tract, leading to bacterial invasion, triggering immune responses, and initiating IBD [149]. It has been shown that exposure to PM2.5 increases the concentrations of oxidized low-density lipoproteins [151]. Furthermore, exposure to particulate matter and ozone modifies intestinal permeability by damaging the intercellular barriers [152]. Kaplan et al. showed that residential exposures to sulfur dioxide (SO_2) and nitric oxide (NO_2) might increase the risk of early-onset UC and CD, respectively [148]. Such exposures also seem to influence the course of the disease; an increase in the density of pollutant emission by 1-log was associated with a 40% increase in the rate of IBD hospitalizations (incidence RR = 1.40; 95% CI: 1.31–1.50, for both UC and CD hospitalization) [153]. Finally, in a large Italian study, long-term exposure to PM2.5 levels above 20 $\mu g/m^3$ was associated with a significant increase in the development of IBD (adjusted OR of 1.21 95% CI: 1.03–1.42) compared to those below 20 $\mu g/m^3$ [154]. Liu et al. analyzed (455,210 people aged 40–69 years) the long-term associations between exposure to air pollution and the risk of IBD [155]. They found significant associations for UC with PM2.5, PM2.5–10, PM10, NO_2, and Nox. In contrast, Okafor et al. found no associations between PM2.5, O_3, diesel PM, traffic density, and IBD [156].

Besides air, the ingestion of pollutants via water sources has also been recently investigated as a relevant factor for the incidence and course of IBD [157,158]. The presence of antagonists of steroid receptors, endocrine-disrupting chemicals (EDCs), and the interaction with the glucocorticoid receptor and peroxisome-proliferator-activated receptor gamma (PPAR-γ) may play an important role in the pathogenesis of IBD through in vitro studies. However, there are no supporting in vivo studies. Concerning metal elements and disinfectants in drinking water, they have been associated with alterations in the microbial environment in the intestinal tract and exacerbate immune system responses [159]. Some observational studies have shown that iron nitrate and sulfite in drinking water is associated with a higher incidence of IBD [160–162]. A recent large Chinese study found an association between increased concentrations of manganese, mercury, selenium, sulfur tetraoxide (SO_4), chlorine, and nitrate nitrogen (NO_3-N) and a higher risk of IBD [163].

Among environmental risk factors, cigarette smoking stands out as one of the most well-established, with distinct effects on UC and CD [99,164]. In UC, smoking seems to modulate the immune system and reduce the production of TNF-α through the action of nicotine on the nicotinic acetylcholine receptor. However, the mechanism by which it exerts its protective effect in UC has not been clearly defined [164]. In CD, smoking can increase carbon monoxide (CO), causing an alteration of the vasodilation capacity in microvessels, resulting in ischemia and perpetuation of ulceration and fibrosis [165]. In CD, smoking has been associated with both the development of the disease and its course, particularly for CD. A prospective study including 229,111 women, showed that smoking increases the risk of developing CD among current smokers with a HR of 1.90 (95% CI: 1.42–2.53) [166]. The increased risk is associated with the number of packs smoked. It also seems to increase the risk of penetrating intestinal complications, as well as the need for surgery [99,167]. Notably, smoking cessation has been associated with a reduction in disease risk, as former smokers show a lower HR of 1.35 (95% CI: 1.05–1.73) compared to active smokers (HR 1.90, 95% CI: 1.42–2.53) [166]. Additionally, smoking cessation positively impacts disease progression, leading to improvements such as a reduction in disease flares, decreased reliance on steroids, and less frequent need for immunosuppressive therapy [168,169].

In this context of pathogenic environmental factors in IBD, sleep disorders have been investigated and are emerging as potential risk factors (OR: 3.09) for IBD development, exacerbation, and diminished quality of life [170]. Sleep disorders were observed in 59.6% of patients with IBD, which was significantly higher than in healthy individuals [171]. It has been hypothesized that they may not only be a result but rather a cause of chronic inflammatory diseases. In support of this hypothesis, alterations in some non-rapid eye movement (NREM) sleep stages, where the greatest impact of immune regulation and the decrease in colonic contractility occurs, can lead to a reduction in mucosal integrity [172]. Furthermore, in healthy young volunteers with disturbed sleep, increases in key cytokines involved in the pathological processes of IBDs, such as interleukins IL-1β, TNF-α, and IL-6, have been found [171]. However, there is a scarcity of longitudinal studies that investigate sleep disorders in the pathogenesis of IBD.

Regarding diet, it has been shown that diet can induce epigenetic changes related to IBD. The human diet is influenced by environmental and cultural practices and can influence intestinal inflammation through various pathways. They seem to be related to the alteration of the expression of miRNAs, the alteration of the composition of the intestinal microbiome and metabolome, and the influence of the integrity and permeability of the gastrointestinal barrier [173]. The elements of the Western diet, characterized by a low content of fiber, fruits, and vegetables, and a lack of micronutrients, as well as a diet high in fat, seem to be associated with epigenetic changes, such as a decrease in certain miRNAs (miR-143/145a, miR-148a, and miR-152) in colonocytes, increasing the aggravation of colitis [174]. Furthermore, a high-fat diet can modify the miRNA profile of visceral adipose exosomes towards a pro-inflammatory phenotype, predisposing the intestine to inflammation through the promotion of M1 macrophage polarization [175]. A diet high in fat has been associated with an increased risk of developing UC with a high intake of total fat, polyunsaturated fatty acids (PUFAs), and omega-6 fatty acids, as well as an increased risk of CD with a high intake of PUFAs, omega-6 fatty acids, and saturated fats [176]. From animal studies, the mechanism could be due to a possible increase in colonic epithelial natural killer T cells and a reduction in circulating Tregs [177]. In addition, a diet high in saturated fats can alter the composition of bile acids, which can favor the proliferation of sulfate-reducing bacteria, leading to an increase in hydrogen sulfide, which is toxic to the mucosa. A diet low or deficient in methyl donors can contribute to intestinal inflammation by reducing the expression of histone deacetylase (SIRT1). This reduction promotes endoplasmic reticulum stress and abnormal intestinal expression of CEA Cell Adhesion Molecule 6 (CEACAM6), facilitating the colonization of adherent-invasive *Escherichia coli* and subsequent inflammation [178].

Fewer data are available on the consumption of animal proteins and food additives. Some recent data report a greater exposure of CD patients to a larger number of processed foods and food additives compared to control groups, which could predispose to the development of CD and ongoing inflammation [179]. Food additives such as aluminum, titanium dioxide (TiO2), and microparticles/nanoparticles have been implicated in murine models of colitis [180,181]. TiO2 can be absorbed by intestinal epithelial cells and can exacerbate inflammation in predisposed individuals [179]. Furthermore, there are studies in the literature that have associated the consumption of meat with the risk of IBDs, although human studies in this area are still rather heterogeneous [182,183]. Regarding alcohol, chronic exposure can increase the expression of miR-122a and miR-155 in the intestine, decreasing the expression of occludins, leading to increased intestinal permeability, activation of TNF-α and NF-κB in the intestine, respectively [184]. In contrast, polyphenols, present mainly in fruits and vegetables [185–187], can reduce the risk of intestinal inflammation, mainly by modifying the miR profile and inhibiting HDACs. Furthermore, in humans, a high intake of dietary fiber, particularly from cruciferous fruits and vegetables, has been associated with a reduced risk of CD (HR = 0.59; 95% CI: 0.39–0.90) [188,189]. The protective effect of fiber was observed as statistically significant in those who consumed more than 22.1 g/day. A high intake of fruit has also been associated with a 73–80% reduction in the risk of CD in the same study [190]. The role of environmental exposures across childhood, cumulative lifetime, and adulthood in IBD pathogenesis is summarized in Figure 3.

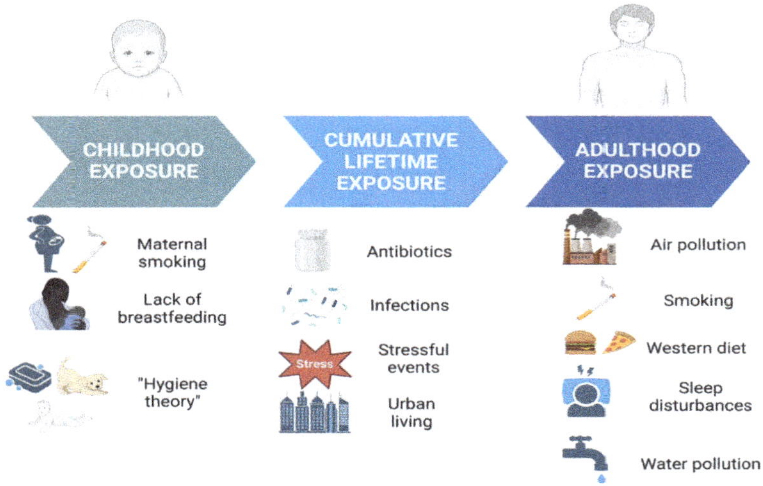

Figure 3. Environmental exposures contributing to IBD pathogenesis across the lifespan. The figure highlights risk factors at different life stages—childhood exposure, including maternal smoking, lack of breastfeeding, and reduced microbial diversity associated with the "hygiene theory"; cumulative lifetime exposure, such as antibiotic use, infections, stressful events, and urban living; and adulthood exposure, including air and water pollution, smoking, Western diets, and sleep disturbances. These exposures may influence immune responses and gut microbiome composition, increasing susceptibility to inflammation and IBD development.

6. Conclusions

Our findings from the most recent research confirm that IBDs are complex disorders driven by the intricate interplay between genetic predisposition, immune dysregulation, gut microbiota alterations, and environmental exposures. Although knowledge on this topic continues to grow, much remains to be understood. More in depth, the intersection of these pathogenic mechanisms and the relative contribution to disease onset and progression needs to be investigated. Future research is essential to further elucidate these dynamics and improve our understanding of IBD pathogenesis.

In the meantime, preventive strategies during pregnancy and early childhood offer significant potential. Maternal smoking, poor nutrition, and antibiotic exposure in childhood have been associated with increased IBD risk, whereas breastfeeding and diets rich in fiber and polyphenols provide protective effects by fostering healthy immune and microbiota development. These insights underscore the importance of addressing modifiable factors during these critical life stages.

Therapeutically, efforts to restore microbial diversity, repair epithelial barrier function, and modulate immune responses represent promising approaches. Advances in multi-omics technologies and exploration of neglected microbiome components, such as the virome and mycobiome, will further enhance our understanding and open new avenues for precision medicine. Thanks to these scientific advancements, the next objectives will focus on reducing the burden of IBD, developing effective and personalized treatments and minimizing adverse effects. The ultimate goal will be reducing the incidence of IBD by integrating early-life prevention strategies with innovative therapeutic approaches.

Author Contributions: Conceptualization, V.C., P.P. and F.D.V.; methodology, P.P. and V.C.; writing—original draft preparation, P.P., F.D.V., A.D.G., B.B., E.P., M.M., D.N. and J.I.; figures, P.P., J.I. and M.M., writing—review and editing V.C., P.P. and D.N.; visualization, F.S. and V.C.; supervision, F.S., D.P. and A.G. All authors have read and agreed to the published version of the manuscript.

Funding: This research received no external funding.

Acknowledgments: Thanks to Fondazione Roma for the continuous support of our scientific research.

Conflicts of Interest: No conflict of interest to declare.

References

1. Zhang, Y.-Z. Inflammatory Bowel Disease: Pathogenesis. *World J. Gastroenterol.* **2014**, *20*, 91. [CrossRef] [PubMed]
2. Abdulla, M.; Mohammed, N. A Review on Inflammatory Bowel Diseases: Recent Molecular Pathophysiology Advances. *Biol. Targets Ther.* **2022**, *16*, 129–140. [CrossRef] [PubMed]
3. Annese, V. Genetics and Epigenetics of IBD. *Pharmacol. Res.* **2020**, *159*, 104892. [CrossRef] [PubMed]
4. Aden, K.; Reindl, W. The Gut Microbiome in Inflammatory Bowel Diseases: Diagnostic and Therapeutic Implications. *Visc. Med.* **2019**, *35*, 332–337. [CrossRef]
5. Ho, S.-M.; Lewis, J.D.; Mayer, E.A.; Bernstein, C.N.; Plevy, S.E.; Chuang, E.; Rappaport, S.M.; Croitoru, K.; Korzenik, J.R.; Krischer, J.; et al. Challenges in IBD Research: Environmental Triggers. *Inflamm. Bowel Dis.* **2019**, *25*, S13–S23. [CrossRef] [PubMed]
6. Guan, Q. A Comprehensive Review and Update on the Pathogenesis of Inflammatory Bowel Disease. *J. Immunol. Res.* **2019**, *2019*, 7247238. [CrossRef] [PubMed]
7. Baumgart, D.C.; Carding, S.R. Inflammatory Bowel Disease: Cause and Immunobiology. *Lancet* **2007**, *369*, 1627–1640. [CrossRef] [PubMed]
8. Kong, L.; Pokatayev, V.; Lefkovith, A.; Carter, G.T.; Creasey, E.A.; Krishna, C.; Subramanian, S.; Kochar, B.; Ashenberg, O.; Lau, H.; et al. The Landscape of Immune Dysregulation in Crohn's Disease Revealed through Single-Cell Transcriptomic Profiling in the Ileum and Colon. *Immunity* **2023**, *56*, 444–458.e5. [CrossRef]
9. Okumura, R.; Takeda, K. Roles of Intestinal Epithelial Cells in the Maintenance of Gut Homeostasis. *Exp. Mol. Med.* **2017**, *49*, e338. [CrossRef]
10. Kim, Y.S.; Ho, S.B. Intestinal Goblet Cells and Mucins in Health and Disease: Recent Insights and Progress. *Curr. Gastroenterol. Rep.* **2010**, *12*, 319–330. [CrossRef] [PubMed]
11. Wei, J.; Chen, C.; Feng, J.; Zhou, S.; Feng, X.; Yang, Z.; Lu, H.; Tao, H.; Li, L.; Xv, H.; et al. Muc2 Mucin O-Glycosylation Interacts with Enteropathogenic Escherichia Coli to Influence the Development of Ulcerative Colitis Based on the NF-kB Signaling Pathway. *J. Transl. Med.* **2023**, *21*, 793. [CrossRef] [PubMed]
12. Ashton, J.J.; Boukas, K.; Davies, J.; Stafford, I.S.; Vallejo, A.F.; Haggarty, R.; Coelho, T.A.F.; Batra, A.; Afzal, N.A.; Vadgama, B.; et al. Ileal Transcriptomic Analysis in Paediatric Crohn's Disease Reveals *IL17-* and *NOD*-Signalling Expression Signatures in Treatment-Naïve Patients and Identifies Epithelial Cells Driving Differentially Expressed Genes. *J. Crohns Colitis* **2021**, *15*, 774–786. [CrossRef] [PubMed]
13. Bennstein, S.B.; Uhrberg, M. Circulating Innate Lymphoid Cells (cILCs): Unconventional Lymphocytes with Hidden Talents. *J. Allergy Clin. Immunol.* **2024**, *154*, 523–536. [CrossRef]
14. Krämer, B.; Goeser, F.; Lutz, P.; Glässner, A.; Boesecke, C.; Schwarze-Zander, C.; Kaczmarek, D.; Nischalke, H.D.; Branchi, V.; Manekeller, S.; et al. Compartment-Specific Distribution of Human Intestinal Innate Lymphoid Cells Is Altered in HIV Patients under Effective Therapy. *PLoS Pathog.* **2017**, *13*, e1006373. [CrossRef]
15. Srivastava, R.K.; Sapra, L.; Bhardwaj, A.; Mishra, P.K.; Verma, B.; Baig, Z. Unravelling the Immunobiology of Innate Lymphoid Cells (ILCs): Implications in Health and Disease. *Cytokine Growth Factor Rev.* **2023**, *74*, 56–75. [CrossRef] [PubMed]
16. Bao, B.; Wang, Y.; Boudreau, P.; Song, X.; Wu, M.; Chen, X.; Patik, I.; Tang, Y.; Ouahed, J.; Ringel, A.; et al. Bacterial Sphingolipids Exacerbate Colitis by Inhibiting ILC3-Derived IL-22 Production. *Cell. Mol. Gastroenterol. Hepatol.* **2024**, *18*, 101350. [CrossRef] [PubMed]
17. Eken, A.; Singh, A.K.; Treuting, P.M.; Oukka, M. IL-23R+ Innate Lymphoid Cells Induce Colitis via Interleukin-22-Dependent Mechanism. *Mucosal Immunol.* **2014**, *7*, 143–154. [CrossRef] [PubMed]
18. Mazzurana, L.; Bonfiglio, F.; Forkel, M.; D'Amato, M.; Halfvarson, J.; Mjösberg, J. Crohn's Disease Is Associated With Activation of Circulating Innate Lymphoid Cells. *Inflamm. Bowel Dis.* **2021**, *27*, 1128–1138. [CrossRef] [PubMed]
19. Hunter, M.M.; Wang, A.; Parhar, K.S.; Johnston, M.J.G.; Van Rooijen, N.; Beck, P.L.; McKay, D.M. In Vitro-Derived Alternatively Activated Macrophages Reduce Colonic Inflammation in Mice. *Gastroenterology* **2010**, *138*, 1395–1405. [CrossRef] [PubMed]
20. Zhang, K.; Guo, J.; Yan, W.; Xu, L. Macrophage Polarization in Inflammatory Bowel Disease. *Cell Commun. Signal.* **2023**, *21*, 367. [CrossRef]
21. Lissner, D.; Schumann, M.; Batra, A.; Kredel, L.-I.; Kühl, A.A.; Erben, U.; May, C.; Schulzke, J.-D.; Siegmund, B. Monocyte and M1 Macrophage-Induced Barrier Defect Contributes to Chronic Intestinal Inflammation in IBD. *Inflamm. Bowel Dis.* **2015**, *21*, 1297–1305. [CrossRef] [PubMed]
22. Ma, S.; Zhang, J.; Liu, H.; Li, S.; Wang, Q. The Role of Tissue-Resident Macrophages in the Development and Treatment of Inflammatory Bowel Disease. *Front. Cell Dev. Biol.* **2022**, *10*, 896591. [CrossRef] [PubMed]

23. Zhang, M.; Li, X.; Zhang, Q.; Yang, J.; Liu, G. Roles of Macrophages on Ulcerative Colitis and Colitis-Associated Colorectal Cancer. *Front. Immunol.* **2023**, *14*, 1103617. [CrossRef]
24. Garrido-Trigo, A.; Corraliza, A.M.; Veny, M.; Dotti, I.; Melón-Ardanaz, E.; Rill, A.; Crowell, H.L.; Corbí, Á.; Gudiño, V.; Esteller, M.; et al. Macrophage and Neutrophil Heterogeneity at Single-Cell Spatial Resolution in Human Inflammatory Bowel Disease. *Nat. Commun.* **2023**, *14*, 4506. [CrossRef] [PubMed]
25. Azramezani Kopi, T.; Amini Kadijani, A.; Parsian, H.; Shahrokh, S.; Asadzadeh Aghdaei, H.; Mirzaei, A.; Balaii, H.; Zali, M.R. The Value of mRNA Expression of S100A8 and S100A9 as Blood-Based Biomarkers of Inflammatory Bowel Disease. *Arab J. Gastroenterol.* **2019**, *20*, 135–140. [CrossRef]
26. Okada, K.; Itoh, H.; Ikemoto, M. Circulating S100A8/A9 Is Potentially a Biomarker That Could Reflect the Severity of Experimental Colitis in Rats. *Heliyon* **2020**, *6*, e03470. [CrossRef] [PubMed]
27. Luo, X.; Wang, R.; Zhang, X.; Wen, X.; Deng, S.; Xie, W. Identification CCL2,CXCR2,S100A9 of the Immune-Related Gene Markers and Immune Infiltration Characteristics of Inflammatory Bowel Disease and Heart Failure via Bioinformatics Analysis and Machine Learning. *Front. Cardiovasc. Med.* **2023**, *10*, 1268675. [CrossRef]
28. Poggi, A.; Benelli, R.; Venè, R.; Costa, D.; Ferrari, N.; Tosetti, F.; Zocchi, M.R. Human Gut-Associated Natural Killer Cells in Health and Disease. *Front. Immunol.* **2019**, *10*, 961. [CrossRef] [PubMed]
29. Zaiatz Bittencourt, V.; Jones, F.; Tosetto, M.; Doherty, G.A.; Ryan, E.J. Dysregulation of Metabolic Pathways in Circulating Natural Killer Cells Isolated from Inflammatory Bowel Disease Patients. *J. Crohns Colitis* **2021**, *15*, 1316–1325. [CrossRef] [PubMed]
30. Geremia, A.; Biancheri, P.; Allan, P.; Corazza, G.R.; Di Sabatino, A. Innate and Adaptive Immunity in Inflammatory Bowel Disease. *Autoimmun. Rev.* **2014**, *13*, 3–10. [CrossRef]
31. Kałużna, A.; Olczyk, P.; Komosińska-Vassev, K. The Role of Innate and Adaptive Immune Cells in the Pathogenesis and Development of the Inflammatory Response in Ulcerative Colitis. *J. Clin. Med.* **2022**, *11*, 400. [CrossRef] [PubMed]
32. Mitsialis, V.; Wall, S.; Liu, P.; Ordovas-Montanes, J.; Parmet, T.; Vukovic, M.; Spencer, D.; Field, M.; McCourt, C.; Toothaker, J.; et al. Single-Cell Analyses of Colon and Blood Reveal Distinct Immune Cell Signatures of Ulcerative Colitis and Crohn's Disease. *Gastroenterology* **2020**, *159*, 591–608.e10. [CrossRef] [PubMed]
33. Medina, T.S.; Murison, A.; Smith, M.; Kinker, G.S.; Chakravarthy, A.; Vitiello, G.A.F.; Turpin, W.; Shen, S.Y.; Yau, H.L.; Sarmento, O.F.; et al. The Chromatin and Single-Cell Transcriptional Landscapes of CD4 T Cells in Inflammatory Bowel Disease Link Risk Loci with a Proinflammatory Th17 Cell Population. *Front. Immunol.* **2023**, *14*, 1161901. [CrossRef] [PubMed]
34. Cao, M.; Chen, P.; Peng, B.; Cheng, Y.; Xie, J.; Hou, Z.; Chen, H.; Ye, L.; Li, H.; Wang, H.; et al. The Transcription Factor ELF4 Alleviates Inflammatory Bowel Disease by Activating IL1RN Transcription, Suppressing Inflammatory TH17 Cell Activity, and Inducing Macrophage M2 Polarization. *Front. Immunol.* **2023**, *14*, 1270411. [CrossRef]
35. Tanemoto, S.; Sujino, T.; Miyamoto, K.; Moody, J.; Yoshimatsu, Y.; Ando, Y.; Koya, I.; Harada, Y.; Tojo, A.O.; Ono, K.; et al. Single-Cell Transcriptomics of Human Gut T Cells Identifies Cytotoxic $CD4^{+}CD8A^{+}$ T Cells Related to Mouse CD4 Cytotoxic T Cells. *Front. Immunol.* **2022**, *13*, 977117. [CrossRef] [PubMed]
36. Casalegno Garduño, R.; Däbritz, J. New Insights on $CD8^{+}$ T Cells in Inflammatory Bowel Disease and Therapeutic Approaches. *Front. Immunol.* **2021**, *12*, 738762. [CrossRef] [PubMed]
37. Corridoni, D.; Antanaviciute, A.; Gupta, T.; Fawkner-Corbett, D.; Aulicino, A.; Jagielowicz, M.; Parikh, K.; Repapi, E.; Taylor, S.; Ishikawa, D.; et al. Single-Cell Atlas of Colonic $CD8^{+}$ T Cells in Ulcerative Colitis. *Nat. Med.* **2020**, *26*, 1480–1490. [CrossRef] [PubMed]
38. Globig, A.-M.; Mayer, L.S.; Heeg, M.; Andrieux, G.; Ku, M.; Otto-Mora, P.; Hipp, A.V.; Zoldan, K.; Pattekar, A.; Rana, N.; et al. Exhaustion of CD39-Expressing $CD8^{+}$ T Cells in Crohn's Disease Is Linked to Clinical Outcome. *Gastroenterology* **2022**, *163*, 965–981.e31. [CrossRef] [PubMed]
39. Mayne, C.G.; Williams, C.B. Induced and Natural Regulatory T Cells in the Development of Inflammatory Bowel Disease: *Inflamm. Bowel Dis.* **2013**, *19*, 1772–1788. [CrossRef]
40. Yan, J.; Zeng, Y.; Guan, Z.; Li, Z.; Luo, S.; Niu, J.; Zhao, J.; Gong, H.; Huang, T.; Li, Z.; et al. Inherent Preference for Polyunsaturated Fatty Acids Instigates Ferroptosis of Treg Cells That Aggravates High-Fat-Diet-Related Colitis. *Cell Rep.* **2024**, *43*, 114636. [CrossRef] [PubMed]
41. Boland, B.S.; He, Z.; Tsai, M.S.; Olvera, J.G.; Omilusik, K.D.; Duong, H.G.; Kim, E.S.; Limary, A.E.; Jin, W.; Milner, J.J.; et al. Heterogeneity and Clonal Relationships of Adaptive Immune Cells in Ulcerative Colitis Revealed by Single-Cell Analyses. *Sci. Immunol.* **2020**, *5*, eabb4432. [CrossRef]
42. Zhang, Q.; Zeng, Z.; Wei, N.; Su, Y.; Wang, J.; Ni, Q.; Wang, Y.; Yang, J.; Liu, X.; Xu, H.; et al. Mesenteric Lymph Nodes: A Critical Site for the up-Regulatory Effect of hUC-MSCs on Treg Cells by Producing TGF-β1 in Colitis Treatment. *Stem Cell Res. Ther.* **2024**, *15*, 190. [CrossRef]
43. Eiro, N.; Fraile, M.; González-Jubete, A.; González, L.O.; Vizoso, F.J. Mesenchymal (Stem) Stromal Cells Based as New Therapeutic Alternative in Inflammatory Bowel Disease: Basic Mechanisms, Experimental and Clinical Evidence, and Challenges. *Int. J. Mol. Sci.* **2022**, *23*, 8905. [CrossRef] [PubMed]

44. Stavely, R.; Robinson, A.M.; Fraser, S.; Filippone, R.T; Stojanovska, V.; Eri, R.; Apostolopoulos, V.; Sakkal, S.; Nurgali, K. Bone Marrow-Derived Mesenchymal Stem Cells Mitigate Chronic Colitis and Enteric Neuropathy via Anti-Inflammatory and Anti-Oxidative Mechanisms. *Sci. Rep.* **2024**, *14*, 6649. [CrossRef]
45. Dave, M.; Dev, A.; Somoza, R.A.; Zhao, N.; Viswanath, S.; Mina, P.R.; Chirra, P.; Obmann, V.C.; Mahabeleshwar, G.H.; Menghini, P.; et al. MSCs Mediate Long-Term Efficacy in a Crohn's Disease Model by Sustained Anti-Inflammatory Macrophage Programming via Efferocytosis. *npj Regen. Med.* **2024**, *9*, 6. [CrossRef]
46. Scanu, M.; Toto, F.; Petito, V.; Masi, L.; Fidaleo, M.; Puca, P.; Baldelli, V.; Reddel, S.; Vernocchi, P.; Pani, G.; et al. An Integrative Multi-Omic Analysis Defines Gut Microbiota, Mycobiota, and Metabolic Fingerprints in Ulcerative Colitis Patients. *Front. Cell. Infect. Microbiol.* **2024**, *14*, 1366192. [CrossRef]
47. Luchen, C.C.; Chibuye, M.; Spijker, R.; Simuyandi, M.; Chisenga, C.; Bosomprah, S.; Chilengi, R.; Schultsz, C.; Mende, D.R.; Harris, V.C. Impact of Antibiotics on Gut Microbiome Composition and Resistome in the First Years of Life in Low- to Middle-Income Countries: A Systematic Review. *PLoS Med.* **2023**, *20*, e1004235. [CrossRef] [PubMed]
48. Pan, R.; He, Y.; Yuan, J.; Zhao, S.; Ma, M.; Chai, Z.; Ji, X.; Hu, X.; He, C.; Zhou, D.; et al. The Role of Antibiotic Exposure as Risk Factor for IBD Epidemic: An Updated Meta-Analysis. *J. Gastroenterol. Hepatol.* **2024**, *39*, 2561–2571. [CrossRef]
49. Mårild, K.; Lerchova, T.; Östensson, M.; Imberg, H.; Størdal, K.; Ludvigsson, J. Early-Life Infections, Antibiotics and Later Risk of Childhood and Early Adult-Onset Inflammatory Bowel Disease: Pooled Analysis of Two Scandinavian Birth Cohorts. *Aliment. Pharmacol. Ther.* **2024**, *61*, 323–334. [CrossRef]
50. Pascal, V.; Pozuelo, M.; Borruel, N.; Casellas, F.; Campos, D.; Santiago, A.; Martinez, X.; Varela, E.; Sarrabayrouse, G.; Machiels, K.; et al. A Microbial Signature for Crohn's Disease. *Gut* **2017**, *66*, 813–822. [CrossRef] [PubMed]
51. Abdel-Rahman, L.I.H.; Morgan, X.C. Searching for a Consensus Among Inflammatory Bowel Disease Studies: A Systematic Meta-Analysis. *Inflamm. Bowel Dis.* **2023**, *29*, 125–139. [CrossRef]
52. Alam, M.T.; Amos, G.C.A.; Murphy, A.R.J.; Murch, S.; Wellington, E.M.H.; Arasaradnam, R.P. Microbial Imbalance in Inflammatory Bowel Disease Patients at Different Taxonomic Levels. *Gut Pathog.* **2020**, *12*, 1. [CrossRef] [PubMed]
53. Amos, G.C.A.; Sergaki, C.; Logan, A.; Iriarte, R.; Bannaga, A.; Chandrapalan, S.; Wellington, E.M.H.; Rijpkema, S.; Arasaradnam, R.P. Exploring How Microbiome Signatures Change across Inflammatory Bowel Disease Conditions and Disease Locations. *Sci. Rep.* **2021**, *11*, 18699. [CrossRef]
54. Britton, G.J.; Contijoch, E.J.; Mogno, I.; Vennaro, O.H.; Llewellyn, S.R.; Ng, R.; Li, Z.; Mortha, A.; Merad, M.; Das, A.; et al. Microbiotas from Humans with Inflammatory Bowel Disease Alter the Balance of Gut Th17 and RORγt$^+$ Regulatory T Cells and Exacerbate Colitis in Mice. *Immunity* **2019**, *50*, 212–224.e4. [CrossRef]
55. Sugihara, K.; Kamada, N. Metabolic Network of the Gut Microbiota in Inflammatory Bowel Disease. *Inflamm. Regen.* **2024**, *44*, 11. [CrossRef] [PubMed]
56. Dong, D.; Su, T.; Chen, W.; Wang, D.; Xue, Y.; Lu, Q.; Jiang, C.; Ni, Q.; Mao, E.; Peng, Y. *Clostridioides Difficile* Aggravates Dextran Sulfate Solution (DSS)-Induced Colitis by Shaping the Gut Microbiota and Promoting Neutrophil Recruitment. *Gut Microbes* **2023**, *15*, 2192478. [CrossRef] [PubMed]
57. Leon-Coria, A.; Kumar, M.; Workentine, M.; Moreau, F.; Surette, M.; Chadee, K. Muc2 Mucin and Nonmucin Microbiota Confer Distinct Innate Host Defense in Disease Susceptibility and Colonic Injury. *Cell. Mol. Gastroenterol. Hepatol.* **2021**, *11*, 77–98. [CrossRef]
58. Li, M.; Ding, Y.; Wei, J.; Dong, Y.; Wang, J.; Dai, X.; Yan, J.; Chu, F.; Zhang, K.; Meng, F.; et al. Gut Microbiota Metabolite Indole-3-Acetic Acid Maintains Intestinal Epithelial Homeostasis Through Mucin Sulfation. *Gut Microbes* **2024**, *16*, 2377576. [CrossRef]
59. Leibovitzh, H.; Lee, S.-H.; Xue, M.; Raygoza Garay, J.A.; Hernandez-Rocha, C.; Madsen, K.L.; Meddings, J.B.; Guttman, D.S.; Espin-Garcia, O.; Smith, M.I.; et al. Altered Gut Microbiome Composition and Function Are Associated with Gut Barrier Dysfunction in Healthy Relatives of Patients With Crohn's Disease. *Gastroenterology* **2022**, *163*, 1364–1376.e10. [CrossRef] [PubMed]
60. Luchetti, M.M.; Ciccia, F.; Avellini, C.; Benfaremo, D.; Rizzo, A.; Spadoni, T.; Svegliati, S.; Marzioni, D.; Santinelli, A.; Costantini, A.; et al. Gut Epithelial Impairment, Microbial Translocation and Immune System Activation in Inflammatory Bowel Disease–Associated Spondyloarthritis. *Rheumatology* **2021**, *60*, 92–102. [CrossRef] [PubMed]
61. Alexander, K.L.; Zhao, Q.; Reif, M.; Rosenberg, A.F.; Mannon, P.J.; Duck, L.W.; Elson, C.O. Human Microbiota Flagellins Drive Adaptive Immune Responses in Crohn's Disease. *Gastroenterology* **2021**, *161*, 522–535.e6. [CrossRef] [PubMed]
62. Vujkovic-Cvijin, I.; Welles, H.C.; Ha, C.W.Y.; Huq, L.; Mistry, S.; Brenchley, J.M.; Trinchieri, G.; Devkota, S.; Belkaid, Y. The Systemic Anti-Microbiota IgG Repertoire Can Identify Gut Bacteria That Translocate Across Gut Barrier Surfaces. *Sci. Transl. Med.* **2022**, *14*, eabl3927. [CrossRef] [PubMed]
63. Gallagher, K.; Catesson, A.; Griffin, J.L.; Holmes, E.; Williams, H.R.T. Metabolomic Analysis in Inflammatory Bowel Disease: A Systematic Review. *J. Crohns Colitis* **2021**, *15*, 813–826. [CrossRef] [PubMed]

64. Ning, L.; Zhou, Y.-L.; Sun, H.; Zhang, Y.; Shen, C.; Wang, Z.; Xuan, B.; Zhao, Y.; Ma, Y.; Yan, Y.; et al. Microbiome and Metabolome Features in Inflammatory Bowel Disease via Multi-Omics Integration Analyses across Cohorts. *Nat. Commun.* **2023**, *14*, 7135. [CrossRef]
65. Zhao, H.; Zhou, Y.; Xu, J.; Zhang, Y.; Wang, H.; Zhao, C.; Huang, H.; Yang, J.; Huang, C.; Li, Y.; et al. Short-Chain Fatty Acid-Producing Bacterial Strains Attenuate Experimental Ulcerative Colitis by Promoting M2 Macrophage Polarization via JAK/STAT3/FOXC3 Axis Inactivation. *J. Transl. Med.* **2024**, *22*, 369. [CrossRef]
66. Tian, X.; Li, S.; Wang, C.; Zhang, Y.; Feng, X.; Yan, Q.; Guo, R.; Wu, F.; Wu, C.; Wang, Y.; et al. Gut Virome-Wide Association Analysis Identifies Cross-Population Viral Signatures for Inflammatory Bowel Disease. *Microbiome* **2024**, *12*, 130. [CrossRef] [PubMed]
67. Ungaro, F.; Massimino, L.; Furfaro, F.; Rimoldi, V.; Peyrin-Biroulet, L.; D'Alessio, S.; Danese, S. Metagenomic Analysis of Intestinal Mucosa Revealed a Specific Eukaryotic Gut Virome Signature in Early-Diagnosed Inflammatory Bowel Disease. *Gut Microbes* **2019**, *10*, 149–158. [CrossRef]
68. Bernardi, F.; Ungaro, F.; D'Amico, F.; Zilli, A.; Parigi, T.L.; Massimino, L.; Allocca, M.; Danese, S.; Furfaro, F. The Role of Viruses in the Pathogenesis of Immune-Mediated Gastro-Intestinal Diseases. *Int. J. Mol. Sci.* **2024**, *25*, 8301. [CrossRef] [PubMed]
69. Carasso, S.; Zaatry, R.; Hajjo, H.; Kadosh-Kariti, D.; Ben-Assa, N.; Naddaf, R.; Mandelbaum, N.; Pressman, S.; Chowers, Y.; Gefen, T.; et al. Inflammation and Bacteriophages Affect DNA Inversion States and Functionality of the Gut Microbiota. *Cell Host Microbe* **2024**, *32*, 322–334.e9. [CrossRef] [PubMed]
70. Yu, M.; Ding, H.; Gong, S.; Luo, Y.; Lin, H.; Mu, Y.; Li, H.; Li, X.; Zhong, M. Fungal Dysbiosis Facilitates Inflammatory Bowel Disease by Enhancing CD4$^+$ T Cell Glutaminolysis. *Front. Cell. Infect. Microbiol.* **2023**, *13*, 1140757. [CrossRef]
71. Iliev, I.D.; Funari, V.A.; Taylor, K.D.; Nguyen, Q.; Reyes, C.N.; Strom, S.P.; Brown, J.; Becker, C.A.; Fleshner, P.R.; Dubinsky, M.; et al. Interactions Between Commensal Fungi and the C-Type Lectin Receptor Dectin-1 Influence Colitis. *Science* **2012**, *336*, 1314–1317. [CrossRef]
72. Zhang, W.; Lyu, M.; Bessman, N.J.; Xie, Z.; Arifuzzaman, M.; Yano, H.; Parkhurst, C.N.; Chu, C.; Zhou, L.; Putzel, G.G.; et al. Gut-Innervating Nociceptors Regulate the Intestinal Microbiota to Promote Tissue Protection. *Cell* **2022**, *185*, 4170–4189.e20. [CrossRef] [PubMed]
73. Lopetuso, L.R.; Deleu, S.; Godny, L.; Petito, V.; Puca, P.; Facciotti, F.; Sokol, H.; Ianiro, G.; Masucci, L.; Abreu, M.; et al. The First International Rome Consensus Conference on Gut Microbiota and Faecal Microbiota Transplantation in Inflammatory Bowel Disease. *Gut* **2023**, *72*, 1642–1650. [CrossRef] [PubMed]
74. Costello, S.P.; Soo, W.; Bryant, R.V.; Jairath, V.; Hart, A.L.; Andrews, J.M. Systematic Review with Meta-Analysis: Faecal Microbiota Transplantation for the Induction of Remission for Active Ulcerative Colitis. *Aliment. Pharmacol. Ther.* **2017**, *46*, 213–224. [CrossRef] [PubMed]
75. Caldeira, L.d.F.; Borba, H.H.; Tonin, F.S.; Wiens, A.; Fernandez-Llimos, F.; Pontarolo, R. Fecal Microbiota Transplantation in Inflammatory Bowel Disease Patients: A Systematic Review and Meta-Analysis. *PLoS ONE* **2020**, *15*, e0238910. [CrossRef] [PubMed]
76. Loddo, I.; Romano, C. Inflammatory Bowel Disease: Genetics, Epigenetics, and Pathogenesis. *Front. Immunol.* **2015**, *6*, 551. [CrossRef] [PubMed]
77. Liu, T.-C.; Stappenbeck, T.S. Genetics and Pathogenesis of Inflammatory Bowel Disease. *Annu. Rev. Pathol. Mech. Dis.* **2016**, *11*, 127–148. [CrossRef]
78. Palmieri, O.; Latiano, A.; Valvano, R.; D'Incà, R.; Vecchi, M.; Sturniolo, G.C.; Saibeni, S.; Peyvandi, F.; Bossa, F.; Zagaria, C.; et al. Variants of OCTN1–2 Cation Transporter Genes Are Associated with Both Crohn's Disease and Ulcerative Colitis. *Aliment. Pharmacol. Ther.* **2005**, *23*, 497–506. [CrossRef] [PubMed]
79. Hu, S.; Vich Vila, A.; Gacesa, R.; Collij, V.; Stevens, C.; Fu, J.M.; Wong, I.; Talkowski, M.E.; Rivas, M.A.; Imhann, F.; et al. Whole Exome Sequencing Analyses Reveal Gene–Microbiota Interactions in the Context of IBD. *Gut* **2020**, *70*, 285–296. [CrossRef]
80. Galluccio, M.; Tripicchio, M.; Pochini, L. The Human OCTN Sub-Family: Gene and Protein Structure, Expression, and Regulation. *Int. J. Mol. Sci.* **2024**, *25*, 8743. [CrossRef]
81. Del Chierico, F.; Masi, L.; Petito, V.; Baldelli, V.; Puca, P.; Benvenuto, R.; Fidaleo, M.; Palucci, I.; Lopetuso, L.R.; Caristo, M.E.; et al. Solute Transporter OCTN1/Slc22a4 Affects Disease Severity and Response to Infliximab in Experimental Colitis: Role of Gut Microbiota and Immune Modulation. *Inflamm. Bowel Dis.* **2024**, *30*, 2259–2270. [CrossRef] [PubMed]
82. Luo, P.; Yang, Z.; Chen, B.; Zhong, X. The Multifaceted Role of CARD9 in Inflammatory Bowel Disease. *J. Cell. Mol. Med.* **2020**, *24*, 34–39. [CrossRef] [PubMed]
83. Danne, C.; Michaudel, C.; Skerniskyte, J.; Planchais, J.; Magniez, A.; Agus, A.; Michel, M.-L.; Lamas, B.; Da Costa, G.; Spatz, M.; et al. CARD9 in Neutrophils Protects from Colitis and Controls Mitochondrial Metabolism and Cell Survival. *Gut* **2023**, *72*, 1081–1092. [CrossRef] [PubMed]

84. Danne, C.; Lamas, B.; Lavelle, A.; Michel, M.-L.; Da Costa, G.; Pham, H.-P.; Lefevre, A.; Bridonneau, C.; Bredon, M.; Planchais, J.; et al. Dissecting the Respective Roles of Microbiota and Host Genetics in the Susceptibility of *Card9*$^{-/-}$ Mice to Colitis. *Microbiome* **2024**, *12*, 76. [CrossRef] [PubMed]
85. Valatas, V.; Kolios, G.; Bamias, G. TL1A (TNFSF15) and DR3 (TNFRSF25): A Co-Stimulatory System of Cytokines With Diverse Functions in Gut Mucosal Immunity. *Front. Immunol.* **2019**, *10*, 583. [CrossRef]
86. Sun, R.; Hedl, M.; Abraham, C. TNFSF15 Promotes Antimicrobial Pathways in Human Macrophages and These Are Modulated by TNFSF15 Disease-Risk Variants. *Cell. Mol. Gastroenterol. Hepatol.* **2021**, *11*, 249–272. [CrossRef] [PubMed]
87. Kakuta, Y.; Ichikawa, R.; Fuyuno, Y.; Hirano, A.; Umeno, J.; Torisu, T.; Watanabe, K.; Asakura, A.; Nakano, T.; Izumiyama, Y.; et al. An Integrated Genomic and Transcriptomic Analysis Reveals Candidates of Susceptibility Genes for Crohn's Disease in Japanese Populations. *Sci. Rep.* **2020**, *10*, 10236. [CrossRef]
88. Zhou, Y.; Zhu, Y.; Jiang, H.; Chen, Z.; Lu, B.; Li, J.; Shen, X. Polymorphism Rs6478109 in the *TNFSF15* Gene Contributes to the Susceptibility to Crohn's Disease but Not Ulcerative Colitis: A Meta-Analysis. *J. Int. Med. Res.* **2020**, *48*, 0300060520961675. [CrossRef] [PubMed]
89. Muise, A.M.; Snapper, S.B.; Kugathasan, S. The Age of Gene Discovery in Very Early Onset Inflammatory Bowel Disease. *Gastroenterology* **2012**, *143*, 285–288. [CrossRef]
90. Uhlig, H.H.; Schwerd, T.; Koletzko, S.; Shah, N.; Kammermeier, J.; Elkadri, A.; Ouahed, J.; Wilson, D.C.; Travis, S.P.; Turner, D.; et al. The Diagnostic Approach to Monogenic Very Early Onset Inflammatory Bowel Disease. *Gastroenterology* **2014**, *147*, 990–1007.e3. [CrossRef]
91. Nambu, R.; Warner, N.; Mulder, D.J.; Kotlarz, D.; McGovern, D.P.B.; Cho, J.; Klein, C.; Snapper, S.B.; Griffiths, A.M.; Iwama, I.; et al. A Systematic Review of Monogenic Inflammatory Bowel Disease. *Clin. Gastroenterol. Hepatol.* **2022**, *20*, e653–e663. [CrossRef] [PubMed]
92. Arnadottir, G.A.; Norddahl, G.L.; Gudmundsdottir, S.; Agustsdottir, A.B.; Sigurdsson, S.; Jensson, B.O.; Bjarnadottir, K.; Theodors, F.; Benonisdottir, S.; Ivarsdottir, E.V.; et al. A Homozygous Loss-of-Function Mutation Leading to CYBC1 Deficiency Causes Chronic Granulomatous Disease. *Nat. Commun.* **2018**, *9*, 4447. [CrossRef] [PubMed]
93. Abdel-Motal, U.M.; Hubrack, S.Z.; Bullock, A.N.; Al-Marri, A.A.; Agrebi, N.; Al-Subaiey, A.A.; Ibrahim, N.A.; Charles, A.K.; Al-Kaabi, S.R.; Al-Mohannadi, M.J.; et al. Human AGR2 Deficiency Causes Mucus Barrier Dysfunction and Infantile Inflammatory Bowel Disease. *Cell. Mol. Gastroenterol. Hepatol.* **2021**, *12*, 1809–1830. [CrossRef]
94. Neehus, A.-L.; Moriya, K.; Nieto-Patlán, A.; Le Voyer, T.; Lévy, R.; Özen, A.; Karakoc-Aydiner, E.; Baris, S.; Yildiran, A.; Altundag, E.; et al. Impaired Respiratory Burst Contributes to Infections in PKCδ-Deficient Patients. *J. Exp. Med.* **2021**, *218*, e20210501. [CrossRef] [PubMed]
95. Ozen, A.; Comrie, W.A.; Ardy, R.C.; Conde, C.D.; Dalgic, B.; Beser, F.; Morawski, A.R.; Karakoc-Aydiner, E.; Tutar, E.; Baris, S.; et al. CD55 Deficiency, Early-Onset Protein-Losing Enteropathy, and Thrombosis. *N. Engl. J. Med.* **2017**, *377*, 52–61. [CrossRef] [PubMed]
96. Azabdaftari, A.; Jones, K.D.J.; Kammermeier, J.; Uhlig, H.H. Monogenic Inflammatory Bowel Disease-Genetic Variants, Functional Mechanisms and Personalised Medicine in Clinical Practice. *Hum. Genet.* **2023**, *142*, 599–611. [CrossRef] [PubMed]
97. Sudhakar, P.; Andrighetti, T.; Verstockt, S.; Caenepeel, C.; Ferrante, M.; Sabino, J.; Verstockt, B.; Vermeire, S. Integrated Analysis of Microbe-Host Interactions in Crohn's Disease Reveals Potential Mechanisms of Microbial Proteins on Host Gene Expression. *iScience* **2022**, *25*, 103963. [CrossRef] [PubMed]
98. Ng, S.C.; Bernstein, C.N.; Vatn, M.H.; Lakatos, P.L.; Loftus, E.V.; Tysk, C.; O'Morain, C.; Moum, B.; Colombel, J.-F. Epidemiology and Natural History Task Force of the International Organization of Inflammatory Bowel Disease (IOIBD) Geographical Variability and Environmental Risk Factors in Inflammatory Bowel Disease. *Gut* **2013**, *62*, 630–649. [CrossRef] [PubMed]
99. Mahid, S.S.; Minor, K.S.; Soto, R.E.; Hornung, C.A.; Galandiuk, S. Smoking and Inflammatory Bowel Disease: A Meta-Analysis. *Mayo Clin. Proc.* **2006**, *81*, 1462–1471. [CrossRef] [PubMed]
100. Dunford, A.R.; Sangster, J.M. Maternal and Paternal Periconceptional Nutrition as an Indicator of Offspring Metabolic Syndrome Risk in Later Life through Epigenetic Imprinting: A Systematic Review. *Diabetes Metab. Syndr.* **2017**, *11* (Suppl. S2), S655–S662. [CrossRef]
101. Zong, D.; Liu, X.; Li, J.; Ouyang, R.; Chen, P. The Role of Cigarette Smoke-Induced Epigenetic Alterations in Inflammation. *Epigenet. Chromatin* **2019**, *12*, 65. [CrossRef] [PubMed]
102. Marciniak, A.; Patro-Małysza, J.; Kimber-Trojnar, Ż.; Marciniak, B.; Oleszczuk, J.; Leszczyńska-Gorzelak, B. Fetal Programming of the Metabolic Syndrome. *Taiwan. J. Obstet. Gynecol.* **2017**, *56*, 133–138. [CrossRef] [PubMed]
103. Grossniklaus, U.; Kelly, W.G.; Kelly, B.; Ferguson-Smith, A.C.; Pembrey, M.; Lindquist, S. Transgenerational Epigenetic Inheritance: How Important Is It? *Nat. Rev. Genet.* **2013**, *14*, 228–235. [CrossRef]
104. Ventham, N.T.; Kennedy, N.A.; Nimmo, E.R.; Satsangi, J. Beyond Gene Discovery in Inflammatory Bowel Disease: The Emerging Role of Epigenetics. *Gastroenterology* **2013**, *145*, 293–308. [CrossRef]

105. Schaible, T.D.; Harris, R.A.; Dowd, S.E.; Smith, C.W.; Kellermayer, R. Maternal Methyl-Donor Supplementation Induces Prolonged Murine Offspring Colitis Susceptibility in Association with Mucosal Epigenetic and Microbiomic Changes. *Hum. Mol. Genet.* **2011**, *20*, 1687–1696. [CrossRef] [PubMed]
106. Lim, A.I.; McFadden, T.; Link, V.M.; Han, S.-J.; Karlsson, R.-M.; Stacy, A.; Farley, T.K.; Lima-Junior, D.S.; Harrison, O.J.; Desai, J.V.; et al. Prenatal Maternal Infection Promotes Tissue-Specific Immunity and Inflammation in Offspring. *Science* **2021**, *373*, eabf3002. [CrossRef] [PubMed]
107. Van Der Sloot, K.W.J.; Weersma, R.K.; Alizadeh, B.Z.; Dijkstra, G. Identification of Environmental Risk Factors Associated With the Development of Inflammatory Bowel Disease. *J. Crohns Colitis* **2020**, *14*, 1662–1671. [CrossRef]
108. Wiklund, P.; Karhunen, V.; Richmond, R.C.; Parmar, P.; Rodriguez, A.; De Silva, M.; Wielscher, M.; Rezwan, F.I.; Richardson, T.G.; Veijola, J.; et al. DNA Methylation Links Prenatal Smoking Exposure to Later Life Health Outcomes in Offspring. *Clin. Epigenet.* **2019**, *11*, 97. [CrossRef] [PubMed]
109. Fragou, D.; Pakkidi, E.; Aschner, M.; Samanidou, V.; Kovatsi, L. Smoking and DNA Methylation: Correlation of Methylation with Smoking Behavior and Association with Diseases and Fetus Development Following Prenatal Exposure. *Food Chem. Toxicol.* **2019**, *129*, 312–327. [CrossRef]
110. McLean, C.; Jun, S.; Kozyrskyj, A. Impact of Maternal Smoking on the Infant Gut Microbiota and Its Association with Child Overweight: A Scoping Review. *World J. Pediatr.* **2019**, *15*, 341–349. [CrossRef] [PubMed]
111. Xu, L.; Lochhead, P.; Ko, Y.; Claggett, B.; Leong, R.W.; Ananthakrishnan, A.N. Systematic Review with Meta-Analysis: Breastfeeding and the Risk of Crohn's Disease and Ulcerative Colitis. *Aliment. Pharmacol. Ther.* **2017**, *46*, 780–789. [CrossRef] [PubMed]
112. Klement, E.; Cohen, R.V.; Boxman, J.; Joseph, A.; Reif, S. Breastfeeding and Risk of Inflammatory Bowel Disease: A Systematic Review with Meta-Analysis. *Am. J. Clin. Nutr.* **2004**, *80*, 1342–1352. [CrossRef]
113. Gordon, H.; Blad, W.; Trier Møller, F.; Orchard, T.; Steel, A.; Trevelyan, G.; Ng, S.; Harbord, M. UK IBD Twin Registry: Concordance and Environmental Risk Factors of Twins with IBD. *Dig. Dis. Sci.* **2022**, *67*, 2444–2450. [CrossRef]
114. Penders, J.; Thijs, C.; van den Brandt, P.A.; Kummeling, I.; Snijders, B.; Stelma, F.; Adams, H.; van Ree, R.; Stobberingh, E.E. Gut Microbiota Composition and Development of Atopic Manifestations in Infancy: The KOALA Birth Cohort Study. *Gut* **2007**, *56*, 661–667. [CrossRef]
115. M'Rabet, L.; Vos, A.P.; Boehm, G.; Garssen, J. Breast-Feeding and Its Role in Early Development of the Immune System in Infants: Consequences for Health Later in Life1. *J. Nutr.* **2008**, *138*, 1782S–1790S. [CrossRef]
116. Keag, O.E.; Norman, J.E.; Stock, S.J. Long-Term Risks and Benefits Associated with Cesarean Delivery for Mother, Baby, and Subsequent Pregnancies: Systematic Review and Meta-Analysis. *PLoS Med.* **2018**, *15*, e1002494. [CrossRef]
117. Li, Y.; Tian, Y.; Zhu, W.; Gong, J.; Gu, L.; Zhang, W.; Guo, Z.; Li, N.; Li, J. Cesarean Delivery and Risk of Inflammatory Bowel Disease: A Systematic Review and Meta-Analysis. *Scand. J. Gastroenterol.* **2014**, *49*, 834–844. [CrossRef]
118. Bruce, A.; Black, M.; Bhattacharya, S. Mode of Delivery and Risk of Inflammatory Bowel Disease in the Offspring: Systematic Review and Meta-Analysis of Observational Studies. *Inflamm. Bowel Dis.* **2014**, *20*, 1217–1226. [CrossRef] [PubMed]
119. Kostic, A.D.; Xavier, R.J.; Gevers, D. The Microbiome in Inflammatory Bowel Disease: Current Status and the Future Ahead. *Gastroenterology* **2014**, *146*, 1489–1499. [CrossRef] [PubMed]
120. Dethlefsen, L.; Huse, S.; Sogin, M.L.; Relman, D.A. The Pervasive Effects of an Antibiotic on the Human Gut Microbiota, as Revealed by Deep 16S rRNA Sequencing. *PLoS Biol.* **2008**, *6*, e280. [CrossRef] [PubMed]
121. Pérez-Cobas, A.E.; Gosalbes, M.J.; Friedrichs, A.; Knecht, H.; Artacho, A.; Eismann, K.; Otto, W.; Rojo, D.; Bargiela, R.; von Bergen, M.; et al. Gut Microbiota Disturbance during Antibiotic Therapy: A Multi-Omic Approach. *Gut* **2013**, *62*, 1591–1601. [CrossRef] [PubMed]
122. Ungaro, R.; Bernstein, C.N.; Gearry, R.; Hviid, A.; Kolho, K.-L.; Kronman, M.P.; Shaw, S.; Van Kruiningen, H.; Colombel, J.-F.; Atreja, A. Antibiotics Associated with Increased Risk of New-Onset Crohn's Disease but Not Ulcerative Colitis: A Meta-Analysis. *Am. J. Gastroenterol.* **2014**, *109*, 1728–1738. [CrossRef] [PubMed]
123. Manichanh, C.; Borruel, N.; Casellas, F.; Guarner, F. The Gut Microbiota in IBD. *Nat. Rev. Gastroenterol. Hepatol.* **2012**, *9*, 599–608. [CrossRef]
124. Gevers, D.; Kugathasan, S.; Denson, L.A.; Vázquez-Baeza, Y.; Van Treuren, W.; Ren, B.; Schwager, E.; Knights, D.; Song, S.J.; Yassour, M.; et al. The Treatment-Naive Microbiome in New-Onset Crohn's Disease. *Cell Host Microbe* **2014**, *15*, 382–392. [CrossRef]
125. Cholapranee, A.; Ananthakrishnan, A.N. Environmental Hygiene and Risk of Inflammatory Bowel Diseases: A Systematic Review and Meta-Analysis. *Inflamm. Bowel Dis.* **2016**, *22*, 2191–2199. [CrossRef]
126. Michaux, M.; Chan, J.M.; Bergmann, L.; Chaves, L.F.; Klinkenberg, B.; Jacobson, K. Spatial Cluster Mapping and Environmental Modeling in Pediatric Inflammatory Bowel Disease. *World J. Gastroenterol.* **2023**, *29*, 3688–3702. [CrossRef]
127. Song, C.; Yang, J.; Ye, W.; Zhang, Y.; Tang, C.; Li, X.; Zhou, X.; Xie, Y. Urban-Rural Environmental Exposure during Childhood and Subsequent Risk of Inflammatory Bowel Disease: A Meta-Analysis. *Expert Rev. Gastroenterol. Hepatol.* **2019**, *13*, 591–602. [CrossRef]

128. Wu, X.-W.; Ji, H.-Z.; Yang, M.-F.; Wu, L.; Wang, F.-Y. Helicobacter Pylori Infection and Inflammatory Bowel Disease in Asians: A Meta-Analysis. *World J. Gastroenterol.* **2015**, *21*, 4750–4756. [CrossRef]
129. Castaño-Rodríguez, N.; Kaakoush, N.O.; Lee, W.S.; Mitchell, H.M. Dual Role of Helicobacter and Campylobacter Species in IBD: A Systematic Review and Meta-Analysis. *Gut* **2017**, *66*, 235–249. [CrossRef] [PubMed]
130. Luther, J.; Dave, M.; Higgins, P.D.R.; Kao, J.Y. Association between Helicobacter Pylori Infection and Inflammatory Bowel Disease: A Meta-Analysis and Systematic Review of the Literature. *Inflamm. Bowel Dis.* **2010**, *16*, 1077–1084. [CrossRef] [PubMed]
131. Rokkas, T.; Gisbert, J.P.; Niv, Y.; O'Morain, C. The Association between Helicobacter Pylori Infection and Inflammatory Bowel Disease Based on Meta-Analysis. *United Eur. Gastroenterol. J.* **2015**, *3*, 539–550. [CrossRef] [PubMed]
132. Codolo, G.; Mazzi, P.; Amedei, A.; Del Prete, G.; Berton, G.; D'Elios, M.M.; de Bernard, M. The Neutrophil-Activating Protein of Helicobacter Pylori down-Modulates Th2 Inflammation in Ovalbumin-Induced Allergic Asthma. *Cell. Microbiol.* **2008**, *10*, 2355–2363. [CrossRef]
133. Luther, J.; Owyang, S.Y.; Takeuchi, T.; Cole, T.S.; Zhang, M.; Liu, M.; Erb-Downward, J.; Rubenstein, J.H.; Chen, C.-C.; Pierzchala, A.V.; et al. Helicobacter Pylori DNA Decreases Pro-Inflammatory Cytokine Production by Dendritic Cells and Attenuates Dextran Sodium Sulphate-Induced Colitis. *Gut* **2011**, *60*, 1479–1486. [CrossRef]
134. Arnold, I.C.; Hitzler, I.; Müller, A. The Immunomodulatory Properties of Helicobacter Pylori Confer Protection against Allergic and Chronic Inflammatory Disorders. *Front. Cell. Infect. Microbiol.* **2012**, *2*, 10. [CrossRef]
135. Okada, H.; Kuhn, C.; Feillet, H.; Bach, J.-F. The "hygiene Hypothesis" for Autoimmune and Allergic Diseases: An Update. *Clin. Exp. Immunol.* **2010**, *160*, 1–9. [CrossRef]
136. Schaub, B.; Liu, J.; Höppler, S.; Schleich, I.; Huehn, J.; Olek, S.; Wieczorek, G.; Illi, S.; von Mutius, E. Maternal Farm Exposure Modulates Neonatal Immune Mechanisms through Regulatory T Cells. *J. Allergy Clin. Immunol.* **2009**, *123*, 774–782.e5. [CrossRef]
137. Hasosah, M.; Alhashmi, W.; Abualsaud, R.; Alamoudi, A.; Aljawad, A.; Tunkar, M.; Felemban, N.; Basalim, A.; Khan, M.; Alanazi, A.; et al. Environmental Risk Factors for Childhood Inflammatory Bowel Diseases: A Multicenter Case-Control Study. *Children* **2022**, *9*, 438. [CrossRef]
138. Strisciuglio, C.; Giugliano, F.; Martinelli, M.; Cenni, S.; Greco, L.; Staiano, A.; Miele, E. Impact of Environmental and Familial Factors in a Cohort of Pediatric Patients With Inflammatory Bowel Disease. *J. Pediatr. Gastroenterol. Nutr.* **2017**, *64*, 569–574. [CrossRef] [PubMed]
139. Piovani, D.; Danese, S.; Peyrin-Biroulet, L.; Nikolopoulos, G.K.; Lytras, T.; Bonovas, S. Environmental Risk Factors for Inflammatory Bowel Diseases: An Umbrella Review of Meta-Analyses. *Gastroenterology* **2019**, *157*, 647–659.e4. [CrossRef]
140. Jakobsen, C.; Paerregaard, A.; Munkholm, P.; Wewer, V. Environmental Factors and Risk of Developing Paediatric Inflammatory Bowel Disease—A Population Based Study 2007–2009. *J. Crohns Colitis* **2013**, *7*, 79–88. [CrossRef]
141. Sidik, S. Chronic Stress Can Inflame the Gut—Now Scientists Know Why. *Nature* **2023**, *618*, 221–222. [CrossRef]
142. Schneider, K.M.; Blank, N.; Alvarez, Y.; Thum, K.; Lundgren, P.; Litichevskiy, L.; Sleeman, M.; Bahnsen, K.; Kim, J.; Kardo, S.; et al. The Enteric Nervous System Relays Psychological Stress to Intestinal Inflammation. *Cell* **2023**, *186*, 2823–2838.e20. [CrossRef]
143. Bayrer, J.R.; Castro, J.; Venkataraman, A.; Touhara, K.K.; Rossen, N.D.; Morrie, R.D.; Maddern, J.; Hendry, A.; Braverman, K.N.; Garcia-Caraballo, S.; et al. Gut Enterochromaffin Cells Drive Visceral Pain and Anxiety. *Nature* **2023**, *616*, 137–142. [CrossRef] [PubMed]
144. Karl, J.P.; Hatch, A.M.; Arcidiacono, S.M.; Pearce, S.C.; Pantoja-Feliciano, I.G.; Doherty, L.A.; Soares, J.W. Effects of Psychological, Environmental and Physical Stressors on the Gut Microbiota. *Front. Microbiol.* **2018**, *9*, 2013. [CrossRef] [PubMed]
145. Oligschlaeger, Y.; Yadati, T.; Houben, T.; Condello Oliván, C.M.; Shiri-Sverdlov, R. Inflammatory Bowel Disease: A Stressed "Gut/Feeling". *Cells* **2019**, *8*, 659. [CrossRef] [PubMed]
146. Konturek, P.C.; Brzozowski, T.; Konturek, S.J. Stress and the Gut: Pathophysiology, Clinical Consequences, Diagnostic Approach and Treatment Options. *J. Physiol. Pharmacol.* **2011**, *62*, 591–599. [PubMed]
147. Hu, D.; Ren, J.; Wang, G.; Gu, G.; Liu, S.; Wu, X.; Chen, J.; Ren, H.; Hong, Z.; Li, J. Geographic Mapping of Crohn's Disease and Its Relation to Affluence in Jiangsu Province, an Eastern Coastal Province of China. *Gastroenterol. Res. Pract.* **2014**, *2014*, 1–6. [CrossRef] [PubMed]
148. Kaplan, G.G.; Hubbard, J.; Korzenik, J.; Sands, B.E.; Panaccione, R.; Ghosh, S.; Wheeler, A.J.; Villeneuve, P.J. The Inflammatory Bowel Diseases and Ambient Air Pollution: A Novel Association. *Am. J. Gastroenterol.* **2010**, *105*, 2412–2419. [CrossRef] [PubMed]
149. Sahoo, D.K.; Heilmann, R.M.; Paital, B.; Patel, A.; Yadav, V.K.; Wong, D.; Jergens, A.E. Oxidative Stress, Hormones, and Effects of Natural Antioxidants on Intestinal Inflammation in Inflammatory Bowel Disease. *Front. Endocrinol.* **2023**, *14*, 1217165. [CrossRef] [PubMed]
150. Tian, T.; Wang, Z.; Zhang, J. Pathomechanisms of Oxidative Stress in Inflammatory Bowel Disease and Potential Antioxidant Therapies. *Oxid. Med. Cell. Longev.* **2017**, *2017*, 4535194. [CrossRef]
151. Qin, J.; Xia, W.; Liang, G.; Xu, S.; Zhao, X.; Wang, D.; Sun, X.; Li, Y.; Liu, H. Association of Fine Particulate Matter with Glucose and Lipid Metabolism: A Longitudinal Study in Young Adults. *Occup. Environ. Med.* **2021**, *78*, 448–453. [CrossRef] [PubMed]

152. Rivas-Arancibia, S.; Miranda-Martínez, A.; Rodríguez-Martínez, E.; Hernández-Orozco, E.; Valdés-Fuentes, M.; De La Rosa-Sierra, R. Ozone Environmental Pollution: Relationship between the Intestine and Neurodegenerative Diseases. *Antioxidants* **2023**, *12*, 1323. [CrossRef] [PubMed]
153. Ananthakrishnan, A.N.; McGinley, E.L.; Binion, D.G.; Saeian, K. Ambient Air Pollution Correlates with Hospitalizations for Inflammatory Bowel Disease: An Ecologic Analysis. *Inflamm. Bowel Dis.* **2011**, *17*, 1138–1145. [CrossRef]
154. Adami, G.; Pontalti, M.; Cattani, G.; Rossini, M.; Viapiana, O.; Orsolini, G.; Benini, C.; Bertoldo, E.; Fracassi, E.; Gatti, D.; et al. Association between Long-Term Exposure to Air Pollution and Immune-Mediated Diseases: A Population-Based Cohort Study. *RMD Open* **2022**, *8*, e002055. [CrossRef] [PubMed]
155. Liu, Y.; Wang, T.; Si, B.; Du, H.; Liu, Y.; Waqas, A.; Huang, S.; Zhao, G.; Chen, S.; Xu, A. Intratracheally Instillated Diesel $PM_{2.5}$ Significantly Altered the Structure and Composition of Indigenous Murine Gut Microbiota. *Ecotoxicol. Environ. Saf.* **2021**, *210*, 111903. [CrossRef]
156. Okafor, P.N.; Dahlen, A.; Youssef, M.; Olayode, A.; Sonu, I.; Neshatian, L.; Nguyen, L.; Charu, V. Environmental Pollutants Are Associated With Irritable Bowel Syndrome in a Commercially Insured Cohort of California Residents. *Clin. Gastroenterol. Hepatol.* **2023**, *21*, 1617–1626.e9. [CrossRef] [PubMed]
157. Soares, A.; Guieysse, B.; Jefferson, B.; Cartmell, E.; Lester, J.N. Nonylphenol in the Environment: A Critical Review on Occurrence, Fate, Toxicity and Treatment in Wastewaters. *Environ. Int.* **2008**, *34*, 1033–1049. [CrossRef]
158. Wagner, M.; Schlüsener, M.P.; Ternes, T.A.; Oehlmann, J. Identification of Putative Steroid Receptor Antagonists in Bottled Water: Combining Bioassays and High-Resolution Mass Spectrometry. *PLoS ONE* **2013**, *8*, e72472. [CrossRef]
159. Perl, D.P.; Fogarty, U.; Harpaz, N.; Sachar, D.B. Bacterial-Metal Interactions: The Potential Role of Aluminum and Other Trace Elements in the Etiology of Chrohn's Disease. *Inflamm. Bowel Dis.* **2004**, *10*, 881–883. [CrossRef]
160. Jowett, S.L. Influence of Dietary Factors on the Clinical Course of Ulcerative Colitis: A Prospective Cohort Study. *Gut* **2004**, *53*, 1479–1484. [CrossRef] [PubMed]
161. Aamodt, G.; Bukholm, G.; Jahnsen, J.; Moum, B.; Vatn, M.H.; The IBSEN Study Group. The Association Between Water Supply and Inflammatory Bowel Disease Based on a 1990–1993 Cohort Study in Southeastern Norway. *Am. J. Epidemiol.* **2008**, *168*, 1065–1072. [CrossRef] [PubMed]
162. Jädert, C.; Petersson, J.; Massena, S.; Ahl, D.; Grapensparr, L.; Holm, L.; Lundberg, J.O.; Phillipson, M. Decreased Leukocyte Recruitment by Inorganic Nitrate and Nitrite in Microvascular Inflammation and NSAID-Induced Intestinal Injury. *Free Radic. Biol. Med.* **2012**, *52*, 683–692. [CrossRef] [PubMed]
163. Zhou, S.; Chai, P.; Dong, X.; Liang, Z.; Yang, Z.; Li, J.; Teng, G.; Sun, S.; Xu, M.; Zheng, Z.-J.; et al. Drinking Water Quality and Inflammatory Bowel Disease: A Prospective Cohort Study. *Environ. Sci. Pollut. Res.* **2023**, *30*, 71171–71183. [CrossRef]
164. Johnson, G.J.; Cosnes, J.; Mansfield, J.C. Review Article: Smoking Cessation as Primary Therapy to Modify the Course of Crohn's Disease. *Aliment. Pharmacol. Ther.* **2005**, *21*, 921–931. [CrossRef]
165. Rozich, J.J.; Holmer, A.; Singh, S. Effect of Lifestyle Factors on Outcomes in Patients With Inflammatory Bowel Diseases. *Am. J. Gastroenterol.* **2020**, *115*, 832–840. [CrossRef]
166. Higuchi, L.M.; Khalili, H.; Chan, A.T.; Richter, J.M.; Bousvaros, A.; Fuchs, C.S. A Prospective Study of Cigarette Smoking and the Risk of Inflammatory Bowel Disease in Women. *Am. J. Gastroenterol.* **2012**, *107*, 1399–1406. [CrossRef]
167. Nasr, S.; Nsiri, I.; Fredj, M.B. Effectiveness of Smoking Cessation Interventions for Smokers with Crohn's Disease: A Systematic Review. *Future Sci. OA* **2023**, *9*, FSO870. [CrossRef] [PubMed]
168. Nunes, T.; Etchevers, M.J.; Merino, O.; Gallego, S.; García-Sánchez, V.; Marín-Jiménez, I.; Menchén, L.; Barreiro-de Acosta, M.; Bastida, G.; García, S.; et al. High Smoking Cessation Rate in Crohn's Disease Patients after Physician Advice—The TABACROHN Study. *J. Crohns Colitis* **2013**, *7*, 202–207. [CrossRef] [PubMed]
169. Cosnes, J.; Beaugerie, L.; Carbonnel, F.; Gendre, J. Smoking Cessation and the Course of Crohn's Disease: An Intervention Study. *Gastroenterology* **2001**, *120*, 1093–1099. [CrossRef] [PubMed]
170. Sofia, M.A.; Lipowska, A.M.; Zmeter, N.; Perez, E.; Kavitt, R.; Rubin, D.T. Poor Sleep Quality in Crohn's Disease Is Associated With Disease Activity and Risk for Hospitalization or Surgery. *Inflamm. Bowel Dis.* **2020**, *26*, 1251–1259. [CrossRef]
171. Zhang, J.-Z.; Song, X.-Z.; Song, X.-N.; Shen, Y.-L.; Tang, H.; Li, H. Prevalence and Risk Factors of Sleep Disorders in Inflammatory Bowel Disease: A Cross-Sectional Study. *Int. J. Colorectal Dis.* **2024**, *39*, 140. [CrossRef] [PubMed]
172. Ali, T.; Orr, W.C. Sleep Disturbances and Inflammatory Bowel Disease. *Inflamm. Bowel Dis.* **2014**, *20*, 1986–1995. [CrossRef]
173. Vieujean, S.; Caron, B.; Haghnejad, V.; Jouzeau, J.-Y.; Netter, P.; Heba, A.-C.; Ndiaye, N.C.; Moulin, D.; Barreto, G.; Danese, S.; et al. Impact of the Exposome on the Epigenome in Inflammatory Bowel Disease Patients and Animal Models. *Int. J. Mol. Sci.* **2022**, *23*, 7611. [CrossRef] [PubMed]
174. Dougherty, U.; Mustafi, R.; Zhu, H.; Zhu, X.; Deb, D.; Meredith, S.C.; Ayaloglu-Butun, F.; Fletcher, M.; Sanchez, A.; Pekow, J.; et al. Upregulation of Polycistronic microRNA-143 and microRNA-145 in Colonocytes Suppresses Colitis and Inflammation-Associated Colon Cancer. *Epigenetics* **2021**, *16*, 1317–1334. [CrossRef]

175. Wei, M.; Gao, X.; Liu, L.; Li, Z.; Wan, Z.; Dong, Y.; Chen, X.; Niu, Y.; Zhang, J.; Yang, G. Visceral Adipose Tissue Derived Exosomes Exacerbate Colitis Severity via Pro-Inflammatory MiRNAs in High Fat Diet Fed Mice. *ACS Nano* **2020**, *14*, 5099–5110. [CrossRef] [PubMed]
176. Timms, V.J.; Daskalopoulos, G.; Mitchell, H.M.; Neilan, B.A. The Association of Mycobacterium Avium Subsp. Paratuberculosis with Inflammatory Bowel Disease. *PLoS ONE* **2016**, *11*, e0148731. [CrossRef]
177. Guo, Z.; Cai, X.; Guo, X.; Xu, Y.; Gong, J.; Li, Y.; Zhu, W. Let-7b Ameliorates Crohn's Disease-Associated Adherent-Invasive E Coli Induced Intestinal Inflammation via Modulating Toll-Like Receptor 4 Expression in Intestinal Epithelial Cells. *Biochem. Pharmacol.* **2018**, *156*, 196–203. [CrossRef]
178. Melhem, H.; Hansmannel, F.; Bressenot, A.; Battaglia-Hsu, S.-F.; Billioud, V.; Alberto, J.M.; Gueant, J.L.; Peyrin-Biroulet, L. Methyl-Deficient Diet Promotes Colitis and SIRT1-Mediated Endoplasmic Reticulum Stress. *Gut* **2016**, *65*, 595–606. [CrossRef]
179. Trakman, G.L.; Lin, W.Y.Y.; Hamilton, A.L.; Wilson-O'Brien, A.L.; Stanley, A.; Ching, J.Y.; Yu, J.; Mak, J.W.Y.; Sun, Y.; Niu, J.; et al. Processed Food as a Risk Factor for the Development and Perpetuation of Crohn's Disease—The ENIGMA Study. *Nutrients* **2022**, *14*, 3627. [CrossRef]
180. De Chambrun, G.P.; Body-Malapel, M.; Frey-Wagner, I.; Djouina, M.; Deknuydt, F.; Atrott, K.; Esquerre, N.; Altare, F.; Neut, C.; Arrieta, M.C.; et al. Aluminum Enhances Inflammation and Decreases Mucosal Healing in Experimental Colitis in Mice. *Mucosal Immunol.* **2014**, *7*, 589–601. [CrossRef]
181. Becker, H.M.; Bertschinger, M.M.; Rogler, G. Microparticles and Their Impact on Intestinal Immunity. *Dig. Dis.* **2012**, *30*, 47–54. [CrossRef] [PubMed]
182. Rappaport, S.M. Implications of the Exposome for Exposure Science. *J. Expo. Sci. Environ. Epidemiol.* **2011**, *21*, 5–9. [CrossRef]
183. Vel Szic, K.S.; Declerck, K.; Vidaković, M.; Vanden Berghe, W. From Inflammaging to Healthy Aging by Dietary Lifestyle Choices: Is Epigenetics the Key to Personalized Nutrition? *Clin. Epigenet.* **2015**, *7*, 33. [CrossRef]
184. Lippai, D.; Bala, S.; Catalano, D.; Kodys, K.; Szabo, G. Micro-RNA-155 Deficiency Prevents Alcohol-Induced Serum Endotoxin Increase and Small Bowel Inflammation in Mice. *Alcohol. Clin. Exp. Res.* **2014**, *38*, 2217–2224. [CrossRef] [PubMed]
185. Lv, Q.; Xing, Y.; Liu, J.; Dong, D.; Liu, Y.; Qiao, H.; Zhang, Y.; Hu, L. Lonicerin Targets EZH2 to Alleviate Ulcerative Colitis by Autophagy-Mediated NLRP3 Inflammasome Inactivation. *Acta Pharm. Sin. B* **2021**, *11*, 2880–2899. [CrossRef]
186. Galleggiante, V.; De Santis, S.; Liso, M.; Verna, G.; Sommella, E.; Mastronardi, M.; Campiglia, P.; Chieppa, M.; Serino, G. Quercetin-Induced miR-369-3p Suppresses Chronic Inflammatory Response Targeting C/EBP-β. *Mol. Nutr. Food Res.* **2019**, *63*, 1801390. [CrossRef]
187. James, S.; Aparna, J.S.; Babu, A.; Paul, A.M.; Lankadasari, M.B.; Athira, S.R.; Kumar, S.S.; Vijayan, Y.; Namitha, N.N.; Mohammed, S.; et al. Cardamonin Attenuates Experimental Colitis and Associated Colorectal Cancer. *Biomolecules* **2021**, *11*, 661. [CrossRef]
188. Qiao, C.-X.; Xu, S.; Wang, D.-D.; Gao, S.-Y.; Zhao, S.-F.; Zhang, M.-L.; Yu, B.; Yin, Q.; Zhao, G. MicroRNA-19b Alleviates Lipopolysaccharide-Induced Inflammatory Injury in Human Intestinal Cells by up-Regulation of Runx3. *Eur. Rev. Med. Pharmacol. Sci.* **2018**, *22*, 5284–5294. [CrossRef] [PubMed]
189. Ananthakrishnan, A.N.; Khalili, H.; Konijeti, G.G.; Higuchi, L.M.; de Silva, P.; Korzenik, J.R.; Fuchs, C.S.; Willett, W.C.; Richter, J.M.; Chan, A.T. A Prospective Study of Long-Term Intake of Dietary Fiber and Risk of Crohn's Disease and Ulcerative Colitis. *Gastroenterology* **2013**, *145*, 970–977. [CrossRef] [PubMed]
190. Hou, J.K.; Abraham, B.; El-Serag, H. Dietary Intake and Risk of Developing Inflammatory Bowel Disease: A Systematic Review of the Literature. *Am. J. Gastroenterol.* **2011**, *106*, 563–573. [CrossRef]

biomedicines

MDPI

Review

Bile Acids in Inflammatory Bowel Disease: From Pathophysiology to Treatment

Samantha H. Bai, Arun Chandnani and Siyan Cao *

Division of Gastroenterology, Department of Medicine, Washington University School of Medicine, St. Louis, MO 63110, USA; s.bai@wustl.edu (S.H.B.); arunc@wustl.edu (A.C.)
* Correspondence: caos@wustl.edu

Abstract: Inflammatory bowel disease (IBD) is a chronic condition that affects about 7 million people worldwide, and new therapies are needed. Understanding the complex roles that bile acids (BAs) play in IBD may lead to the development of novel IBD treatments independent of direct immunosuppression. This review discusses the latest discoveries in the roles BAs play in IBD pathogenesis and explores how these discoveries offer promising new therapeutic targets to treat IBD and improve patient outcomes. Several therapies discussed include specific BA receptor (BAR) agonists, dietary therapies, supplements, probiotics, and mesenchymal stem cell therapies that have all been shown to decrease IBD disease activity.

Keywords: bile acids; inflammatory bowel disease; ulcerative colitis; Crohn's disease; pathogenesis; new therapies

1. Introduction

Inflammatory bowel disease (IBD), which includes ulcerative colitis (UC) and Crohn's disease (CD), is a chronic, relapsing disease that affects about 7 million people worldwide [1,2]. IBD is a multifactorial disease with complex interactions between the diet, genetics, environment, gut microbiome, and the immune system, although the mechanisms remain poorly understood [3]. Current IBD treatments include biological and small molecule therapies that target the immune system. These medications can have significant side effects, including infection, malignancy, and thromboembolism. In addition, they only achieve sustained remission in a subset of patients [4], underscoring the need for new therapeutic approaches.

Recent advances have shown that gut metabolites such as bile acids (BAs) are also critical in IBD. BAs are amphipathic molecules derived from cholesterol to form primary BAs. These primary BAs undergo enterohepatic cycling and can be deconjugated by the gut microbiota to form secondary BAs. BAs exert their effects on the intestine by operating as signaling molecules that activate a variety of BA receptors (BARs), thereby regulating intestinal homeostasis [5].

A deeper understanding of the role of BAs in IBD may identify previously unknown pathogenesis and unveil novel therapies for IBD. In this review, we provide a comprehensive overview of the most recent studies elucidating the synthesis and function of BAs and their multifactorial roles in IBD pathogenesis, discuss several potential BA-based treatments for IBD, and identify areas of further research to advance our understanding of the complex interplay between BAs and IBD.

A comprehensive search of the PubMed, Embase, and Scopus databases from January 2020 until October 2024 was conducted to identify English-language articles regarding the role of bile acids in IBD. The specific search terms employed were the following: "bile acid", "bile salt", "Inflammatory Bowel Diseases", "IBD", "Crohn's disease", "CD", "ulcerative colitis", "UC", and "colitis". The screening process involved two independent reviewers (S.H.B. and S.C.) who first assessed titles and abstracts to identify potentially relevant studies. The full texts of these articles were examined to determine if they were eligible for inclusion as well as their reference lists to ensure relevant studies were included. The ultimate decision to include abstracts and articles was based on their relevance to the research objectives.

2. Overview of BAs and Their Emerging Roles in IBD

2.1. Synthesis of BAs

BAs are amphiphilic steroid molecules that play important roles in a variety of physiological processes, including dietary absorption of lipids and vitamins, protection against microbes, and regulation of the gut microbiota and intestinal inflammation [3,6–8]. Primary BAs are derived from cholesterol in the liver via two pathways: classic and alternative pathways [9,10]. Via a series of cytochrome P450 enzymes, cholesterol is converted to cholic acid (CA) or chenodeoxycholic acid (CDCA) in the classical pathway and CDCA in the alternative pathway [11]. CA and CDCA are the most common primary BAs in humans, while mice and infants generate 6-hydroxylated versions of CA and CDCA, known as muricholic acid (MCA) [12–15]. CA and CDCA are subsequently conjugated with glycine or taurine via BA-CoA synthase and BA-CoA amino acid N-acetyltransferase [16,17]. The conjugated BAs are secreted from the liver to the gallbladder and released into the duodenum after meals [18]. In the small intestine, 95% of BAs are reabsorbed in the ileum via the apical sodium-dependent bile acid transporter (ASBT) and returned to the liver via the portal vein [19–21]. This enterohepatic circulation occurs between 4 and 12 times per day in humans [22,23]. The remaining 5% of BAs that are not reabsorbed enter the colon, where they are excreted in the feces and undergo biotransformation by the intestinal microbiota to form secondary BAs [24–26]. The main microbial biotransformation reactions include deconjugation by bile salt hydrolases (BSHs), $7\alpha/\beta$-dehydroxylation by bacterial BA-inducible (*bai*) genes, and oxidation and epimerization by pyridine nucleotide-dependent hydroxysteroid dehydrogenases (HSDHs) [17,27,28]. The two major secondary BAs in humans are lithocholic acid (LCA) and deoxycholic acid (DCA), which are produced from CDCA and CA, respectively [29–31].

BAs exert their biological effects primarily by serving as ligands for BARs [32]. The main BARs are the nuclear receptors farnesoid X receptor (FXR), retinoid-related orphan receptor γt (RORγt), vitamin D receptor (VDR), pregnane X receptor (PXR), and constitutive androstane receptor (CAR), as well as the membrane-bound receptors G protein-coupled BAR 1, also known as Takeda G protein-coupled receptor 5, (GPBAR1 or TGR5), and sphingosine-1-phosphate receptor 2 (S1PR2) [5,33,34]. BAs also regulate BA synthesis via feedback mechanisms. The BA pool that returns to the liver from the ileum directly suppresses the production of new BAs in hepatocytes via FXR, which increases fibroblast growth factor expression (FGF-15 in mice and FGF-19 in humans) and suppresses BA synthesis [35,36]. Understanding these complex interactions and feedback mechanisms is crucial for elucidating how BAs influence the development of IBD.

2.2. BA Alterations in Patients with IBD

Patients with IBD develop an altered BA composition [37] characterized by an increase in primary BAs and a decrease in secondary BAs [38–40]. While most studies were conducted on adult patients with IBD, similar trends have been found in pediatric patients [41]. Recent analyses of pooled samples of patients with CD and UC revealed an increase in the primary BA glycocholic acid (GCA) [37] and decreases in the secondary BAs DCA [38], LCA [38], glycodeoxycholic acid (GDCA) [38], glycolithocholic acid (GLCA) [38], isolithocholic acid (isoLCA) [39], 3-oxolithocholic acid (3-oxoLCA) [39], taurodeoxycholic acid (TDCA) [38], and taurolithocholic acid (TLCA) [38]. The reduction in secondary BAs is thought to result from gut dysbiosis in IBD patients, which reduces primary BA deconjugation and 7α-dehydroxylation by the gut microbiota, leading to the depletion of secondary BAs [40,41]. However, there is some conflicting data as another study showed that both UC and CD patients had a decrease in the primary BA CDCA [38]. Both CD [42,43] and

UC [42] patients also had increases in the total fecal BAs compared to healthy controls. It remains to be determined whether disease duration and activity, location of inflammation, and past and current treatments affect the BA pool in IBD patients.

Patients with CD showed increased levels of the primary BAs CA [44,45], CDCA [44], and GCA [46,47], and decreased levels of the secondary BAs DCA [48,49] and LCA [46,48,49]. Secondary BAs were even lower in patients with active CD compared to patients with CD in remission [48]. Yet other studies have found decreased levels of the primary BAs glycochenodeoxycholic acid (GCDCA) [46], glycohyodeoxycholic acid (GHDCA) [50], and taurocholic acid (TCA) [46], and increased levels of the secondary BAs DCA [47,51], GDCA [46,47], isoLCA [47], and TDCA [47] in CD patients. Patients with ileal CD exhibited increased levels of primary BAs and secondary BAs compared to those with colonic CD [52]. Surgeries have also been shown to skew BA species in the intestine. Compared to CD patients who did not undergo surgery, CD patients who underwent ileal resection had more CA [53] and less isoLCA [54], although other studies found an increase in DCA [53]. These changes in BAs with ileal resection are thought to be due to alterations in the gut microbiota [54]. CD patients who underwent ileocecectomy were more susceptible to ileitis and those who developed ileitis exhibited elevated CA and CDCA levels, reduced microbial diversity, and decreased abundance of *Faecalibacterium prausnitzii* compared to those without ileitis [53]. In addition to intestinal inflammation, altered BAs have been linked to psychological disorders in CD, although the underlying mechanisms are unknown. The self-rated depression scale positively correlated with 7-dehydrocholic acid (7-DHCA) and negatively correlated with hyodeoxycholic acid (HDCA) and 12-DHCA, while the self-rated anxiety scale positively correlated with TDCA, TLCA, and tauro-β-MCA (TβMCA) [49].

Similarly, UC patients have also exhibited an altered BA composition in the digestive tract, such as increased levels in the primary BAs CA [55,56], CDCA [56], GCA [56], GCDCA [55,57], TCA [55,56], and taurochenodeoxycholic acid (TCDCA) [55,57], and decreased levels in the secondary BAs DCA [50,55,56], LCA [50,55,56], GDCA [55], GLCA [55], HDCA [56], isoLCA [56], 12-ketolithocholic acid (12-KLCA) [56], and TLCA [55]. Patients with more severe UC exhibited greater decreases in secondary BAs than those with less severe UC [56,58]. Ethnicity may also influence BA composition as Hispanics and South Asians with UC have higher levels of primary BAs [59] and LCA [60] than Caucasians. UC patients who underwent a total proctocolectomy with ileal pouch-anal anastomosis (IPAA) had lower levels of DCA and LCA [61], as well as decreased secondary BA-producing bacteria, such as Ruminococcaceae and those with *bai* genes, further suggesting that gut dysbiosis in IBD patients leads to secondary BA deficiency [62]. BAs may also explain the differential effects of smoking on UC versus CD. The 3-beta-hydroxysteroid dehydrogenase enzyme, which is involved in BA metabolism, was upregulated in CD patients who never smoked and was downregulated in UC patients who currently smoke [63]. In support of the connection between altered BAs and psychological disorders in UC, UC patients with high-stress reactivity had decreased levels of CDCA, GCA, GCDCA, and LCA than those with lower stress reactivity [64].

While there is a general association between increased primary BAs and decreased secondary BAs in IBD patients, some studies have conflicting results regarding specific BAs (Table 1), which raises concerns regarding the roles specific BAs play in IBD pathogenesis. However, several key differences between studies may contribute to the contradictory results. For example, one study measured BAs in fecal samples, while another used serum samples [43,49]. Differences in patient populations and sample collection timings may also contribute to these results.

In addition to intestinal inflammation, BA dysregulation may contribute to higher risks of primary sclerosing cholangitis (PSC) and colorectal cancer in IBD patients. IBD-PSC patients exhibited decreased sulfated BAs, increased conjugated secondary BAs, and elevated liver fibrosis compared to IBD-only patients [65]. This may be partly due to differences in the gut microbiota as PSC-IBD patients exhibited increased microbial genes involved in secondary BA metabolism with enrichment in *Veillonella atypica*, *Veillonella dispar*, and *Clostridium scindens* [65]. Patients with UC and PSC who underwent IPAA and later developed chronic pouchitis exhibited lower levels of LCA and decreased microbiota α-diversity than those with a normal pouch [66]. Abnormal BA metabolism and gut dysbiosis may also contribute to colitis-associated cancer. Mice with azoxymethane (AOM) and dextran sulfate sodium (DSS)-induced colon cancer exhibited a reduction in *Clostridium XIV* and *Lactobacillus*, decreased secondary BAs, downregulation of the FXR-FGF15 axis, and upregulation of TGR5 [67].

Table 1. Alterations in BAs in IBD patients.

Bile Acids	Pooled IBD Samples	Crohn's Disease	Ulcerative Colitis
Primary Bile Acids			
CA		↑ [44,45]	↑ [55,56]
CDCA		↑ [44] ↓ [38]	↑ [56] ↓ [38,64]
GCA	↑ [37]	↑ [46,47]	↑ [56] ↓ [64]
GCDCA		↓ [46]	↑ [55,57] ↓ [64]
GHDCA		↓ [50]	
TCA		↓ [46]	↑ [55,56]
TCDCA			↑ [55,57]
Secondary Bile Acids			
DCA	↓ [38]	↑ [47,51] ↓ [48,49]	↓ [50,55,56]
GDCA	↓ [38]	↑ [46,47]	↓ [55]
GLCA	↓ [38]		↓ [55]
HDCA			↓ [56]
isoLCA	↓ [39]	↑ [47]	↓ [56]
12-KLCA			↓ [56]
LCA	↓ [38]	↓ [46,48,49]	↓ [50,55,56,64]
3-oxoLCA	↓ [39]		
TDCA	↓ [38]	↑ [47]	
TLCA	↓ [38]		↓ [55]

2.3. Roles of BAs in IBD Pathogenesis

Studies in the past decade suggest that BAs impact the pathogenesis of IBD through dysregulation of the gut microbiome, immune system, BARs, intestinal epithelium, gut–liver axis, diet, environment, and other metabolites (Figure 1). IBD patients are known to develop gut dysbiosis, which may contribute to the BA changes in IBD by skewing BA metabolism [68]. BSH gene abundance was associated with CD and UC [69]. IBD patients exhibited reductions in BA-related genes, including *cbh* and *baiN* in the gut microbiota, especially in *Alistipes* [70], *Blautia* [70], *Butyricicoccus* [55], *Clostridium IV* [55], *Clostridium XIV* [55], *Collinsella* [70], *Faecalibacterium* [55,70], and *Roseburia* [55]. Several studies in animal models of IBD also demonstrated that a shift in BAs correlated with changes in the gut microbiome. *Fusobacterium nucleatum* worsened DSS-induced colitis, partially by dysregulating BA metabolism [71]. Yorkshire pigs with DSS-induced colitis exhibited decreased BAs, possibly due to increases in *Bilophila* and *Alistipes* [72]. Yorkshire Terrier dogs with chronic enteropathy exhibited reduced UDCA as well as *Fusobacterium* and *Clostridium Hiranonis* compared to healthy controls, which only partially improved with clinical remission [73]. CD patients with the manganese transporter ZIP8 A391T mutation, which increases the risk of CD, exhibited lower levels of *Veillonella* and FGF19, suggesting that ZIP8 alters the gut microbiome and BA metabolism [74]. Microbial biofilms may also play an important role in the BA regulation of IBD as UC patients with mucosal biofilms had less bacterial diversity and more primary BAs compared to those without biofilms [75]. In addition, mucous-colonizing bacteria in IBD patients positively correlated with endoplasmic reticulum (ER) stress-related BA signals [76]. Overall, the studies suggest that there are identifiable microbial genetic differences involved in BA metabolism that are found in the gut microbiota of patients with IBD and that there are specific bacteria involved in BA metabolism that are associated with IBD. This suggests that microbiota-targeted therapies that modulate BA metabolism may be potential IBD treatments. However, there is variability in several factors between the aforementioned studies, such as varying diets and environments of the respective patient populations, which may affect the composition of the gut microbiome. Thus, it remains unclear if there are specific bacteria or genetic differences that are most implicated in IBD pathogenesis, and more studies are needed to further explore this relationship.

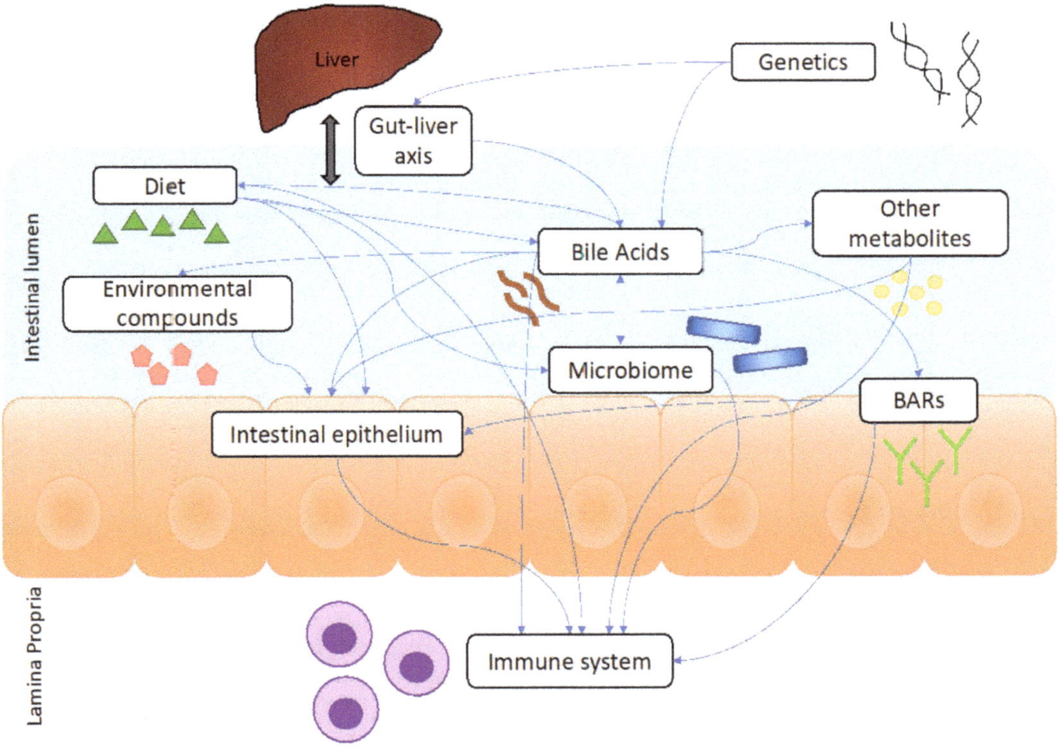

Figure 1. Overview of complex interactions that BAs have with factors that contribute to IBD. BAs contribute to IBD pathogenesis through numerous interactions displayed by arrows with the diet, environment, genetics, gut–liver axis, microbiome, other metabolites, BARs, intestinal epithelium, and the immune system. The figure shows several ways that BAs interact with various factors that contribute to IBD. IBD: inflammatory bowel disease; BAR: bile acid receptor.

Modulating the immune system is another key role BAs may play in IBD pathogenesis [77]. Primary BAs are generally pro-inflammatory while secondary BAs have anti-inflammatory properties. In UC patients, the primary BAs GCA, GCDCA, and TCA positively correlated with IL-1α and TNF-α while the secondary BAs DCA, GDCA, LCA, and TLCA negatively correlated with these pro-inflammatory cytokines [55]. BAs also regulate specific immune cell subsets that control intestinal homeostasis. One good example is the T_H17-T_{reg} cell balance, which is essential for mucosal homeostasis [78]. For example, 3-oxoLCA bound to RORγt, leading to the suppression of T_H17 cell differentiation, while isoallolithocholic acid (isoalloLCA) promoted the differentiation of T_{reg} cells through FOXP3 induction mediated by mitochondrial reactive oxygen species [79]. The primary BA CA was increased by an inulin fiber diet, leading to IL-33 upregulation and worsening DSS-induced murine colitis and human IBD, which are likely mediated by group 2 innate lymphoid cells (ILC2s) and eosinophils [80]. In DSS-induced colitis, CA, CDCA, and LCA regulated RORγt$^+$ T_{reg} levels via VDR [81], and UDCA, isoalloLCA, and 3-oxoLCA increased the proportion of ILC3s in the intestine [82], thereby improving epithelial barrier integrity and alleviating colitis. Other metabolites, including short-chain fatty acids, also work with the immune system to regulate BAs; for example, tumor necrosis factor (TNF-α), interferon-γ (IFN-γ), and butyrate-inhibited TCA uptake by Caco-2 cells, possibly through the PI3K and JAK/STAT1 pathways [83].

BA signaling via BARs is likely another important regulator of IBD [84]. Pediatric IBD patients exhibited reduced expression of FXR, PXR, and TGR5 [85]. UC patients exhibited increased TGR5 and decreased VDR compared to healthy controls [55]. FXR and PXR were less activated in CD patients [46]. In addition, mice with *Tgr5* disruption in intestinal stem cells developed more severe DSS-induced colitis than wild-type mice [86]. Genetics, including mutations in BAR genes, have also been shown to affect BA metabolism and IBD. The *FXR-1GT* single nucleotide variation, which leads to decreased activation of FXR targets, is associated with earlier onset and more frequent surgeries in women with CD, possibly through estrogen-mediated ER attenuation of FXR activation [87]. BARs, including FXR, PXR, VDR, and GPBAR1, are highly expressed in innate and adaptive immune cells that impact IBD pathophysiology [79,88–93], e.g., TGR5R-dependent protein kinase A activation drove the ubiquitination and phosphorylation of NLRP3, a key regulator of innate immune response in the intestinal mucosa. BAs and TGR5 activation were shown to inhibit NLRP3 inflammasome activation and inflammation in vivo [90]. A later study revealed that FXR directly interacted with NLRP3 and caspase 1, leading to the suppression of NLRP3 inflammasome. Consequently, $Fxr^{-/-}$ mice were more susceptible to endotoxemia shock [91]. BARs also control lymphocyte activation in inflammation. CXCR6$^+$ natural killer T (NKT) cells mediated tumor suppression in the liver, which relied on the primary BA-to-secondary BA conversion by the intestinal microbiome [94]. Future studies should determine how the BAR-regulated immune responses orchestrate IBD pathogenesis.

Impaired gut barrier function is an essential contributing factor to IBD. The regulation of intestinal epithelial tight junctions by BAs may also impact the development of IBD. DCA has been shown to increase the mRNA expression of occludin and zonula occludens-1 (ZO-1) in tight junctions, which are essential for preserving the integrity of tight junctions [95]. Knocking out *Fxr* in mice improved the intestinal barrier through improved maintenance of tight junctions and downregulated inflammatory cytokines, leading to decreased intestinal inflammation in several mouse models of colitis [96].

The gut–liver axis may play a significant role in the BA modulation of IBD. IBD patients have exhibited higher levels of hepatic FGF19, an inhibitor of BA production, during remission than in active disease [97]. The hepatic RelA/STAT3-CYP enzyme pathway increased primary BAs and exacerbated DSS-induced colitis [98]. Knocking out the gene encoding for G protein guanine nucleotide-binding protein subunit alpha 13 in the liver reversed the increases in CA and CDCA by upregulating the BA transporter ABCB11 in mice with DSS-induced colitis, further demonstrating that hepatic modulation of BAs is important for IBD pathogenesis [99]. BAs are also key modulators in patients with both IBD and liver disease. PSC-UC patients exhibited elevated BA signaling pathways and altered microbiota compared to patients with UC alone [100]. Mice with DSS-induced colitis developed metabolic dysfunction-associated steatotic liver disease (MASLD), partly due to BA dysregulation [101]. Cholestatic liver disease was also attenuated by suppressing BA synthesis in an IBD-PSC model with $Mdr2^{-/-}$ mice treated with DSS [102]. In two mouse models of MASLD and colitis, MASLD induced gut dysbiosis and increased secondary BAs in the ileum, leading to ileitis via CD8$^+$ T cells and the TGR5/mTOR/oxidative phosphorylation signaling pathway [103]. Ileitis then inhibited hepatic FXR activation and worsened MASLD, suggesting that secondary BAs may be a critical link between MASLD and IBD [103].

The interplay between BAs and diet may be another crucial regulator of IBD. Mice with active colitis on a high-fat diet exhibited increased ferroptosis compared to those with a normal diet, which was likely caused by increased DCA levels driven by upregulated hypoxia-inducible factor-2α and divalent metal transporter-1 [104]. Multiple studies have demonstrated that western-style diets worsen DSS- and 2,4,6-trinitrobenzene sulfonic acid (TNBS)-induced colitis by dysregulating BA metabolism, including increasing DCA and LCA and decreasing the spatial distribution of TCA. A high-fat/high-sugar maternal diet elevated offspring susceptibility to TNBS-induced colitis by increasing Bacteroidetes, thereby promoting gasdermin D (GSDMD)-mediated pyroptosis and IL-1β production in macrophages [105]. Transition feeding of a high-fat diet induced BA accumulation in the ER by TNF-α and exacerbated intestinal epithelial apoptosis via the activation of the ER stress sensor IRE1α [106]. Those diets were also shown to skew macrophages toward M1 polarization and pro-inflammatory cytokine production [107], and decrease *Clostridium scindens* and secondary Bas, including isoalloLCA, leading to dysregulation of T_H17/T_{reg} cells [108]. Moreover, a ketogenic diet, which is also high in fats, also worsened DSS-induced colitis, partly by increasing BAs, including CA, GCA, and TCDCA [109]. A study by Liu et al. found that Paneth cell dysregulation, which contributes to CD, was induced by a Western-style diet via upregulation of DCA by *baiCD*-expressing *Clostridium* spp., which increased FXR activation and type I IFNs [110]. In contrast, another study showed that a lard-based high-fat diet protected against DSS-induced colitis and colitis-associated cancer by increasing gut microbial diversity, including Firmicutes and *Clostridium* cluster XIVa abundance, upregulating secondary BAs and modulating the VDR pathway [111]. This discrepancy may be because these studies used high-fat diets from different manufacturers, which have different compositions.

IBD activity may also be modulated by interactions between BAs, the environment, and other metabolites. One study suggested that UC patients exhibited increased environmental exposures to perfluoroalkyl substance perfluorooctanoic acid compared to CD patients and controls [112]. This exposure may contribute to colitis by altering the intestinal barrier, decreasing LCA and DCA, altering the T_H17/T_{reg} balance [113], increasing IL-17A, and downregulating IL-10 [112,113]. Aflatoxin B_1 exposure decreased BAs, including CDCA, and induced a similar gut dysbiosis in rats to those found in IBD patients [114]. BAs may also modulate IBD by altering short-chain fatty acid metabolism. Butyrate is downregulated in IBD, which may be partly due to DCA and CDCA inhibition of butyrate uptake [115]. These findings highlight the intricate relationship between BAs and IBD through interactions with the environment, gut metabolome, diet, genetics, gut–liver axis, intestinal epithelium, BARs, immune system, and the microbiome. This dynamic interplay has revealed several potential clinical applications for BAs in IBD, and further studies are needed to facilitate the development of novel BA-based IBD therapies.

2.4. BAs as Biomarkers of IBD

Studies have suggested that BAs may serve as biomarkers of IBD disease activity and treatment response. Elevated fecal calprotectin, elevated C-reactive protein (CRP), and diarrhea correlated with BA levels in UC but not CD patients [50]. Specifically, elevated fecal calprotectin was associated with decreased levels of GLCA, and HDCA; increased CRP correlated with decreases in DCA, TDCA, LCA, TLCA, ursodeoxycholic acid (UDCA), and HDCA; and worsening diarrhea was associated with decreased levels of DCA, GDCA, and LCA [50]. The ratio of primary BAs to secondary BAs also stratified IBD activity, further demonstrating that BAs may be potential biomarkers for IBD activity [116].

BAs may be used to predict and monitor response to IBD treatment. Pediatric CD patients who achieved and sustained remission with exclusive enteral nutrition (EEN) exhibited increased secondary BAs (DCA and LCA), while those who did not sustain remission exhibited increased primary BAs (CA and CDCA) [117]. UC patients who responded to mesalamine had more secondary BAs, especially 12-KLCA [118]. The enrichment of GLCA, GDCA, and UDCA, as well as the abundance of microbial *bai* genes, predicted early remission in IBD patients undergoing anti-cytokine therapy [119]. Non-responsiveness to anti-TNFs was associated with higher levels of sulfate- and glycine-conjugated primary BAs in CD patients [120] and elevated CA in UC patients [106]. CD patients who responded to anti-$\alpha 4\beta 7$ integrin therapy exhibited elevated secondary BAs, including LCA and DCA [121,122]. In addition to stratifying IBD severity and therapeutic response, BAs have been identified as markers in IBD patients for BA malabsorption [123], more aggressive PSC [65], and poorer response to anti-SARS-CoV-2 vaccination [124]. BAs may also serve as response biomarkers for fecal microbiota transplantation (FMT) in UC, as patients with active UC who achieved clinical response and remission with FMT showed an increase in primary BA biosynthesis [125], while another study showed that FMT restored secondary BAs [126]. Children with IBD and *Clostridioides difficile* infection (CDI) treated with FMT normalized their BAs to donor levels with a decrease in primary BAs and an increase in secondary BAs 6 months post-FMT [127]. These studies underscore the potential of BAs as valuable tools that clinicians can use to manage IBD by serving as promising biomarkers for IBD disease activity, treatment choice, and management of complications.

2.5. BA-Based IBD Therapies

Recent studies have shown that BAs play a role in enhancing the efficacy of existing treatments of IBD, which suggests that BA-based therapies could potentially be effective as both monotherapies and/or used as adjunct therapy with existing IBD treatments. Recent studies have also revealed novel BA-based therapies. These therapies include dietary modifications, herbal medications, probiotics, BA supplementation, BAR agonists, modulators of the microbiota, gut–liver axis, and other BA-mediated pathways, as well as the use of mesenchymal stem cells (Figure 2). In this section, we will highlight current IBD treatments that involve BA-mediated pathways and discuss promising BA-based therapies.

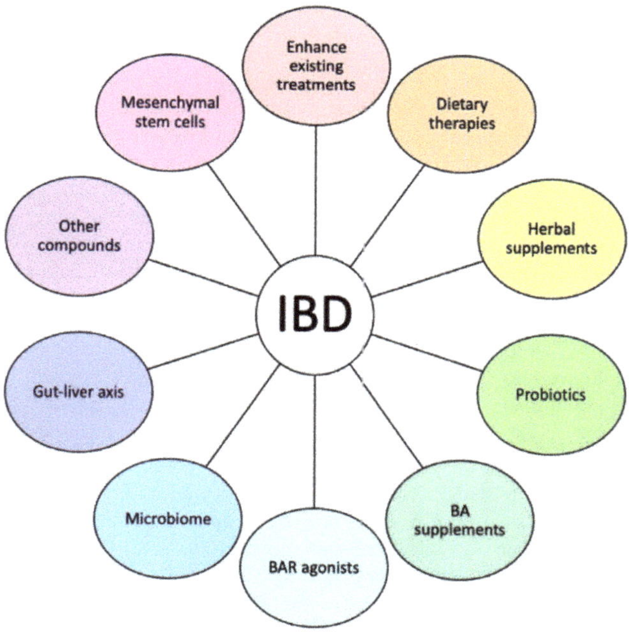

Figure 2. Potential BA-based treatments for IBD. Possible BA-directed therapies to improve IBD treatment include augmenting existing IBD treatments, new dietary treatments, probiotics, BA supplementation, BAR agonists, targeting the gut microbiome and the gut–liver axis, regulating other BA pathways with other compounds, and mesenchymal stem cells. IBD: inflammatory bowel disease; BA: bile acid; BAR: bile acid receptor.

2.5.1. Enhancement of Existing IBD Treatments

BAs may play a critical role in enhancing the efficacy of existing treatments for IBD [12]. BAs contribute to the therapeutic effects of immunomodulators in IBD treatment. In addition to suppressing TNF, infliximab has been shown to inhibit inflammation by enriching BSH-producing bacteria and restoring BA metabolism. CD patients on infliximab exhibited increased BSH-producing bacteria *Blautia* and *Collinsella*, elevated unconjugated BAs [128], decreased primary BAs [128], and increased FGF19 [129]. BAs are also important in anti-$\alpha4\beta7$ integrin therapy. Mice with TNBS-induced colitis who were given an FMT from CD patients who achieved remission with vedolizumab exhibited elevated CDCA and LCA levels, leading to increased stimulation of FXR and TGR5, and ultimately alleviating colitis [122]. The most recent literature suggests that BAs play an important role in augmenting the efficacy of current treatments for IBD. New research exploring the mechanisms of action and interactions between BAs and existing therapies may reveal new treatment strategies for IBD.

2.5.2. Diets That Modify BAs

The multifaceted role of BAs in IBD has been shown to enhance existing dietary therapies as well as reveal potential new BA-based therapies. BAs have been shown to be key mediators in existing dietary therapies for IBD. Remission in pediatric CD patients by EEN may be mediated by BAs as responders later develop normalization of BA hydrophobicity, which may activate TGR5 receptors and reduce intestinal inflammation [130]. EEN was also found to improve BA dysmetabolism in pediatric CD patients. Enrichment in BAs, including hyocholic acid (HCA) and α-muricholic acid (αMCA), was associated with decreased CD symptoms and increased abundances of *Clostridium innocuum* and *Hungatella hathewayi* [131]. Another study found EEN improved expressions of the Firmicutes phylum and genus Flavonifractor and Clostridium V and upregulation of secondary BAs in pediatric CD patients [132]. In addition to mediating existing dietary therapies, new BA-based therapies include dietary modifications, herbal medications, probiotics, BA supplementation, BAR agonists, modulators of the microbiota, gut–liver axis, and other BA-mediated pathways, as well as the use of mesenchymal stem cells. Recent studies have highlighted several promising dietary therapies for IBD. Western diets exacerbated colitis in pre-clinical models, suggesting that low-fat and low-sugar diets may be beneficial for IBD [105,107,108]. Intermittent fasting ameliorated DSS-induced colitis, partially through decreasing Akkermansia, increasing LCA, and downregulating pro-inflammatory IL-1α, IL-6, keratinocyte-derived chemokine, and the granulocyte colony-stimulating factor [133]. Oral fucose ameliorated DSS-induced colitis by lowering taurine-β-MCA (an FXR antagonist) and TCA, restoring the FXR-FGF15-CYP7A1 pathway, and increasing *Lactobacillus*. Those findings suggest that dietary fucose mitigates colitis by regulating BAs via the gut microbiota [134]. Psyllium improved DSS and T cell transfer-induced colitis by activating FXR and increasing fecal BA [135]. Insoluble dietary fiber alleviated DSS-induced colitis, partly by increasing BA absorption, suppressing the TLR4/NF-KB signaling pathway [136], decreasing *Akkermansia*, increasing *Parasutterella*, *Erysipelatoclostridium*, and *Alistipes*, reversing the DSS-induced decline in secondary BAs, and protecting against DSS-induced intestinal barrier damage [137].

2.5.3. Herbal/Natural Supplements

Herbal supplements are part of another potential IBD treatment that has been shown to improve murine colitis by modulating BAs. Several traditional Chinese medicines, including fermented Wallace melon juice [138], Scutellaria baicalensis Georgi [139], Lizhong [140], Huankuile [141], Dahuang-Mudan [142], *Auricularia polytricha* [143], and *Flammulina velutipes* [143], mitigated DSS- and TNBS-induced colitis via BA regulation. CA, CDCA, DCA, and tauroursodeoxycholic acid (TUDCA) were restored to normal levels by *Pleurotus eryngii* [144], *Indigo Naturalis* [145], *Atractylodes macrocephala* Koidz [146], and Sijunzi [147], respectively. Of note, TUDCA is a key component of black bear bile, a traditional Chinese medicine used to treat many inflammatory diseases [148]. Additional studies showed that Si-Ni-San reversed the shift of BA synthesis to the acidic pathway [149], while Gegen Qinlian [150,151] and curcumin enriched the production of secondary BAs [152]. *Rosmarinus officinalis* L. polyphenols increased primary BAs and secondary BAs, which promoted goblet cell proliferation and mucus secretion, thus strengthening the intestinal epithelial barrier [153].

Natural supplements have also been shown to alleviate DSS-induced colitis by regulating the gut microbiota-BA-immune axis. *Dendrobium officinale* increased the abundance of Lactobacillales and total BAs [154], while crocetin enriched *Akkermansia* and *Mediterraneibacter* and decreased the levels of primary BAs and secondary BAs [155]. Qingchang Huashi reversed gut dysbiosis and normalized the ratio of deconjugated to conjugated BAs [156]. Alginate promoted *Bifidobacterium animalis* and HDCA synthesis [157]. Apple polyphenol extract decreased HDCA, increased β-MCA, and enriched Verrucomicrobia, Bacteroides, and Akkermansia [158]. Dietary carvacrol and thymol supplementation enhanced the abundance of *Bifidobacterium pseudolongum*, HDCA, and 12-ketodeoxycholic acid, thereby altering the cGMP-PKG-mTORC1 pathway [159]. The grape seed proanthocyanidin improved mild IBD in dogs by enriching anti-inflammatory bacteria CA and LCA [160]. A synthesized metal-phenolic nanozyme with iron and curcumin also enhanced anti-inflammatory gut bacteria as well as LCA and TDCA [161]. *Schistosoma* soluble egg antigen upregulated *Prevotellaceae_UCG-001*, downregulated *Helicobacter*, *Lachnoclostridium*, and *Enterococcus*, and increased BAs [162]. *Sophora alopecuroides* L. increased Firmicutes, Tenericutes, and TM7, decreased Bacteroides and Deferribacteres, and lowered α-, β-, and ω-MCA, CA, transforming growth factor-β1 and IL-1β [163]. N-ethyl-L-glutamine from tea increased DCA, CA, and TCA and decreased the MHC-II-dependent presentation of microbiota antigens by the immune system [164]. Gallic acid alleviates colitis by regulating the gut microbiota, increasing ILC3s, and boosting levels of UDCA, isoalloLCA, and 3-oxoLCA [82]. Yiyi Fuzi Baijiant modulated primary BA biosynthesis and the balance of T_H17/T_{reg} [165]. Herba Origani upregulated Bacteriodota, reversed the decrease in nutriacholic acid, DCA, and HDCA, and downregulated IL-1β and TNF-α to maintain intestinal immune homeostasis [166].

Many medicinal plants modulate BA signaling to ameliorate DSS-induced colitis [94]. Fuzhuan brick tea [167], moxibustin [168], and nigakinone [169] regulated BA enterohepatic circulation by activating FXR and inhibiting the TLR4 and NLRP3 pathways. In contrast, sedanolide [170] and trans-anethole decreased FXR by inhibiting the sphingomyelin phosphodiesterase 3 pathway [170] and upregulating FGF15, ASBT, and the bile salt export pump [171]. FXR and TGR5 were upregulated by dihydromyricetin via increased Lactobacillus [172], Akkermansia, CDCA, and LCA. Fucoidan upregulated FXR and TGR5 by increasing CA, UDCA, DCA, and LCA and decreasing β-MCA [173]. Baitouweng Tang normalized BA levels and increased Bacteroidetes, Firmicutes, Proteobacteria, Actinobacteria, Tenericutes, and TM7 [174]. *Eucommia ulmoides* leaves also upregulated TGR5 expression by restoring CA, β-MCA, and DCA to normal levels; increased TCA and TUDCA; and promoted the expression of tight junction proteins [175]. Patrinia villosa improved TNBS-induced colitis by regulating BA metabolism, activating VDR, and inhibiting nuclear factor kappa B (NF-κB) signaling pathways [176].

2.5.4. Probiotics

Probiotics have shown potential as effective therapies for IBD through their regulation of the gut microbiota and BA metabolism. DSS-induced colitis was alleviated by the probiotic strain GR-4 through the upregulation of bacteria that metabolize BAs, by *Bifidobacterium pseudocatenulatum* G7 through an increase in the BA pool size [177], and by *Bifidobacterium longum* (*B. longum*) FGDLZ8M1 by enhancing tolerance to bile salts [178]. *Lactobacillus plantarum* 550 augmented tacrolimus' improvement in DSS-induced colitis, partially by increasing TCDCA [179]. Probiotics can also exert anti-inflammatory effects by regulating BAs in DSS-induced colitis in mice. The *Lactobacillus casei* strain Shirota increased TCA, TCDCA, TDCA, and TUDCA and decreased α-MCA and β-MCA, inhibiting IFN-γ and upregulated IL-10 via NF-κB suppression [180]. Bacteroides uniformis JCM5828 inhibited T_H17 differentiation by increasing α-MCA, HDCA, and isoLCA and decreasing UDCA and HDCA [181]. Several probiotic consortiums have been shown to modulate BAs and ameliorate mouse models of colitis. A consortium of *Clostridium* AP sp000509125, Bacteroides ovatus, and Eubacterium limosum, mitigated DSS-induced colitis by restoring secondary BA metabolism to increase UDCA and LCA, which upregulated TGR5 and strengthened the intestinal barrier [182]. An 11-member microbiota consortium GUT-108 reversed colitis in *Il10*$^{-/-}$ mice by increasing LCA and DCA, decreasing colitogenic *Enterobacteriaceae*, and increasing beneficial resident *Clostridium* (Clusters IV and XIVa) species, including *Lachnospiraceae* [183]. A mixture of *Lactobacillus rhamnosus* dm905 and *Lactococcus lactis* mitigated colitis in *Il10*$^{-/-}$ mice, partly by decreasing PXR, TGR5, VDR, CAR, the NLRP3 inflammasome, and pro-inflammatory cytokines [184]. Probiotics may even improve the clinical response to anti-TNF agents. *B. longum* CECT 7894 enhanced the efficacy of infliximab in DSS-mediated colitis by increasing bacteria with BSH and 7α-dehydroxylases genes and upregulating secondary BAs, including LCA, UDCA, and isoLCA [185].

2.5.5. BA Supplements

BA supplementation is another promising treatment avenue for IBD. UDCA is FDA-approved for cholestatic liver disorders and may also benefit IBD patients by decreasing dysbiosis and mitigating intestinal inflammation. Recent studies showed that UDCA ameliorated TNBS-induced colitis in rats [186] and attenuated colitis in a PSC-IBD mouse model by downregulating mucosal addressin cell adhesion molecule-1 [187]. A dihydroartemisinin-UDCA conjugate also improved DSS-induced colitis by inhibiting T_H1/T_H17 differentiation [188]. In a prospective, single-center study, UC patients given UDCA and mesalazine had improved disease compared to the mesalazine-only group, possibly due to upregulation of Firmicutes, downregulation of Proteobacteria, and decreased IL-23 and IL-17 [189]. LCA supplementation reduced intestinal inflammation in DSS−, TNBS−, and CD45RB^{hi} T cell transfer models of colitis via TGR5 [62] and VDR [190], as well as through the mitigation of epithelial cell apoptosis [191]. DSS-induced colitis was also attenuated by administering other BAs. Oral 12-KLCA upregulated VDR and downregulated IL-17A secretion from colonic ILC3s [56]. HDCA potentiated FXR and TGR5 activation [192] and impeded monocyte/macrophage recruitment [193]. HCA decreased TNF-α production by CD4$^+$ T cells [131]. A mix of α-MCA and HDCA inhibited T_H17 differentiation [181]. TUDCA was shown to alleviate inflammation-induced ER stress in intestinal epithelial cells and improve acute and chronic colitis in mice [194]. TUDCA also restored the integrity of the intestinal barrier via claudin-1 and ZO-1 [195]. Recently, oral TUDCA led to significant clinical, endoscopic, and histological improvements in a phase I trial in patients with symptomatic UC by reducing ER stress [196]. Randomized control trials of TUDCA are needed to further evaluate its efficacy in IBD patients. Taurohyodeoxycholic acid alleviated TNBS-induced colitis by restoring the T_H1/T_H2 and T_H17/T_{reg} balance [197]. IsoalloLCA and 3β-hydroxydeoxycholic acid may also have anti-inflammatory properties as they enhance T_{reg} differentiation by inducing the transcription factor forkhead box P3 [198,199]. DCA inhibitors are other potential IBD treatments. Several studies have shown that DCA supplementation worsened mouse models of colitis by inducing gut dysbiosis [200], downregulating the FXR-FGF15 axis [200], increasing intestinal T_H17 infiltration [201] and the proportion of CD3$^+$ and CD4$^+$ T cells [202], and decreasing intestinal tuft cells [202]. DCA was also found to delay wound healing through AKT activation, suggesting that AKT inhibitors could be another possible approach for IBD treatment [175]. Improvements to increase the specificity of BA analogs are ongoing. One study designing gut-restricted analogs found that incorporating an N-methyl-D-glucamine group into CDCA increased TGR5 receptor potency with low oral exposure [203].

BA supplementation may also improve IBD-associated disease and complications. Many IBD patients also develop PSC. Treatment with UDCA improved PSC in one case study of a pediatric patient with UC and PSC [204]. IBD patients have a higher risk of developing colorectal cancer than the general population. UDCA has been shown to reduce colitis and tumor growth in AOM/DSS-induced colorectal cancer by facilitating *Akkermansia* colonization [186], activating FXR via synergistic effects with intestinal epithelial cells and T_H17 and ILC3s [205], increasing 3′-phosphoadenosine 5′-phosphosulfate synthase 2 by preventing BA accumulation and increasing the formation of BA sulfates [206], and inducing suppressor of cytokine signaling 1 via TGR5 in macrophages [207]. Patients with PSC-UC have an even greater risk of colon cancer compared to UC patients, which may be due to GDCA inducing microRNA-506 and downregulating p53 [208] as well as due to the increased oncomir microRNA-356 expression downregulating VDR and TNF-α [209]. These studies suggest that targeting BA pathways may be important in preventing colitis-associated colon cancer. Another study found no association between BAs and colorectal cancer in IBD patients, but this study was limited by cohort size as it only had six patients with IBD-associated cancers [210]. The risk of CDI is increased in IBD patients. Pediatric UC patients with CDI had decreased LCA, UDCA, and gut microbial genes for BSH, 7α-hydroxysteroid dehydrogenase, and 7α/β-dehydroxylation compared to those with UC alone, suggesting that BAs could also be potential treatments for CDI in IBD patients [211].

2.5.6. BAR Agonists

In addition to BAs, BAR agonists can be another option for IBD treatment. BARs are one of the primary ways BAs exert their biological effects. BARs are found in a variety of cell types involved in IBD. GPBAR1, FXR, and PXR are highly expressed in innate and adaptive immune systems. Several recent studies have identified various BAR agonists, explored their mechanisms of action, and further elucidated their impact on IBD disease activity. PBT002—a dual GPBAR1 agonist and RORγt inverse agonist—was designed to target both innate and adaptive immunity. GPBAR1 is widely expressed in intestinal epithelial cells, myeloid cells, and NKT cells, while RORγt is expressed in T_H17, regulatory T cells (T_{reg}), and type 3 innate lymphoid cells (ILC3). PBT002 was shown to mitigate disease activity in TNBS−, DSS−, and DSS + IL-23 models of colitis by decreasing pro-inflammatory cytokines [212]. Further, the relative abundance of *Clostridium* spp. (which is reduced by colitis) was reversed in mice treated with PBT002. Given that *Clostridium* spp. is a known BSH-producing bacteria, the results suggest that BAR agonists also play a role in reversing gut dysbiosis associated with IBD. Several other BAR agonists are also described in the recent literature. CAR activation suppressed BA-driven ileitis in a mouse model, suggesting that CAR agonists may be a possible treatment for small bowel CD [213]. Several FXR agonists have shown promise in improving colitis in mouse models. Fexaramine improved DCA-induced intestinal inflammation by restoring FXR activity, activating FGF15, normalizing BA metabolism, and increasing SCFA-producing bacteria [214]. Nelumal A mitigated DSS-induced colitis and AOM/DSS-induced tumorigenesis by increasing FXR expression and tight junctions and decreasing BA synthesis [215]. Moreover, the global FXR agonist obeticholic acid, as well as a PPARα agonist, improved DSS-induced colitis [216]. Interestingly, *Fxr* ablation specifically in the mouse liver ameliorated DSS-induced colitis by enhancing the colon mucus barrier. This may be due to differing regulations of FXR in the liver versus globally [217]. The numerous BAR agonists and their respective mechanisms of action and impacts on IBD disease activity demonstrate the need for future research in this domain. Future research that evaluates the mechanistic pathways of BAR agonists, explores their long-term safety and efficacy, identifies their impact on the gut microbiome, and clarifies their potential interactions with current IBD treatments are necessary.

2.5.7. Microbiome and the Gut–Liver Axis

Modulation of BA metabolism via the microbiota and the gut–liver axis is another promising strategy for IBD. Patients with IBD lost the microbial *baiCD* regulation of the host angiopoietin-like 4 gene that has been shown to ameliorate DSS-induced colitis [218]. Selectively deleting the *baiH* gene in *Faecalicatena contorta* S122 in a complex microbiome protected against DSS-induced colitis, likely by diminishing Erysipelotrichaceae [212]. These studies suggest that targeting specific microbial genes involved in BA metabolism could be an effective treatment for IBD. Administering microbes with anti-inflammatory properties may be another potential IBD treatment as FMT of Roseburia bacteria in sheep with DSS-induced colitis mitigated intestinal inflammation [219]. FGF19-M52, an engineered FGF19 variant without hepatic pro-mitogenic capacity protected mice from DSS-induced colitis by regulating BA metabolism [220]. Another study showed that deficiency of the Rela/Stat3-CYP enzyme pathway in mouse liver led to a decrease in primary BAs and ameliorated colitis, suggesting that inhibitors of this pathway could offer a novel mechanism to control inflammation in IBD through the gut–liver axis [98].

2.5.8. Other BA-Related Therapeutic Targets

Recent studies have identified other potential therapeutic targets of IBD mediated by BAs. Low-dose insulin alleviated DSS-induced colitis in mice by increasing the abundance of *Blautia*, *Enterorhadus*, *Rumi-NK4A214_group*, and LCA, which activated TGR5 and polarization of M1 macrophages [221]. P-glycoprotein was decreased in UC patients, possibly due to lower secondary BA production, and may be a potential UC treatment target [222]. The antimicrobial peptide cecropin A ameliorated DSS-induced colitis, partly by normalizing BA metabolism [217]. Recombinant fibrinogen-like protein 2 improved DSS-induced colitis by reversing the decline in gut microbiota diversity and restoring BA homeostasis by decreasing total BA, increasing FXR and FGF15, and downregulating CYP7A1 [223]. An inhibitor of zinc metallopeptidase glutamate carboxypeptidase II, which was upregulated in IBD patients, was conjugated to DCA and alleviated inflammation in DSS-induced and *Il10*$^{-/-}$ models of colitis by lowering intestinal barrier permeability, normalizing tight junction protein expression, and suppressing procaspase-3 activation [224]. Hyperbaric oxygen also showed promise in improving UC by reducing neutrophil STAT3, increasing Firmicutes, decreasing Akkermansia, and increasing LCA [225]. Clinical trials are ongoing to further evaluate the efficacy of hyperbaric oxygen in IBD patients.

2.5.9. Mesenchymal Stem Cells

Mesenchymal stem cells may be another novel therapy for IBD by restoring BA homeostasis [226]. Administering mesenchymal stem cells improved TNBS-induced colitis by increasing gut microbiota α-diversity, enriching Bacteroides, Firmicutes, and Tenericutes, and decreasing Proteobacteria, partially through upregulating secondary BA synthesis [227]. Mesenchymal stem cell-derived exosomes also improved DSS-induced colitis by increasing colonic FXR and improving gut dysbiosis [228]. It remains unclear whether restoring BA levels and composition is required for the efficacy of mesenchymal stem cell transplant.

Recent studies have enhanced the understanding of BAs and their roles in IBD. To date, approximately 692 different BAs have been discovered, and it is predicted that tens of thousands of new BAs remain to be discovered [77]. Advances in technology and the development of innovative methodologies, including mass spectrometry processes and metabolomics analysis tools, will likely lead to the discovery of new BAs with unique physiological functions and potential therapeutic applications [229,230].

3. Conclusions

BAs are critical players in IBD pathogenesis and recent studies have furthered the understanding of the many roles they play in the gut microbiome, immune system, BARs, intestinal epithelium, gut–liver axis, diet, genetics, environment, and other modalities. Studies have demonstrated that patients with IBD exhibit alterations in their BA composition, and both CD and UC patients have generally been found to have an increase in primary BAs and a decrease in secondary BAs. BAs have been found to contribute to intestinal inflammation via several mechanisms, including via BARs, modulation of the immune system via regulation of specific immune cells and inflammatory cytokines, and exerting effects on gut barrier function via regulation of intestinal epithelial tight junctions. The latest research exploring the complex roles BAs play in IBD pathogenesis has revealed several promising targets for therapeutic interventions. Emerging BA-based therapies include new dietary treatments, probiotics, BA supplementation, BAR agonists, mesenchymal stem cells, and targeting the gut microbiome and gut–liver axis. For example, BAR agonist PBT002 has been shown to mitigate disease activity in TNBS−, DSS−, and DSS + IL-23 models of colitis by decreasing pro-inflammatory cytokines [212] and is associated with increased levels of *Clostridium* spp. Diet therapies such as intermittent fasting and oral fructose were shown to decrease DSS-induced colitis via modulating BAs such as LCA and TCA. Probiotic therapies such as *Lactobacillus plantarum* 550 and *Clostridium* AP sp000509125 were shown to improve DSS-induced colitis via the regulation of BAs. Mesenchymal stem cells similarly improved TNBS-induced colitis by influencing the gut microbiota α-diversity partially via upregulation of secondary BAs. BA-directed therapies may be used as standalone treatments or as adjuvants to augment existing therapeutic regimens. Additionally, the altered composition of BAs in patients with IBD shows potential as a promising biomarker for assessing IBD disease activity, as well as predicting and monitoring response to treatment. While the literature reviewed shows promise for new treatment modalities and uses of BAs, there are several limitations. Several of the studies show contradictions in the composition of specific BAs, likely a result of differences in methodologies between studies. Furthermore, while current studies have expanded knowledge of the role of BAs in IBD pathogenesis, especially regarding specific mechanisms of action, it is difficult to ascertain the magnitude of the impact of each individual mechanism of action. Therefore, future studies should define the mechanistic roles of BA-based therapies on a variety of cell types and signaling pathways in the digestive tract and beyond. Controlled clinical trials are also needed to determine their therapeutic potential. Leveraging technological advancements to discover new BAs and enhancing knowledge of the myriad of functions they play in IBD may lead to new classes of therapeutics for IBD that ultimately improve patient outcomes.

Author Contributions: S.H.B. and S.C. conceived the study, wrote the article, and created the tables and figures. A.C. performed the revisions, edited the figures, and created the abbreviations list. All authors have read and agreed to the published version of the manuscript.

Funding: The work was funded by a Crohn's and Colitis Foundation Career Development Award (CCF1062472; S.C.) and an NIH/NIDDK K08 Clinical Investigator Award (1K08DK140612-01, S.C.). S.H.B. and S.C. were supported by an NIH T32 Institutional Research Training Grant. S.C. was also supported by an American Gastroenterological Association Fellowship-to-Faculty Transition Award (AGA2023-32-03), Digestive Disease Research Core Center (DDRCC) Pilot and Feasibility Award (P30 DK052574), Doris Duke COVID-19 Fund to Retain Clinical Scientists Program (CFRCS), Lawrence C. Pakula, MD IBD Education & Innovation Fund (IA-2022-IBD-1), Washington University Clinical and Translational Research Funding Program (CTRFP1714), Washington University Precision Health Innovation Award (PHIA 101), and Washington University DDRCC (NIDDK P30 DK052574).

Institutional Review Board Statement: Not applicable.

Informed Consent Statement: Not applicable.

Data Availability Statement: No new data were generated or analyzed in support of this research.

Conflicts of Interest: S.H.B., A.C. and S.C. declare no conflicts of interest.

References

1. Thomas, J.P.; Modos, D.; Rushbrook, S.M.; Powell, N.; Korcsmaros, T. The Emerging Role of Bile Acids in the Pathogenesis of Inflammatory Bowel Disease. *Front. Immunol.* **2022**, *13*, 829525. [CrossRef] [PubMed]
2. GBD 2017 Inflammatory Bowel Disease Collaborators. The global, regional, and national burden of inflammatory bowel disease in 195 countries and territories, 1990–2017: A systematic analysis for the Global Burden of Disease Study 2017. *Lancet Gastroenterol. Hepatol.* **2020**, *5*, 17–30. [CrossRef] [PubMed]
3. Kriaa, A.; Mariaule, V.; Jablaoui, A.; Rhimi, S.; Mkaouar, H.; Hernandez, J.; Korkmaz, B.; Lesner, A.; Maguin, E.; Aghdassi, A.; et al. Bile Acids: Key Players in Inflammatory Bowel Diseases? *Cells* **2022**, *11*, 901. [CrossRef] [PubMed]

4. Syed, S.; Boland, B.S.; Bourke, L.T.; Chen, L.A.; Churchill, L.; Dobes, A.; Greene, A.; Heller, C.; Jayson, C.; Kostiuk, B.; et al. Challenges in IBD Research 2024: Precision Medicine. *Inflamm. Bowel Dis.* **2024**, *30* (Suppl. 2), S39–S54. [CrossRef]
5. Long, X.Q.; Liu, M.Z.; Liu, Z.H.; Xia, L.Z.; Lu, S.P.; Xu, X.P.; Wu, M.H. Bile acids and their receptors: Potential therapeutic targets in inflammatory bowel disease. *World J. Gastroenterol.* **2023**, *29*, 4252–4270. [CrossRef]
6. Di Ciaula, A.; Bonfrate, L.; Khalil, M.; Portincasa, P. The interaction of bile acids and gut inflammation influences the pathogenesis of inflammatory bowel disease. *Intern. Emerg. Med.* **2023**, *18*, 2181–2197. [CrossRef]
7. Pratt, M.; Forbes, J.D.; Knox, N.C.; Bernstein, C.N.; Van Domselaar, G. Microbiome-Mediated Immune Signaling in Inflammatory Bowel Disease and Colorectal Cancer: Support from Meta-omics Data. *Front. Cell Dev. Biol.* **2021**, *9*, 716604. [CrossRef]
8. Camilleri, M. Bile acid detergency: Permeability, inflammation, and effects of sulfation. *Am. J. Physiol. Gastrointest. Liver Physiol.* **2022**, *322*, G480–G488. [CrossRef]
9. Xiang, D.; Yang, J.; Liu, L.; Yu, H.; Gong, X.; Liu, D. The regulation of tissue-specific farnesoid X receptor on genes and diseases involved in bile acid homeostasis. *Biomed. Pharmacother.* **2023**, *168*, 115606. [CrossRef]
10. Kwon, S.J.; Khan, M.S.; Kim, S.G. Intestinal Inflammation and Regeneration-Interdigitating Processes Controlled by Dietary Lipids in Inflammatory Bowel Disease. *Int. J. Mol. Sci.* **2024**, *25*, 1311. [CrossRef]
11. Thibaut, M.M.; Bindels, L.B. Crosstalk between bile acid-activated receptors and microbiome in entero-hepatic inflammation. *Trends Mol. Med.* **2022**, *28*, 223–236. [CrossRef] [PubMed]
12. Pan, Y.; Zhang, H.; Li, M.; He, T.; Guo, S.; Zhu, L.; Tan, J.; Wang, B. Novel approaches in IBD therapy: Targeting the gut microbiota-bile acid axis. *Gut Microbes* **2024**, *16*, 2356284. [CrossRef] [PubMed]
13. Li, L.; Liu, T.; Gu, Y.; Wang, X.; Xie, R.; Sun, Y.; Wang, B.; Cao, H. Regulation of gut microbiota-bile acids axis by probiotics in inflammatory bowel disease. *Front. Immunol.* **2022**, *13*, 974305. [CrossRef] [PubMed]
14. Fiorucci, S.; Carino, A.; Baldoni, M.; Santucci, L.; Costanzi, E.; Graziosi, L.; Distrutti, E.; Biagioli, M. Bile Acid Signaling in Inflammatory Bowel Diseases. *Dig. Dis. Sci.* **2021**, *66*, 674–693. [CrossRef]
15. Poland, J.C.; Flynn, C.R. Bile Acids, Their Receptors, and the Gut Microbiota. *Physiology* **2021**, *36*, 235–245. [CrossRef]
16. Zhang, J.; Lyu, A.; Wang, C. The molecular insights of bile acid homeostasis in host diseases. *Life Sci.* **2023**, *330*, 121919. [CrossRef]
17. Cai, J.; Sun, L.; Gonzalez, F.J. Gut microbiota-derived bile acids in intestinal immunity, inflammation, and tumorigenesis. *Cell Host Microbe* **2022**, *30*, 289–300. [CrossRef]
18. Gadaleta, R.M.; Cariello, M.; Crudele, L.; Moschetta, A. Bile Salt Hydrolase-Competent Probiotics in the Management of IBD: Unlocking the "Bile Acid Code". *Nutrients* **2022**, *14*, 3212. [CrossRef]
19. Guo, X.; Okpara, E.S.; Hu, W.; Yan, C.; Wang, Y.; Liang, Q.; Chiang, J.Y.L.; Han, S. Interactive Relationships between Intestinal Flora and Bile Acids. *Int. J. Mol. Sci.* **2022**, *23*, 8343. [CrossRef]
20. Bromke, M.A.; Krzystek-Korpacka, M. Bile Acid Signaling in Inflammatory Bowel Disease. *Int. J. Mol. Sci.* **2021**, *22*, 9096. [CrossRef]
21. Sun, R.; Xu, C.; Feng, B.; Gao, X.; Liu, Z. Critical roles of bile acids in regulating intestinal mucosal immune responses. *Ther. Adv. Gastroenterol.* **2021**, *14*, 17562848211018098. [CrossRef] [PubMed]
22. Kumar, A.; Al-Hassi, H.O.; Steed, H.; Phipps, O.; Brookes, M.J. Bile Acids and the Microbiome: Making Sense of This Dynamic Relationship in Their Role and Management in Crohn's Disease. *Can. J. Gastroenterol. Hepatol.* **2022**, *2022*, 8416578. [CrossRef] [PubMed]
23. Fuchs, C.D.; Trauner, M. Role of bile acids and their receptors in gastrointestinal and hepatic pathophysiology. *Nat. Rev. Gastroenterol. Hepatol.* **2022**, *19*, 432–450. [CrossRef] [PubMed]
24. Fitzpatrick, L.R.; Jenabzadeh, P. IBD and Bile Acid Absorption: Focus on Pre-clinical and Clinical Observations. *Front. Physiol.* **2020**, *11*, 564. [CrossRef]
25. Li, M.; Yang, L.; Mu, C.; Sun, Y.; Gu, Y.; Chen, D.; Liu, T.; Cao, H. Gut microbial metabolome in inflammatory bowel disease: From association to therapeutic perspectives. *Comput. Struct. Biotechnol. J.* **2022**, *20*, 2402–2414. [CrossRef]
26. Guzior, D.V.; Quinn, R.A. Review: Microbial transformations of human bile acids. *Microbiome* **2021**, *9*, 140. [CrossRef]
27. Fu, Y.; Lyu, J.; Wang, S. The role of intestinal microbes on intestinal barrier function and host immunity from a metabolite perspective. *Front. Immunol.* **2023**, *14*, 1277102. [CrossRef]
28. Di Vincenzo, F.; Puca, P.; Lopetuso, L.R.; Petito, V.; Masi, L.; Bartocci, B.; Murgiano, M.; De Felice, M.; Petronio, L.; Gasbarrini, A.; et al. Bile Acid-Related Regulation of Mucosal Inflammation and Intestinal Motility: From Pathogenesis to Therapeutic Application in IBD and Microscopic Colitis. *Nutrients* **2022**, *14*, 2664. [CrossRef]
29. Su, X.; Gao, Y.; Yang, R. Gut microbiota derived bile acid metabolites maintain the homeostasis of gut and systemic immunity. *Front. Immunol.* **2023**, *14*, 1127743. [CrossRef]
30. Gasaly, N.; de Vos, P.; Hermoso, M.A. Impact of Bacterial Metabolites on Gut Barrier Function and Host Immunity: A Focus on Bacterial Metabolism and Its Relevance for Intestinal Inflammation. *Front. Immunol.* **2021**, *12*, 658354. [CrossRef]
31. Funabashi, M.; Grove, T.L.; Wang, M.; Varma, Y.; McFadden, M.E.; Brown, L.C.; Guo, C.; Higginbottom, S.; Almo, S.C.; Fischbach, M.A. A metabolic pathway for bile acid dehydroxylation by the gut microbiome. *Nature* **2020**, *582*, 566–570. [CrossRef] [PubMed]
32. Ning, S.; Zhang, Z.; Zhou, C.; Wang, B.; Liu, Z.; Feng, B. Cross-talk between macrophages and gut microbiota in inflammatory bowel disease: A dynamic interplay influencing pathogenesis and therapy. *Front. Med.* **2024**, *11*, 1457218. [CrossRef] [PubMed]
33. Lin, S.; Wang, S.; Wang, P.; Tang, C.; Wang, Z.; Chen, L.; Luo, G.; Chen, H.; Liu, Y.; Feng, B.; et al. Bile acids and their receptors in regulation of gut health and diseases. *Prog. Lipid Res.* **2023**, *89*, 101210. [CrossRef] [PubMed]

34. Zhou, M.; Wang, D.; Li, X.; Cao, Y.; Yi, C.; Wiredu Ocansey, D.K.; Zhou, Y.; Mao, F. Farnesoid-X receptor as a therapeutic target for inflammatory bowel disease and colorectal cancer. *Front. Pharmacol.* **2022**, *13*, 1016836. [CrossRef] [PubMed]
35. Calzadilla, N.; Comiskey, S.M.; Dudeja, P.K.; Saksena, S.; Gill, R.K.; Alrefai, W.A. Bile acids as inflammatory mediators and modulators of intestinal permeability. *Front. Immunol.* **2022**, *13*, 1021924. [CrossRef]
36. Lavelle, A.; Sokol, H. Gut microbiota-derived metabolites as key actors in inflammatory bowel disease. *Nat. Rev. Gastroenterol. Hepatol.* **2020**, *17*, 223–237. [CrossRef]
37. Quinn, R.A.; Melnik, A.V.; Vrbanac, A.; Fu, T.; Patras, K.A.; Christy, M.P.; Bodai, Z.; Belda-Ferre, P.; Tripathi, A.; Chung, L.K.; et al. Global chemical effects of the microbiome include new bile-acid conjugations. *Nature* **2020**, *579*, 123–129. [CrossRef]
38. Xu, R.H.; Shen, J.N.; Lu, J.B.; Liu, Y.J.; Song, Y.; Cao, Y.; Wang, Z.H.; Zhang, J. Bile acid profiles and classification model accuracy for inflammatory bowel disease diagnosis. *Medicine* **2024**, *103*, e38457. [CrossRef]
39. Paik, D.; Yao, L.; Zhang, Y.; Bae, S.; D'Agostino, G.D.; Zhang, M.; Kim, E.; Franzosa, E.A.; Avila-Pacheco, J.; Bisanz, J.E.; et al. Human gut bacteria produce Tau(Eta)17-modulating bile acid metabolites. *Nature* **2022**, *603*, 907–912. [CrossRef]
40. Jangi, S.; Zhao, N.; Hsia, K.; Park, Y.S.; Michaud, D.S.; Yoon, H. Specific bacterial co-abundance groups are associated with inflammatory status in patients with ulcerative colitis. *J. Crohns Colitis* **2024**, jjae125. [CrossRef]
41. Yang, M.; Gu, Y.; Li, L.; Liu, T.; Song, X.; Sun, Y.; Cao, X.; Wang, B.; Jiang, K.; Cao, H. Bile Acid-Gut Microbiota Axis in Inflammatory Bowel Disease: From Bench to Bedside. *Nutrients* **2021**, *13*, 3143. [CrossRef] [PubMed]
42. Vijayvargiya, P.; Gonzalez Izundegui, D.; Calderon, G.; Tawfic, S.; Batbold, S.; Saifuddin, H.; Duggan, P.; Melo, V.; Thomas, T.; Heeney, M.; et al. Increased Fecal Bile Acid Excretion in a Significant Subset of Patients with Other Inflammatory Diarrheal Diseases. *Dig. Dis. Sci.* **2022**, *67*, 2413–2419. [CrossRef] [PubMed]
43. Effinger, A.; McAllister, M.; Tomaszewska, I.; O'Driscoll, C.M.; Taylor, M.; Gomersall, S.; Heaton, J.; Smith, K.L.; Sarcevica, I.; Young, S.L.; et al. Investigating the Impact of Crohn's Disease on the Bioaccessibility of a Lipid-Based Formulation with an In Vitro Dynamic Gastrointestinal Model. *Mol. Pharm.* **2021**, *18*, 1530–1543. [CrossRef] [PubMed]
44. Gentry, E.C.; Collins, S.L.; Panitchpakdi, M.; Belda-Ferre, P.; Stewart, A.K.; Carrillo Terrazas, M.; Lu, H.H.; Zuffa, S.; Yan, T.; Avila-Pacheco, J.; et al. Reverse metabolomics for the discovery of chemical structures from humans. *Nature* **2024**, *626*, 419–426. [CrossRef]
45. Reiter, S.; Dunkel, A.; Metwaly, A.; Panes, J.; Salas, A.; Haller, D.; Hofmann, T. Development of a Highly Sensitive Ultra-High-Performance Liquid Chromatography Coupled to Electrospray Ionization Tandem Mass Spectrometry Quantitation Method for Fecal Bile Acids and Application on Crohn's Disease Studies. *J. Agric. Food Chem.* **2021**, *69*, 5238–5251. [CrossRef]
46. Wilson, A.; Almousa, A.; Teft, W.A.; Kim, R.B. Attenuation of bile acid-mediated FXR and PXR activation in patients with Crohn's disease. *Sci. Rep.* **2020**, *10*, 1866. [CrossRef]
47. Liu, C.; Zhan, S.; Li, N.; Tu, T.; Lin, J.; Li, M.; Chen, M.; Zeng, Z.; Zhuang, X. Bile acid alterations associated with indolent course of inflammatory bowel disease. *Scand. J. Gastroenterol.* **2023**, *58*, 988–997. [CrossRef]
48. Kiasat, A.; Prast-Nielsen, S.; Rautiainen, S.; Engstrand, L.; Andersson, F.; Lindberg, J.; Schuppe-Koistinen, I.; Lof Granstrom, A.; Gustafsson, U.O. Plasma bile acids in association with Crohn's disease. *Scand. J. Gastroenterol.* **2024**, *59*, 674–682. [CrossRef]
49. Feng, L.; Zhou, N.; Li, Z.; Fu, D.; Guo, Y.; Gao, X.; Liu, X. Co-occurrence of gut microbiota dysbiosis and bile acid metabolism alteration is associated with psychological disorders in Crohn's disease. *FASEB J.* **2022**, *36*, e22100. [CrossRef]
50. Sommersberger, S.; Gunawan, S.; Elger, T.; Fererberger, T.; Loibl, J.; Huss, M.; Kandulski, A.; Krautbauer, S.; Muller, M.; Liebisch, G.; et al. Altered fecal bile acid composition in active ulcerative colitis. *Lipids Health Dis.* **2023**, *22*, 199. [CrossRef]
51. Liu, H.; Xu, M.; He, Q.; Wei, P.; Ke, M.; Liu, S. Untargeted serum metabolomics reveals specific metabolite abnormalities in patients with Crohn's disease. *Front. Med.* **2022**, *9*, 814839. [CrossRef] [PubMed]
52. Gonzalez, C.G.; Mills, R.H.; Zhu, Q.; Sauceda, C.; Knight, R.; Dulai, P.S.; Gonzalez, D.J. Location-specific signatures of Crohn's disease at a multi-omics scale. *Microbiome* **2022**, *10*, 133. [CrossRef] [PubMed]
53. Battat, R.; Scherl, E.J.; Lukin, D.; Charilaou, P.; Mahtani, P.; Gerber, J.; Gandara, J.A.; Consortium, J.I.L.C.B.; Dundar, F.; Zumbo, P.; et al. Increased Primary Bile Acids with Ileocolonic Resection Impact Ileal Inflammation and Gut Microbiota in Inflammatory Bowel Disease. *J. Crohns Colitis* **2023**, *17*, 795–803. [CrossRef] [PubMed]
54. Lewis, J.D.; Daniel, S.G.; Li, H.; Hao, F.; Patterson, A.D.; Hecht, A.L.; Brensinger, C.M.; Wu, G.D.; Bittinger, K.; Dine, C.D.; et al. Surgery for Crohn's Disease Is Associated with a Dysbiotic Microbiome and Metabolome: Results from Two Prospective Cohorts. *Cell Mol. Gastroenterol. Hepatol.* **2024**, *18*, 101357. [CrossRef] [PubMed]
55. Yang, Z.H.; Liu, F.; Zhu, X.R.; Suo, F.Y.; Jia, Z.J.; Yao, S.K. Altered profiles of fecal bile acids correlate with gut microbiota and inflammatory responses in patients with ulcerative colitis. *World J. Gastroenterol.* **2021**, *27*, 3609–3629. [CrossRef]
56. Li, N.; Ma, P.; Li, Y.; Shang, X.; Nan, X.; Shi, L.; Han, X.; Liu, J.; Hong, Y.; Li, Q.; et al. Gut microbiota-derived 12-ketolithocholic acid suppresses the IL-17A secretion from colonic group 3 innate lymphoid cells to prevent the acute exacerbation of ulcerative colitis. *Gut Microbes* **2023**, *15*, 2290315. [CrossRef]
57. Nystrom, N.; Prast-Nielsen, S.; Correia, M.; Globisch, D.; Engstrand, L.; Schuppe-Koistinen, I.; Halfvarson, J. Mucosal and Plasma Metabolomes in New-onset Paediatric Inflammatory Bowel Disease: Correlations with Disease Characteristics and Plasma Inflammation Protein Markers. *J. Crohns Colitis* **2023**, *17*, 418–432. [CrossRef]
58. Schirmer, M.; Strazar, M.; Avila-Pacheco, J.; Rojas-Tapias, D.F.; Brown, E.M.; Temple, E.; Deik, A.; Bullock, K.; Jeanfavre, S.; Pierce, K.; et al. Linking microbial genes to plasma and stool metabolites uncovers host-microbial interactions underlying ulcerative colitis disease course. *Cell Host Microbe* **2024**, *32*, 209–226.e7. [CrossRef]

59. Misra, R.; Sarafian, M.; Pechlivanis, A.; Ding, N.; Miguens-Blanco, J.; McDonald, J.; Holmes, E.; Marchesi, J.; Arebi, N. Ethnicity Associated Microbial and Metabonomic Profiling in Newly Diagnosed Ulcerative Colitis. *Clin. Exp. Gastroenterol.* **2022**, *15*, 199–212. [CrossRef]
60. Aboud Syriani, L.; Parsana, R.; Durazo-Arvizu, R.A.; Michail, S. Differences in gut microbiota and fecal bile acids between Caucasian and Hispanic children and young adults with ulcerative colitis. *Physiol. Rep.* **2023**, *11*, e15752. [CrossRef]
61. Dubinsky, V.; Reshef, L.; Rabinowitz, K.; Yadgar, K.; Godny, L.; Zonensain, K.; Wasserberg, N.; Dotan, I.; Gophna, U. Dysbiosis in Metabolic Genes of the Gut Microbiomes of Patients with an Ileo-anal Pouch Resembles That Observed in Crohn's Disease. *mSystems* **2021**, *6*, e00984-20. [CrossRef] [PubMed]
62. Sinha, S.R.; Haileselassie, Y.; Nguyen, L.P.; Tropini, C.; Wang, M.; Becker, L.S.; Sim, D.; Jarr, K.; Spear, E.T.; Singh, G.; et al. Dysbiosis-Induced Secondary Bile Acid Deficiency Promotes Intestinal Inflammation. *Cell Host Microbe* **2020**, *27*, 659–670.e5. [CrossRef] [PubMed]
63. Yan Ang, Q.; Plichta, D.; Kim, S.; Hyun, A.K.I.; Gregory, S.; Xia, Y.; Lau, H.; Xavier, R.; Ananthakrishnan, A.N. Differential Impact of Smoking on Methylome and Transcriptome in Crohn's Disease and Ulcerative Colitis. *Inflamm. Bowel Dis.* **2024**, *30*, 981–991. [CrossRef] [PubMed]
64. Jacobs, J.P.; Sauk, J.S.; Ahdoot, A.I.; Liang, F.; Katzka, W.; Ryu, H.J.; Khandadash, A.; Lagishetty, V.; Labus, J.S.; Naliboff, B.D.; et al. Microbial and Metabolite Signatures of Stress Reactivity in Ulcerative Colitis Patients in Clinical Remission Predict Clinical Flare Risk. *Inflamm. Bowel Dis.* **2024**, *30*, 336–346. [CrossRef]
65. Leibovitzh, H.; Nayeri, S.; Borowski, K.; Hernandez-Rocha, C.; Lee, S.H.; Turpin, W.; Stempak, J.M.; Sandhu, I.; Milgrom, R.; Smith, M.I.; et al. Inflammatory bowel disease associated with primary sclerosing cholangitis is associated with an altered gut microbiome and bile acid profile. *J. Crohns Colitis* **2024**, *18*, 1957–1966. [CrossRef]
66. Santiago, P.; Quinn, K.P.; Chen, J.; Friton, J.J.; Rypstra, C.R.; Kashyap, P.C.; Raffals, L.E. Altered Bile Acid and Pouch Microbiota Composition in Patients with Chronic Pouchitis. *Inflamm. Bowel Dis.* **2024**, *30*, 1062–1070. [CrossRef]
67. Liu, L.; Yang, M.; Dong, W.; Liu, T.; Song, X.; Gu, Y.; Wang, S.; Liu, Y.; Abla, Z.; Qiao, X.; et al. Gut Dysbiosis and Abnormal Bile Acid Metabolism in Colitis-Associated Cancer. *Gastroenterol. Res. Pract.* **2021**, *2021*, 6645970. [CrossRef]
68. Collins, S.L.; Stine, J.G.; Bisanz, J.E.; Okafor, C.D.; Patterson, A.D. Bile acids and the gut microbiota: Metabolic interactions and impacts on disease. *Nat. Rev. Microbiol.* **2023**, *21*, 236–247. [CrossRef]
69. Jia, B.; Park, D.; Hahn, Y.; Jeon, C.O. Metagenomic analysis of the human microbiome reveals the association between the abundance of gut bile salt hydrolases and host health. *Gut Microbes* **2020**, *11*, 1300–1313. [CrossRef]
70. Deng, Z.L.; Pieper, D.H.; Stallmach, A.; Steube, A.; Vital, M.; Reck, M.; Wagner-Dobler, I. Engraftment of essential functions through multiple fecal microbiota transplants in chronic antibiotic-resistant pouchitis-a case study using metatranscriptomics. *Microbiome* **2023**, *11*, 269. [CrossRef]
71. Lin, S.; Zhang, X.; Zhu, X.; Jiao, J.; Wu, Y.; Li, Y.; Zhao, L. Fusobacterium nucleatum aggravates ulcerative colitis through promoting gut microbiota dysbiosis and dysmetabolism. *J. Periodontol.* **2023**, *94*, 405–418. [CrossRef] [PubMed]
72. Zhao, X.; Jiang, L.; Fang, X.; Guo, Z.; Wang, X.; Shi, B.; Meng, Q. Host-microbiota interaction-mediated resistance to inflammatory bowel disease in pigs. *Microbiome* **2022**, *10*, 115. [CrossRef] [PubMed]
73. Galler, A.I.; Suchodolski, J.S.; Steiner, J.M.; Sung, C.H.; Hittmair, K.M.; Richter, B.; Burgener, I.A. Microbial dysbiosis and fecal metabolomic perturbations in Yorkshire Terriers with chronic enteropathy. *Sci. Rep.* **2022**, *12*, 12977. [CrossRef] [PubMed]
74. Briggs, K.; Tomar, V.; Ollberding, N.; Haberman, Y.; Bourgonje, A.R.; Hu, S.; Chaaban, L.; Sunuwar, L.; Weersma, R.K.; Denson, L.A.; et al. Crohn's Disease-Associated Pathogenic Mutation in the Manganese Transporter ZIP8 Shifts the Ileal and Rectal Mucosal Microbiota Implicating Aberrant Bile Acid Metabolism. *Inflamm. Bowel Dis.* **2024**, *30*, 1379–1388. [CrossRef] [PubMed]
75. Baumgartner, M.; Lang, M.; Holley, H.; Crepaz, D.; Hausmann, B.; Pjevac, P.; Moser, D.; Haller, F.; Hof, F.; Beer, A.; et al. Mucosal Biofilms Are an Endoscopic Feature of Irritable Bowel Syndrome and Ulcerative Colitis. *Gastroenterology* **2021**, *161*, 1245–1256.e20. [CrossRef]
76. Wang, W.; Liu, Z.; Yue, W.; Zhu, L.; Zhong, H.; Yang, C.; He, T.; Wan, P.; Geng, J. Mucosa-Colonizing Microbiota Correlate with Host Autophagy Signaling in Patients with Inflammatory Bowel Disease. *Front. Microbiol.* **2022**, *13*, 875238. [CrossRef]
77. Mohanty, I.; Allaband, C.; Mannochio-Russo, H.; El Abiead, Y.; Hagey, L.R.; Knight, R.; Dorrestein, P.C. The changing metabolic landscape of bile acids—Keys to metabolism and immune regulation. *Nat. Rev. Gastroenterol. Hepatol.* **2024**, *21*, 493–516. [CrossRef]
78. Zhang, S.; Zhong, R.; Tang, S.; Chen, L.; Zhang, H. Metabolic regulation of the Th17/Treg balance in inflammatory bowel disease. *Pharmacol. Res.* **2024**, *203*, 107184. [CrossRef]
79. Hang, S.; Paik, D.; Yao, L.; Kim, E.; Trinath, J.; Lu, J.; Ha, S.; Nelson, B.N.; Kelly, S.P.; Wu, L.; et al. Bile acid metabolites control T(H)17 and T(reg) cell differentiation. *Nature* **2019**, *576*, 143–148. [CrossRef]
80. Arifuzzaman, M.; Won, T.H.; Yano, H.; Uddin, J.; Emanuel, E.R.; Hu, E.; Zhang, W.; Li, T.T.; Jin, W.B.; Grier, A.; et al. Dietary fiber is a critical determinant of pathologic ILC2 responses and intestinal inflammation. *J. Exp. Med.* **2024**, *221*, e20232148. [CrossRef]
81. Song, X.; Sun, X.; Oh, S.F.; Wu, M.; Zhang, Y.; Zheng, W.; Geva-Zatorsky, N.; Jupp, R.; Mathis, D.; Benoist, C.; et al. Microbial bile acid metabolites modulate gut RORgamma(+) regulatory T cell homeostasis. *Nature* **2020**, *577*, 410–415. [CrossRef] [PubMed]
82. Leng, Y.; Zhang, X.; Zhang, Q.; Xia, J.; Zhang, Y.; Ma, C.; Liu, K.; Li, H.; Hong, Y.; Xie, Z. Gallic acid attenuates murine ulcerative colitis by promoting group 3 innate lymphocytes, affecting gut microbiota, and bile acid metabolism. *J. Nutr. Biochem.* **2024**, *131*, 109677. [CrossRef] [PubMed]

83. Couto, M.; Andrade, N.; Magro, F.; Martel, F. Taurocholate uptake by Caco-2 cells is inhibited by pro-inflammatory cytokines and butyrate. *Cytokine* **2023**, *169*, 156307. [CrossRef] [PubMed]
84. Biagioli, M.; Marchiano, S.; Carino, A.; Di Giorgio, C.; Santucci, L.; Distrutti, E.; Fiorucci, S. Bile Acids Activated Receptors in Inflammatory Bowel Disease. *Cells* **2021**, *10*, 1281. [CrossRef] [PubMed]
85. Negroni, A.; Fiaschini, N.; Palone, F.; Vitali, R.; Colantoni, E.; Laudadio, I.; Oliva, S.; Aloi, M.; Cucchiara, S.; Stronati, L. Intestinal Inflammation Alters the Expression of Hepatic Bile Acid Receptors Causing Liver Impairment. *J. Pediatr. Gastroenterol. Nutr.* **2020**, *71*, 189–196. [CrossRef]
86. Sorrentino, G.; Perino, A.; Yildiz, E.; El Alam, G.; Bou Sleiman, M.; Gioiello, A.; Pellicciari, R.; Schoonjans, K. Bile Acids Signal via TGR5 to Activate Intestinal Stem Cells and Epithelial Regeneration. *Gastroenterology* **2020**, *159*, 956–968.e8. [CrossRef]
87. Wilson, A.; Wang, Q.; Almousa, A.A.; Jansen, L.E.; Choi, Y.H.; Schwarz, U.I.; Kim, R.B. Genetic variation in the farnesoid X-receptor predicts Crohn's disease severity in female patients. *Sci. Rep.* **2020**, *10*, 11725. [CrossRef]
88. Cheung, K.C.P.; Ma, J.; Loiola, R.A.; Chen, X.; Jia, W. Bile acid-activated receptors in innate and adaptive immunity: Targeted drugs and biological agents. *Eur. J. Immunol.* **2023**, *53*, e2250299. [CrossRef]
89. Ma, C.; Han, M.; Heinrich, B.; Fu, Q.; Zhang, Q.; Sandhu, M.; Agdashian, D.; Terabe, M.; Berzofsky, J.A.; Fako, V.; et al. Gut microbiome-mediated bile acid metabolism regulates liver cancer via NKT cells. *Science* **2018**, *360*, eaan5931. [CrossRef]
90. Guo, C.; Xie, S.; Chi, Z.; Zhang, J.; Liu, Y.; Zhang, L.; Zheng, M.; Zhang, X.; Xia, D.; Ke, Y.; et al. Bile Acids Control Inflammation and Metabolic Disorder through Inhibition of NLRP3 Inflammasome. *Immunity* **2016**, *45*, 802–816, Erratum in *Immunity* **2016**, *45*, 944. [CrossRef]
91. Hao, H.; Cao, L.; Jiang, C.; Che, Y.; Zhang, S.; Takahashi, S.; Wang, G.; Gonzalez, F.J. Farnesoid X Receptor Regulation of the NLRP3 Inflammasome Underlies Cholestasis-Associated Sepsis. *Cell Metab.* **2017**, *25*, 856–867.e5. [CrossRef] [PubMed]
92. Mendler, A.; Pierzchalski, A.; Bauer, M.; Roder, S.; Sattler, A.; Standl, M.; Borte, M.; von Bergen, M.; Rolle-Kampczyk, U.; Herberth, G. MAIT cell activation in adolescents is impacted by bile acid concentrations and body weight. *Clin. Exp. Immunol.* **2020**, *200*, 199–213. [CrossRef]
93. Fu, T.; Li, Y.; Oh, T.G.; Cayabyab, F.; He, N.; Tang, Q.; Coulter, S.; Truitt, M.; Medina, P.; He, M.; et al. FXR mediates ILC-intrinsic responses to intestinal inflammation. *Proc. Natl. Acad. Sci. USA* **2022**, *119*, e2213041119. [CrossRef] [PubMed]
94. Ma, Y.; Yang, H.; Wang, X.; Huang, Y.; Li, Y.; Pan, G. Bile acids as signaling molecules in inflammatory bowel disease: Implications for treatment strategies. *J. Ethnopharmacol.* **2024**, *337 Pt 3*, 118968. [CrossRef] [PubMed]
95. Tang, X.; Chen, X.; Ferrari, M.; Walvoort, M.T.C.; de Vos, P. Gut Epithelial Barrier Function is Impacted by Hyperglycemia and Secondary Bile Acids In Vitro: Possible Rescuing Effects of Specific Pectins. *Mol. Nutr. Food Res.* **2024**, *68*, e2300910. [CrossRef]
96. O'Guinn, M.L.; Handler, D.A.; Hsieh, J.J.; Mallicote, M.U.; Feliciano, K.; Gayer, C.P. FXR deletion attenuates intestinal barrier dysfunction in murine acute intestinal inflammation. *Am. J. Physiol. Gastrointest. Liver Physiol.* **2024**, *327*, G175–G187. [CrossRef]
97. Lukawska, A.; Mulak, A. Serum fibroblast growth factor 19 level correlates inversely with clinical and endoscopic activity of inflammatory bowel disease. *Adv. Clin. Exp. Med.* **2024**. [CrossRef]
98. Jyotsna; Sarkar, B.; Yadav, M.; Deka, A.; Markandey, M.; Sanyal, P.; Nagarajan, P.; Gaikward, N.; Ahuja, V.; Mohanty, D.; et al. A hepatocyte-specific transcriptional program driven by Rela and Stat3 exacerbates experimental colitis in mice by modulating bile synthesis. *Elife* **2024**, *12*, RP93273. [CrossRef]
99. Kwon, S.J.; Kim, Y.S.; Tak, J.; Lee, S.G.; Lee, E.B.; Kim, S.G. Hepatic Galpha13 ablation shifts region-specific colonic inflammatory status by modulating the bile acid synthetic pathway in mice. *Sci. Rep.* **2024**, *14*, 19580. [CrossRef]
100. Quraishi, M.N.; Acharjee, A.; Beggs, A.D.; Horniblow, R.; Tselepis, C.; Gkoutos, G.; Ghosh, S.; Rossiter, A.E.; Loman, N.; van Schaik, W.; et al. A Pilot Integrative Analysis of Colonic Gene Expression, Gut Microbiota, and Immune Infiltration in Primary Sclerosing Cholangitis-Inflammatory Bowel Disease: Association of Disease with Bile Acid Pathways. *J. Crohns Colitis* **2020**, *14*, 935–947. [CrossRef]
101. Kwon, J.; Lee, C.; Heo, S.; Kim, B.; Hyun, C.K. DSS-induced colitis is associated with adipose tissue dysfunction and disrupted hepatic lipid metabolism leading to hepatosteatosis and dyslipidemia in mice. *Sci. Rep.* **2021**, *11*, 5283. [CrossRef]
102. Gui, W.; Hole, M.J.; Molinaro, A.; Edlund, K.; Jorgensen, K.K.; Su, H.; Begher-Tibbe, B.; Gassler, N.; Schneider, C.V.; Muthukumarasamy, U.; et al. Colitis ameliorates cholestatic liver disease via suppression of bile acid synthesis. *Nat. Commun.* **2023**, *14*, 3304. [CrossRef] [PubMed]
103. Zheng, C.; Wang, L.; Zou, T.; Lian, S.; Luo, J.; Lu, Y.; Hao, H.; Xu, Y.; Xiang, Y.; Zhang, X.; et al. Ileitis promotes MASLD progression via bile acid modulation and enhanced TGR5 signaling in ileal CD8(+) T cells. *J. Hepatol.* **2024**, *80*, 764–777. [CrossRef] [PubMed]
104. Wang, C.; Chu, Q.; Dong, W.; Wang, X.; Zhao, W.; Dai, X.; Liu, W.; Wang, B.; Liu, T.; Zhong, W.; et al. Microbial metabolite deoxycholic acid-mediated ferroptosis exacerbates high-fat diet-induced colonic inflammation. *Mol. Metab.* **2024**, *84*, 101944. [CrossRef] [PubMed]
105. Huang, C.; Tan, H.; Song, M.; Liu, K.; Liu, H.; Wang, J.; Shi, Y.; Hou, F.; Zhou, Q.; Huang, R.; et al. Maternal Western diet mediates susceptibility of offspring to Crohn's-like colitis by deoxycholate generation. *Microbiome* **2023**, *11*, 96. [CrossRef]
106. Zheng, M.; Zhai, Y.; Yu, Y.; Shen, J.; Chu, S.; Focaccia, E.; Tian, W.; Wang, S.; Liu, X.; Yuan, X.; et al. TNF compromises intestinal bile-acid tolerance dictating colitis progression and limited infliximab response. *Cell Metab.* **2024**, *36*, 2086–2103.e9. [CrossRef]
107. Wang, L.; Gong, Z.; Zhang, X.; Zhu, F.; Liu, Y.; Jin, C.; Du, X.; Xu, C.; Chen, Y.; Cai, W.; et al. Gut microbial bile acid metabolite skews macrophage polarization and contributes to high-fat diet-induced colonic inflammation. *Gut Microbes* **2020**, *12*, 1–20. [CrossRef]

108. Zhou, M.; Liu, X.; He, J.; Xu, X.; Ju, C.; Luo, S.; Lu, X.; Du, P.; Chen, Y. High-fructose corn syrup aggravates colitis via microbiota dysbiosis-mediated Th17/Treg imbalance. *Clin. Sci.* **2023**, *137*, 1619–1635. [CrossRef]
109. Li, S.; Zhuge, A.; Wang, K.; Lv, L.; Bian, X.; Yang, L.; Xia, J.; Jiang, X.; Wu, W.; Wang, S.; et al. Ketogenic diet aggravates colitis, impairs intestinal barrier and alters gut microbiota and metabolism in DSS-induced mice. *Food Funct.* **2021**, *12*, 10210–10225. [CrossRef]
110. Liu, T.C.; Kern, J.T.; Jain, U.; Sonnek, N.M.; Xiong, S.; Simpson, K.F.; VanDussen, K.L.; Winkler, E.S.; Haritunians, T.; Malique, A.; et al. Western diet induces Paneth cell defects through microbiome alterations and farnesoid X receptor and type I interferon activation. *Cell Host Microbe* **2021**, *29*, 988–1001.e6. [CrossRef]
111. O'Mahony, C.; Clooney, A.; Clarke, S.F.; Aguilera, M.; Gavin, A.; Simnica, D.; Ahern, M.; Fanning, A.; Stanley, M.; Rubio, R.C.; et al. Dietary-Induced Bacterial Metabolites Reduce Inflammation and Inflammation-Associated Cancer via Vitamin D Pathway. *Int. J. Mol. Sci.* **2023**, *24*, 1864. [CrossRef] [PubMed]
112. Fart, F.; Salihovic, S.; McGlinchey, A.; Gareau, M.G.; Oresic, M.; Halfvarson, J.; Hyotylainen, T.; Schoultz, I. Perfluoroalkyl substances are increased in patients with late-onset ulcerative colitis and induce intestinal barrier defects ex vivo in murine intestinal tissue. *Scand. J. Gastroenterol.* **2021**, *56*, 1286–1295. [CrossRef] [PubMed]
113. Liu, Y.; Wang, Y.; Ren, T.; Yu, G.; Meng, X.; Feng, L.; Li, F.; Zhang, J.; Wang, C. Unraveling the long-term gastrointestinal impact of perinatal perfluorobutane sulfonate exposure on rat offspring: Intestinal barrier dysfunction and Th17/Treg imbalance. *Sci. Total Environ.* **2024**, *955*, 176858. [CrossRef] [PubMed]
114. Zhou, J.; Tang, L.; Wang, J.S. Aflatoxin B1 Induces Gut-Inflammation-Associated Fecal Lipidome Changes in F344 Rats. *Toxicol. Sci.* **2021**, *183*, 363–377. [CrossRef]
115. Couto, M.R.; Andrade, N.; Magro, F.; Martel, F. Bile salts and proinflammatory cytokines inhibit MCT1-mediated cellular uptake of butyrate and interfere with its antiproliferative properties. *Exp. Cell Res.* **2023**, *429*, 113670. [CrossRef]
116. Chen, W.; Wang, D.; Deng, X.; Zhang, H.; Dong, D.; Su, T.; Lu, Q.; Jiang, C.; Ni, Q.; Cui, Y.; et al. Bile acid profiling as an effective biomarker for staging in pediatric inflammatory bowel disease. *Gut Microbes* **2024**, *16*, 2323231. [CrossRef]
117. Connors, J.; Dunn, K.A.; Allott, J.; Bandsma, R.; Rashid, M.; Otley, A.R.; Bielawski, J.P.; Van Limbergen, J. The relationship between fecal bile acids and microbiome community structure in pediatric Crohn's disease. *ISME J.* **2020**, *14*, 702–713. [CrossRef]
118. Sun, Q.; Tang, Y.; Dai, L.; Tang, Z.; Zhou, W.; Wu, T.; Ji, G. Serum Bile Acid Metabolites Predict the Therapeutic Effect of Mesalazine in Patients with Ulcerative Colitis. *J. Proteome Res.* **2023**, *22*, 1287–1297. [CrossRef]
119. Lee, J.W.J.; Plichta, D.; Hogstrom, L.; Borren, N.Z.; Lau, H.; Gregory, S.M.; Tan, W.; Khalili, H.; Clish, C.; Vlamakis, H.; et al. Multi-omics reveal microbial determinants impacting responses to biologic therapies in inflammatory bowel disease. *Cell Host Microbe* **2021**, *29*, 1294–1304.e4. [CrossRef]
120. Ding, N.S.; McDonald, J.A.K.; Perdones-Montero, A.; Rees, D.N.; Adegbola, S.O.; Misra, R.; Hendy, P.; Penez, L.; Marchesi, J.R.; Holmes, E.; et al. Metabonomics and the Gut Microbiome Associated with Primary Response to Anti-TNF Therapy in Crohn's Disease. *J. Crohns Colitis* **2020**, *14*, 1090–1102. [CrossRef]
121. Han, B.; Tang, D.; Lv, X.; Fan, J.; Li, S.; Zhu, H.; Zhang, J.; Xu, S.; Xu, X.; Huang, Z.; et al. Integrated multi-omics reveal gut microbiota-mediated bile acid metabolism alteration regulating immunotherapy responses to anti-alpha4beta7-integrin in Crohn's disease. *Gut Microbes* **2024**, *16*, 2310894. [CrossRef] [PubMed]
122. Han, B.; Lv, X.; Liu, G.; Li, S.; Fan, J.; Chen, L.; Huang, Z.; Lin, G.; Xu, X.; Huang, Z.; et al. Gut microbiota-related bile acid metabolism-FXR/TGR5 axis impacts the response to anti-alpha4beta7-integrin therapy in humanized mice with colitis. *Gut Microbes* **2023**, *15*, 2232143. [CrossRef] [PubMed]
123. Lyutakov, I.; Lozanov, V.; Sugareva, P.; Valkov, H.; Penchev, P. Serum 7-alfa-hydroxy-4-cholesten-3-one and fibroblast growth factor-19 as biomarkers diagnosing bile acid malabsorption in microscopic colitis and inflammatory bowel disease. *Eur. J. Gastroenterol. Hepatol.* **2021**, *33*, 380–387. [CrossRef] [PubMed]
124. Alexander, J.L.; Mullish, B.H.; Danckert, N.P.; Liu, Z.; Olbei, M.L.; Saifuddin, A.; Torkizadeh, M.; Ibraheim, H.; Blanco, J.M.; Roberts, L.A.; et al. The gut microbiota and metabolome are associated with diminished COVID-19 vaccine-induced antibody responses in immunosuppressed inflammatory bowel disease patients. *eBioMedicine* **2023**, *88*, 104430. [CrossRef]
125. Wu, X.; Li, P.; Wang, W.; Xu, J.; Ai, R.; Wen, Q.; Cui, B.; Zhang, F. The Underlying Changes in Serum Metabolic Profiles and Efficacy Prediction in Patients with Extensive Ulcerative Colitis Undergoing Fecal Microbiota Transplantation. *Nutrients* **2023**, *15*, 3340. [CrossRef]
126. Ramos, R.J.; Zhu, C.; Joseph, D.F.; Thaker, S.; Lacomb, J.F.; Markarian, K.; Lee, H.J.; Petrov, J.C.; Monzur, F.; Buscaglia, J.M.; et al. Metagenomic and bile acid metabolomic analysis of fecal microbiota transplantation for recurrent Clostridiodes difficile and/or inflammatory bowel diseases. *Med. Res. Arch.* **2022**, *10*. [CrossRef]
127. Chen, L.A.; Oliva-Hemker, M.; Radin, A.; Weidner, M.; O'Laughlin, B.D.; Sears, C.L.; Javitt, N.B.; Hourigan, S.K. Longitudinal Bile Acid Composition Changes Following Faecal Microbiota Transplantation for Clostridioides difficile Infection in Children with and Without Underlying Inflammatory Bowel Disease. *J. Crohns Colitis* **2023**, *17*, 1364–1368. [CrossRef]
128. Wang, Y.; Gao, X.; Zhang, X.; Xiao, F.; Hu, H.; Li, X.; Dong, F.; Sun, M.; Xiao, Y.; Ge, T.; et al. Microbial and metabolic features associated with outcome of infliximab therapy in pediatric Crohn's disease. *Gut Microbes* **2021**, *13*, 1–18. [CrossRef]
129. Manka, P.; Sydor, S.; Wase, N.; Best, J.; Brandenburg, M.; Hellbeck, A.; Schanzer, J.; Vilchez-Vargas, R.; Link, A.; Figge, A.; et al. Anti-TNFalpha treatment in Crohn's disease: Impact on hepatic steatosis, gut-derived hormones and metabolic status. *Liver Int.* **2021**, *41*, 2646–2658. [CrossRef]

130. Diederen, K.; Li, J.V.; Donachie, G.E.; de Meij, T.G.; de Waart, D.R.; Hakvoort, T.B.M.; Kindermann, A.; Wagner, J.; Auyeung, V.; Te Velde, A.A.; et al. Exclusive enteral nutrition mediates gut microbial and metabolic changes that are associated with remission in children with Crohn's disease. *Sci. Rep.* **2020**, *10*, 18879. [CrossRef]
131. Xiao, F.; Gao, X.; Hu, H.; Le, J.; Chen, Y.; Shu, X.; Liang, Z.; Xu, Y.; Wang, Y.; Zhang, T. Exclusive Enteral Nutrition Exerts Anti-Inflammatory Effects through Modulating Microbiota, Bile Acid Metabolism, and Immune Activities. *Nutrients* **2022**, *14*, 4463. [CrossRef] [PubMed]
132. Lv, Y.; Lou, Y.; Liu, A.; Cheng, Q.; Yang, G.; Xu, C.; Luo, Y.; Lou, J.; Yu, J.; Fang, Y.; et al. The impact of exclusive enteral nutrition on the gut microbiome and bile acid metabolism in pediatric Crohn's disease. *Clin. Nutr.* **2023**, *42*, 116–128. [CrossRef] [PubMed]
133. Wu, J.; Man, D.; Shi, D.; Wu, W.; Wang, S.; Wang, K.; Li, Y.; Yang, L.; Bian, X.; Wang, Q.; et al. Intermittent Fasting Alleviates Risk Markers in a Murine Model of Ulcerative Colitis by Modulating the Gut Microbiome and Metabolome. *Nutrients* **2022**, *14*, 5311. [CrossRef] [PubMed]
134. Ke, J.; Li, Y.; Han, C.; He, R.; Lin, R.; Qian, W.; Hou, X. Fucose Ameliorate Intestinal Inflammation Through Modulating the Crosstalk Between Bile Acids and Gut Microbiota in a Chronic Colitis Murine Model. *Inflamm. Bowel Dis.* **2020**, *26*, 863–873. [CrossRef]
135. Bretin, A.; Zou, J.; San Yeoh, B.; Ngo, V.L.; Winer, S.; Winer, D.A.; Reddivari, L.; Pellizzon, M.; Walters, W.A.; Patterson, A.D.; et al. Psyllium Fiber Protects Against Colitis Via Activation of Bile Acid Sensor Farnesoid X Receptor. *Cell Mol. Gastroenterol. Hepatol.* **2023**, *15*, 1421–1442. [CrossRef]
136. Yang, L.; Lin, Q.; Han, L.; Wang, Z.; Luo, M.; Kang, W.; Liu, J.; Wang, J.; Ma, T.; Liu, H. Soy hull dietary fiber alleviates inflammation in BALB/C mice by modulating the gut microbiota and suppressing the TLR-4/NF-kappaB signaling pathway. *Food Funct.* **2020**, *11*, 5965–5975. [CrossRef]
137. Tian, M.; Li, D.; Ma, C.; Feng, Y.; Hu, X.; Chen, F. Barley Leaf Insoluble Dietary Fiber Alleviated Dextran Sulfate Sodium-Induced Mice Colitis by Modulating Gut Microbiota. *Nutrients* **2021**, *13*, 846. [CrossRef]
138. Zhang, J.; Zhong, Y.; Wang, D.; Zhu, J.; Deng, Y.; Li, Y.; Liu, C.; Wang, J.L.; Zhang, M. Wallace melon juice fermented with Lactobacillus alleviates dextran sulfate sodium-induced ulcerative colitis in mice through modulating gut microbiota and the metabolism. *J. Food Sci.* **2024**, *89*, 2450–2464. [CrossRef]
139. Zhang, L.; Miao, C.; Wang, Z.; Guan, X.; Ma, Y.; Song, J.; Shen, S.; Song, H.; Li, M.; Liu, C. Preparation and characterisation of baicalin magnesium and its protective effect in ulcerative colitis via gut microbiota-bile acid axis modulation. *Phytomedicine* **2024**, *126*, 155416. [CrossRef]
140. Wang, L.; Tao, J.H.; Chen, Y.F.; Shen, Y.M.; Jiang, S. Lizhong Decoction Ameliorates Ulcerative Colitis in Mice via Regulation of Plasma and Urine Metabolic Profiling. *Chin. J. Integr. Med.* **2022**, *28*, 1015–1022. [CrossRef]
141. Han, Z.; Wang, H.; Guo, D.; Zhang, J. Integrative transcriptomic and metabonomic profiling analyses reveal the molecular mechanism of Chinese traditional medicine huankuile suspension on TNBS-induced ulcerative colitis. *Aging* **2021**, *13*, 5087–5103. [CrossRef] [PubMed]
142. Nong, F.; Luo, S.; Liang, Y.; Zhao, Z.; Xing, S.; Wen, B.; Zhou, L. Evaluation of the effect of Dahuang-Mudan decoction on TNBS-induced colitis using UPLC-QTOF/MS-based metabolomic analysis. *Biomed. Chromatogr.* **2021**, *35*, e5003. [CrossRef] [PubMed]
143. Nguepi Tsopmejio, I.S.; Yuan, J.; Diao, Z.; Fan, W.; Wei, J.; Zhao, C.; Li, Y.; Song, H. Auricularia polytricha and Flammulina velutipes reduce liver injury in DSS-induced Inflammatory Bowel Disease by improving inflammation, oxidative stress, and apoptosis through the regulation of TLR4/NF-kappaB signaling pathways. *J. Nutr. Biochem.* **2023**, *111*, 109190. [CrossRef] [PubMed]
144. Ma, G.; Tao, Q.; Li, X.; Han, Y.; Du, H.; Hu, Q.; Xiao, H. Metabolomics study of dietary Pleurotus eryngii beta-type glycosidic polysaccharide on colitis induced by dextran sodium sulfate in mice—Exploration for the potential metabolic indicators in urine and serum. *Food Chem.* **2024**, *458*, 140195. [CrossRef]
145. Fan, A.; Hou, B.L.; Tang, Z.; Wang, T.; Zhang, D.; Liang, Y.; Wang, Z. Liquid Chromatography-Tandem Mass Spectrometry-Based Metabolomics Analysis of Indigo Naturalis Treatment of Ulcerative Colitis in Mice. *J. Med. Food* **2023**, *26*, 877–889. [CrossRef]
146. Cheng, H.; Zhang, D.; Wu, J.; Liu, J.; Tan, Y.; Feng, W.; Peng, C. Atractylodes macrocephala Koidz. volatile oil relieves acute ulcerative colitis via regulating gut microbiota and gut microbiota metabolism. *Front. Immunol.* **2023**, *14*, 1127785. [CrossRef]
147. Wu, Y.; Zheng, Y.; Wang, X.; Tang, P.; Guo, W.; Ma, H.; Zhang, A.; Li, D.; Xie, Y.; Wang, C.Z.; et al. Ginseng-Containing Sijunzi Decoction Ameliorates Ulcerative Colitis by Orchestrating Gut Homeostasis in Microbial Modulation and Intestinal Barrier Integrity. *Am. J. Chin. Med.* **2023**, *51*, 677–699. [CrossRef]
148. Li, S.; Tan, H.Y.; Wang, N.; Hong, M.; Li, L.; Cheung, F.; Feng, Y. Substitutes for Bear Bile for the Treatment of Liver Diseases: Research Progress and Future Perspective. *Evid. Based Complement. Altern. Med.* **2016**, *2016*, 4305074. [CrossRef]
149. Wang, A.; Yang, X.; Lin, J.; Wang, Y.; Yang, J.; Zhang, Y.; Tian, Y.; Dong, H.; Zhang, Z.; Song, R. Si-Ni-San alleviates intestinal and liver damage in ulcerative colitis mice by regulating cholesterol metabolism. *J. Ethnopharmacol.* **2025**, *336*, 118715. [CrossRef]
150. Huang, J.; Zhang, J.; Wang, F.; Tang, X. Modified Gegen Qinlian Decoction modulated the gut microbiome and bile acid metabolism and restored the function of goblet cells in a mouse model of ulcerative colitis. *Front. Immunol.* **2024**, *15*, 1445838. [CrossRef]
151. Li, Q.; Cui, Y.; Xu, B.; Wang, Y.; Lv, F.; Li, Z.; Li, H.; Chen, X.; Peng, X.; Chen, Y.; et al. Main active components of Jiawei Gegen Qinlian decoction protects against ulcerative colitis under different dietary environments in a gut microbiota-dependent manner. *Pharmacol. Res.* **2021**, *170*, 105694. [CrossRef] [PubMed]

152. Zhou, F.; Mai, T.; Wang, Z.; Zeng, Z.; Shi, J.; Zhang, F.; Kong, N.; Jiang, H.; Guo, L.; Xu, M.; et al. The improvement of intestinal dysbiosis and hepatic metabolic dysfunction in dextran sulfate sodium-induced colitis mice: Effects of curcumin. *J. Gastroenterol. Hepatol.* **2023**, *38*, 1333–1345. [CrossRef] [PubMed]
153. Wang, Q.; Xu, K.; Cai, X.; Wang, C.; Cao, Y.; Xiao, J. Rosmarinic Acid Restores Colonic Mucus Secretion in Colitis Mice by Regulating Gut Microbiota-Derived Metabolites and the Activation of Inflammasomes. *J. Agric. Food Chem.* **2023**, *71*, 4571–4585. [CrossRef] [PubMed]
154. Zeng, X.; Tang, S.; Dong, X.; Dong, M.; Shao, R.; Liu, R.; Li, T.; Zhang, X.; Wong, Y.H.; Xie, Q. Analysis of metagenome and metabolome disclosed the mechanisms of Dendrobium officinale polysaccharide on DSS-induced ulcerative colitis-affected mice. *Int. J. Biol. Macromol.* **2024**, *277 Pt 2*, 134229. [CrossRef]
155. Feng, P.; Li, Q.; Liu, L.; Wang, S.; Wu, Z.; Tao, Y.; Huang, P.; Wang, P. Crocetin Prolongs Recovery Period of DSS-Induced Colitis via Altering Intestinal Microbiome and Increasing Intestinal Permeability. *Int. J. Mol. Sci.* **2022**, *23*, 3832. [CrossRef]
156. Hu, J.; Huang, H.; Che, Y.; Ding, C.; Zhang, L.; Wang, Y.; Hao, H.; Shen, H.; Cao, L. Qingchang Huashi Formula attenuates DSS-induced colitis in mice by restoring gut microbiota-metabolism homeostasis and goblet cell function. *J. Ethnopharmacol.* **2021**, *266*, 113394. [CrossRef]
157. Pi, Y.; Zhang, X.; Wu, Y.; Wang, Z.; Bai, Y.; Liu, X.; Han, D.; Zhao, J.; Tobin, I.; Zhao, J.; et al. Alginate Alleviates Dextran Sulfate Sodium-Induced Colitis by Promoting Bifidobacterium animalis and Intestinal Hyodeoxycholic Acid Synthesis in Mice. *Microbiol. Spectr.* **2022**, *10*, e0297922. [CrossRef]
158. Liu, F.; Wang, X.; Li, D.; Cui, Y.; Li, X. Apple polyphenols extract alleviated dextran sulfate sodium-induced ulcerative colitis in C57BL/6 male mice by restoring bile acid metabolism disorder and gut microbiota dysbiosis. *Phytother. Res.* **2021**, *35*, 1468–1485. [CrossRef]
159. Zhang, K.; Xu, Y.; Zheng, Y.; Zhang, T.; Wu, Y.; Yan, Y.; Lei, Y.; Cao, X.; Wang, X.; Yan, F.; et al. Bifidobacterium pseudolongum-Derived Bile Acid from Dietary Carvacrol and Thymol Supplementation Attenuates Colitis via cGMP-PKG-mTORC1 Pathway. *Adv. Sci.* **2024**, *11*, e2406917. [CrossRef]
160. Zhang, M.; Mo, R.; Wang, H.; Liu, T.; Zhang, G.; Wu, Y. Grape seed proanthocyanidin improves intestinal inflammation in canine through regulating gut microbiota and bile acid compositions. *FASEB J.* **2023**, *37*, e23285. [CrossRef]
161. Zhu, Y.; Huang, X.; Deng, Z.; Bai, T.; Gao, B.; Xu, C.; Fu, J.; Zhao, Y.; Zhang, Y.; Zhang, M.; et al. Orally biomimetic metal-phenolic nanozyme with quadruple safeguards for intestinal homeostasis to ameliorate ulcerative colitis. *J. Nanobiotechnol.* **2024**, *22*, 545. [CrossRef] [PubMed]
162. Zhu, T.; Xue, Q.; Liu, Y.; Xu, Y.; Xiong, C.; Lu, J.; Yang, H.; Zhang, Q.; Huang, Y. Analysis of Intestinal Microflora and Metabolites from Mice with DSS-Induced IBD Treated with Schistosoma Soluble Egg Antigen. *Front. Cell Dev. Biol.* **2021**, *9*, 777218. [CrossRef] [PubMed]
163. Jia, Y.Q.; Yuan, Z.W.; Zhang, X.S.; Dong, J.Q.; Liu, X.N.; Peng, X.T.; Yao, W.L.; Ji, P.; Wei, Y.M.; Hua, Y.L. Total alkaloids of *Sophora alopecuroides* L. ameliorated murine colitis by regulating bile acid metabolism and gut microbiota. *J. Ethnopharmacol.* **2020**, *255*, 112775. [CrossRef] [PubMed]
164. Xu, W.; Liu, A.X.; Liu, K.H.; Zhang, S.; Gong, Z.H.; Xiao, W.J. l-Theanine Alleviates Ulcerative Colitis by Regulating Colon Immunity via the Gut Microbiota in an MHC-II-Dependent Manner. *J. Agric. Food Chem.* **2024**, *72*, 19852–19868. [CrossRef]
165. Liu, M.; Wang, Z.; Liu, X.; Xiao, H.; Liu, Y.; Wang, J.; Chen, C.; Wang, X.; Liu, W.; Xiang, Z.; et al. Therapeutic effect of Yiyi Fuzi Baijiang formula on TNBS-induced ulcerative colitis via metabolism and Th17/Treg cell balance. *J. Ethnopharmacol.* **2023**, *309*, 116301. [CrossRef]
166. Yu, Z.; Li, D.; Sun, H. Herba Origani alleviated DSS-induced ulcerative colitis in mice through remolding gut microbiota to regulate bile acid and short-chain fatty acid metabolisms. *Biomed. Pharmacother.* **2023**, *161*, 114409. [CrossRef]
167. Wang, X.; Liu, J.; Wei, J.; Zhang, Y.; Xu, Y.; Yue, T.; Yuan, Y. Protective Mechanism of Eurotium amstelodami from Fuzhuan Brick Tea against Colitis and Gut-Derived Liver Injury Induced by Dextran Sulfate Sodium in C57BL/6 Mice. *Nutrients* **2024**, *16*, 1178. [CrossRef]
168. Shen, J.C.; Qi, Q.; Han, D.; Lu, Y.; Huang, R.; Zhu, Y.; Zhang, L.S.; Qin, X.D.; Zhang, F.; Wu, H.G.; et al. Moxibustion improves experimental colitis in rats with Crohn's disease by regulating bile acid enterohepatic circulation and intestinal farnesoid X receptor. *J. Integr. Med.* **2023**, *21*, 194–204. [CrossRef]
169. Liu, F.; Yao, Y.; Wang, Q.; Zhang, F.; Wang, M.; Zhu, C.; Lin, C. Nigakinone alleviates DSS-induced experimental colitis via regulating bile acid profile and FXR/NLRP3 signaling pathways. *Phytother. Res.* **2023**, *37*, 15–34. [CrossRef]
170. Li, S.; Zhuge, A.; Chen, H.; Han, S.; Shen, J.; Wang, K.; Xia, J.; Xia, H.; Jiang, S.; Wu, Y.; et al. Sedanolide alleviates DSS-induced colitis by modulating the intestinal FXR-SMPD3 pathway in mice. *J. Adv. Res.* **2024**. [CrossRef]
171. Li, X.H.; Liu, L.; Wu, W.Z. Trans-Anethole Alleviates DSS-Induced Ulcerative Colitis by Remodeling the Intestinal Flora to Regulate Immunity and Bile Acid Metabolism. *Mediat. Inflamm.* **2023**, *2023*, 4188510. [CrossRef] [PubMed]
172. Dong, S.; Zhu, M.; Wang, K.; Zhao, X.; Hu, L.; Jing, W.; Lu, H.; Wang, S. Dihydromyricetin improves DSS-induced colitis in mice via modulation of fecal-bacteria-related bile acid metabolism. *Pharmacol. Res.* **2021**, *171*, 105767. [CrossRef] [PubMed]
173. Liu, X.; Zhang, Y.; Li, W.; Zhang, B.; Yin, J.; Liuqi, S.; Wang, J.; Peng, B.; Wang, S. Fucoidan Ameliorated Dextran Sulfate Sodium-Induced Ulcerative Colitis by Modulating Gut Microbiota and Bile Acid Metabolism. *J. Agric. Food Chem.* **2022**, *70*, 14864–14876. [CrossRef] [PubMed]

174. Hua, Y.L.; Jia, Y.Q.; Zhang, X.S.; Yuan, Z.W.; Ji, P.; Hu, J.J.; Wei, Y.M. Baitouweng Tang ameliorates DSS-induced ulcerative colitis through the regulation of the gut microbiota and bile acids via pathways involving FXR and TGR5. *Biomed. Pharmacother.* **2021**, *137*, 111320. [CrossRef]
175. Zhai, Z.; Niu, K.M.; Liu, Y.; Lin, C.; Wu, X. The Gut Microbiota-Bile Acids-TGR5 Axis Mediates Eucommia ulmoides Leaf Extract Alleviation of Injury to Colonic Epithelium Integrity. *Front. Microbiol.* **2021**, *12*, 727681. [CrossRef]
176. Wang, J.; Wang, X.; Ma, X.; Xu, B.; Chen, L.; Chen, C.; Liu, W.; Liu, Y.; Xiang, Z. Therapeutic effect of Patrinia villosa on TNBS-induced ulcerative colitis via metabolism, vitamin D receptor and NF-kappaB signaling pathways. *J. Ethnopharmacol.* **2022**, *288*, 114989. [CrossRef]
177. Sun, Y.; Zhou, J.; Du, H.; Zhou, Z.; Han, Y.; Luo, M.; Guo, X.; Gu, M.; Yang, H.; Xiao, H. The Anti-inflammatory Potential of a Strain of Probiotic Bifidobacterium pseudocatenulatum G7: In Vitro and In Vivo Evidence. *J. Agric. Food Chem.* **2024**, *72*, 10355–10365. [CrossRef]
178. Zhang, C.; Zhao, Y.; Jiang, J.; Yu, L.; Tian, F.; Zhao, J.; Zhang, H.; Chen, W.; Zhai, Q. Identification of the key characteristics of Bifidobacterium longum strains for the alleviation of ulcerative colitis. *Food Funct.* **2021**, *12*, 3476–3492. [CrossRef]
179. Lv, W.; Zhang, D.; He, T.; Liu, Y.; Shao, L.; Lv, Z.; Pu, X.; Wang, Y.; Liu, L. Combination of Lactobacillus plantarum improves the effects of tacrolimus on colitis in a mouse model. *Front. Cell Infect. Microbiol.* **2023**, *13*, 1130820. [CrossRef]
180. Wong, W.Y.; Chan, B.D.; Sham, T.T.; Lee, M.M.; Chan, C.O.; Chau, C.T.; Mok, D.K.; Kwan, Y.W.; Tai, W.C. Lactobacillus casei Strain Shirota Ameliorates Dextran Sulfate Sodium-Induced Colitis in Mice by Increasing Taurine-Conjugated Bile Acids and Inhibiting NF-kappaB Signaling via Stabilization of IkappaBalpha. *Front. Nutr.* **2022**, *9*, 816836. [CrossRef]
181. Yan, Y.; Lei, Y.; Qu, Y.; Fan, Z.; Zhang, T.; Xu, Y.; Du, Q.; Brugger, D.; Chen, Y.; Zhang, K.; et al. Bacteroides uniformis-induced perturbations in colonic microbiota and bile acid levels inhibit TH17 differentiation and ameliorate colitis developments. *NPJ Biofilms Microbiomes* **2023**, *9*, 56. [CrossRef] [PubMed]
182. Zhou, C.; Wang, Y.; Li, C.; Xie, Z.; Dai, L. Amelioration of Colitis by a Gut Bacterial Consortium Producing Anti-Inflammatory Secondary Bile Acids. *Microbiol. Spectr.* **2023**, *11*, e0333022. [CrossRef] [PubMed]
183. Van der Lelie, D.; Oka, A.; Taghavi, S.; Umeno, J.; Fan, T.J.; Merrell, K.E.; Watson, S.D.; Ouellette, L.; Liu, B.; Awoniyi, M.; et al. Rationally designed bacterial consortia to treat chronic immune-mediated colitis and restore intestinal homeostasis. *Nat. Commun.* **2021**, *12*, 3105. [CrossRef] [PubMed]
184. Liu, Z.; Wang, H. Probiotics alleviate inflammatory bowel disease in mice by regulating intestinal microorganisms-bile acid-NLRP3 inflammasome pathway. *Acta Biochim. Pol.* **2021**, *68*, 687–693. [CrossRef]
185. Xiao, F.; Dong, F.; Li, X.; Li, Y.; Yu, G.; Liu, Z.; Wang, Y.; Zhang, T. Bifidobacterium longum CECT 7894 Improves the Efficacy of Infliximab for DSS-Induced Colitis via Regulating the Gut Microbiota and Bile Acid Metabolism. *Front. Pharmacol.* **2022**, *13*, 902337. [CrossRef]
186. He, Q.; Wu, J.; Ke, J.; Zhang, Q.; Zeng, W.; Luo, Z.; Gong, J.; Chen, Y.; He, Z.; Lan, P. Therapeutic role of ursodeoxycholic acid in colitis-associated cancer via gut microbiota modulation. *Mol. Ther.* **2023**, *31*, 585–598. [CrossRef]
187. Gao, R.Y.; Shearn, C.T.; Orlicky, D.J.; Battista, K.D.; Alexeev, E.E.; Cartwright, I.M.; Lanis, J.M.; Kostelecky, R.E.; Ju, C.; Colgan, S.P.; et al. Bile acids modulate colonic MAdCAM-1 expression in a murine model of combined cholestasis and colitis. *Mucosal Immunol.* **2021**, *14*, 479–490. [CrossRef]
188. Yu, J.; Sheng, S.; Zou, X.; Shen, Z. Dihydroartemisinin-ursodeoxycholic acid conjugate is a potential treatment agent for inflammatory bowel disease. *Int. Immunopharmacol.* **2023**, *117*, 109918. [CrossRef]
189. Wang, Z.; Chen, J.; Chen, Z.; Xie, L.; Wang, W. Clinical effects of ursodeoxycholic acid on patients with ulcerative colitis may improve via the regulation of IL-23-IL-17 axis and the changes of the proportion of intestinal microflora. *Saudi J. Gastroenterol.* **2021**, *27*, 149–157. [CrossRef]
190. Kubota, H.; Ishizawa, M.; Kodama, M.; Nagase, Y.; Kato, S.; Makishima, M.; Sakurai, K. Vitamin D Receptor Mediates Attenuating Effect of Lithocholic Acid on Dextran Sulfate Sodium Induced Colitis in Mice. *Int. J. Mol. Sci.* **2023**, *24*, 3517. [CrossRef]
191. Lajczak-McGinley, N.K.; Porru, E.; Fallon, C.M.; Smyth, J.; Curley, C.; McCarron, P.A.; Tambuwala, M.M.; Roda, A.; Keely, S.J. The secondary bile acids, ursodeoxycholic acid and lithocholic acid, protect against intestinal inflammation by inhibition of epithelial apoptosis. *Physiol. Rep.* **2020**, *8*, e14456. [CrossRef] [PubMed]
192. Watanabe, S.; Chen, Z.; Fujita, K.; Nishikawa, M.; Ueda, H.; Iguchi, Y.; Une, M.; Nishida, T.; Imura, J. Hyodeoxycholic Acid (HDCA) Prevents Development of Dextran Sulfate Sodium (DSS)-Induced Colitis in Mice: Possible Role of Synergism between DSS and HDCA in Increasing Fecal Bile Acid Levels. *Biol. Pharm. Bull.* **2022**, *45*, 1503–1509. [CrossRef] [PubMed]
193. Liu, Y.; Xu, J.; Ren, X.; Zhang, Y.; Ke, Z.; Zhou, J.; Wang, Y.; Zhang, Y.; Liu, Y. Cholecystectomy-induced secondary bile acids accumulation ameliorates colitis through inhibiting monocyte/macrophage recruitment. *Gut Microbes* **2022**, *14*, 2107387. [CrossRef] [PubMed]
194. Cao, S.S.; Zimmermann, E.M.; Chuang, B.M.; Song, B.; Nwokoye, A.; Wilkinson, J.E.; Eaton, K.A.; Kaufman, R.J. The unfolded protein response and chemical chaperones reduce protein misfolding and colitis in mice. *Gastroenterology* **2013**, *144*, 989–1000.e6. [CrossRef]
195. Zhao, J.; Hao, S.; Chen, Y.; Ye, X.; Fang, P.; Hu, H. Tauroursodeoxycholic acid liposome alleviates DSS-induced ulcerative colitis through restoring intestinal barrier and gut microbiota. *Colloids Surf. B Biointerfaces* **2024**, *236*, 113798. [CrossRef]

196. Huang, K.; Deng, F.S.; Liu, T.C.; Wang, M.; Gremida, A.K.; Deepak, P.; Chen, C.H.; Davidson, N.O.; Kaufman, R.J.; Ciorba, M.A. A Translational Phase I Study of Tauroursodeoxycholic Acid (Tudca) to Reduce Symptoms and Er Stress in Active Ulcerative Colitis. *Gastroenterology* **2021**, *160*, S707–S708. [CrossRef]
197. Lv, L.; Chen, Z.; Bai, W.; Hao, J.; Heng, Z.; Meng, C.; Wang, L.; Luo, X.; Wang, X.; Cao, Y.; et al. Taurohyodeoxycholic acid alleviates trinitrobenzene sulfonic acid induced ulcerative colitis via regulating Th1/Th2 and Th17/Treg cells balance. *Life Sci.* **2023**, *318*, 121501. [CrossRef]
198. Li, W.; Hang, S.; Fang, Y.; Bae, S.; Zhang, Y.; Zhang, M.; Wang, G.; McCurry, M.D.; Bae, M.; Paik, D.; et al. A bacterial bile acid metabolite modulates T(reg) activity through the nuclear hormone receptor NR4A1. *Cell Host Microbe* **2021**, *29*, 1366–1377.e9. [CrossRef]
199. Campbell, C.; McKenney, P.T.; Konstantinovsky, D.; Isaeva, O.I.; Schizas, M.; Verter, J.; Mai, C.; Jin, W.B.; Guo, C.J.; Violante, S.; et al. Bacterial metabolism of bile acids promotes generation of peripheral regulatory T cells. *Nature* **2020**, *581*, 475–479. [CrossRef]
200. Xu, M.; Cen, M.; Shen, Y.; Zhu, Y.; Cheng, F.; Tang, L.; Hu, W.; Dai, N. Deoxycholic Acid-Induced Gut Dysbiosis Disrupts Bile Acid Enterohepatic Circulation and Promotes Intestinal Inflammation. *Dig. Dis. Sci.* **2021**, *66*, 568–576. [CrossRef]
201. Li, D.; Zhou, J.; Wang, L.; Gong, Z.; Le, H.; Huang, Y.; Xu, C.; Tian, C.; Cai, W.; Wu, J. Gut microbial metabolite deoxycholic acid facilitates Th17 differentiation through modulating cholesterol biosynthesis and participates in high-fat diet-associated colonic inflammation. *Cell Biosci.* **2023**, *13*, 186. [CrossRef] [PubMed]
202. Ju, J.; Zhang, C.; Yang, J.; Yang, Q.; Yin, P.; Sun, X. Deoxycholic acid exacerbates intestinal inflammation by modulating interleukin-1beta expression and tuft cell proportion in dextran sulfate sodium-induced murine colitis. *PeerJ* **2023**, *11*, e14842. [CrossRef] [PubMed]
203. Nakhi, A.; Wong, H.L.; Weldy, M.; Khoruts, A.; Sadowsky, M.J.; Dosa, P.I. Structural modifications that increase gut restriction of bile acid derivatives. *RSC Med. Chem.* **2021**, *12*, 394–405. [CrossRef] [PubMed]
204. Fujita, Y.; Sugaya, T.; Inui, A.; Yoshihara, S. Effectiveness of Ursodeoxycholic Acid in the Treatment of Primary Sclerosing Cholangitis with Ulcerative Colitis: A Pediatric Case. *Tohoku J. Exp. Med.* **2021**, *253*, 109–112. [CrossRef] [PubMed]
205. Dong, X.; Qi, M.; Cai, C.; Zhu, Y.; Li, Y.; Coulter, S.; Sun, F.; Liddle, C.; Uboha, N.V.; Halberg, R.; et al. Farnesoid X receptor mediates macrophage-intrinsic responses to suppress colitis-induced colon cancer progression. *JCI Insight* **2024**, *9*, 170428. [CrossRef]
206. Xu, P.; Xi, Y.; Zhu, J.; Zhang, M.; Luka, Z.; Stolz, D.B.; Cai, X.; Xie, Y.; Xu, M.; Ren, S.; et al. Intestinal Sulfation Is Essential to Protect Against Colitis and Colonic Carcinogenesis. *Gastroenterology* **2021**, *161*, 271–286.e11. [CrossRef]
207. Fathima, A.; Jamma, T. UDCA ameliorates inflammation driven EMT by inducing TGR5 dependent SOCS1 expression in mouse macrophages. *Sci. Rep.* **2024**, *14*, 24285. [CrossRef]
208. Kempinska-Podhorodecka, A.; Adamowicz, M.; Ostrycharz, E.; Chmielarz, M.; Wojcicki, M.; Milkiewicz, P.; Milkiewicz, M. Role of miR-506 in ulcerative colitis associated with primary sclerosing cholangitis. *Sci. Rep.* **2021**, *11*, 10134. [CrossRef]
209. Kempinska-Podhorodecka, A.; Blatkiewicz, M.; Wunsch, E.; Krupa, L.; Gutkowski, K.; Milkiewicz, P.; Milkiewicz, M. Oncomir MicroRNA-346 Is Upregulated in Colons of Patients with Primary Sclerosing Cholangitis. *Clin. Transl. Gastroenterol.* **2020**, *11*, e00112. [CrossRef]
210. Lavelle, A.; Nancey, S.; Reimund, J.M.; Laharie, D.; Marteau, P.; Treton, X.; Allez, M.; Roblin, X.; Malamut, G.; Oeuvray, C.; et al. Fecal microbiota and bile acids in IBD patients undergoing screening for colorectal cancer. *Gut Microbes* **2022**, *14*, 2078620. [CrossRef]
211. Rotondo-Trivette, S.; Wang, B.; Gayer, C.; Parsana, R.; Luan, Y.; Sun, F.; Michail, S. Decreased secondary faecal bile acids in children with ulcerative colitis and Clostridioides difficile infection. *Aliment. Pharmacol. Ther.* **2021**, *54*, 792–804. [CrossRef] [PubMed]
212. Jin, W.B.; Li, T.T.; Huo, D.; Qu, S.; Li, X.V.; Arifuzzaman, M.; Lima, S.F.; Shi, H.Q.; Wang, A.; Putzel, G.G.; et al. Genetic manipulation of gut microbes enables single-gene interrogation in a complex microbiome. *Cell* **2022**, *185*, 547–562.e22. [CrossRef] [PubMed]
213. Chen, M.L.; Huang, X.; Wang, H.; Hegner, C.; Liu, Y.; Shang, J.; Eliason, A.; Diao, H.; Park, H.; Frey, B.; et al. CAR directs T cell adaptation to bile acids in the small intestine. *Nature* **2021**, *593*, 147–151. [CrossRef] [PubMed]
214. Xu, M.; Shen, Y.; Cen, M.; Zhu, Y.; Cheng, F.; Tang, L.; Zheng, X.; Kim, J.J.; Dai, N.; Hu, W. Modulation of the Gut Microbiota-farnesoid X Receptor Axis Improves Deoxycholic Acid-induced Intestinal Inflammation in Mice. *J. Crohns Colitis* **2021**, *15*, 1197–1210. [CrossRef] [PubMed]
215. Miyazaki, T.; Shirakami, Y.; Mizutani, T.; Maruta, A.; Ideta, T.; Kubota, M.; Sakai, H.; Ibuka, T.; Genovese, S.; Fiorito, S.; et al. Novel FXR agonist nelumal A suppresses colitis and inflammation-related colorectal carcinogenesis. *Sci. Rep.* **2021**, *11*, 492. [CrossRef]
216. Chen, L.; Jiao, T.; Liu, W.; Luo, Y.; Wang, J.; Guo, X.; Tong, X.; Lin, Z.; Sun, C.; Wang, K.; et al. Hepatic cytochrome P450 8B1 and cholic acid potentiate intestinal epithelial injury in colitis by suppressing intestinal stem cell renewal. *Cell Stem Cell* **2022**, *29*, 1366–1381.e9. [CrossRef]
217. Xin, Z.; Zhai, Z.; Long, H.; Zhang, F.; Ni, X.; Deng, J.; Yi, L.; Deng, B. Metabolic Profiling by UPLC-Orbitrap-MS/MS of Liver from C57BL/6 Mice with DSS-Induced Inflammatory Bowel Disease. *Mediat. Inflamm.* **2020**, *2020*, 6020247. [CrossRef]
218. Hernandez-Rocha, C.; Borowski, K.; Turpin, W.; Filice, M.; Nayeri, S.; Raygoza Garay, J.A.; Stempak, J.M.; Silverberg, M.S. Integrative Analysis of Colonic Biopsies from Inflammatory Bowel Disease Patients Identifies an Interaction Between Microbial Bile Acid-inducible Gene Abundance and Human Angiopoietin-like 4 Gene Expression. *J. Crohns Colitis* **2021**, *15*, 2078–2087. [CrossRef]

219. Yan, S.; Du, R.; Yao, W.; Zhang, H.; Xue, Y.; Teligun; Li, Y.; Bao, H.; Zhao, Y.; Cao, S.; et al. Host-microbe interaction-mediated resistance to DSS-induced inflammatory enteritis in sheep. *Microbiome* **2024**, *12*, 208. [CrossRef]
220. Gadaleta, R.M.; Garcia-Irigoyen, O.; Cariello, M.; Scialpi, N.; Peres, C.; Vetrano, S.; Fiorino, G.; Danese, S.; Ko, B.; Luo, J.; et al. Fibroblast Growth Factor 19 modulates intestinal microbiota and inflammation in presence of Farnesoid X Receptor. *eBioMedicine* **2020**, *54*, 102719. [CrossRef]
221. He, S.; Li, J.; Yao, Z.; Gao, Z.; Jiang, Y.; Chen, X.; Peng, L. Insulin alleviates murine colitis through microbiome alterations and bile acid metabolism. *J. Transl. Med.* **2023**, *21*, 498. [CrossRef]
222. Foley, S.E.; Tuohy, C.; Dunford, M.; Grey, M.J.; De Luca, H.; Cawley, C.; Szabady, R.L.; Maldonado-Contreras, A.; Houghton, J.M.; Ward, D.V.; et al. Gut microbiota regulation of P-glycoprotein in the intestinal epithelium in maintenance of homeostasis. *Microbiome* **2021**, *9*, 183. [CrossRef]
223. Zhao, Y.; Xiang, Z.; Pan, H.; Huang, X.; Chen, W.; Huang, Z. FGL2 improves experimental colitis related to gut microbiota structure and bile acid metabolism by regulating macrophage autophagy and apoptosis. *Heliyon* **2024**, *10*, e34349. [CrossRef]
224. Peters, D.E.; Norris, L.D.; Tenora, L.; Snajdr, I.; Ponti, A.K.; Zhu, X.; Sakamoto, S.; Veeravalli, V.; Pradhan, M.; Alt, J.; et al. A gut-restricted glutamate carboxypeptidase II inhibitor reduces monocytic inflammation and improves preclinical colitis. *Sci. Transl. Med.* **2023**, *15*, eabn7491. [CrossRef]
225. Gonzalez, C.G.; Mills, R.H.; Kordahi, M.C.; Carrillo-Terrazas, M.; Secaira-Morocho, H.; Widjaja, C.E.; Tsai, M.S.; Mittal, Y.; Yee, B.A.; Vargas, F.; et al. The Host-Microbiome Response to Hyperbaric Oxygen Therapy in Ulcerative Colitis Patients. *Cell Mol. Gastroenterol. Hepatol.* **2022**, *14*, 35–53. [CrossRef]
226. Liu, A.; Li, C.; Wang, C.; Liang, X.; Zhang, X. Impact of Mesenchymal Stem Cells on the Gut Microbiota and Microbiota Associated Functions in Inflammatory Bowel Disease: A Systematic Review of Preclinical Evidence on Animal Models. *Curr. Stem Cell Res. Ther.* **2024**, *19*, 981–992. [CrossRef]
227. Yang, F.; Ni, B.; Liu, Q.; He, F.; Li, L.; Zhong, X.; Zheng, X.; Lu, J.; Chen, X.; Lin, H.; et al. Human umbilical cord-derived mesenchymal stem cells ameliorate experimental colitis by normalizing the gut microbiota. *Stem Cell Res. Ther.* **2022**, *13*, 475. [CrossRef]
228. Ocansey, D.K.W.; Zhang, Z.; Xu, X.; Liu, L.; Amoah, S.; Chen, X.; Wang, B.; Zhang, X.; Mao, F. Mesenchymal stem cell-derived exosome mitigates colitis via the modulation of the gut metagenomics-metabolomics-farnesoid X receptor axis. *Biomater. Sci.* **2022**, *10*, 4822–4836. [CrossRef]
229. Mohanty, I.; Mannochio-Russo, H.; Schweer, J.V.; El Abiead, Y.; Bittremieux, W.; Xing, S.; Schmid, R.; Zuffa, S.; Vasquez, F.; Muti, V.B.; et al. The underappreciated diversity of bile acid modifications. *Cell* **2024**, *187*, 1801–1818.e20. [CrossRef]
230. Vich Vila, A.; Zhang, J.; Liu, M.; Faber, K.N.; Weersma, R.K. Untargeted faecal metabolomics for the discovery of biomarkers and treatment targets for inflammatory bowel diseases. *Gut* **2024**, *73*, 1909–1920. [CrossRef]

biomedicines

MDPI

Article

Characteristics of Mucosa-Associated Microbiota in Ulcerative Colitis Patients with 5-Aminosalicylic Acid Intolerance

Hiroshi Matsumoto [1,*], Momoyo Sasahira [1], Tei Tei Go [1], Shogen Yo [1], Takehiro Ninomiya [1], Motoyasu Osawa [1], Osamu Handa [1], Eiji Umegami [1], Ryo Inoue [2] and Akiko Shiotani [1]

[1] Department of Gastroenterology, Kawasaki Medical School, Okayama 701-0192, Japan; momomo0318@gmail.com (M.S.); gutingting0529@med.kawasaki-m.ac.jp (T.T.G.); yoshogen@med.kawasaki-m.ac.jp (S.Y.); takehiro.nino0614@gmail.com (T.N.); o.m1976-1017@med.kawasaki-m.ac.jp (M.O.); handao@med.kawasaki-m.ac.jp (O.H.); eumegaki@med.kawasaki-m.ac.jp (E.U.); shiotani@med.kawasaki-m.ac.jp (A.S.)

[2] Faculty of Agriculture, Setsunan University, 45-1 Nagaotoge-cho, Hirakata 573-0101, Japan; ryo.inoue@setsunan.ac.jp

* Correspondence: hmatsumoto0311@gmail.com; Tel.: +81-86-462-1111

Abstract: Background/Objectives: 5-Aminosalicylic acid (5-ASA) is a first-line therapy for ulcerative colitis (UC). This study examined the mucosa-associated microbiota (MAM) in UC patients, distinguishing between those who were 5-ASA tolerant and intolerant. Methods: Brushing samples were collected from the sigmoid and ileal end of patients with UC during endoscopic procedures. The samples were profiled by using the Illumina MiSeq platform. The V3–V4 regions of the 16S rRNA gene (460 bp) were amplified by using tailed PCR. Results: A total of 15 patients with 5-ASA intolerance, 38 patients with 5-ASA tolerance, and 19 healthy controls were recruited in this study. The α-diversity indices were remarkably different among the three groups in the ileum mucosa but not in the sigmoid colon. In the ileum mucosa, Alistipes, Ruminococcaceae, and Odoribacter were less abundant in the 5-ASA-intolerant group than in the control and 5-ASA-tolerant groups. On the contrary, Merdibacter, Brevundimonas, and Porphyromonas were more abundant in the 5-ASA-intolerant group than in other groups. Conclusions: The present study showed that the changes in MAM were characterized by a decrease in mucoprotective bacteria rather than an increase in harmful bacteria.

Keywords: gut microbiota; mucosa-associated microbiota; ulcerative colitis; 5-ASA intolerance; dysbiosis

1. Introduction

Ulcerative colitis (UC) is a chronic inflammatory disease that impacts the colon and rectum [1]. In genetically susceptible individuals, intestinal inflammation occurs due to an overactive immune response and imbalanced intestinal microbiota. However, the mechanism of UC remains unclear [2–4]. Bacterial dysbiosis in IBD is characterized by a reduction in bacterial diversity, a decrease in the Firmicutes phylum (Faecalibacterium, Blautia, Roseburia, et al.), and an increase in the Proteobacteria phylum (Enterobacteriaceae, including Eschrichia) [5–7]. Compared with healthy subjects, an increase in fecal Proteobacteria and a decrease in Firmicutes have been observed in IBD patients; additionally, compared with patients in remission, the mucosa of patients in an active stage were colonized with a higher abundance of Proteobacteria and a lower abundance of Firmicutes.

Treatments for UC are based on the severity of the symptoms and may include corticosteroids, biological therapies, small molecular drugs, adhesion molecule inhibitors, azathioprine or 6-mercaptopurine, and 5-aminosalicylic acid (5-ASA). For patients with mild-moderate UC, 5-ASA is the conventional treatment for the induction of remission. A 5-ASA-containing preparation is the first-line option for induction and maintenance therapy in patients with mild-to-moderate UC. 5-ASA-containing preparations have two major types, namely, mesalazine/5-ASA and sulfasalazine (SASP), which are currently used as first-line therapy for UC [8–10]. SASP is composed of 5-ASA linked to sulfapyridine by a diazo bond, and this bond is readily cleaved by bacterial azoreductases in the colon [11]. 5-ASA is absorbed by intestinal epithelial cells, providing anti-inflammatory benefits to the intestinal mucosa. 5-ASA may neutralize oxidative stress inflicted by macrophages and neutrophils, preventing leukotriene synthesis and the recruitment of inflammatory cells [12]. Mehta R et al. reported that the gut microbial metabolism of 5-ASA diminishes its clinical efficacy in inflammatory bowel disease (IBD) [13]. Twelve uncharacterized microbial acetyltransferases, which belong to thiolases and acyl-CoA N-acyltransferase superfamilies, are linked to 5-ASA inactivation.

Recent experimental data suggest that the gut microbiome plays a role in the pharmacokinetics of several medications [14–16]. For example, gut microbial enzymes were recently identified and characterized in vitro to metabolize digoxin and L-dopa, medications for heart failure and Parkinson's disease, respectively. In humans, association studies suggest a role of the microbiome in modulating the drug efficacy of anti-cytokine biologics and cardiometabolic drugs [17,18]. In addition, it focused on reports that the intestinal microbiota plays a significant role in the efficacy of immune checkpoint inhibitors, anti-programmed cell death protein 1 receptor (PD-1) therapy and cytotoxic T-lymphocyte-antigen (CTLA-4), against cancer [19,20]. Although they generally lack mechanistic explanations, drug metabolism by gut microbiota is associated with the effects and adverse events of 5-ASA and other drugs and may also be related to the clinical outcomes of the disease stage.

5-ASA and SASP are effective and safe, but some patients may become intolerant to 5-ASA [21,22]. 5-ASA can cause intolerance in up to 15% of patients, despite having few serious side effects [23–25]. Headache, skin rash, nausea, abdominal pain, and diarrhea comprise the list of mild adverse events. More severe adverse events include nephrotoxicity, hepatic dysfunction, pancreatitis, pericarditis, pneumonitis, severe skin reaction, toxic epidermal necrolysis, and acute gastroenteropathy, which is often referred to as "acute 5-ASA intolerance syndrome [26]". 5-ASA intolerance mechanisms include allergic reactions, chemical toxicity, and dysbiosis [27,28]. Mizuno S et al. reported that the 5-ASA-intolerant group had more fecal bacteria in the genera *Faecalibacterium*, *Streptococcus*, and *Clostridium* than the 5-ASA-tolerant group [29]. However, there are only reports about the association between 5-ASA intolerance and mucosa-associated microbiota (MAM).

Most studies on the gut microbiome have focused on fecal microbiota, which is predominantly found in the lumen. Meanwhile, stable MAM has received increased attention [30,31]. The precise and accurate evaluation of MAM is crucial for comprehending and distinguishing host–microbe interactions contributing to health promotion and diseases. In previous studies, we found differences in bacterial community profiles between endoscopic brushing samples and fecal samples. During colonoscopic procedures, brushing samples may replace the need for fecal samples in analyzing MAM [32].

The relationship between UC and MAM has already been reported [33]. The reduction in the abundance of butyric acid-producing bacteria, *Odoribacter*, in ileal MAM may play an important role in the pathophysiology of UC. In this study, the characteristics of MAM of 5-ASA intolerance in patients with UC were investigated. The relationship between 5-ASA intolerance and MAM was also examined to devise a therapeutic strategy for addressing 5-ASA intolerance. This study aims to characterize MAM in UC patients with 5-ASA-intolerant patients.

2. Materials and Methods

2.1. Ethics

Ethical approval was obtained from Kawasaki Medical School Ethic and Medical Research Committee (no.3087; Ethics Committee approval date is 18 May 2020, specific dates for study period 27 June 2020–21 June 2024). Written informed consent was achieved from each research subject before enrollment. All patients were enrolled at the Division of

Gastroenterology of Kawasaki Medical School Hospital. This study was registered at the University Hospital Medical Information Network Center.

2.2. Patients and Sample Collection

The enrolled subjects were as follows: healthy controls (HCs) undergoing routine medical checkups and patients with UC. The diagnosis of UC is based on a combination of clinical, biochemical, stool, endoscopic, and histological investigations [34]. As HCs, those who received any medication or complained of any gastrointestinal symptoms and patients with tumor lesions or inflammatory lesions found by colonoscopy were excluded. Only patients without antibiotic use within 3 months, colon cancer, history of colectomy, active GI bleeding, or hospital admission in the preceding 6 months were included. Samples were gathered from the terminal ileum and sigmoid colon using an endoscopic microbiology brush (COOK, Bloomington, IN, USA), following the standard polyethylene glycol preparation for colonoscopy. We analyzed the ileal mucus because we have previously reported that the ileal MAM is associated with severity and disease type in patients with UC [33]. Disease severity was evaluated on the basis of the Mayo endoscopic sub-score consisting of a four-point scoring system.

2.3. Definition of 5-ASA Intolerance

As defined in previous reports [23,24,35], 5-ASA intolerance is diagnosed when individuals have exhibited at least one symptom—headache, digestive symptoms, skin symptoms, or fever—upon 5-ASA administration.

2.4. DNA Extraction, PCR Amplification, Library Preparation, and 16SrRNA Sequencing

16SrRNA gene amplicon library was prepared and sequenced using previously reported methods for DNA extraction, amplicon generation, and sequencing [32]. A library of amplicons encoding the 16S rRNA gene was prepared, and sequencing was conducted as previously described [36]. The samples were profiled by high-throughput amplicon sequencing with dual-index barcoding using the Illumina Miseq platform (Illumina, San Diego, CA, USA). 16S rDNA's V3–V4 regions, spanning 460 base pairs, were amplified using tailed PCR [37]. Afterward, PCR amplicons were purified using SPRI select beads (Beckman Coulter, Brea, CA, USA). The DNA concentration of purified amplicons was measured using a Quantus Fluorometer and the QuantiFluor® dsDNA System (Promega, Madison, WI, USA), and an approximately equal amount of their DNA was pooled. The pooled sample was sequenced using the Miseq Reagent Kit V3 (600 cycles; Illumina, San Diego, CA, USA) on the Miseq system in accordance with the manufacturer's instructions.

2.5. Bioinformatics Analysis

Sequence data processing, consisting of quality filtering, chimera checking, operational taxonomic unit (OTU) definition, and taxonomic assignment, was accomplished using the combination of QIIME 1.9.0 (https://qiime2.org/), USEARCH 9.2.4 (https://cryptick-lab.github.io/NGS-Analysis/_site/usearch-previous.html), UCHIME 4.2.40 (https://www.drive5.com/usearch/), and VSEARCH 2.4.3 (https://github.com/torognes/vsearch/releases/tag/v2.28.1). Singletons were eliminated, and 97% sequence similarity OTUs were taxonomically assigned using the RDP classifier v2.10.2 with the Greengenes database version 13.8.

2.6. Alpha-Diversity

The observed features, Shannon entropy, and Chao 1 diversity indices were calculated by using the phyloseq package of R software (version 4.4.1). It was visualized by principal coordinate analysis and statistically analyzed using permutational multivariate analysis of variance (PERMANOVA) using R software. PERMANOVA was performed by using the vegan package (version 2.6-2).

2.7. Statistical Analysis

The differences in families among the lines were analyzed using the Statistical Analysis of Metagenomic Profiles (STAMP) software (version 2.1.3) [38]. The diversity and relative abundance of bacterial genera indices were compared among three groups by the Kruskal–Wallis analysis and compared between the two groups by the Mann–Whitney U test. The category data were analyzed using chi-square test. Statistical analyses were performed using SPSS (version 25 for Windows, IBM Japan, Ltd., Tokyo, Japan). Statistical significance was set at a p value of <0.05.

3. Results

3.1. Patient Background

Samples were obtained from 15 patients with UC who exhibited intolerance to 5-ASA (six men, mean age 48.1 years old), 38 patients with UC who demonstrated tolerance to 5-ASA (16 men, mean age 44.5 years old), and 19 controls (seven men, mean age 56.2 years old). The mean age was significantly older in the controls than in the UC group (Table 1). No significant difference in disease duration, disease type, type of 5-ASA, and endoscopic activity was found between the 5-ASA-tolerant and -intolerant groups. However, significant differences in biologics use were found; the 5-ASA-intolerant group used biologics more than the 5-ASA-tolerant group. In the 5-ASA-intolerant group, six patients showed negative results in the drug-induced lymphocyte stimulation test.

Table 1. Patient background.

	Control **19**	**5-ASA Tolerance Group** **38**	**5-ASA Intolerance Group** **15**	*p*
Age [mean ± SD]	56.2 ± 13.7	44.5 ± 16.1	48.1 ± 13.4	0.018
Gender (Male/Female)	7/12	16/22	6/9	NS
Disease duration (yr)	-	14.0 ± 9.1	14.1 ± 16.6	NS
Disease type Pan-colitis/Left side colitis/proctitis	-	18/16/4	11/4/0	NS
Type of 5ASA Time-dependant/pH-dependant/MMX/SASP	-	7/11/18/2	4/3/5/3	NS
Biologics TNFα/IL12-23/VED/JAK	-	7(18.4%) [3/1/3/0]	11(100%) [1/0/1/9]	<0.01
Endoscopic activity Mayo 0/1/2/3	-	29/7(95%)/2/0	7/2(82%)/2/0	NS
DLST Positive/negative/not inspected	-	-	0/6/5	

3.2. Analysis of Mucosa Samples

3.2.1. The α-Diversity Indices among the Three Groups Using Ileum Mucus

The median indices of observed features and chao1 were significantly lower ($p < 0.01$) in the 5-ASA-intolerant group than in the controls. Moreover, significant differences in the observed features, Shannon entropy, and Chao1 indices were found among the three groups (Figure 1). However, no statistically significant difference in β-diversity was found in the ileum.

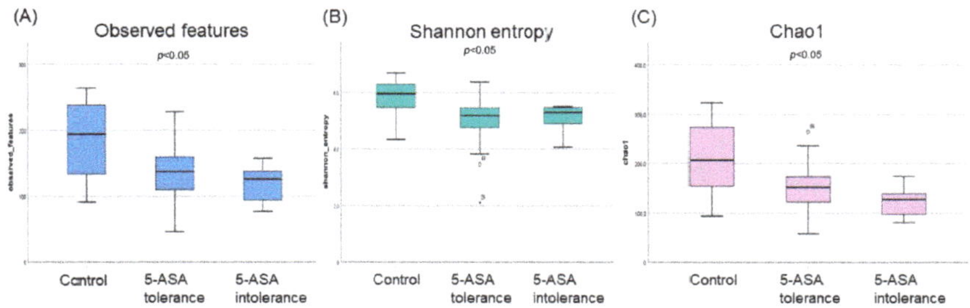

Figure 1. α-Diversity of ileal mucosa-associated microbiota (MAM); (**A**) observed features, (**B**) Shannon entropy, (**C**) Chao1.

3.2.2. Comparative Analyses of the Taxonomic Composition of the Ileum Microbial Community

Comparative analysis of the taxonomic composition at the genus level among the three groups was performed (Figure 2). In the 5-ASA-intolerant group, *Bacteroidota* were less abundant compared with the control group. On the contrary, *Firmicutes* were more abundant compared with the control group. *Lachnospiraceae*, *Oscillibacter*, and *Odoribacter* were less abundant in the 5-ASA-intolerant group than in the 5-ASA-tolerant group. In addition, *Methylobacterium* and *Brevundimonas* were more abundant in the 5-ASA-intolerant group than in the 5-ASA-tolerant group (Figures 3A–C and 4A–E).

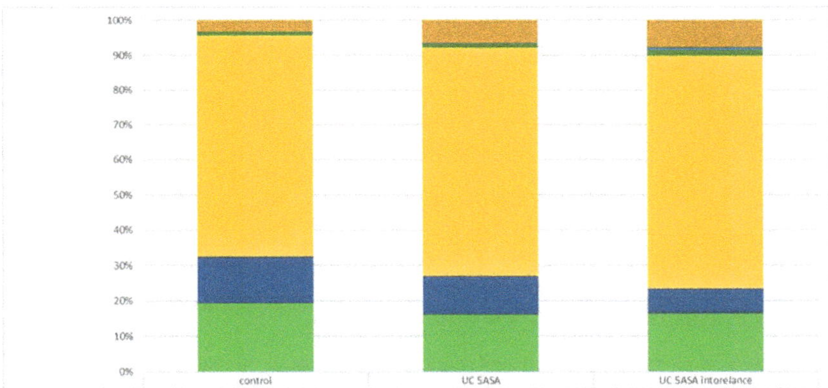

	control	UC 5ASA	UC 5ASA intorelance
p__Verrucomicrobiota	36	4.8	0.6
p__Synergistota	37	0	0
p__Spirochaetota	0.6	7.6	0
p__Proteobacteria	1,677	3,818	2,156
p__Patescibacteria	76	161	179
p__Fusobacteriota	478	629	443
p__Firmicutes	33,832	38,283	18,373
p__Desulfobacterota	119	28	12
p__Chloroflexi	0	0	0
p__Campilobacterota	29	2	0
p__Bacteroidota	6,959	6,458	1,929
p__Bdellovibrionota	0	0	0
p__Ascomycota	0	0	0
p__Aquificota	0	0	0
p__Actinobacteriota	10,363	9,414	4,532

Figure 2. Taxonomic analysis of mucosa-associated microbiota (MAM) analysis using ileum mucus.

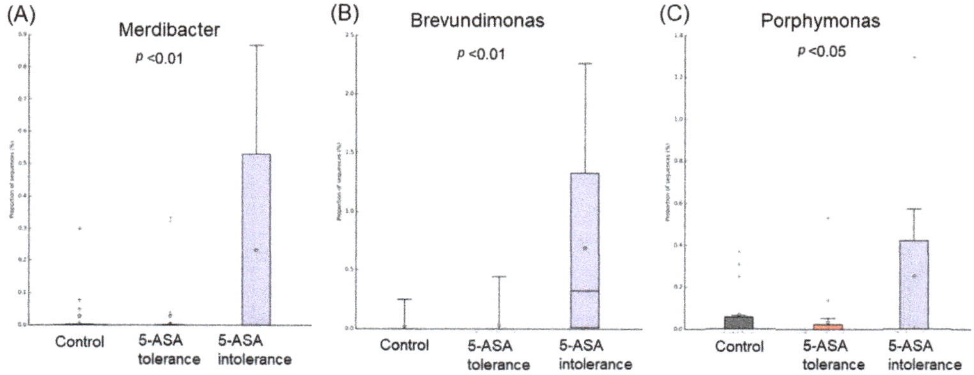

Figure 3. Comparison of three groups of ileal MAM: list of bacterial species that showed significant differences among three groups. The abundance of five intolerance groups was lower than the other two groups. (**A**) Merdibacter, (**B**) Brevundimonas, and (**C**) Porphymonas.

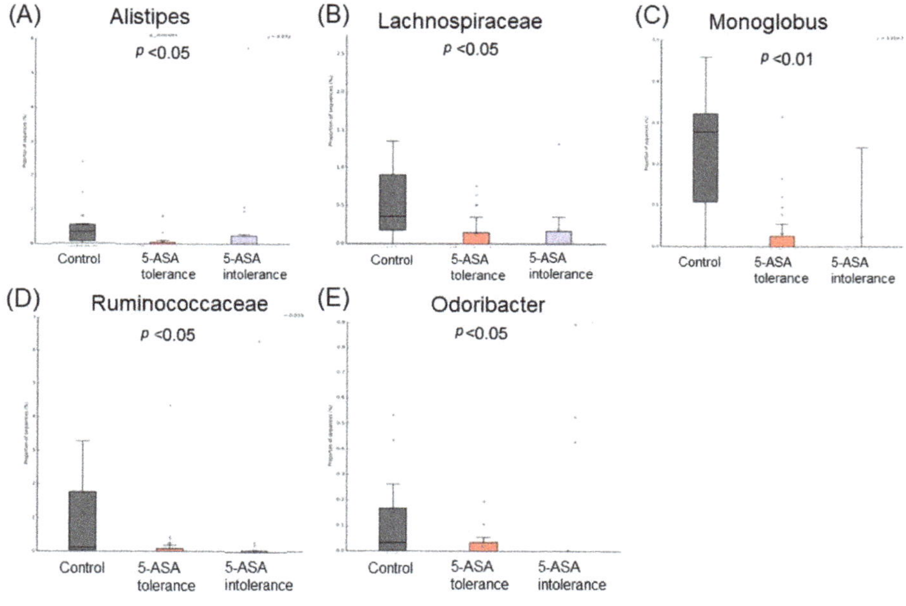

Figure 4. Comparison of three groups of ileal MAM: list of bacterial species that showed significant differences among three groups. The abundance of five intolerance groups was higher than the other two groups. (**A**) Alistipes, (**B**) Lachnospiraceae, (**C**) Monogiobus, (**D**) Ruminococcaceae, and (**E**) Odribacter.

3.2.3. Comparison between Two Groups of Ileal MAM (Figure 5)

Lachnospiraceae ND3007 and *Monoglobus* were significantly more abundant in the control group, while *Ruminococcus gravus* and *Veillonella* were substantially more abundant in the 5-ASA-resistant group (Figure 5A). *Blautis, Fusicatenibacter, Ruminococcus torques, Ruminococcus, Butyrucicoccaceae,* and *Lachnociostridium* were significantly more abundant in the control group than in the 5-ASA intolerance group (Figure 5B). *Lachnospiraceae, Fusicatenibacter, Ruminococcus torques, Lachnospiraceae UCG-004, Dorea, Lachnoclostridium,* and *Ruminococcus gauvreauii* were significantly more abundant in the 5-ASA intolerance group than in the 5-ASA tolerance group (Figure 5C).

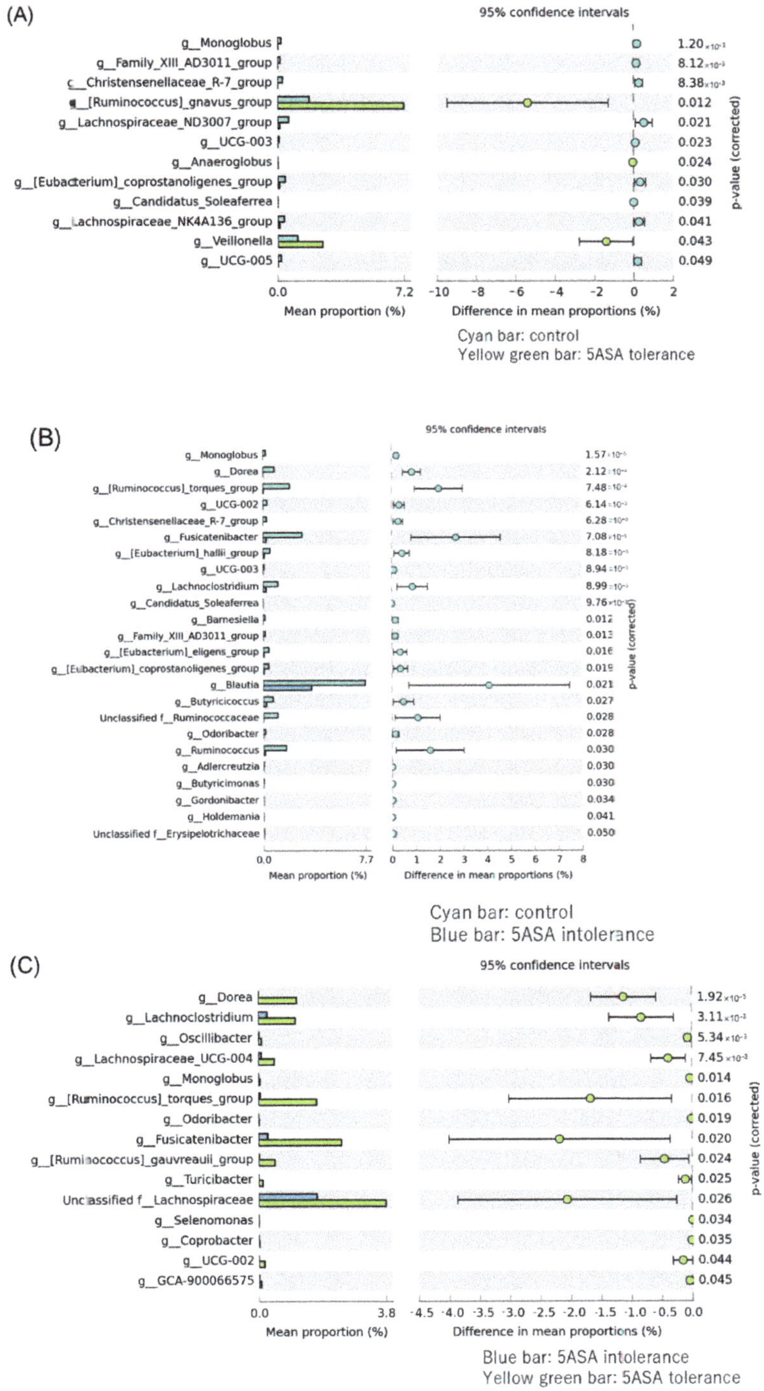

Figure 5. Comparison between two groups of ileal MAM. Bacteria species that showed significant differences between the two groups of (**A**) control (cyan bar) and 5-ASA tolerance (yellow green bar), (**B**) control and 5-ASA intolerance (blue bar), (**C**) 5-ASA intolerance and tolerance.

3.2.4. The α-Diversity Indices among the Three Groups Using Sigmoid Colonic Mucus

The median indices of the observed features and Chao1r were significantly lower ($p < 0.01$) in the 5-ASA-intolerant group than in the controls. Moreover, significant differences in the observed features, Shannon entropy, and Chao1 indices were observed among the three groups (Figure 6).

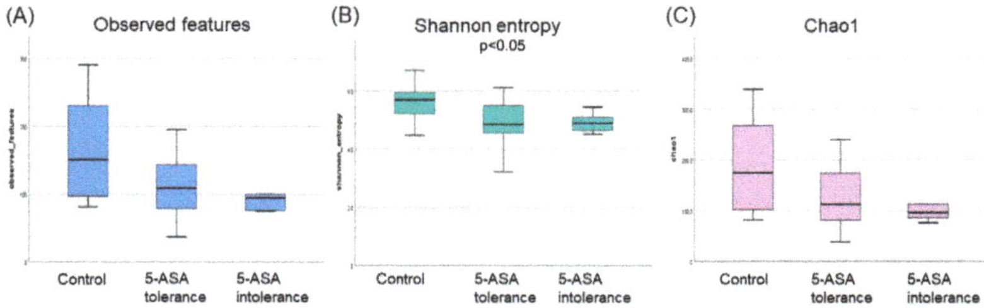

Figure 6. α-Diversity of colonic mucosa-associated microbiota (MAM): (**A**) observed features, (**B**) Shannon entropy, and (**C**) Chao 1.

3.2.5. Comparative Analyses of the Taxonomic Composition of the Microbial Community

Comparative analysis of the taxonomic composition at the genus level among the three groups was performed (Figure 7). *Proteobacteria* were less abundant in the 5-ASA-intolerant group than in HCs. *Actinobacteria* were more abundant in the 5-ASA-intolerant group than in HCs. *Oscillibacter* in the 5-ASA-intolerant group were more abundant than that in the 5-ASA-tolerant group (Figures 8A–C and 9A,B).

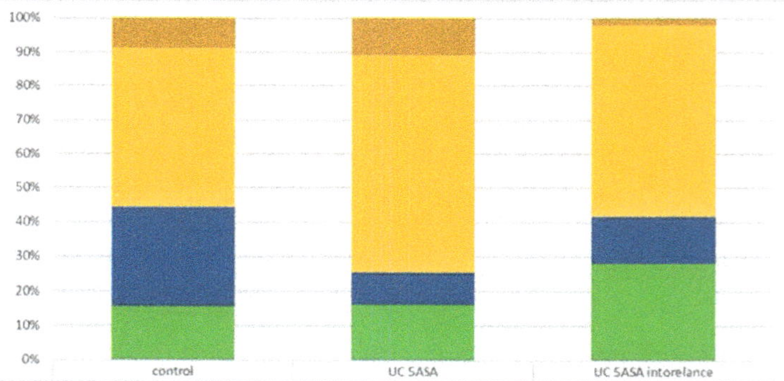

	control	UC 5ASA	UC 5ASA intorelance
p__Verrucomicrobiota	6	0.3	0
p__Synergistota	0	0	0
p__Spirochaetota	0	0.4	0
p__Proteobacteria	3,693	4,474	1,524
p__Patescibacteria	4.5	13.5	2.5
p__Fusobacteriota	1.5	79.7	0
p__Firmicutes	19,722	26,369	42,434
p__Desulfobacterota	145	0	58
p__Chloroflexi	0	0	0
p__Campilobacterota	0	19.8	0
p__Bacteroidota	11,955	3,809	10,201
p__Bdellovibrionota	0	0	0
p__Ascomycota	0	0	0
p__Aquificota	0	0	0
p__Actinobacteriota	6,648	6,752	21,137

Figure 7. Taxonomic analysis of mucosa-associated microbiota (MAM) analysis using colonic mucus.

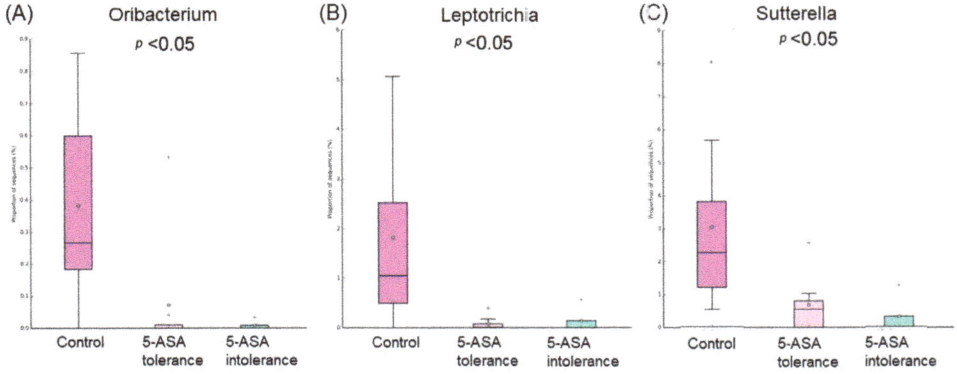

Figure 8. Comparison of three groups of colonic MAM: list of bacterial species that showed significant differences among three groups. The abundance of five intolerance groups was lower than the other two groups. (**A**) Oribacterium, (**B**) Laptotrichia, and (**C**) Sutterella.

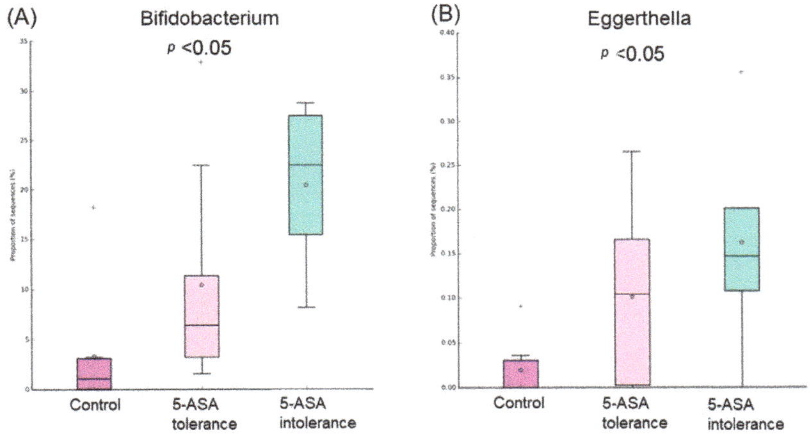

Figure 9. Comparison of three groups of colonic MAM: list of bacterial species that showed significant differences among three groups. The abundance of five intolerance groups was higher than the other two groups. (**A**) Bifidobacterium and (**B**) Eggerthella.

3.2.6. Comparison between Two Groups of Sigmoid Colonic MAM

Ruminococcus gnavus and *Incetrae sedis* were significantly more abundant in the 5-ASA tolerance group (purple group), while Prevotella, Sutterella, Leptotrichiam and Ruminococcaceae were substantially more abundant in the control group (red group) (Figure 10A). *Bifidobacterium* were significantly more abundant in the 5-ASA intolerance group, while Prevotella, Sutterella, Ruminococcaceae and Oribacterium were substantially more abundant in the control group (B). Anaerostipes and Lactobillus were significantly more abundant in the 5-ASA intolerance group, while *Incetae, Oscillibacter* and *Eubacterium nodatum* were substantially more abundant in the 5-ASA-resistant group (C).

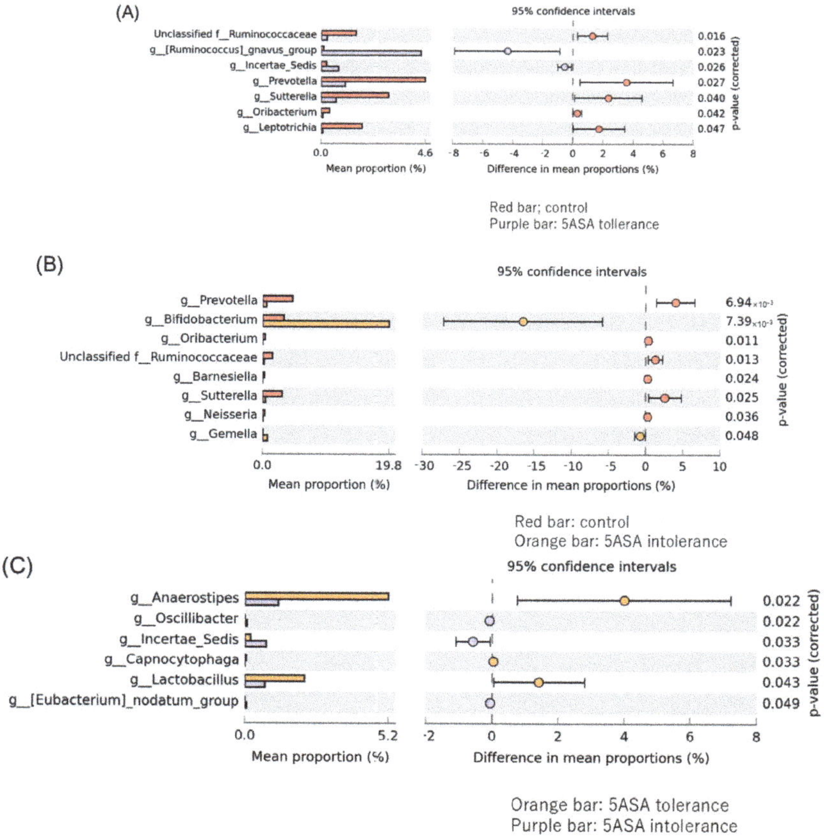

Figure 10. Comparison between two groups of sigmoid colonic MAM. Bacteria species that showed significant differences between the two groups of (**A**) control (red bar) and 5-ASA tolerance (purple bar), (**B**) control and 5-ASA intolerance (orange bar), (**C**) 5-ASA intolerance and tolerance.

4. Discussion

This study is the first to describe the relationship between 5-ASA intolerance UC and MAM. In addition, the result of MAM analysis using ileal and sigmoid colon samples was different in the 5-ASA-intolerant group. In particular, this was the first time that ileal samples were analyzed, and fewer bacteria, such as Oribacterium and Alistipes, in the 5-ASA-intolerant group were found to be effective for UC–fecal microbiota transplantation (FMT). Furthermore, fewer short fatty acid-producing bacteria, such as Lachnospiraceae and Ruminococcus, were found.

5-ASA intolerance development mechanisms are linked to an allergic reaction to 5-ASA preparations. Previous studies have revealed that the pathogenesis of UC involves many factors, such as immunological function, environmental factors, genetic predisposition, and intestinal microbiota, and suggested that the disturbance of the intestinal microbiota (dysbiosis) may be involved in 5-ASA intolerance [27,28].

Several studies have discussed beneficial butyrate-producing bacteria such as *Faecalibacterium prausnitzii* and Ruminococcaceae in 5-ASA-intolerant ulcerative colitis patients [39]. On the other hand, there are other reports of an increase in potentially harmful bacteria such as Enterobacteriaceae, Streptococcus, Veillonella, and Klebsiella in 5-ASA-intolerant UC patients [29]. These changes are in the feces, and our study used mucus. The present study examined changes in mucus and was characterized by a decrease in mucoprotective bacteria rather than an increase in harmful bacteria; the genera Ruminococcus and Lachnospiraceae were more abundant in healthy subjects and in UC long-term remission than in UC short-term remission and relapse patients. The abundance of *F. praegeri* was higher in healthy subjects and UC long-term remission than in UC short-term remission and relapse patients. *F. prausnitzii* and Lactobacillus were inversely proportional to UC disease severity, while Bacteroides, Hemophilus, and Veillonella were directly proportional [40].

In the 5-ASA-intolerant group, the abundance of Odoribacter and Alistipes, which are the key bacteria to effective FMT, was low in the ileal mucosa samples. An anaerobic Gram-negative bacterium, *Odoribacter splanchnicus*, generates SCFAs, including acetate, propionate, and butyric acid. SCFAs directly impact epithelial cells and influence Treg responses. The decrease in *O. splanchnicus* in IBD patients might stem from lower intestinal SCFA levels [41]. In a study by Lima et al., patients with UC who received FMT and had high levels of *O. splanchnicus* in their immunoglobulin A-coated microbiota had better clinical responses [42].

Alistipes may have defensive impacts against some illnesses, including liver fibrosis, colitis, cancer immunotherapy, and cardiovascular diseases [43]. *A. finegoldii* may be a protective species against colitis because *A. finegoldii* is diminished in mice with colitis. Thus, a study was performed in which microbiota-depleted mice were treated with oral DSS to induce colitis. The administration of *A. finegoldii* to mice resulted in a colitis severity comparable to that observed in wild-type mice [44]. In addition, previous studies have shown a common trend in Alistipes abundance in NOD2 knock-out murine microbiota profiles [45].

In fecal microbiota transplantation (FMT), fecal microbiota extracted from a healthy donor is placed into a patient's intestine to rectify microbiome imbalance [46]. Several investigations, encompassing randomized controlled trials [47–50], systematic reviews, and meta-analyses [51–53], have indicated that fecal microbiota transplantation (FMT) is a viable treatment option for patients with active ulcerative colitis (UC). Evidence suggests that FMT may demonstrate greater efficacy compared to alternative microbial modulation strategies, such as the use of antibiotics, probiotics, and prebiotics.

Intestinal microbiota related to the gut–kidney axis were abundant in the sigmoid colon. Renal dysfunction is an adverse event of 5-ASA. The relationship between 5-ASA and gut bacteria is intricate, but it is not directly associated with kidney damage. 5-ASA can alter the gut microbiota composition, as shown in a study where it increased the relative abundance of Firmicutes and Actinobacteria, which include beneficial bacteria, and decreased the abundance of Bacteroidetes. This alteration in gut microbiota could contribute to various physiological effects, including impacts on the immune system. However, this study did not directly associate these changes with kidney damage. Alternatively, this study focused on the general effects of 5-ASA on gut bacteria and the potential implications for intestinal health and inflammation control. The detailed effects of these microbiota changes on kidney function or potential damage are not explicitly outlined in this study; thus, further research is necessary to establish any direct link.

The relationship between commonly used drugs and changes in the gut microbiome has been extensively studied, and several key findings are considered. One study showed that alimentary tract drugs such as proton pump inhibitors, osmotically acting laxatives, aminosalicylic acid, and similar agents can markedly alter the gut microbiome [54]. In this study, compared with the controls, the 5-ASA-intolerant group showed reduced ileal MAM diversity despite sampling in the absence of 5-ASA medication. Different results were observed when the administration of the current 5-ASA medication in the 5-ASA-intolerant group. Therefore, further research must be conducted to clarify the MAM of the 5-ASA-intolerant group during 5-ASA current medication.

This study also has some limitations. First, the number of cases studied is small for a single-center study. Second, fecal microbiota and metabolites have not been studied. Third, this study has a large number of inactive UC, and changes during the active phase are unknown. Moreover, the types of 5-ASA, pH-dependent, time-dependent, MMX, and

SASP have not been studied. No 5-ASA intolerance symptom-specific studies have been conducted. Thus, further research must be conducted to clarify these limitations.

In this study, the relationship between 5-ASA intolerance and MAM was investigated. Interestingly, ileal MAM is different from sigmoid colon MAM in the 5-ASA-intolerant group. The present study showed changes in MAM and was characterized by a decrease in mucoprotective bacteria rather than an increase in harmful bacteria in 5-ASA intolerance patients.

Author Contributions: Conceptualization, H.M. and A.S.; methodology, T.T.G. and R.I.; validation, M.S., S.Y., T.T.G., T.N., M.O. and O.H.; formal analysis, T.T.G. and M.S.; investigation, H.M. and R.I.; resources, T.T.G.; data curation, T.T.G.; writing—original draft preparation, H.M. and S.Y.; writing—review and editing, A.S. and E.U.; visualization, H.M.; supervision, A.S.; project administration, H.M.; funding acquisition, H.M. All authors have read and agreed to the published version of the manuscript.

Funding: This research was funded by the project funding of Kawasaki Medical School.

Institutional Review Board Statement: Ethical approval was obtained from Kawasaki Medical School Ethic and Medical Research Committee (no.3087; Ethics Committee approval date is 18 May 2020, specific dates for study period 27 June 2020–21 June 2024).

Informed Consent Statement: Informed consent was obtained from all subjects involved in the study.

Data Availability Statement: The raw data supporting the conclusions of this article will be made available by the authors upon request. The data are restricted due to privacy reasons.

Acknowledgments: During the preparation of this work, Hiroshi Matsumoto used Grammarly, [free version; date of use: 14 September 2024] in order to check the English check. After using this tool/service, the author(s) reviewed and edited the content as needed and take(s) full responsibility for the content of the publication.

Conflicts of Interest: The authors declare no conflicts of interest.

References

1. Kobayashi, T.; Siegmund, B.; Le Berre, C.; Wei, S.C.; Ferrante, M.; Shen, B.; Bernstein, C.N.; Danese, S.; Peyrin-Biroulet, L.; Hibi, T. Ulcerative Colitis. *Nat. Rev. Dis. Primers* **2020**, *6*, 74. [CrossRef] [PubMed]
2. Chu, H.; Khosravi, A.; Kusumawardhani, I.P.; Kwon, A.H.K.; Vasconcelos, A.C.; Cunha, L.D.; Mayer, A.E.; Shen, Y.; Wu, W.-L.; Kambal, A.; et al. Gene-Microbiota Interactions Contribute to the Pathogenesis of Inflammatory Bowel Disease. *Science* **2016**, *352*, 1116–1120. [CrossRef] [PubMed]
3. Hu, S.; Vich Vila, A.; Gacesa, R.; Collij, V.; Stevens, C.; Fu, J.M.; Wong, I.; Talkowski, M.E.; Rivas, M.A.; Imhann, F.; et al. Whole Exome Sequencing Analyses Reveal Gene-Microbiota Interactions in the Context of IBD. *Gut* **2021**, *70*, 285–296. [CrossRef] [PubMed]
4. Qiu, P.; Ishimoto, T.; Fu, L.; Zhang, J.; Zhang, Z.; Liu, Y. The Gut Microbiota in Inflammatory Bowel Disease. *Front. Cell. Infect. Microbiol.* **2022**, *12*, 733992. [CrossRef] [PubMed]
5. Andoh, A.; Nishida, A. Alteration of the Gut Microbiome in Inflammatory Bowel Disease. *Digestion* **2023**, *104*, 16–23. [CrossRef]
6. Meade, S.; Liu Chen Kiow, J.; Massaro, C.; Kaur, G.; Squirell, E.; Bressler, B.; Lunken, G. Gut Microbiome-Associated Predictors as Biomarkers of Response to Advanced Therapies in Inflammatory Bowel Disease: A Systematic Review. *Gut Microbes* **2023**, *15*, 2287073. [CrossRef]
7. Shan, Y.; Lee, M.; Chang, E.B. The Gut Microbiome and Inflammatory Bowel Diseases. *Annu. Rev. Med.* **2022**, *73*, 455–468. [CrossRef]
8. Browne, A.S.; Kelly, C.R. Fecal Transplant in Inflammatory Bowel Disease. *Gastroenterol. Clin. N. Am.* **2017**, *46*, 825–837. [CrossRef]
9. Matsuoka, K.; Kobayashi, T.; Ueno, F.; Matsui, T.; Hirai, F.; Inoue, N.; Kato, J.; Kobayashi, K.; Kobayashi, K.; Koganei, K.; et al. Evidence-Based Clinical Practice Guidelines for Inflammatory Bowel Disease. *J. Gastroenterol.* **2018**, *53*, 305–353. [CrossRef]
10. Harbord, M.; Eliakim, R.; Bettenworth, D.; Karmiris, K.; Katsanos, K.; Kopylov, U.; Kucharzik, T.; Molnár, T.; Raine, T.; Sebastian, S.; et al. Third European Evidence-Based Consensus on Diagnosis and Management of Ulcerative Colitis. Part 2: Current Management. *J. Crohns Colitis* **2017**, *11*, 769–784. [CrossRef]
11. Peppercorn, M.A.; Goldman, P. The Role of Intestinal Bacteria in the Metabolism of Salicylazosulfapyridine. *J. Pharmacol. Exp. Ther.* **1972**, *181*, 555–562. [PubMed]

12. Ko, C.W.; Singh, S.; Feuerstein, J.D.; Falck-Ytter, C.; Falck-Ytter, Y.; Cross, R.K.; American Gastroenterological Association Institute Clinical Guidelines Committee. AGA Clinical Practice Guidelines on the Management of Mild-to-Moderate Ulcerative Colitis. *Gastroenterology* **2019**, *156*, 748–764. [CrossRef] [PubMed]
13. Nakase, H.; Uchino, M.; Shinzaki, S.; Matsuura, M.; Matsuoka, K.; Kobayashi, T.; Saruta, M.; Hirai, F.; Hata, K.; Hiraoka, S.; et al. Evidence-Based Clinical Practice Guidelines for Inflammatory Bowel Disease 2020. *J. Gastroenterol.* **2021**, *56*, 489–526. [CrossRef] [PubMed]
14. Javdan, B.; Lopez, J.G.; Chankhamjon, P.; Lee, Y.-C.J.; Hull, R.; Wu, Q.; Wang, X.; Chatterjee, S.; Donia, M.S. Personalized Mapping of Drug Metabolism by the Human Gut Microbiome. *Cell* **2020**, *181*, 1661–1679.e22. [CrossRef] [PubMed]
15. Zimmermann, M.; Zimmermann-Kogadeeva, M.; Wegmann, R.; Goodman, A.L. Mapping Human Microbiome Drug Metabolism by Gut Bacteria and Their Genes. *Nature* **2019**, *570*, 462–467. [CrossRef]
16. Koppel, N.; Maini Rekdal, V.; Balskus, E.P. Chemical Transformation of Xenobiotics by the Human Gut Microbiota. *Science* **2017**, *356*, eaag2770. [CrossRef]
17. Lee, J.W.J.; Plichta, D.; Hogstrom, L.; Borren, N.Z.; Lau, H.; Gregory, S.M.; Tan, W.; Khalili, H.; Clish, C.; Vlamakis, H.; et al. Multi-Omics Reveal Microbial Determinants Impacting Responses to Biologic Therapies in Inflammatory Bowel Disease. *Cell Host Microbe* **2021**, *29*, 1294–1304.e4. [CrossRef]
18. Forslund, S.K.; Chakaroun, R.; Zimmermann-Kogadeeva, M.; Markó, L.; Aron-Wisnewsky, J.; Nielsen, T.; Moitinho-Silva, L.; Schmidt, T.S.B.; Falony, G.; Vieira-Silva, S.; et al. Combinatorial, Additive and Dose-Dependent Drug-Microbiome Associations. *Nature* **2021**, *600*, 500–505. [CrossRef]
19. Gopalakrishnan, V.; Spencer, C.N.; Nezi, L.; Reuben, A.; Andrews, M.C.; Karpinets, T.V.; Prieto, P.A.; Vicente, D.; Hoffman, K.; Wei, S.C.; et al. Gut Microbiome Modulates Response to Anti-PD-1 Immunotherapy in Melanoma Patients. *Science* **2018**, *359*, 97–103. [CrossRef]
20. Vétizou, M.; Pitt, J.M.; Daillère, R.; Lepage, P.; Waldschmitt, N.; Flament, C.; Rusakiewicz, S.; Routy, B.; Roberti, M.P.; Duong, C.P.M.; et al. Anticancer Immunotherapy by CTLA-4 Blockade Relies on the Gut Microbiota. *Science* **2015**, *350*, 1079–1084. [CrossRef]
21. Donald, I.P.; Wilkinson, S.P. The Value of 5-Aminosalicylic Acid in Inflammatory Bowel Disease for Patients Intolerant or Allergic to Sulphasalazine. *Postgrad. Med. J.* **1985**, *61*, 1047–1048. [CrossRef] [PubMed]
22. Mikami, Y.; Tsunoda, J.; Suzuki, S.; Mizushima, I.; Kiyohara, H.; Kanai, T. Significance of 5-Aminosalicylic Acid Intolerance in the Clinical Management of Ulcerative Colitis. *Digestion* **2023**, *104*, 58–65. [CrossRef] [PubMed]
23. Di Paolo, M.C.; Paoluzi, O.A.; Pica, R.; Iacopini, F.; Crispino, P.; Rivera, M.; Spera, G.; Paoluzi, P. Sulphasalazine and 5-Aminosalicylic Acid in Long-Term Treatment of Ulcerative Colitis: Report on Tolerance and Side-Effects. *Dig. Liver Dis.* **2001**, *33*, 563–569. [CrossRef] [PubMed]
24. Ransford, R.A.J.; Langman, M.J.S. Sulphasalazine and Mesalazine: Serious Adverse Reactions Re-Evaluated on the Basis of Suspected Adverse Reaction Reports to the Committee on Safety of Medicines. *Gut* **2002**, *51*, 536–539. [CrossRef]
25. Dignass, A.; Van Assche, G.; Lindsay, J.O.; Lémann, M.; Söderholm, J.; Colombel, J.F.; Danese, S.; D'Hoore, A.; Gassull, M.; Gomollón, F.; et al The Second European Evidence-Based Consensus on the Diagnosis and Management of Crohn's Disease: Current Management. *J. Crohns Colitis* **2010**, *4*, 28–62. [CrossRef]
26. Wang, Y.; Parker, C.E.; Feagan, B.G.; MacDonald, J.K. Oral 5-Aminosalicylic Acid for Maintenance of Remission in Ulcerative Colitis. *Cochrane Database Syst. Rev.* **2016**, *2016*, CD000544. [CrossRef]
27. Miyoshi, J.; Matsuoka, K.; Yoshida, A.; Naganuma, M.; Hisamatsu, T.; Yajima, T.; Inoue, N.; Okamoto, S.; Iwao, Y.; Ogata, H.; et al. 5-Aminosalicylic Acid Aggravates Colitis Mimicking Exacerbation of Ulcerative Colitis. *Intest Res* **2018**, *16*, 635–640. [CrossRef]
28. Bernstein, C.N.; Forbes, J.D. Gut Microbiome in Inflammatory Bowel Disease and Other Chronic Immune-Mediated Inflammatory Diseases. *Inflamm. Intest. Dis.* **2017**, *2*, 116–123. [CrossRef]
29. Zhang, M.; Sun, K.; Wu, Y.; Yang, Y.; Tso, P.; Wu, Z. Interactions between Intestinal Microbiota and Host Immune Response in Inflammatory Bowel Disease. *Front. Immunol.* **2017**, *8*, 942. [CrossRef]
30. Mizuno, S.; Ono, K.; Mikami, Y.; Naganuma, M.; Fukuda, T.; Minami, K.; Masaoka, T.; Terada, S.; Yoshida, T.; Saigusa, K.; et al. 5-Aminosalicylic Acid Intolerance Is Associated with a Risk of Adverse Clinical Outcomes and Dysbiosis in Patients with Ulcerative Colitis. *Intest. Res.* **2020**, *18*, 69–78. [CrossRef]
31. Carstens, A.; Annika, R.; Anna, A.; Anders, M.; Lars, A.; Jonas, H.; Lars, E. Differential Clustering of Fecal and Mucosa-Associated Microbiota in 'healthy' Individuals. *J. Dig. Dis.* **2018**, *19*, 745–752. [CrossRef] [PubMed]
32. Juge, N. Relationship between Mucosa-Associated Gut Microbiota and Human Diseases. *Biochem. Soc. Trans.* **2020**, *50*, 1225–1236. [CrossRef] [PubMed]
33. Matsumoto, H.; Kuroki, Y.; Higashi, S.; Goda, K.; Fukushima, S.; Katsumoto, R.; Oosawa, M.; Murao, T.; Ishii, M.; Oka, K.; et al. Analysis of the colonic mucosa associated microbiota(MAM) using brushing samples during colonic endoscopic procedures. *J. Clin. Biochem. Nutr.* **2019**, *65*, 132–137. [CrossRef] [PubMed]
34. Osawa, M.; Handa, O.; Fukushima, S.; Matsumoto, H.; Umegaki, E.; Inoue, R.; Naito, Y.; Shiotani, A. Reduced Abundance of Butyric Acid-Producing Bacteria in the Ileal Mucosa-Associated Microbiota of Ulcerative Colitis Patients. *J. Clin. Biochem. Nutr.* **2023**, *73*, 77–83. [CrossRef] [PubMed]

35. Maaser, C.; Sturm, A.; Vavricka, S.R.; Kucharzik, T.; Fiorino, G.; Annese, V.; Calabrese, E.; Baumgart, D.C.; Bettenworth, D.; Borralho Nunes, P.; et al. ECCO-ESGAR Guideline for Diagnostic Assessment in IBD Part 1: Initinal diagnosis, monitoring of known IBD, detection of complication. *J. Crohns Colitis* **2019**, *13*, 144–164. [CrossRef]
36. Shimizu, H.; Arai, K.; Tang, J.; Hosoi, K.; Funayama, R. 5-Aminosalicylate Intolerance Causing Exacerbation in Pediatric Ulcerative Colitis. *Pediatr. Int.* **2017**, *59*, 583–587. [CrossRef]
37. Hayashi, A.; Mikami, Y.; Miyamoto, K.; Kamada, N.; Sato, T.; Mizuno, S.; Naganuma, M.; Teratani, T.; Aoki, R.; Fukuda, S.; et al. Intestinal Dysbiosis and Biotin Deprivation Induce Alopecia through Overgrowth of Lactobacillus Murinus in Mice. *Cell Rep.* **2017**, *20*, 1513–1524. [CrossRef]
38. Klindworth, A.; Pruesse, E.; Schweer, T.; Peplies, J.; Quast, C.; Horn, M.; Glöckner, F.O. Evaluation of General 16S Ribosomal RNA Gene PCR Primers for Classical and next-Generation Sequencing-Based Diversity Studies. *Nucleic Acids Res.* **2013**, *41*, e1. [CrossRef]
39. Parks, D.H.; Tyson, G.W.; Hugenholtz, P.; Beiko, R.G. STAMP: Statistical analysis of taxonomic and functional profiles. *Bioinformatics* **2014**, *30*, 3123–3124. [CrossRef]
40. Herrera-deGuise, C.; Varela, E.; Sarrabayrouse, G.; Pozuelo del Río, M.; Alonso, V.R.; Sainz, N.B.; Casellas, F.; Mayorga, L.F.; Manichanh, C.; Vidaur, F.A.; et al. Gut Microbiota Composition in Long-Remission Ulcerative Colitis in Close to Healthy Gut Microbiota. *Inflamm. Bowel Dis.* **2023**, *29*, 1362–1369. [CrossRef]
41. Basha, O.M.; Hafez, A.H.; Salem, S.M.; Anis, R.H.; Hanafy, A.S. Impact of gut Microbiome alteration in Ulcerative Colitis patients on disease severity and outcom. *Clin. Exp. Med.* **2023**, *23*, 1763–1772. [CrossRef] [PubMed]
42. Zhang, Z.; Zhang, H.; Chen, T.; Shi, L.; Wang, D.; Tang, D. Regulatory Role of Short-Chain Fatty Acids in Inflammatory Bowel Disease. *Cell Commun. Signal.* **2022**, *20*, 64. [CrossRef] [PubMed]
43. Lima, S.F.; Gogokhia, L.; Viladomiu, M.; Chou, L.; Putzel, G.; Jin, W.-B.; Pires, S.; Guo, C.-J.; Gerardin, Y.; Crawford, C.V.; et al. Transferable Immunoglobulin A–Coated Odoribacter Splanchnicus in Responders to Fecal Microbiota Transplantation for Ulcerative Colitis Limits Colonic Inflammation. *Gastroenterology* **2022**, *162*, 166–178. [CrossRef] [PubMed]
44. Parker, B.J.; Wearsch, P.A.; Veloo, A.C.M.; Rodriguez-Palacios, A. The Genus Alistipes: Gut Bacteria with Emerging Implications to Inflammation, Cancer, and Mental Health. *Front. Immunol.* **2020**, *11*, 906. [CrossRef] [PubMed]
45. Dziarski, R.; Park, S.Y.; Kashyap, D.R.; Dowd, S.E.; Gupta, D. *Pglyrp*-Regulated Gut Microflora *Prevotella falsenii, Parabacteroides distasonis* and *Bacteroides eggerthii* Enhance and *Alistipes finegoldii* Attenuates Colitis in Mice. *PLoS ONE* **2016**, *11*, e0146162. [CrossRef]
46. Frank, D.N.; St Amand, A.L.; Feldman, R.A.; Boedeker, E.C.; Harpaz, N.; Pace, N.R. Molecular-Phylogenetic Characterization of Microbial Community Imbalances in Human Inflammatory Bowel Diseases. *Proc. Natl. Acad. Sci. USA* **2007**, *104*, 13780–13785. [CrossRef]
47. Gupta, A.; Khanna, S. Fecal Microbiota Transplantation. *JAMA* **2017**, *318*, 102. [CrossRef]
48. Moayyedi, P.; Surette, M.G.; Kim, P.T.; Libertucci, J.; Wolfe, M.; Onischi, C.; Armstrong, D.; Marshall, J.K.; Kassam, Z.; Reinisch, W.; et al. Fecal Microbiota Transplantation Induces Remission in Patients With Active Ulcerative Colitis in a Randomized Controlled Trial. *Gastroenterology* **2015**, *149*, 102–109.e6. [CrossRef]
49. Paramsothy, S.; Kamm, M.A.; Kaakoush, N.O.; Walsh, A.J.; van den Bogaerde, J.; Samuel, D.; Leong, R.W.L.; Connor, S.; Ng, W.; Paramsothy, R.; et al. Multidonor Intensive Faecal Microbiota Transplantation for Active Ulcerative Colitis: A Randomised Placebo-Controlled Trial. *Lancet* **2017**, *389*, 1218–1228. [CrossRef]
50. Costello, S.P.; Hughes, P.A.; Waters, O.; Bryant, R.V.; Vincent, A.D.; Blatchford, P.; Katsikeros, R.; Makanyanga, J.; Campaniello, M.A.; Mavrangelos, C.; et al. Effect of Fecal Microbiota Transplantation on 8-Week Remission in Patients with Ulcerative Colitis: A Randomized Clinical Trial. *JAMA* **2019**, *321*, 156–164. [CrossRef]
51. Paramsothy, S.; Paramsothy, R.; Rubin, D.T.; Kamm, M.A.; Kaakoush, N.O.; Mitchell, H.M.; Castaño-Rodríguez, N. Faecal Microbiota Transplantation for Inflammatory Bowel Disease: A Systematic Review and Meta-Analysis. *J. Crohns Colitis* **2017**, *11*, 1180–1199. [CrossRef] [PubMed]
52. Costello, S.P.; Soo, W.; Bryant, R.V.; Jairath, V.; Hart, A.L.; Andrews, J.M. Systematic Review with Meta-Analysis: Faecal Microbiota Transplantation for the Induction of Remission for Active Ulcerative Colitis. *Aliment. Pharmacol. Ther.* **2017**, *46*, 213–224. [CrossRef] [PubMed]
53. Allegretti, J.; Eysenbach, L.M.; El-Nachef, N.; Fischer, M.; Kelly, C.; Kassam, Z. The Current Landscape and Lessons from Fecal Microbiota Transplantation for Inflammatory Bowel Disease: Past, Present, and Future. *Inflamm. Bowel Dis.* **2017**, *23*, 1710–1717. [CrossRef] [PubMed]
54. Nagata, N.; Nishijima, S.; Miyoshi-Akiyama, T.; Kojima, Y.; Kimura, M.; Aoki, R.; Ohsugi, M.; Ueki, K.; Miki, K.; Iwata, E.; et al. Population-Level Metagenomics Uncovers Distinct Effects of Multiple Medications on the Human Gut Microbiome. *Gastroenterology* **2022**, *163*, 1038–1052. [CrossRef]

biomedicines

MDPI

Article

The Effect of Drugs on the Intestinal Microbiota in Crohn's Disease

Xue Yang †, Yinghui Zhang †, Caiping Gao , Yan Pan, Shan Du, Shiyu Xiao *,‡ and Zhou Zhou *,‡

Department of Gastroenterology, Sichuan Provincial People's Hospital, School of Medicine, University of Electronic Science and Technology of China, Chengdu 610054, China; yangxue_2001@163.com (X.Y.); zhangyinghui530@163.com (Y.Z.); gaocaip@126.com (C.G.); panyan_08@163.com (Y.P.); constantship@163.com (S.D.)

* Correspondence: xiaoshiyu57@163.com (S.X.); doublezhou2006@163.com (Z.Z.); Tel.: +86-028-87394213 (Z.Z.)

† These authors contributed equally to this work.

‡ These authors contributed equally to this work.

Abstract: Objective: We took advantage of a single-center cross-sectional study to investigate the effect of different drugs on intestinal microbiota and function in Crohn's disease. Methods: We studied the difference in fecal microbiota of Crohn's disease patients treated with mesalazine, azathioprine, and infliximab, as well as untreated patients, by metagenome and screened for differential microbiota. Further, we investigated functional differences in intestinal microbiota among the four groups. Results: Through metagenomic sequencing, we found that there was no difference between the four groups in ACE and Chao1 indices, but IFX and mesalazine improved species diversity and homogeneity compared to the untreated group, as evidenced by statistically significant differences in the Shannon index, Simpson index, and pielou_evenness. In addition, beta diversity suggested a difference between groups, but the difference was not significant. Non-parametric tests revealed differences between the four groups at the phylum level, class level, and genus level. Further analysis by LEfSe analysis revealed that the level of short-chain fatty acid-producing microbiota was increased in the treated groups, while there was no difference between the treated groups when compared to each other. Finally, the KEGG database and EggNOG database revealed that there were functional differences in intestinal microbiota among the four groups, including microbial metabolism pathway, cysteine and methionine metabolism pathway, cytoskeleton, etc. Conclusions: Mesalazine, azathioprine, and infliximab can all affect the intestinal microbiota and function in patients with Crohn's disease, and the drugs may alleviate intestinal inflammation in patients with Crohn's disease by modulating the intestinal microbiota.

Keywords: Crohn's disease; mesalazine; azathioprine; infliximab; fecal microbiota; metagenomic analysis

1. Introduction

Crohn's disease (CD) is a chronic, recurrent intestinal inflammatory disease with increasing incidence in the clinic; repeated inflammation of the intestinal tract can further lead to intestinal mucosal injury, bleeding, perforation and other symptoms, which seriously affects the quality of life of patients [1]. Recent research showed that the development of CD was related to the interactions of intestinal microecology, intestinal epithelial barrier, and immune function [2].

In terms of treatment, mesalazine, azathioprine, hormones, methotrexate, and biologics, such as infliximab, vedolizumab, ustekinumab, and small molecules, are commonly used for the treatment of CD. However, little research has been done on whether the use of drugs affects the intestinal microbiota, and whether there are differences in the effects of different drugs on the intestinal microbiota.

Although there are many drugs that have been developed and are under development, there is no drug that can cure CD. At the same time, each drug has its own advantages and limitations, and the treatment of CD in the future may be more inclined to individual precision therapy, which requires us to have a deeper understanding of the effects of drugs on the disease, on the internal environment of the organism, and especially on the intestinal microbiota. Based on this, our study investigated the effects of different drugs on intestinal microbiota through metagenomic sequencing, which lays the foundation for exploring the mechanism of drug action.

2. Materials and Methods

2.1. Study Population and Sample Collection

Sixty patients with CD were recruited from the Department of Gastroenterology, Sichuan Provincial People's Hospital, between April 2020 and November 2023. Inclusion criteria were (1) ileal, colonic, or ileocolonic CD diagnosed by clinical, laboratory, radiological, endoscopic, and histological evidence; (2) no antibiotics, probiotics, prebiotics, etc., received within the previous 4 weeks. Exclusion criteria were (1) pregnancy or lactation status; (2) combination of other malignant tumors. To categorise the location and behaviour of the disease, the Montreal classification was used. All patients provided their written informed consent to participate in this study. After the patients were enrolled, we collected fecal samples in a sterile cup, froze it at −80 °C, and then sent it to a third-party institution for metagenomic sequencing.

2.2. Metagenomic Sequencing

Total genomic DNA was extracted from fecal samples using the PowerSoil® DNA Isolation kit (Mo Bio Laboratories, Carlsbad, CA, USA) according to manufacturer's instructions. After the genomic DNA of the samples was qualified, the DNA was interrupted, and then the fragmented DNA was subjected to product purification, library amplification, and product purification to form a sequencing library, and the library was sequenced by Illumina sequencer after passing quality control. The original reads obtained from sequencing were quality controlled and filtered to obtain clean reads, which were spliced and assembled, coding genes were predicted, non-redundant gene sets were constructed, the non-redundant gene sets were functionally annotated and taxonomically analyzed in both general and specialized databases, and the species composition and abundance information of the samples were collected.

Representative sequences of non-redundant gene catalog were aligned to NCBI NR database with e-value cutoff of 1×10^{-5} using Diamond software (version 0.9.29) for taxonomic annotations. KEGG annotation was conducted using Diamond (version 0.9.29) against the Kyoto Encyclopedia of Genes and Genomes database with an e-value cutoff of 1×10^{-5}. EggNOG annotation was conducted using Diamond software (version 0.9.24) with an e-value cutoff of 1×10^{-5}.

2.3. Statistical Analyses

All statistical analyses were performed using SPSS version 21.0 (IBM Corporation, Armonk, NY, USA). Quantitative data were reported as mean ± standard deviation and qualitative variables were expressed as numbers or percentages. Statistical analyses were performed using the two-tailed non-parametric Mann–Whitney test or Wilcoxon rank-sum test. The linear discriminant analysis effect size (LEfSe) pipeline was used to search for biomarkers with statistical differences. All tests for significance were 2-sided, and differences with $p < 0.05$ were considered statistically significant.

3. Results

3.1. Characteristics of the Study Population and Fecal Metagenomic Sequencing

Sixty patients with an established diagnosis were recruited in the study between April 2020 and November 2023, and fecal samples were obtained from 54 patients. One sample was excluded due to unqualified metagenomic sequencing data, seven samples were excluded due to less than five patients enrolled in the treatment modality (the number of cases less than five could not be statistically analyzed, include three cases of Ustekinumab and four cases of Vedolizumab). As a result, 46 fecal samples were included in the study, including 13 cases of infliximab (IFX), 7 cases of azathioprine (AZA), 9 cases of mesalazine (M), and 17 cases of untreated (Pre). Their demographic and clinical characteristics are detailed in Table 1. We found no statistically significant differences between the four groups in terms of age, gender, Montreal classification, and perianal lesions. There was no significant statistical difference in the inflammatory indicators of patients, such as ESR and CRP, but there were significant differences in CDAI among the groups. The untreated group was significantly higher than the treated group, indicating that the untreated patients had a higher overall inflammatory activity.

Table 1. Baseline characteristics of the CD patients.

Characteristics	IFX	AZA	M	Pre	*p*
number	13	7	9	17	
Age (y)	32.92 ± 13.81	37.00 ± 11.73	33.11 ± 16.49	41.71 ± 18.06	0.331
Male/Female (*n*)	6/7	4/11	3/6	12/5	0.169
		Montreal classification			
A1/A2/A3 (*n*)	0/10/3	0/4/3	2/5/2	1/8/8	0.265
B1/B2/B3 (*n*)	6/4/3	3/3/1	6/2/1	6/7/4	0.842
L1/L2/L3 (*n*)	3/7/3	3/1/3	1/3/5	3/5/9	0.391
Perianal lesions	4	1	3	5	0.840
ESR (mm/h)	29.50 (11.25, 48.75)	58.00 (31.00, 90.00)	48.00 (26.50, 108.5)	45.00 (18.50, 81.50)	0.150
CRP (mg/L)	4.64 (1.33, 20.19)	6.18 (1.28, 33.97)	17.53 (4.49, 54.47)	14.97 (5.57, 85.43)	0.258
CDAI	58.4 (28.9, 198.6)	82.4 (69.0, 233.0)	188.9 (90.0, 229.0)	223.0 (152.5, 278.5)	0.026

Age is expressed as mean +/− standard deviation; ESR, CRP, and CDAI are expressed as interquartile range.

3.2. Alpha Diversity and Beta Diversity Analysis between the Groups

We used several methods for alpha diversity assessment of the groups, including ACE index, Chao1 index, Shannon index, Simpson index and pielou_evenness, where the Chao1 index and ACE index were used to measure species richness, Shannon and Simpson indices were used to measure species diversity, and the pielou_evenness index assessed species evenness.

Our study found there were no difference in the Chao1 index and ACE index among the four groups, suggesting that there was no significant difference in species richness (Figure 1A,B). The IFX and M groups were statistically different from the Pre group in Shannon index, Simpson index, and evenness indices (Figure 1C–E), suggesting that infliximab and mesalazine may increase the diversity and homogeneity of intestinal microbiota. Beta diversity analysis was calculated by non-parametric statistical tests. We found difference between groups, but the difference was not significant (R = 0.04, Figure 1F).

3.3. Altered Fecal Microbiota between Different Treatment Groups

To better understand the changes in fecal microbiota between the four groups, we performed the Mann–Whitney U test comparison, on the order through species levels. Detailed information on all taxonomical levels is shown in Figure 2. We found that the fecal microbiota of the treated groups was significantly different from the Pre group. At the phylum level, we found that the different treatment modalities all resulted in a significant reduction in Proteobacteria phylum levels (Figure 2A,C). At the class level, all three treatment modalities resulted in a decrease in Gammaproteobacteria levels when compared to the Pre group (Figure 2B,D). At the genus level, the three treatments increased the abundance of some species, such as Chloroaceticus, Raoultibacter, Ndongoensis, and also increased the abundance of some viruses, such as Saclayviru, Tanisvirus, Rimavirus, and Wanderervirus (Figure 3, Figure 2E).

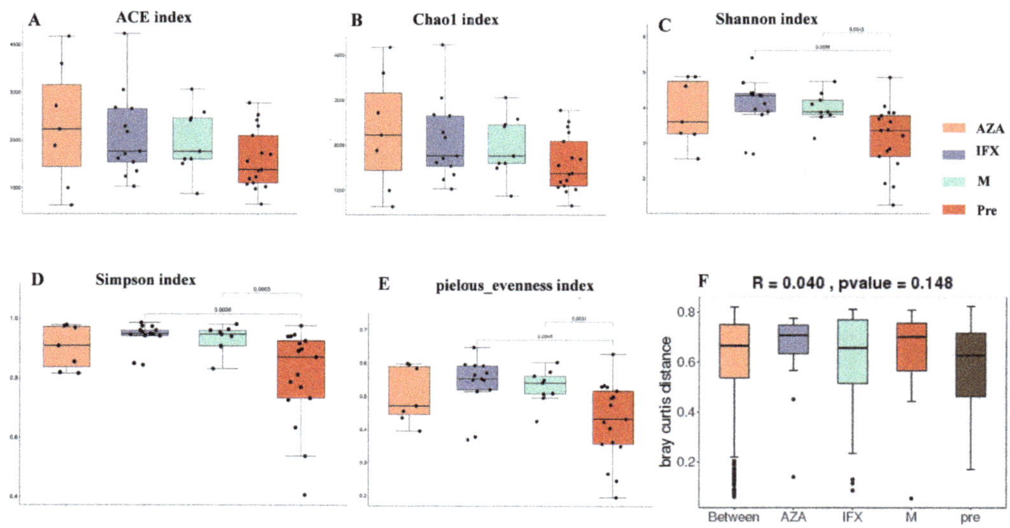

Figure 1. Alpha diversity and beta diversity analysis of fecal microbiota in the four groups. Alpha diversity indices were estimated using the number of observed ACE (**A**), Chao index (**B**), Shannon index (**C**), Simpson index (**D**), and pielou_evenness index (**E**). Beta diversity analysis of fecal microbiota in patients of the four groups (**F**). Significance was determined by the Mann–Whitney U test.

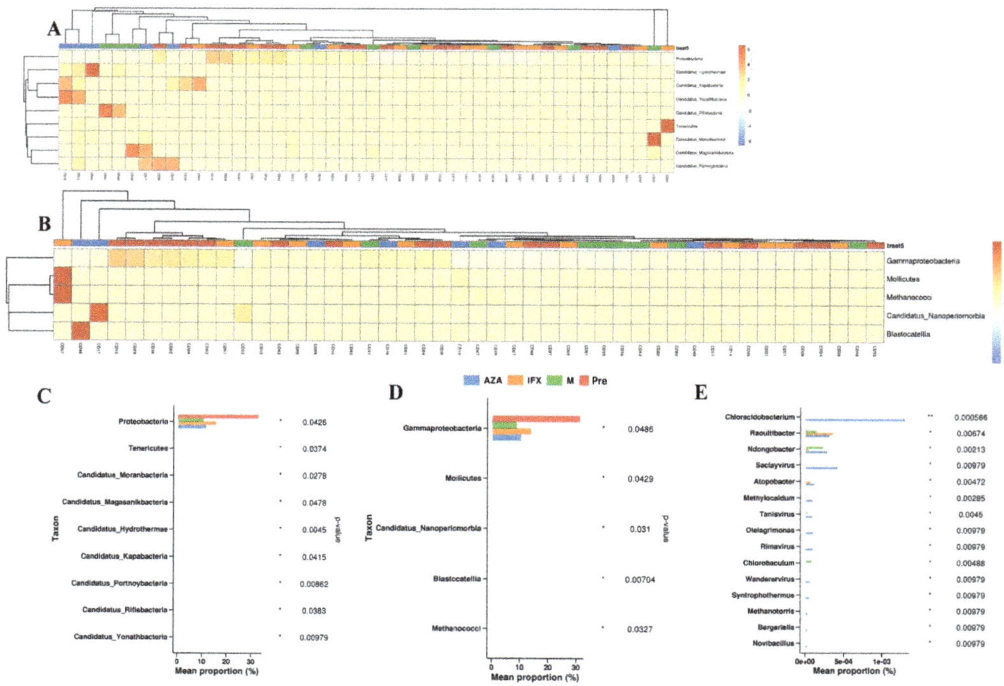

Figure 2. Taxonomic differences in the fecal microbiota in different treatment groups. (**A**) Heatmap of phylum level; (**B**) heatmap of class level; (**C**) bar graph of phylum level; (**D**) bar graph of class level; (**E**) bar graph of genus level. * $p < 0.05$, ** $p < 0.01$.

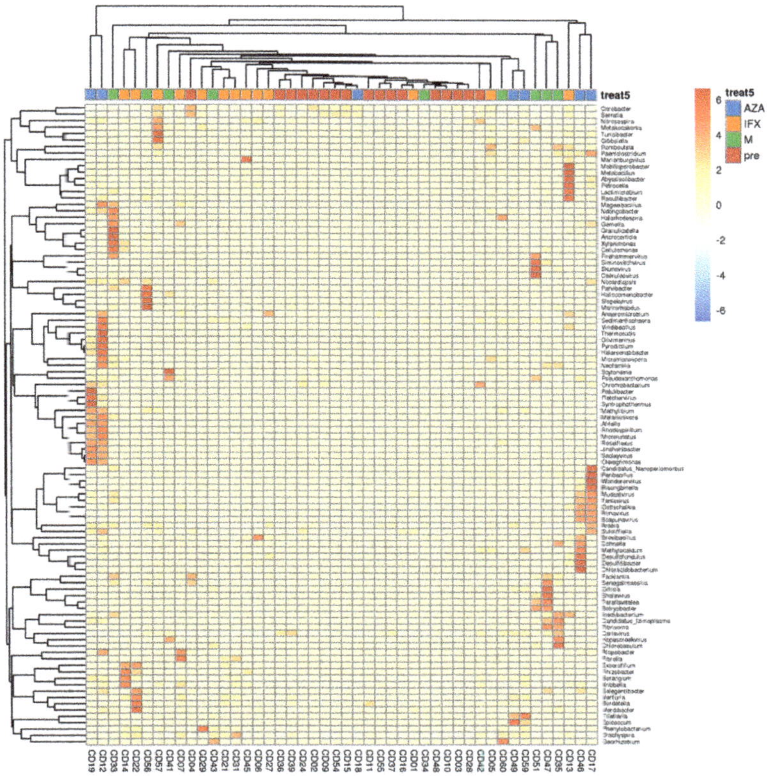

Figure 3. Heatmap of genus level in the fecal microbiota in different treatment groups.

3.4. LEfSe Analysis of Species between Different Treatment Modalities

Considering that alterations in gut microbiota from taxa were found in CD patients with different treatments, we further conducted the LEfSe analysis with a significance *p* value of 0.01 to identify the most significantly enriched taxon between the groups. We compared the fecal microbiota of the three treatment modalities with that of Pre group, and found that IFX increased Firmicutes at the phylum level and Veillonellales at the order and family levels (Figure 4A). AZA increased Firmicutes at the phylum level, Bacillales at the order level, Peptostreptococcaceae at the family level, and Clostridium disporicum and Clostridium saudiense at the species level (Figure 4B). Mesalazine increased Firmicutes at the phylum level, whereas Enterobacterales at the order level and Enterobacteriaceae at the family level were more abundant in the Pre group (Figure 4D). In addition, we compared the fecal microbiota of the three treatment groups and found no differences. Therefore, our study found that untreated CD patients have more intestinal pathogenic bacteria and that different treatments could increase the level of Firmicutes bacteria, Veillonellales, Peptostreptococcaceae, and Clostridium, which are all associated with the production of short-chain fatty acids, suggesting that different treatments might alleviate intestinal inflammation by increasing probiotics and microbiota that improve intestinal metabolism [3–5].

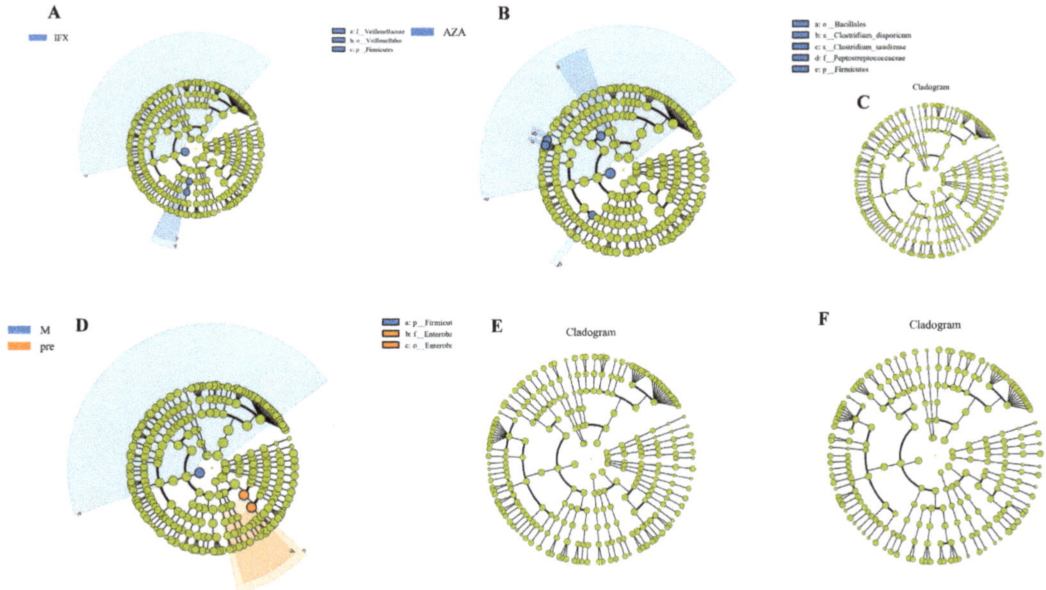

Figure 4. LEfSe analysis of species between different treatment modalities. The circles radiating from the inside to the outside of the evolutionary branching diagram represent the taxonomic levels from kingdom to species; the coloring principle was that the species with no significant differences were uniformly colored in yellow, with significant differences colored in red or blue. (**A**) IFX vs. Pre; (**B**) AZA vs. Pre; (**C**) IFX vs. AZA; (**D**) M vs. Pre; (**E**) IFX vs. M; (**F**) AZA vs. M.

3.5. Functional Profiling with KEGG Pathway and EggNOG

The Kyoto Encyclopedia of Genes and Genomes (KEGG) database is a database that systematically analyzes the metabolic pathways of gene products in cells and the functions of these gene products [6]. The KEGG database helps to study gene and expression information as a whole network. We used the KEGG database to search for differences in four groups (Figure 5A,B). The main differences in the functional composition of the gut bacteria in the four groups were microbial metabolism (p = 0.0288) and cysteine and methionine metabolism (p = 0.0323). Previous studies have found that cysteine and methionine metabolism were closely related to intestinal anti-inflammatory functions and maintenance of barrier functions [7–9]. This suggested that CD patients might alleviate intestinal inflammation by altering the function of intestinal microbiota.

The Evolutionary Genealogy of Genes: Non-supervised Orthologous Groups (EggNOG) database was used to search for and annotate homologous genes, helping to study the evolution and function of homologous genes [10]. We used the EggNOG database to search for differences in homologous genes between the four groups (Figure 6A,B). The main difference in the functional composition of the gut bacteria of the four groups was in the cytoskeleton, which might be involved in intestinal barrier function, inflammation, and fibrosis through the cytoskeleton [11,12].

Functional gene correlation analysis was based on the pathways of KEGG and the pathways of EggNOG. Through KEGG pathways, we screened the top 49 functional genes with the highest abundance (Figure 5C), based on the abundance and changes of each functional gene in each sample. Through EggNOG pathways, we screened the top 229 functional genes with the highest abundance (Figure 6C), based on the abundance and changes of each functional gene in each sample.

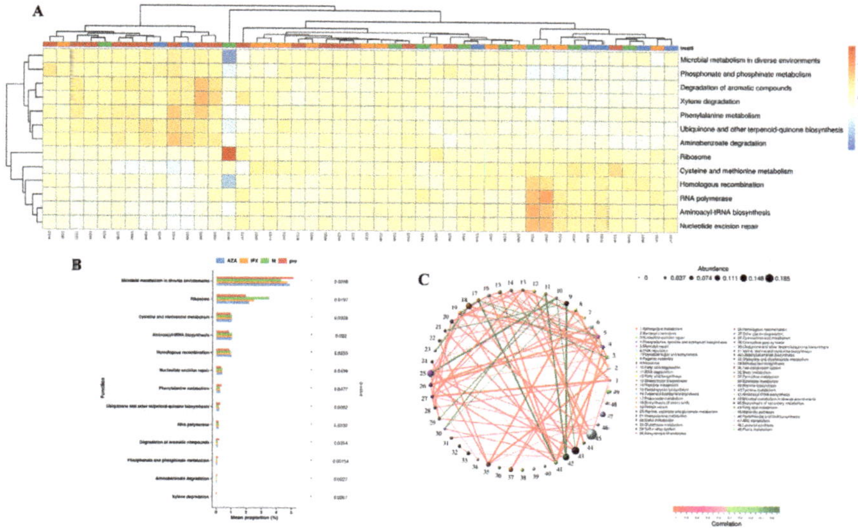

Figure 5. Functional profiling with KEGG pathways. (**A**) Functional genes were tested for non-parametric differences with *p*-values less than 0.05. The right clustering tree is the differential functional gene clustering, the top clustering tree is the sample clustering, and the middle is the heat map. (**B**) Relative abundance of KEGG pathways that were differently distributed in the four group ($p < 0.05$). (**C**) Correlation network diagram is a form of correlation analysis, based on KEGG pathway. * $p < 0.05$.

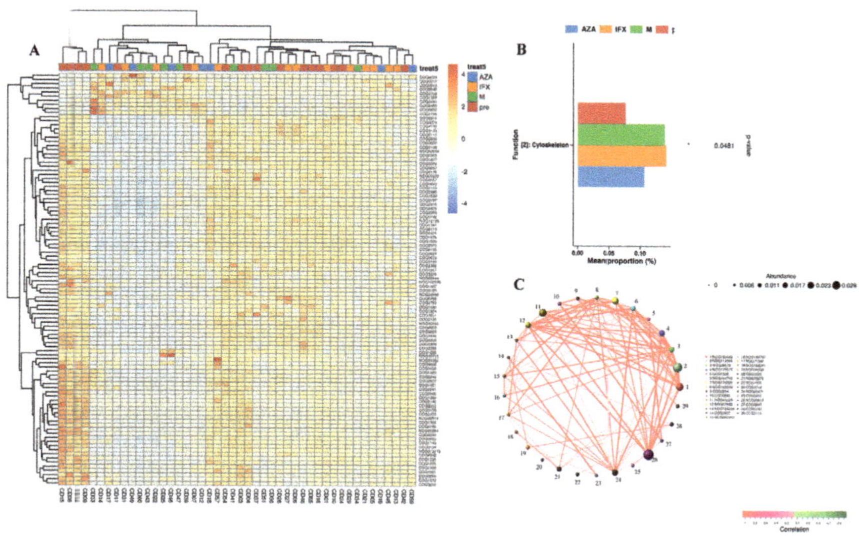

Figure 6. Functional profiling with EggNOG. (**A**) Functional genes were tested for non-parametric differences with *p*-values less than 0.05. The right clustering tree is the differential functional gene clustering, the top clustering tree is the sample clustering, and the middle is the heat map. (**B**) Relative abundance of EggNOG pathways that were differently distributed in the four group ($p < 0.05$). (**C**) Correlation network diagram is a form of correlation analysis, based on EggNOG. * $p < 0.05$.

4. Discussion

CD is a common chronic, inflammatory, recurrent intestinal disease. Patients mainly manifest symptoms as diarrhea, abdominal pain, bloody stools, and other symptoms, and persons in critical condition can form intestinal perforation, intestinal fistula; this disease occurs repeatedly, affecting the quality life of patients [13]. At this stage, there is no drug that can eradicate CD. In clinical practice, we commonly use medications including mesalazine, azathioprine, biological agents, and so on.

Each drug has a different mechanism of action. Mesalazine exerts its anti-inflammatory and antioxidant effects locally in the colonic mucosa mainly through 5-aminosalicylic acid [14]. Glucocorticoids bind to the glucocorticoid receptor in the cytoplasm and regulate the transcription of anti-inflammatory protein genes, inhibit the activation of pro-inflammatory genes, and induce the degradation of pro-inflammatory gene mRNAs through either nuclear receptor-dependent or non-nuclear receptor-dependent pathways, realizing the anti-inflammatory effect [15]. Azathioprine produces immunosuppressive effects by inhibiting DNA synthesis and thus inhibiting lymphocyte proliferation [16]. As for biological agents, infliximab terminates the biological activity and signaling of anti-tumor necrosis factor by forming a stable complex with human anti-tumor necrosis factor [17]. However, whether these drugs affect the intestinal microbiota, and whether they alleviate intestinal inflammation by modulating the intestinal microbiota, has not been studied.

In this study, we analyzed species richness by alpha and beta diversity. We found that there was no difference between the four groups in ACE and Chao1 indices, but IFX and mesalazine improved species diversity and homogeneity compared to the untreated group, as evidenced by statistically significant differences in the Shannon index, Simpson index, and pielou_evenness. In addition, beta diversity suggested a difference between groups, but the difference was not significant. These results suggested that medication might improve the diversity and balance of the intestinal microbiota.

Then, we searched for differences in fecal microbiota among the four groups by non-parametric analysis, and found that the differences among them mainly existed at the phylum level, the class level, and the genus level. Among them, Proteobacteria was the most important differential species at the phylum and the class level, and the abundance of Proteobacteria was significantly reduced in the treatment groups. At the genus level, the three treatment groups increased the abundance of some strains and viruses, for example, Chloroaceticus, Raoultibacter, Ndongoensis, and Saclayviru, which has not been reported in previous studies. Previous studies have found that in the intestines of CD patients, the abundance of Proteobacteria was increased, which may be associated with the development of CD [18]. In the present study, we found that all the drug treatments were able to reduce the abundance of Proteobacteria, suggesting that in addition to their own anti-inflammatory function, drugs might alleviate intestinal inflammation by altering the intestinal microbiota, and that Proteobacteria was an important microbiota target for the action of drugs.

We further analyzed the differences in fecal microbiota between the treated and untreated groups by LEfSe analysis, and two-by-two comparisons revealed an increase in short-chain fatty acid-producing bacteria in all three treatment modalities, including Firmicutes, Veillonellales, Peptostreptococcaceae, Clostridium, etc. Short-chain fatty acids, which are produced by intestinal microbiota through fermentation of dietary plant fibers that are naturally indigestible in humans, are a source of energy for the colonic epithelium and have been shown to play a key role in maintaining intestinal barrier function and regulating intestinal immune homeostasis [19]. Comparisons between treatment groups did not reveal differences in intestinal microbiota, suggesting that CD therapeutic agents might alleviate intestinal mucosal inflammation by altering the microbiota and improving intestinal metabolism.

We explored the effects of different drugs on gut microbiota function through the KEGG database and the EggNOG database. KEGG is a database that integrates genomic, chemical, and systemic functional information to correlate gene catalogs from genomes that have been completely sequenced with systemic functions at the cellular, species, and ecosystem levels [6]. The EggNOG database is a database of direct homologous proteins based on public resource databases for grouping comparisons, annotated with functional descriptions and functional classifications of orthologous homologous taxa [10].

In our study, certain changes in KEGG pathways and EggNOG were observed in the fecal microbiota of CD patients with different treatments. As for the KEGG pathways, we found that many metabolism pathways had statistically significant differences in expression levels, such as microbial metabolism in diverse environments, ribosome, cysteine and methionine metabolism, aminoacyl-tRNA biosynthesis, homologous recombination, etc. Previous studies have found that cysteine and methionine metabolism was strongly associated with gut health, and that it could alleviate intestinal inflammation by reducing oxidative stress, improving energy status, and had also been implicated in a number of intestinal cell-signaling pathways [20]. The role of other metabolic alterations in intestinal inflammation has not been reported. Thereas, through the EggNOG database, we only found differences in cytoskeletal protein function among the four groups. Previous studies have found that the cytoskeleton was associated with intestinal barrier function, inflammation, and fibrosis [21], suggesting that drugs might have the potential to ameliorate intestinal mucosal inflammation by modulating cytoskeletal-related functions through intestinal microbiota.

This study has several limitations. First, this was a single-center cross-sectional study with a relatively small sample size and a lack of a validation dataset. Second, all the results were based on feces-associated microbiota, and no data from the mucosa-associated microbiota were available. Third, this study lacked the intestinal microbiota at baseline levels. Fourth, there were differences in patients' medication regimens. Therefore, subsequent proposed prospective studies may go further to clarify the effects of the drugs on the intestinal microbiota of CD patients.

5. Conclusions

There are numerous drugs for the treatment of CD, but there are few studies related to the effects of drugs on intestinal microbiota. In this study, we found that the intestinal microbiota of CD was altered after treatment with mesalazine, azathioprine, and infliximab by metagenomic sequencing, and further analyzed the effects of the drugs on the function of the intestinal microbiota by functional database, suggesting that drugs may alleviate the intestinal inflammation of CD by regulating the intestinal microbiota.

Author Contributions: Z.Z. and S.X. designed the study plan, edited the manuscript, and contributed equally to this work; X.Y. and Y.Z. diagnosed the patients and collected clinical information from enrolled subjects, and contributed equally; Y.P., S.D., and C.G. collected the fecal samples. All authors have read and agreed to the published version of the manuscript.

Funding: This study was supported by Sichuan Science and Technology Program 2023YFS0289.

Institutional Review Board Statement: The study involving human participants was reviewed and approved by the Institutional Review Board for Clinical Research of Sichuan Provincial People's Hospital (No.20230215) and registered in the Medical Research Registration Information System (MR-51-23-013534) and China Clinical Trial Registration Center (ChiCTR230069727).

Informed Consent Statement: All patients provided written informed consent.

Data Availability Statement: The original contributions presented in the study are included in the article, further inquiries can be directed to the corresponding authors.

Conflicts of Interest: The authors declared that the research was conducted in the absence of any commercial or financial relationships that could be construed as a potential conflict of interest.

Abbreviations

CD, Crohn's disease; LEfSe, the linear discriminant analysis effect size; IFX, infliximab; AZA, azathioprine; ESR, erythrocyte sedimentation rate; CRP, C-reaction protein; CDAI, Crohn's disease activity index; KEGG, The Kyoto Encyclopedia of Genes and Genomes; EggNOG, The Evolutionary Genealogy of Genes: Non-supervised Orthologous Groups.

References

1. Buie, M.J.; Quan, J.; Windsor, J.W.; Coward, S.; Hansen, T.M.; King, J.A.; Kotze, P.G.; Gearry, R.B.; Ng, S.C.; Mak, J.W.Y.; et al. Global Hospitalization Trends for Crohn's Disease and Ulcerative Colitis in the 21st Century: A Systematic Review with Temporal Analyses. *Clin. Gastroenterol. Hepatol.* **2023**, *21*, 2211–2221. [CrossRef] [PubMed]
2. Leibovitzh, H.; Lee, S.H.; Raygoza Garay, J.A.; Espin-Garcia, O.; Xue, M.; Neustaeter, A.; Goethel, A.; Huynh, H.Q.; Griffiths, A.M.; Turner, D.; et al. Immune response and barrier dysfunction-related proteomic signatures in preclinical phase of Crohn's disease highlight earliest events of pathogenesis. *Gut* **2023**, *72*, 1462–1471. [CrossRef] [PubMed]
3. Nishida, A.; Inoue, R.; Inatomi, O.; Bamba, S.; Naito, Y.; Andoh, A. Gut microbiota in the pathogenesis of inflammatory bowel disease. *Clin. J. Gastroenterol.* **2018**, *11*, 1–10. [CrossRef]
4. Gasaly, N.; de Vos, P.; Hermoso, M.A. Impact of Bacterial Metabolites on Gut Barrier Function and Host Immunity: A Focus on Bacterial Metabolism and Its Relevance for Intestinal Inflammation. *Front. Immunol.* **2021**, *12*, 658354. [CrossRef]
5. Shin, Y.; Han, S.; Kwon, J.; Ju, S.; Choi, T.G.; Kang, I.; Kim, S.S. Roles of Short-Chain Fatty Acids in Inflammatory Bowel Disease. *Nutrients* **2023**, *15*, 4466. [CrossRef]
6. Robben, M.; Nasr, M.S.; Das, A.; Veerla, J.P.; Huber, M.; Jaworski, J.; Weidanz, J.; Luber, J. Comparison of the Strengths and Weaknesses of Machine Learning Algorithms and Feature Selection on KEGG Database Microbial Gene Pathway Annotation and Its Effects on Reconstructed Network Topology. *J. Comput. Biol.* **2023**, *30*, 766–782. [CrossRef] [PubMed]
7. Hou, Y.; Wang, L.; Yi, D.; Wu, G. N-acetylcysteine and intestinal health: A focus on its mechanism of action. *Front. Biosci.* **2015**, *20*, 872–891. [CrossRef]
8. Kim, C.J.; Kovacs-Nolan, J.; Yang, C.; Archbold, T.; Fan, M.Z.; Mine, Y. L-cysteine supplementation attenuates local inflammation and restores gut homeostasis in a porcine model of colitis. *Biochim. Biophys. Acta* **2009**, *1790*, 1161–1169. [CrossRef]
9. Liu, G.; Yu, L.; Fang, J.; Hu, C.A.; Yin, J.; Ni, H.; Ren, W.; Duraipandiyan, V.; Chen, S.; Al-Dhabi, N.A.; et al. Methionine restriction on oxidative stress and immune response in dss-induced colitis mice. *Oncotarget* **2017**, *8*, 44511–44520. [CrossRef]
10. Huerta-Cepas, J.; Szklarczyk, D.; Forslund, K.; Cook, H.; Heller, D.; Walter, M.C.; Rattei, T.; Mende, D.R.; Sunagawa, S.; Kuhn, M.; et al. eggNOG 4.5: A hierarchical orthology framework with improved functional annotations for eukaryotic, prokaryotic and viral sequences. *Nucleic Acids Res.* **2016**, *44*, D286–D293. [CrossRef]
11. Lopez-Posadas, R.; Sturzl, M.; Atreya, I.; Neurath, M.F.; Britzen-Laurent, N. Interplay of GTPases and Cytoskeleton in Cellular Barrier Defects during Gut Inflammation. *Front. Immunol.* **2017**, *8*, 1240. [CrossRef] [PubMed]
12. Ivanov, A.I.; Le, H.T.; Naydenov, N.G.; Rieder, F. Novel Functions of the Septin Cytoskeleton: Shaping Up Tissue Inflammation and Fibrosis. *Am. J. Pathol.* **2021**, *191*, 40–51. [CrossRef] [PubMed]
13. Petagna, L.; Antonelli, A.; Ganini, C.; Bellato, V.; Campanelli, M.; Divizia, A.; Efrati, C.; Franceschilli, M.; Guida, A.M.; Ingallinella, S.; et al. Pathophysiology of Crohn's disease inflammation and recurrence. *Biol. Direct* **2020**, *15*, 23. [CrossRef] [PubMed]
14. D'Haens, G.; van Bodegraven, A.A. Mesalazine is safe for the treatment of IBD. *Gut* **2004**, *53*, 155. [CrossRef]
15. Greenhill, C. IBD: Glucocorticoids revealed to augment intestinal epithelial barrier function. *Nat. Rev. Gastroenterol. Hepatol.* **2014**, *11*, 75. [CrossRef]
16. Shaye, O.A.; Yadegari, M.; Abreu, M.T.; Poordad, F.; Simon, K.; Martin, P.; Papadakis, K.A.; Ippoliti, A.; Vasiliauskas, E.; Tran, T.T. Hepatotoxicity of 6-mercaptopurine (6-MP) and Azathioprine (AZA) in adult IBD patients. *Am. J. Gastroenterol.* **2007**, *102*, 2488–2494. [CrossRef]
17. Matsuoka, K.; Kanai, T. Mechanism and therapeutic strategy of secondary failure to anti-tumor necrosis factor-alpha monoclonal antibody treatment for Crohn's disease. *Digestion* **2013**, *88*, 17–19. [CrossRef]
18. Mukhopadhya, I.; Hansen, R.; El-Omar, E.M.; Hold, G.L. IBD-what role do Proteobacteria play? *Nat. Rev. Gastroenterol. Hepatol.* **2012**, *9*, 219–230. [CrossRef] [PubMed]
19. Parada Venegas, D.; De la Fuente, M.K.; Landskron, G.; Gonzalez, M.J.; Quera, R.; Dijkstra, G.; Harmsen, H.J.M.; Faber, K.N.; Hermoso, M.A. Short Chain Fatty Acids (SCFAs)-Mediated Gut Epithelial and Immune Regulation and Its Relevance for Inflammatory Bowel Diseases. *Front. Immunol.* **2019**, *10*, 277. [CrossRef]
20. Ikeda, Y.; Matsuda, S. Gut Protective Effect from D-Methionine or Butyric Acid against DSS and Carrageenan-Induced Ulcerative Colitis. *Molecules* **2023**, *28*, 4392. [CrossRef]
21. Martinez-Sanchez, L.D.C.; Ngo, P.A.; Pradhan, R.; Becker, L.S.; Boehringer, D.; Soteriou, D.; Kubankova, M.; Schweitzer, C.; Koch, T.; Thonn, V.; et al. Epithelial RAC1-dependent cytoskeleton dynamics controls cell mechanics, cell shedding and barrier integrity in intestinal inflammation. *Gut* **2023**, *72*, 275–294. [CrossRef] [PubMed]

biomedicines

MDPI

Article

Oral Microbiota and Inflammatory Bowel Diseases: Detection of Emerging Fungal Pathogens and Herpesvirus

Manoel Marques Evangelista Oliveira [1,*,†], Letícia Bomfim Campos [2], Fernanda Brito [3], Flavia Martinez de Carvalho [4,5], Geraldo Oliveira Silva-Junior [3], Gisela Lara da Costa [1], Tatiane Nobre Pinto [1], Rafaela Moraes Pereira de Sousa [2], Rodrigo Miranda [1], Rodolfo Castro [6,7], Cyrla Zaltman [7] and Vanessa Salete de Paula [2,*,†]

[1] Laboratory of Taxonomy, Biochemistry and Bioprospecting of Fungi, Oswaldo Cruz Institution (IOC), Oswaldo Cruz Foundation (Fiocruz), Rio de Janeiro 21040-360, RJ, Brazil; gisela.costa@fiocruz.br (G.L.d.C.); tatianepinto@aluno.fiocruz.br (T.N.P.); r-prado-miranda@bol.com.br (R.M.)

[2] Laboratory of Molecular Virology and Parasitology, Oswaldo Cruz Institution (IOC), Oswaldo Cruz Foundation (Fiocruz), Rio de Janeiro 21040-360, RJ, Brazil; leticia_bonfim1998@hotmail.com (L.B.C.); rafaelamoraesfiocruz@gmail.com (R.M.P.d.S.)

[3] Department of Periodontology and Diagnostics and Therapeutics, School of Dentistry, Rio de Janeiro State University, Rio de Janeiro 20551-030, RJ, Brazil; fernanda.brito.s@hotmail.com (F.B.); silvajuniorgo@gmail.com (G.O.S.-J.)

[4] Laboratory of Epidemiology of Congenital Malformations, Oswaldo Cruz Institution (IOC), Oswaldo Cruz Foundation (Fiocruz), Rio de Janeiro 21040-360, RJ, Brazil; flavia.carvalho@ioc.fiocruz.br

[5] Post-Graduation Programme in Genetics, Federal University of Rio de Janeiro, Rio de Janeiro 21941-617, RJ, Brazil

[6] Sergio Arouca National School of Public Health, Oswaldo Cruz Foundation, Rio de Janeiro 21040-360, RJ, Brazil; rodolfoalcastro@gmail.com

[7] Institute of Collective Health, Federal University of the State of Rio de Janeiro, Rio de Janeiro 21941-598, RJ, Brazil; c.zaltman@gmail.com

* Correspondence: manoel.marques@fiocruz.br (M.M.E.O.); vdepaula@ioc.fiocruz.br (V.S.d.P.); Tel.: +55-21-3865-8114 (M.M.E.O.); +55-21-2562-1823 (V.S.d.P.)

† These authors contributed equally to this work.

Abstract: Background/Objectives: Ulcerative colitis (UC) and Crohn's disease (CD) are the usual clinical forms of inflammatory bowel disease (IBD). Changes in the oral microbiota, especially the presence of emerging fungi and herpesviruses, have been shown to worsen the clinical aspects of IBD. The aim of this study was to screen for emerging pathogens in the oral yeast microbiota and the presence of herpesvirus in IBD patients. **Methods:** Oral swabs of seven UC or CD patients were collected. The samples were plated on Sabouraud Dextrose Agar and subcultured on CHROMagar Candida and CHROMagar Candida Plus. Polyphasic taxonomy was applied and identified using molecular tools, such as MALDI-TOF MS and ITS partial sequencing. Multiplex qPCR was used to identify the herpesvirus. Results: The mean age was 38.67 ± 14.06 years, 57.14% were female, and two had diabetes. The CD patients presented with *Rhodotorula mucilaginosa, Candida orthopsilosis* and *Kodamaea jinghongensis*, while the UC patients presented with *Cutaneotrichosporon dermatis, Candida glabrata, Candida lusitanea* and *Candida tropicalis*. Two UC individuals had at least one herpesvirus. In the first individual, a co-detection of Herpes Simplex Virus 1 (HSV-1) and *C. lusitaniae* was observed. The second presented with co-infections of Epstein–Barr virus (EBV), Human Herpesvirus 7 (HHV-7) and *C. tropicalis*. **Conclusions:** We identified rarely described yeasts and co-infections in IBD patients, highlighting the need to identify emerging pathogens in the oral microbiota, as they may contribute to opportunistic infections.

 https://doi.org/10.3390/biomedicines13020480

Keywords: oral microbiome; emergent fungi; chronic intestinal inflammation; human herpesvirus; oral dysbiosis

1. Introduction

Inflammatory bowel diseases (IBD), which include Crohn's disease (CD) and ulcerative colitis (UC), are a group of conditions characterized by chronic inflammation at various sites in the gastrointestinal tract [1]. Their etiology and pathogenesis are not well established, but it is speculated to be multifactorial and involves genetic, environmental, immune and microbial factors. The microbiota, which includes a constellation of archaea, bacteria, fungi, viruses, protists and helminths, was associated with IBD susceptibility, clinical aspects, disease activity or remission, and response to treatment [2].

Oral and bowel involvement in CD patients is highly associated with significant reductions in bacterial diversity in both microbiomes, with a decrease in beneficial bacteria, such as *Faecalibacterium prausnitzii*, and an increase in potentially pathogenic species, such as *Escherichia coli* [3,4]. However, the oral cavity is the second largest microbiota in the human body, being colonized by bacteria, but also by fungi and viruses that can lead to the worsening of IBD [5].

The oral cavity is a unique ecosystem that comprises a wide range of habitats, including the teeth, gingival sulcus, tongue, cheeks, tonsils, and the hard and soft palates. The colonization of the human oral microbiome mostly occurs on tooth surfaces, which leads to biofilm formation that is associated with dental plaque [5,6]. This oral microbiota is, in broad terms, similar in all humans, although each person has a characteristic "finger-print" that is unique [7].

Most of the common yeasts found in healthy oral cavities are from the *Candida* group, with *C. albicans* being predominantly found in the superior gastric tract and along the gut [8–10]. In addition, representatives of the *Basidiomycota* and *Ascomycota* clades can still be found [10]. Rivera et al. (2019) measured the profile of yeasts isolated in healthy individuals and 52.0% were identified as *C. albicans*, 43.5% non-*C. albicans* (*C. parapsilosis, C. dubliniensis, C. glabrata, C. tropicalis* and *C. intermedia*) and the least isolated species were *Geotrichum candidum* (1.5%) and *Rhodotorula mucilaginosa* (1.5%) [11].

Although these and other fungal species are part of the healthy oral microbiota, they can cause opportunistic infections that are generally associated with an inflammatory response from the host, which can impact the quality of life of individuals [12]. Above all, some minor yeast species can be found in the oral tract under certain circumstances and can reflect some health and disease statuses [13]. Three species of the genus *Rhodotorula* (*R. mucilaginosa, R. minuta* and *R. glutinis*), commonly described as opportunistic fungi in immunodeficient patients, were found in oral cavity of patients with colorectal cancer [14].

Kodamaea are considered an emergent pathogen, with *K. ohmeri* being the most common pathogen present in nosocomial environments, reported as a causative agent of fungemia mainly in neonatal, elderly and immunocompromised patients [15,16]. In Brazil, saliva and oropharyngeal candidiasis samples from HIV-positive patients presented with *C. albicans* (51.56%), non-*C. albicans* species (43.73%), *Trichosporon mucoides* (3.12%) and *K. ohmeri* (1.56%) [17].

In IBD patients, changes in the oral microbiota, especially the presence of emerging fungi, can be related to disease progression [18]. Studies have shown a significant change in the fungal microbiota of UC or CD patients in comparison to healthy individuals [19–23]. *Trichosporon* is a common fungus present in the mouth of healthy individuals; however, it is being pointed to as a potential emergent fungus in CD patients [24,25].

In addition, according to Mouzan et al. (2017), the fungal microbiome of children with aggravated CD in their mucosal tissues includes the phyla *Basidiomycota* and *Ascomycota*, where there is population-level growth of *Basidiomycota* fungi, such as *Psathyrella*, and a decrease in *Ascomycota* fungi, such as the order *Helotiales* [23]. Therefore, it is important to investigate fungi, especially the presence of emerging fungi in the oral microbiota, to characterize risk factors in individuals with IBD.

As previously mentioned, the oral microbiota is also composed of viruses that are commonly found in this cavity, which are called the oral virome. They form a robust ecosystem with members that are capable of infecting human cells as well as bacterial, and may interfere with the health of the host [5,26]. The most common viruses that infect humans present in the oral microbiota are Human Papilloma Virus (HPV) and Human Herpesvirus (HHV) [27].

The presence of herpesviruses in mucous membranes has been associated with worsening of the inflammatory condition and progression of IBD [28]. Although rare, Herpes Simplex Colitis is associated with exacerbation of UC in immunosuppressed patients [29]. Leal et al. (2022) reported the presence of an opportunistic coinfection by Cytomegalovirus (CMV or HHV-5) and HSV-2 in a steroid/immunomodulator refractory UC patient, leading to the worsening of the clinical aspects and the need for a colectomy even after antiviral treatment [30].

The prevalence of Epstein–Barr virus (EBV or HHV-4) and CMV were higher in UC and CD patients when compared to healthy individuals, and the frequency of herpesviruses also increases with worsening intestinal disease [18]. Altunal et al. (2023) reported that CMV-positive UC patients had a higher frequency of steroid resistance, longer disease duration, longer remission and longer length of hospital stay [31]. All these data show that herpesvirus infections in individuals with IBD may be a risk factor for worsening of the clinical picture.

Although the importance of fungal gut microbiome dysbiosis for IBD has been elucidated, changes in the oral microbiota and their impacts are poorly reported. Furthermore, the risk of herpesvirus infection in UC patients is known, but there was no evidence until now on the impact of coinfection with herpesviruses and emerging fungi in individuals with IBD. Therefore, the main objective of this study was to investigate the presence of fungi and herpesviruses in the oral microbiota of patients with IBD to identify potential risk factors.

2. Materials and Methods

2.1. Sample Collection and Isolation of Yeast

This is a descriptive cross-sectional study, approved by the ethics committee (CAAE: 54235021.7.0000.5259). Informed consent was obtained from all subjects involved in this study, and samples were collected between 25 October 2022 and 25 November 2022. In total, 7 patients with inflammatory bowel disease (ulcerative colitis or Crohn's disease) treated by Crohn's disease outpatient clinic were included. Oral swabs were inserted into a tube with sterile saline solution and then passed through the entire oral cavity for 2 to 3 s and then placed into 5 mL tubes containing 2 mL of a 0.9% saline solution. The samples were then taken to the laboratory within 30 min of the samplings and processed the analysis.

Samples were streaked onto Sabouraud Dextrose Agar (BD Difco™, Franklin Lakes, BD, USA) and incubated at 30 °C for 48 h for morphological assessments. All samples presenting with growth on the SDA medium (Figure 1) were then subcultured onto CHROMagar Candida (BD Difco™, Franklin Lakes, BD, USA) and CHROMagar Candida Plus

(CHROMagar™, Saint-Denis, France) (Figure 2) and colonies were interpreted according to the manufacturer's instructions.

Polyphasic taxonomy was applied with morphologic and phenotypic tests for all isolates obtained and identified using molecular tools, such as MALDI-TOF MS and partial sequencing of the ITS region (Pinto et al., 2022 [32]). Fungal identification at the species level by MALDI-TOF MS was carried out as previously described by Pinto et al. (2022) [32]. Briefly, 10^6 yeast cells were transferred from the culture plate (c.a. 1g) to a 500 μL tube containing 20 μL of 70% formic acid in water (*v*/*v*) and mixed with 10 μL of acetonitrile. The samples (1 μL) were then spotted onto a stainless Bruker MALDI-TOF MS plate (Bruker, Billerica, MA, USA) and covered with 1 μL of a α-cyano-4-hydroxycinnamic acid (CHCA, Fluka, Buchs, Switzerland) used as the matrix. Each sample was analyzed in triplicate. Samples were air-dried at room temperature prior to spectra acquisition. Results are expressed as log values ranging from 0 to 3, where values of 1.7 are generally used for reliable genus identification and values of 2.0 are used for reliable species identification (Stevenson et al., 2010 [33]).

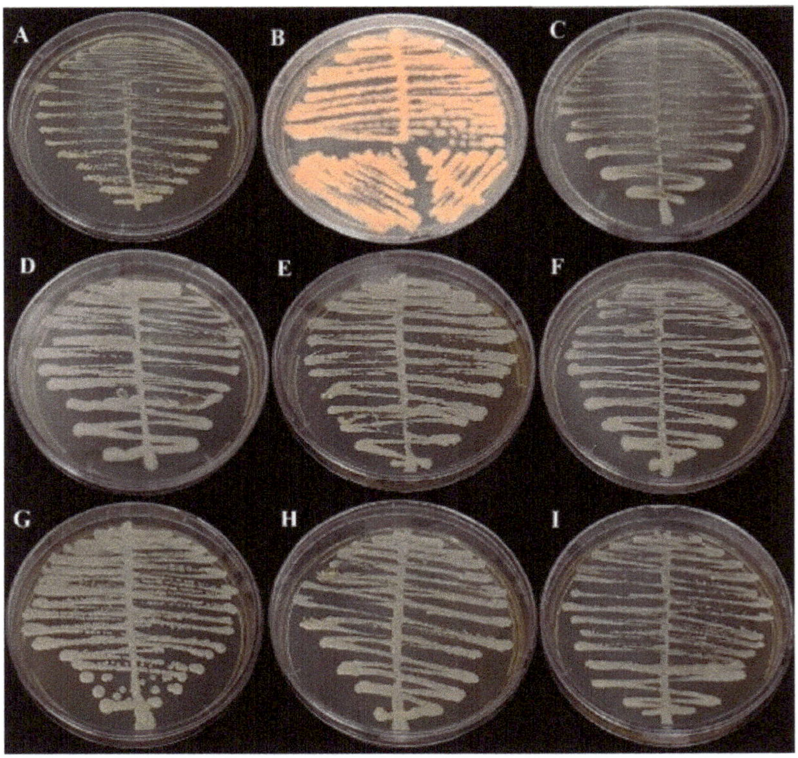

Figure 1. Growth in Sabouraud Dextrose Agar Medium (BD Difco) incubated at 35 °C for 48 h: (**A**) *Cutaneotrichosporon dermatis*, (**B**) *Rhodotorula mucilaginosa*, (**C**) *Candida glabrata*, (**D**) *Candida orthopsilosis*, (**E**) *Kodamaea jinghongensis*, (**F**) *Candida lusitanea*, (**G**) *Kodamaea jinghongensis*, (**H**) *Candida orthopsilosis* and (**I**) *Candida tropicalis*.

The genomic DNA from the yeast, obtained by the extraction of colonies grown on SDA, was performed using Gentra® Puregene® Yeast and G+ Bacteria kits (Qiagen®, Germantown, MD, USA) according to the manufacturer's recommendations. Briefly, the amplification of the ITS1-5.8S-ITS2 ribosomal DNA region was performed in a final volume of 50 μL containing 100 ng of DNA and 10 μL of each primer (Invitrogen™ São Paulo, Brazil),

ITS1 (5′ TCCGTAGGTGAACCTGCGG 3′) and ITS4 (5′TCCTCCGCTTATTGATATGC 3′) (Lindsley et al., 2001 [34]). PCRs were performed employing a Veriti Applied Biosystems thermocycler at an annealing temperature of 58 °C. Automated sequencing was performed using the Fundação Oswaldo Cruz sequencing platform (PDTIS/FIOCRUZ, Rio de Janeiro, Brazil). The sequences were edited using CodonCode Aligner (Genes Code Corporation, Ann Arbor, MI, USA), and phylogenetic analyses were performed using the Blast software (version 2.16.0) for comparison with sequences deposited in the NCBI/GenBank database.

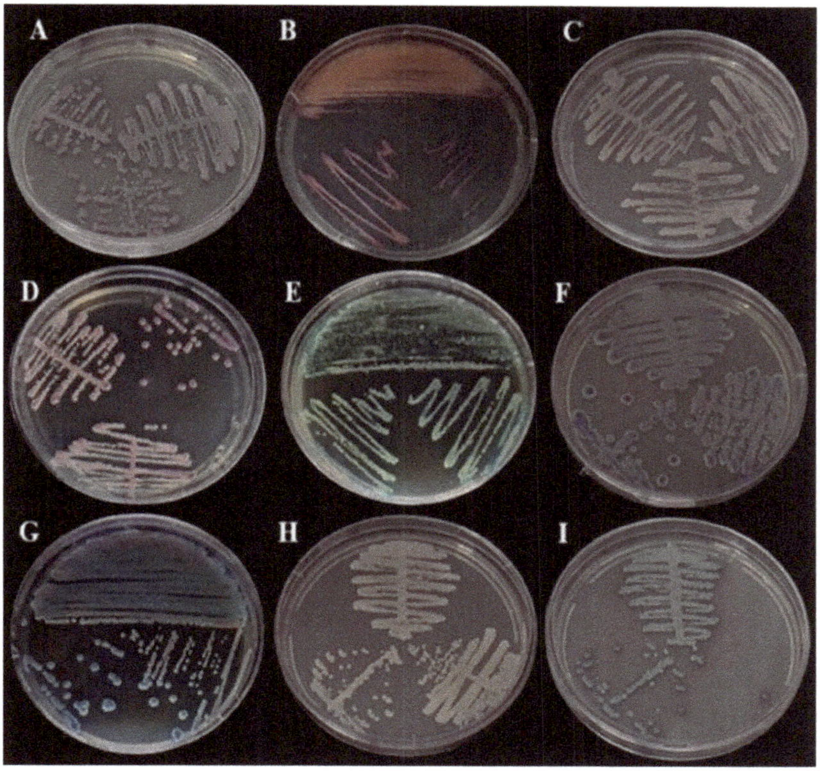

Figure 2. Growth in BDTM CHROMagar^{TM} Candida Medium (BD Difco) incubated at 35 °C for 48 h: (**A**) *Cutaneotrichosporon dermatis*, (**B**) *Rhodotorula mucilaginosa*, (**C**) *Candida glabrata*, (**D**) *Candida orthopsilosis*, (**E**) *Kodamaea jinghongensis*, (**F**) *Candida lusitanea*, (**G**) *Kodamaea jinghongensis*, (**H**) *Candida orthopsilosis* and (**I**) *Candida tropicalis*.

2.2. Phylogenetic Analyses

Evolutionary analyses were conducted in MEGA X [35]. The phylogenetic relationships between the sample isolates and the reference strains from ITS sequences were performed by the Neighbor Joining method [36]. The percentages of replicate trees in which the associated taxa clustered together in the bootstrap test (1000 replicates) are shown next to the branches [37]. The evolutionary distances were computed using the Maximum Composite Likelihood method [38] and are in the units of the number of base substitutions per site.

2.3. Herpesvirus qPCR

For the analysis of the presence and quantification of the viral load of herpesviruses, the samples were extracted using the "QIAamp DNA Mini Kit" (QIAGEN, Hilden, Germany). Then, the samples were analyzed using real-time PCR (qPCR) through the commercial kit AgPath-IDTM One-Step RT-PCR Kit (Life Technologies, Carlsbad, CA, USA). A multiplex real-time PCR (qPCR) was performed for each herpesvirus subfamily (Alphaherpesvirus, Betaherpervirus and Gammaherpesvirus) according to previously established protocols, and synthetic curves were used to quantify the viral load [39–42].

2.4. Data Analisis

Exploratory data analysis (EDA) was used to better observe the results. Initially, the data was organized and cleaned, removing incomplete records and inconsistencies. Then, measures of central tendency (mean) and measures of dispersion (standard deviation) were applied, in addition to establishing frequencies represented in percentages, to summarize the main characteristics of the data. This exploratory approach allowed a deeper understanding of the dataset.

3. Results

3.1. Characteristics of Patients

The basic characteristics of the individuals analyzed in this study are the mean age of the patients, which was 38.67 $\pm$ 14.06 years, and the sex, where 57.14% (4/7) were female. In addition, the mean body mass index (BMI) was 22.46 $\pm$ 5.78, two individuals had diabetes and no patients were smokers. Among the IBD group, 57.14% (4/7) had UC and 42.86% (3/7) had CD, and the average disease duration was 13.7 $\pm$ 5.7 years. Five of these patients showed disease remission (three with UC and two with CD), three of these individuals received biological medication (one with active disease and two in remission), and finally, no patients received corticosteroids. In this study, 85.7% (6/7) of the participants had some level of periodontal disease and the average number of teeth was 20.3 $\pm$ 10.9.

3.2. Detection and Characterization of Fungi

In the polyphasic taxonomy, we observed the presence of three genres of yeast in the oral microbiome, as the partial sequencing of the ITS regions identified species of the genera *Kodamaea, Trichosporon, Rhodotorula* and *Candida*. The Figures 1 and 2 show, respectively, the growth of fungi in Sabouraud Dextrose Agar Medium (BD Difco, Franklin Lakes, NJ, USA) and in BDTM CHROMagar^{TM} Candida Medium (BD Difco, Franklin Lakes, NJ, USA).

Isolation, sequencing and alignment of the ITS region showed a total correspondence between LS11-2, LS17-1 and *K. jinghongensis* (KY213814.1) (Figure 3A). LS3-1 showed a significant correspondence to *R. mucilaginosa* (CBS 11029) (Figure 3B), which is highly related (92%) to *Cystobasidium pallidum*. Isolate LS01-2 showed a significant correspondence to *Cutaneotrichosporon dermatis* (86%) (KY103013.1) (Figure 3C), which is significantly related to the clade composed of *Apiotrichum montevideense* (KY106139.1), *A. domesticum* (NR073239.1), *A. loubieri* (106132.1) and *T. japonicum* (90%) (AF308657.1). Isolates LS11-1 and LS17-3 revealed 70% correspondence to species *C. orthopsilosis* (NR130661.1) (Figure 3D). However, the group formed by isolates LS11-1, LS17-3 and *C. orthopsilosis* were 90% correspondent to *C. metapsilosis* (NR130673.1) (Figure 3D). Isolate ME20 revealed a full correspondence to *C. tropicalis* (MW358908.1), while isolate LE07 corresponded in the same pattern to *C. glabrata* (AM492797.1) (Figure 3D). Isolate LS13 was 97% correspondent to *C. lusitaniae* (AF172262.1) (Figure 3D).

In this study, when the fungi detected according to the etiology of IBD were observed (Table 1), it was found that patients with CD presented with *R. mucilaginosa*, *C. orthopsilosis* and *K. jinghongensis*, while individuals with UC presented with *C. dermatis*, *C. glabrata*, *C. lusitanea* and *C. tropicalis*.

Table 1. Detection and characterization of fungi according to type of inflammatory bowel disease.

Isolate	Sex	Age	Type of IBD	Species of Fungi
LS01-2	Male	51	UC	*Cutaneotrichosporon dermatis*
LS03-1	Female	49	CD	*Rhodotorula mucilaginosa*
LE07	Female	63	UC	*Candida glabrata*
LS11-1/LS11-2	Male	40	CD	*Candida orthopsilosis/Kodamaea jinghongensis*
LS 13	Male	31	UC	*Candida lusitanea*
LE17-1/LS17-3	Female	21	CD	*Kodamaea jinghongensis/Candida orthopsilosis*
ME20	Female	32	UC	*Candida tropicalis*

IBD: Inflammatory bowel disease; CD: Crohn's disease; UC: Ulcerative colitis.

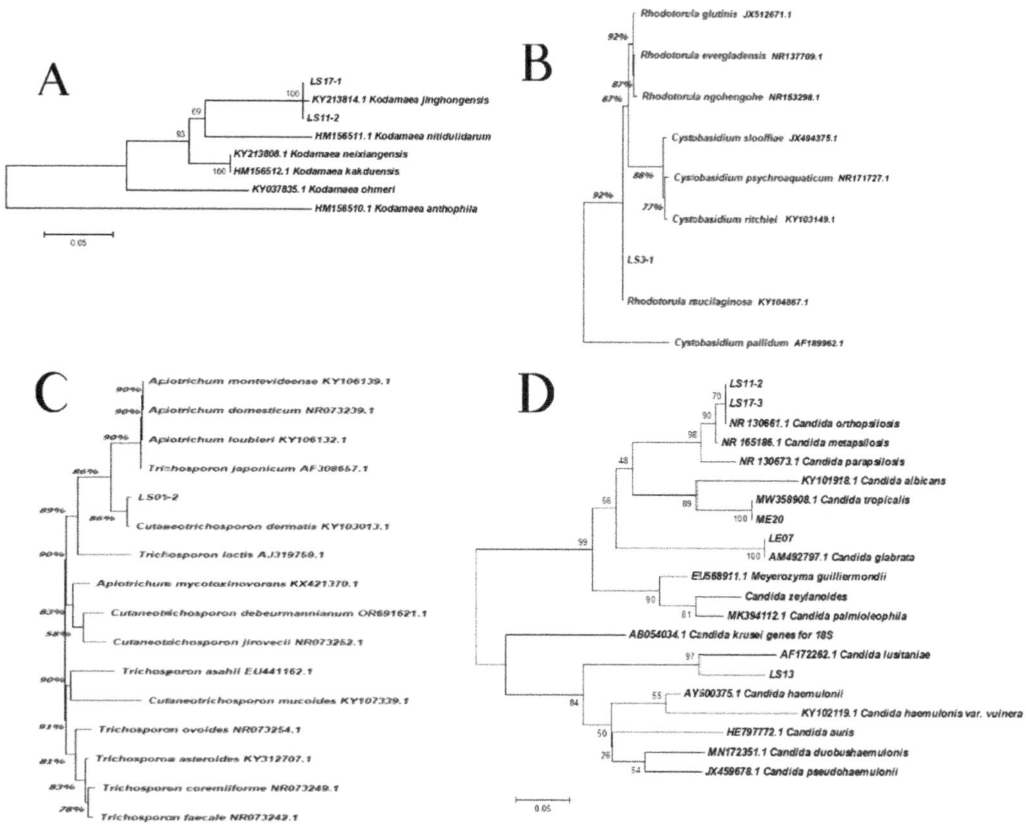

Figure 3. The phylogenetic relationships between the isolates of samples with reference strains inferred from ITS sequences. (**A**) *Kodhamaea* sp.: this analysis involved eight nucleotide sequences, and a total of 263 positions were obtained in the final dataset. (**B**) *Rhodotorula* sp.: this analysis involved nine nucleotide sequences, and a total of 602 positions were obtained in the final dataset. (**C**) *Trichosporon* sp.: this analysis involved 16 nucleotide sequences and a total of 560 positions were obtained in the final dataset. (**D**) *Candida* spp.: this analysis involved 22 nucleotide sequences and a total of 92 positions were obtained in the final dataset.

3.3. Detection and Characterization of Herpesvirus

Of the samples analyzed, two (28.57%) presented with infection by at least one herpesvirus (Table 2). In sample LS13, the presence of HSV-1 was detected (viral load 1.07×10^4). In addition, this patient had UC, and *C. lusitaniae* was detected. While sample ME20 presented with a co-infection of EBV (viral load 7.40×10^4) and HHV-7 (viral load 2.26×10^5), the patient also had UC, and *C. tropicalis* was detected.

Table 2. Detection and quantification of samples with herpesvirus-positivity.

Sample	IBD	Viral Load HSV-1	 EBV	 HHV-7	Fungi Detection
LS13	UC	1.07×10^4	Undetermined	Undetermined	*C. lusitaniae*
ME20	UC	Undetermined	7.40×10^4	2.26×10^5	*C. tropicalis*

All study samples were analyzed for all human herpesviruses; this table shows only those with a detectable viral load. The others were undetermined (no viral load detected). EBV: Epstein–Barr virus; HSV-1: Herpes Simplex Virus 1; HHV-7: Human Herpesvirus 7; IBD: inflammatory bowel disease; UC: ulcerative colitis.

4. Discussion

In this study, different fungal species were observed according to IBD types (CD and UC). *C. dermatis* was identified in an isolate from a UC patient, representing an important yeast associated with rare and opportunistic infections in immunocompromised and even pediatric patients [43–45]. Furthermore, studies show a potential risk of opportunistic infections related to this fungus, due to antifungal resistance and its ability to produce important virulence factors [46,47]. However, there are no studies in IBD patients. In addition to yeasts, the presence of herpesviruses was identified in the oral microbiota of two UC patients.

Many microorganisms present in the human microbiome may serve as a physiological indicator of good health or a potential inflammatory process. The oral mycobiome is predominantly formed by several genera, including *Candida, Cladosporium, Saccharomyces, Fusarium, Aspergillus, Aureobasidium* and *Cryptococcus* [48,49].

R. mucilaginosa, found in this study, is an opportunistic and emerging agent, which can cause infections mainly in immunocompromised patients, and has already been reported in the oral microbiota of patients with colorectal cancer [14,50–54]. Furthermore, in oral *R. mucilaginosa* isolates from patients with chronic kidney disease, all isolates presented with antifungal resistance to azoles and the ability to form biofilms [55]. Therefore, colonization by *R. mucilaginosa* may be a risk factor for serious infection in patients with chronic diseases, such as CD.

K. jinghongensis was found to be present in an oral isolation from a CD patient. *K. jinghongensis* is a yeast species first described by Gao et al. (2017) and to date, there are no studies on the impact of *K. jinghongensis* infection on human health [56,57]. *Kodamaea* is known to be an important opportunistic yeast genus, with *K. ohmeri* being the most reported pathogen for fungemia, and this species was detected in oral samples from patients with head and neck cancer [15,16,58]. Therefore, further studies are needed to evaluate the impact of *K. jinghongensis* infections, especially in individuals with IBD.

The most common yeasts found in the oral microbiota are from the *Candida* genus, and they can switch from commensal to pathogenic depending on host homeostasis [10]. In this study, a *C. orthopsilosis* isolate was found in one CD patient and *C. glabrata, C. lusitanea* and *C. tropicalis* were found in UC individuals. *Candida* species are the most common agents of infection in IBD patients, but the influence of *C. orthopsilosis* and *C. lusitanea* on IBD is not well established [59–61].

The presence of HSV-1 was identified, which has been associated with severe necrotizing tonsillitis and rare cases of Herpes Simplex Colitis, leading to the exacerbation of UC [29]. Additionally, a coinfection between EBV and HHV-7 was identified. EBV infection is more frequent in individuals with IBD and is associated with more severe cases of the disease [18]; however, its association with other herpesviruses, such as HHV-7, can further aggravate the inflammatory condition of these individuals [62,63]. Therefore, identifying possible infections and/or reactivations of herpesviruses in patients with IBD may be important for the differential diagnosis of these individuals. Herpesvirus has been detected in the oral cavities of immunocompromised patients, but the presence of fungal species remains rare [64–67].

Patients with a viral load for herpesvirus were positive for the *Candida* group (*C. lusitaniae* and *C. tropicalis*). In the literature, a mutualistic relationship between Herpes Simplex (HSV-1 and HSV-2) and *C. albicans* is reported, where the viruses can be included in the fungal biofilm, becoming more resistant to pharmacological treatments (acyclovir) [68,69]. In addition, the presence of Herpes Simplex infection increases the adherence and initial formation of *C. albicans* biofilms [70,71], indicating that the interaction between these different species is complex and can influence the dynamics of infection and consequently the health of the individual. However, studies are lacking in determining the association between herpesviruses and other species of *Candida*, as well as other types of herpesviruses besides Herpes Simplex.

Studies have shown that alterations in the fungal microbiota in patients with IBD, especially the presence of emerging fungi, have been shown to be a factor in the worsening of the clinical condition of these individuals [18–23]. Furthermore, the presence of herpesviruses in mucous membranes has been associated with the worsening of the inflammatory condition and exacerbation of IBD [28].

Although CD and UC are both classified as IBD, they have distinct pathogeneses. CD is characterized by segmented inflammation that can affect any part of the gastrointestinal tract, being most common in the ileum, while UC is characterized by continuous inflammation that is predominantly in the colon and rectum [72]. The literature describes that the oral microbiome may present with significant differences between the types of IBD. Xun et al. (2018) described that, in individuals with CD, an enrichment of species from the *Veillonellaceae* family and a decrease in *Neisseriaceae* and *Haemophilus* could be observed. In individuals with UC, an enrichment of the *Streptococcaceae* and *Enterobacteriaceae* family and a decrease in *Lachnospiraceae* and *Prevotella* in the oral microbiota were observed [73]. These differences in the oral microbiomes can be explained by the distinct pathogenesis of IBD and may also influence the development of the disease, since immune responses can vary considerably between CD and UC. However, to date, studies have focused on bacterial differences in the oral microbiome. Further studies are needed to investigate whether there are also differences in the presence of fungi and viruses in the oral cavity of patients with CD and UC.

The severity of the pathogens identified may vary, as they are influenced by the individual's immune status. In general, opportunistic pathogens, such as the fungal species identified in this study, can cause a variety of clinical manifestations and can lead to severe invasive infections, especially in immunocompromised individuals. In addition, some fungal species identified have already been associated with antifungal resistance, which may contribute to greater disease severity and therapeutic challenges.

The infection process is complex and multifactorial, but it generally begins with immunological alterations and the establishment of a proinflammatory environment, which favors dysbiosis of the human microbiome and alters the integrity of mucosal barriers. In other words, a series of conditions occur that will favor the proliferation of microorganisms and the establishment of a local or systemic infection.

In addition, the herpesviruses identified in our study are known for their ability to establish latency and reactivate under conditions of immunosuppression. This reactivation can contribute to the severity of the disease, either through direct effects or by modulating the immune response, facilitating infection by other opportunistic pathogens.

Investigating the presence and co-occurrence of herpesvirus and fungal species in the oral cavity of immunocompromised patients is crucial, as these infections may complicate the clinical management of such patients. Understanding the interactions between viral and fungal pathogens could reveal novel insights into their combined impacts on immune suppression, potentially informing better diagnostic and therapeutic approaches. Additionally, identifying fungal species in these contexts could help anticipate and prevent opportunistic infections, improving patient outcomes and quality of life.

5. Conclusions

It is crucial to investigate the presence of herpesviruses and fungi, particularly emerging fungal species, within the oral microbiota to better understand the risk factors for aggravating IBD in individuals with this disease. To our knowledge, this is the first study to document the presence of the emerging fungi *K. jinghongensis* and *C. dermatis* in the oral microbiota of IBD patients. Additionally, we report the presence of rarely described yeasts, including *R. mucilaginosa, C. orthopsilosis* and *C. lusitaniae*, as well as the coexistence of HSV-1/*C. lusitaniae* and EBV/HHV-7/*C. tropicalis* in UC patients. These findings underscore the importance of identifying emerging pathogens within the oral microbiota and potential opportunistic infections in individuals with chronic intestinal inflammation. The presence of these pathogens could influence inflammatory processes and, consequently, the prognosis of these patients, highlighting the need for continued research into the microbiota's role in IBD development, progression and management.

Author Contributions: Conceptualization, M.M.E.O.; methodology, M.M.E.O. and V.S.d.P.; formal analysis, L.B.C.; investigation, L.B.C., G.L.d.C., T.N.P. and R.M.P.d.S.; writing—original draft preparation, M.M.E.O. and L.B.C.; writing—review and editing, F.B., F.M.d.C., G.O.S.-J., G.L.d.C., T.N.P., R.M.P.d.S., R.M., R.C., C.Z. and V.S.d.P.; visualization, L.B.C.; supervision, M.M.E.O.; project administration, M.M.E.O.; funding acquisition, M.M.E.O. All authors have read and agreed to the published version of the manuscript.

Funding: The LBC was funded by Fundação Coordenação de Aperfeiçoamento de Pessoal de Nível Superior (CAPES—Grant 88887.947447/2024-00). The authors are grateful to Fiocruz, the State Funding Agency Fundação Carlos Chagas Filho de Amparo à Pesquisa do Estado do Rio de Janeiro (FAPERJ—Grants: JCNE E-26/201.433/2021; JCNE E-26/204.581/2024 and E-26/210.114/2023), and Conselho Nacional de Desenvolvimento Científico e Tecnológico (CNPq—Grant Proc. 307007/2022-7).

Institutional Review Board Statement: This study was conducted in accordance with the Declaration of Helsinki and was approved by the Institutional Review Board (or Ethics Committee) of Pedro Ernesto University Hospital/UERJ (CAEE no. 54235021.7.0000.5259, approved in December of 2021).

Informed Consent Statement: Informed consent was obtained from all subjects involved in this study.

Data Availability Statement: The original contributions presented in this study are included in the article. Further inquiries can be directed to the corresponding authors.

Acknowledgments: The authors are grateful to Danielly Corrêa-Moreira for the technical support in the logistics of these samples.

Conflicts of Interest: The authors declare no conflicts of interest.

Abbreviations

The following abbreviations are used in this manuscript:

IBD	Inflammatory Bowel Disease
CD	Crohn's Disease
UC	Ulcerative Colitis
HPV	Human Papilloma Virus
HHV	Human Herpes Virus
CMV	Cytomegalovirus
EBV	Epstein–Barr virus
SDA	Sabouraud Dextrose Agar
PCR	Polymerase Chain Reaction
qPCR	Real-time PCR
EDA	Exploratory Data Analysis

References

1. Alatab, S.; Sepanlou, S.G.; Ikuta, K.; Vahedi, H.; Bisignano, C.; Safiri, S.; Sadeghi, A.; Nixon, M.R.; Abdoli, A.; Abolhassani, H.; et al. The global, regional, and national burden of inflammatory bowel disease in 195 countries and territories, 1990–2017: A systematic analysis for the Global Burden of Disease Study 2017. *Lancet Gastroenterol. Hepatol.* **2020**, *5*, 17–30. [CrossRef] [PubMed] [PubMed Central]
2. Ciorba, M.A.; Konnikova, L.; A Hirota, S.; Lucchetta, E.M.; Turner, J.R.; Slavin, A.; Johnson, K.; Condray, C.D.; Hong, S.; Cressall, B.K.; et al. Challenges in IBD Research 2024: Preclinical Human IBD Mechanisms. *Inflam. Bow Dise* **2024**, *30*, S5–S18. [CrossRef]
3. Pascal, V.; Pozuelo, M.; Borruel, N.; Casellas, F.; Campos, D.; Santiago, A.; Martinez, X.; Varela, E.; Sarrabayrouse, G.; Machiels, K.; et al. A microbial signature for Crohn's disease. *Gut* **2017**, *66*, 813–822. [CrossRef] [PubMed] [PubMed Central]
4. Hu, S.; Mok, J.; Gowans, M.; Ong, D.E.H.; Hartono, J.L.; Lee, J.W.J. Oral Microbiome of Crohn's Disease Patients with and Without Oral Manifestations. *J. Crohns. Colitis.* **2022**, *16*, 1628–1636. [CrossRef] [PubMed] [PubMed Central]
5. Deo, P.N.; Deshmukh, R. Oral microbiome: Unveiling the fundamentals. *J. Oral Maxillofac. Pathol.* **2019**, *23*, 122–128. [CrossRef] [PubMed] [PubMed Central]
6. Dewhirst, F.E.; Chen, T.; Izard, J.; Paster, B.J.; Tanner, A.C.R.; Yu, W.-H.; Lakshmanan, A.; Wade, W.G. The human oral microbiome. *J. Bacteriol.* **2010**, *192*, 5002–5017. [CrossRef] [PubMed] [PubMed Central]
7. Martínez, A.; Kuraji, R.; Kapila, Y.L. The human oral virome: Shedding light on the dark matter. *Periodontol. 2000* **2021**, *87*, 282–298. [CrossRef] [PubMed] [PubMed Central]
8. Kumamoto, C.A. Inflammation and gastrointestinal Candida colonization. *Curr. Opin. Microbiol.* **2011**, *14*, 386–391. [CrossRef] [PubMed] [PubMed Central]
9. Ellepola, K.; Truong, T.; Liu, Y.; Lin, Q.; Lim, T.K.; Lee, Y.M.; Cao, T.; Koo, H.; Seneviratne, C.J. Multi-omics analyses reveal synergistic carbohydrate metabolism in *Streptococcus mutans-Candida albicans* mixed-species biofilms. *Infect. Immun.* **2019**, *87*, e00339-19. [CrossRef]
10. Defta, C.L.; Albu, C.-C.; Albu, Ş.-D.; Bogdan-Andreescu, C.F. Oral Mycobiota: A Narrative Review. *Dent. J.* **2024**, *12*, 115. [CrossRef] [PubMed] [PubMed Central]
11. Rivera, R.E.; Zuluaga, A.; Arango, K.; Kadar, I.; Pinillos, P.A.; Montes, L.F.; Cepeda, E.C.; González, E.; Alfonso, P.A.; Villalba, A.A.; et al. Characterization of oral yeasts isolated from healthy individuals attended in different Colombian dental clinics. *J. Biomed. Res.* **2019**, *33*, 333–342. [CrossRef]
12. D'Enfert, C.; Kaune, A.-K.; Alaban, L.-R.; Chakraborty, S.; Cole, N.; Delavy, M.; Kosmala, D.; Marsaux, B.; Fróis-Martins, R.; Morelli, M.; et al. The impact of the Fungus-Host-Microbiota interplay upon *Candida albicans* infections: Current knowledge and new perspectives. *FEMS Microbiol. Rev.* **2021**, *45*, fuaa060. [CrossRef] [PubMed] [PubMed Central]
13. Deepa, A.; Nair, B.J.; Sivakumar, T.; Joseph, A.P. Uncommon opportunistic fungal infections of oral cavity: A review. *J. Oral Maxillofac. Pathol.* **2014**, *18*, 235–243. [CrossRef] [PubMed] [PubMed Central]
14. Troska, P.; Sucharzewska, E.; Dynowska, M.; Ejdys, E. Fungi of the genus Rhodotorula isolated from the oral cavity of oncologic patients with colorectal cancer. *Ann. Parasitol.* **2017**, *63*, 57–62. [CrossRef] [PubMed]
15. Chakrabarti, A.; Rudramurthy, S.M.; Kale, P.; Hariprasath, P.; Dhaliwal, M.; Singhi, S.; Rao, K.L.N. Epidemiological study of a large cluster of fungaemia cases due to *Kodamaea ohmeri* in an Indian tertiary care centre. *Clin. Microbiol. Infect.* **2014**, *20*, O83–O89. [CrossRef] [PubMed]

16. Zhou, M.; Li, Y.; Kudinha, T.; Xu, Y.; Liu, Z. *Kodamaea ohmeri* as an Emerging Human Pathogen: A Review and Update. *Front. Microbiol.* **2021**, *12*, 736582. [CrossRef]
17. Junqueira, J.C.; Vilela, S.F.G.; Rossoni, R.D.; Barbosa, J.O.; Costa, A.C.B.P.; Rasteiro, V.M.C.; Suleiman, J.M.A.H.; Jorge, A.O.C. Oral colonization by yeasts in HIV-positive patients in Brazil. *Rev. Inst. Med. Trop. Sao Paulo.* **2012**, *54*, 17–24. [CrossRef] [PubMed]
18. Wang, A.; Zhai, Z.; Ding, Y.; Wei, J.; Wei, Z.; Cao, H. The oral-gut microbiome axis in inflammatory bowel disease: From inside to insight. *Front. Immunol.* **2024**, *15*, 1430001. [CrossRef] [PubMed]
19. Underhill, D.M.; Braun, J. Fungal microbiome in inflammatory bowel disease: A critical assessment. *J. Clin. Investig.* **2022**, *132*, e155786. [CrossRef] [PubMed] [PubMed Central]
20. Catalán-Serra, I.; Thorsvik, S.; Beisvag, V.; Bruland, T.; Underhill, D.; Sandvik, A.K.; Granlund, A.v.B. Fungal Microbiota Composition in Inflammatory Bowel Disease Patients: Characterization in Different Phenotypes and Correlation with Clinical Activity and Disease Course. *Inflam. Bow Dis.* **2024**, *30*, 1164–1177. [CrossRef] [PubMed]
21. Yu, M.; Ding, H.; Gong, S.; Luo, Y.; Lin, H.; Mu, Y.; Li, H.; Li, X.; Zhong, M. Fungal dysbiosis facilitates inflammatory bowel disease by enhancing CD4+ T cell glutaminolysis. *Front. Cell Infect. Microbiol.* **2023**, *13*, 1140757. [CrossRef] [PubMed] [PubMed Central]
22. Guzzo, G.L.; Mittinty, M.N.; Llamas, B.; Andrews, J.M.; Weyrich, L.S. Individuals with Inflammatory Bowel Disease Have an Altered Gut Microbiome Composition of Fungi and Protozoa. *Microorganisms.* **2022**, *10*, 1910. [CrossRef] [PubMed] [PubMed Central]
23. El Mouzan, M.; Wang, F.; Al Mofarreh, M.; Menon, R.; Al Barrag, A.; Korolev, K.S.; Al Sarkhy, A.; Al Asmi, M.; Hamed, Y.; Saeed, A.; et al. Fungal Microbiota Profile in Newly Diagnosed Treatment-naïve Children with Crohn's Disease. *J. Crohns Colitis.* **2017**, *11*, 586–592, Erratum in *J. Crohns Colitis.* **2023**, *17*, 149. [CrossRef] [PubMed]
24. Li, Y.; Wang, K.; Zhang, B.; Tu, Q.; Yao, Y.; Cui, B.; Ren, B.; He, J.; Shen, X.; Van Nostrand, J.D.; et al. Salivary mycobiome dysbiosis and its potential impact on bacteriome shifts and host immunity in oral lichen planus. *Int. J. Oral Sci.* **2019**, *11*, 13. [CrossRef] [PubMed] [PubMed Central]
25. Rashed, R.; Valcheva, R.; Dieleman, L.A. Manipulation of Gut Microbiota as a Key Target for Crohn's Disease. *Front. Med.* **2022**, *9*, 887044. [CrossRef] [PubMed] [PubMed Central]
26. Girija, A.S.S.; Ganesh, P.S. Functional biomes beyond the bacteriome in the oral ecosystem. *Jpn. Dent. Sci. Rev.* **2022**, *58*, 217–226. [CrossRef] [PubMed] [PubMed Central]
27. Xiao, X.; Liu, S.; Deng, H.; Song, Y.; Zhang, L.; Song, Z. Advances in the oral microbiota and rapid detection of oral infectious diseases. *Front. Microbiol.* **2023**, *14*, 1121737. [CrossRef] [PubMed] [PubMed Central]
28. Zhang, H.; Zhao, S.; Cao, Z. Impact of Epstein-Barr virus infection in patients with inflammatory bowel disease. *Front. Immunol.* **2022**, *13*, 1001055. [CrossRef] [PubMed] [PubMed Central]
29. Phadke, V.K.; Friedman-Moraco, R.J.; Quigley, B.C.; Farris, A.B.; Norvell, J.P. Concomitant herpes simplex virus colitis and hepatitis in a man with ulcerative colitis: Case report and review of the literature. *Medicine* **2016**, *95*, e5082. [CrossRef] [PubMed] [PubMed Central]
30. Leal, T.; Arroja, B.; Costa, D.; Ferreira, C.; Soares, J.B.; Gonçalves, R. Colitis due to Cytomegalovirus and Herpes Simplex Type 2 as a Complication of a First Presentation of Inflammatory Bowel Disease. *GE Port. J. Gastroenterol.* **2021**, *29*, 56–60. [CrossRef] [PubMed] [PubMed Central]
31. Altunal, L.; Ozel, A.; Ak, C. Cytomegalovirus reactivation in ulcerative colitis patients: Early indicators. *Niger. J. Clin. Pract.* **2023**, *26*, 765–770. [CrossRef] [PubMed]
32. Pinto, T.N.; Kohn, A.; da Costa, G.L.; Oliveira, L.M.A.; Pinto, T.C.A.; Oliveira, M.M.E. Candida guilliermondii as an agent of postpartum subacute mastitis in Rio de Janeiro, Brazil: Case report. *Front. Microbiol.* **2022**, *13*, 964685. [CrossRef] [PubMed] [PubMed Central]
33. Stevenson, L.G.; Drake, S.K.; Shea, Y.R.; Zelazny, A.M.; Murray, P.R. Evaluation of matrix-assisted laser desorption ionization-time of flight mass spectrometry for identification of clinically important yeast species. *J. Clin. Microbiol.* **2010**, *48*, 3482–3486. [CrossRef] [PubMed] [PubMed Central]
34. Lindsley, M.D.; Hurst, S.F.; Iqbal, N.J.; Morrison, C.J. Rapid identification of dimorphic and yeast-like fungal pathogens using specific DNA probes. *J. Clin. Microbiol.* **2001**, *39*, 3505–3511. [CrossRef] [PubMed] [PubMed Central]
35. Kumar, S.; Stecher, G.; Li, M.; Knyaz, C.; Tamura, K. MEGA X: Molecular Evolutionary Genetics Analysis across Computing Platforms. *Mol. Biol. Evol.* **2018**, *35*, 1547–1549. [CrossRef] [PubMed] [PubMed Central]
36. Saitou, N.; Nei, M. The neighbor-joining method: A new method for reconstructing phylogenetic trees. *Mol. Biol. Evol.* **1987**, *4*, 406–425. [CrossRef] [PubMed]
37. Felsenstein, J. Confidence limits on phylogenies: An approach using the bootstrap. *Evolution* **1985**, *39*, 783–791. [CrossRef] [PubMed]
38. Tamura, K.; Nei, M.; Kumar, S. Prospects for inferring very large phylogenies by using the neighbor-joining method. *Proc. Natl. Acad. Sci. USA.* **2004**, *101*, 11030–11035. [CrossRef] [PubMed] [PubMed Central]

39. Lima, L.R.; Silva, A.P.; Schmidt-Chanasit, J.; Paula, V.S. Diagnosis of human herpes virus 1 and 2 (HHV-1 and HHV-2): Use of a synthetic standard curve for absolute quantification by real time polymerase chain reaction. *Mem Inst. Oswaldo. Cruz.* **2017**, *112*, 220–223. [CrossRef] [PubMed] [PubMed Central]
40. Raposo, J.V.; Alves, A.D.R.; Silva, A.d.S.d.; dos Santos, D.C.; Gil Melgaço, J.; Moreira, O.C.; Pinto, M.A.; de Paula, V.S. Multiplex qPCR facilitates identification of betaherpesviruses in patients with acute liver failure of unknown etiology. *BMC Infect. Dis.* **2019**, *19*, 773. [CrossRef] [PubMed] [PubMed Central]
41. Carneiro, V.C.d.S.; Moreira, O.d.C.; Coelho, W.L.d.C.N.P.; Rio, B.C.; Sarmento, D.J.d.S.; Salvio, A.L.; Alves-Leon, S.V.; de Paula, V.S.; Leon, L.A.A. miRNAs in Neurological Manifestation in Patients Co-Infected with SARS-CoV-2 and Herpesvírus 6 (HHV-6). *Int. J. Mol. Sci.* **2023**, *24*, 11201. [CrossRef] [PubMed]
42. Lopes, A.d.O.; Spitz, N.; Martinelli, K.G.; de Paula, A.V.; Toscano, A.L.d.C.C.; Braz-Silva, P.H.; Netto, J.d.S.B.; Tozetto-Mendoza, T.R.; de Paula, V.S. IIntroduction of human gammaherpesvirus 8 genotypes A, B, and C into Brazil from multiple geographic regions. *Virus Res.* **2020**, *276*, 197828. [CrossRef] [PubMed]
43. Fan, Y.-M.; Huang, W.-M.; Yang, Y.-P.; Li, W.; Li, S.-F. Primary cutaneous trichosporonosis caused by *Trichosporon dermatis* in an immunocompetent man. *J. Am. Acad. Dermatol.* **2011**, *65*, 434–436. [CrossRef] [PubMed]
44. Gunn, S.R.; Reveles, X.T.; Hamlington, J.D.; Sadkowski, L.C.; Johnson-Pais, T.L.; Jorgensen, J.H. Use of DNA sequencing analysis to confirm fungemia due to *Trichosporon dermatis* in a pediatric patient. *J. Clin. Microbiol.* **2006**, *44*, 1175–1177. [CrossRef] [PubMed] [PubMed Central]
45. Montoya, A.M.; Luna-Rodríguez, C.E.; Bonifaz, A.; Treviño-Rangel, R.d.J.; Rojas, O.C.; González, G.M. Physiological characterization and molecular identification of some rare yeast species causing onychomycosis. *J. Mycol. Med.* **2021**, *31*, 101121. [CrossRef] [PubMed]
46. Pagani, D.M.; Heidrich, D.; Paulino, G.V.B.; Alves, K.d.O.; Dalbem, P.T.; de Oliveira, C.F.; Andrade, Z.M.M.; Silva, C.; Correia, M.D.; Scroferneker, M.L.; et al. Susceptibility to antifungal agents and enzymatic activity of *Candida haemulonii* and *Cutaneotrichosporon dermatis* isolated from soft corals on the Brazilian reefs. *Arch. Microbiol.* **2016**, *198*, 963–971. [CrossRef] [PubMed]
47. Santo, E.P.T.D.E.; Monteiro, R.C.; da Costa, A.R.F.; Marques-Da-Silva, S.H. Molecular Identification, Genotyping, Phenotyping, and Antifungal Susceptibilities of Medically Important Trichosporon, Apiotrichum, and Cutaneotrichosporon Species. *Mycopathologia* **2020**, *185*, 307–317. [CrossRef] [PubMed]
48. Wade, W.G. The oral microbiome in health and disease. *Pharmacol. Res.* **2013**, *69*, 137–143. [CrossRef] [PubMed]
49. Aggarwal, N.; Kitano, S.; Puah, G.R.Y.; Kittelmann, S.; Hwang, I.Y.; Chang, M.W. Microbiome and Human Health: Current Under-standing, Engineering, and Enabling Technologies. *Chem. Rev.* **2023**, *123*, 31–72. [CrossRef] [PubMed] [PubMed Central]
50. García-Suárez, J.; Gómez-Herruz, P.; Cuadros, J.A.; Burgaleta, C. Epidemiology and outcome of Rhodotorula infection in haematological patients. *Mycoses* **2011**, *54*, 318–324. [CrossRef] [PubMed]
51. Spiliopoulou, A.; Anastassiou, E.D.; Christofidou, M. *Rhodotorula* fungemia of an intensive care unit patient and review of published cases. *Mycopathologia* **2012**, *174*, 301–309. [CrossRef] [PubMed]
52. Kim, H.A.; Hyun, M.; Ryu, S.-Y. Catheter-associated *Rhodotorula mucilaginosa* fungemia in an immunocompetent host. *Infect. Chemother.* **2013**, *45*, 339–342. [CrossRef]
53. Pereira, C.; Ribeiro, S.; Lopes, V.; Mendonça, T. *Rhodotorula mucilaginosa* fungemia and pleural tuberculosis in an immunocompetent patient: An uncommon association. *Mycopathologia* **2016**, *181*, 145–149. [CrossRef] [PubMed]
54. Sundararaju, S.; Salah, H.; Ibrahim, E.B.; Perez-Lopez, A.; Ben Abid, F.; Tsui, C.K.M. Draft Genome Sequence of *Rhodotorula mucilaginosa* from an Adult Patient in Qatar. *Microbiol. Resour. Announc.* **2021**, *10*, e0072521. [CrossRef] [PubMed] [PubMed Central]
55. Jarros, I.C.; Veiga, F.F.; Corrêa, J.L.; Barros, I.L.E.; Gadelha, M.C.; Voidaleski, M.F.; Pieralisi, N.; Pedroso, R.B.; Vicente, V.A.; Negri, M.; et al. Microbiological and virulence aspects of *Rhodotorula mucilaginosa*. *Excli. J.* **2020**, *19*, 687–704. [PubMed] [PubMed Central]
56. Gao, W.-L.; Liu, T.-T.; Zheng, J.; Hui, F.-L. *Kodamaea neixiangensis* f.a.; sp. nov. and *Kodamaea jinghongensis* f.a.; sp. nov.; two yeast species isolated from rotting wood. *Int. J. Syst. Evol. Microbiol.* **2017**, *67*, 3358–3362. [CrossRef] [PubMed]
57. Schoch, C.L.; Ciufo, S.; Domrachev, M.; Hotton, C.L.; Kannan, S.; Khovanskaya, R.; Leipe, D.; Mcveigh, R.; O'neill, K.; Robbertse, B.; et al. NCBI Taxonomy: A comprehensive update on curation, resources and tools. *Database* **2020**, *2020*, baaa062. [CrossRef] [PubMed] [PubMed Central]
58. Wu, J.; Gan, C.; Li, J.; Liu, Y.; Chen, Z.; Zhang, Y.; Yi, G.; Sui, J.; Xu, J. Species Diversity and Antifungal Susceptibilities of Oral Yeasts from Patients with Head and Neck Cancer. *Infect. Drug Resist.* **2021**, *14*, 2279–2288. [CrossRef] [PubMed] [PubMed Central]
59. Stamatiades, G.A.; Ioannou, P.; Petrikkos, G.; Tsioutis, C. Fungal infections in patients with inflammatory bowel disease: A sys-tematic review. *Mycoses* **2018**, *61*, 366–376. [CrossRef] [PubMed] [PubMed Central]

60. Lehman, H.K.; Davé, R. Candida Glabrata Lymphadenitis Following Infliximab Therapy for Inflammatory Bowel Disease in a Patient with Chronic Granulomatous Disease: Case Report and Literature Review. *Front. Pediatr.* **2021**, *9*, 707369. [CrossRef] [PubMed] [PubMed Central]
61. Yoon, H.; Park, S.; Jun, Y.K.; Choi, Y.; Shin, C.M.; Park, Y.S.; Kim, N.; Lee, D.H. Evaluation of Bacterial and Fungal Biomarkers for Dif-ferentiation and Prognosis of Patients with Inflammatory Bowel Disease. *Microorganisms* **2023**, *11*, 2882. [CrossRef] [PubMed] [PubMed Central]
62. Hosomi, S.; Watanabe, K.; Nishida, Y.; Yamagami, H.; Yukawa, T.; Otani, K.; Nagami, Y.; Tanaka, F.; Taira, K.; Kamata, N.; et al. Combined Infection of Human Herpes Viruses: A Risk Factor for Subsequent Colectomy in Ulcerative Colitis. *Inflamm. Bowel Dis.* **2018**, *24*, 1307–1315. [CrossRef] [PubMed]
63. Shimada, T.; Nagata, N.; Okahara, K.; Joya, A.; Hayashida, T.; Oka, S.; Sakurai, T.; Akiyama, J.; Uemura, N.; Gatanaga, H. PCR detection of human herpesviruses in colonic mucosa of individuals with inflammatory bowel disease: Comparison with individuals with immunocompetency and HIV infection. *PLoS ONE* **2017**, *12*, e0184699. [CrossRef] [PubMed] [PubMed Central]
64. Lino, K.; Alves, L.S.; Raposo, J.V.; Medeiros, T.; Souza, C.F.; da Silva, A.A.; de Paula, V.S.; Almeida, J.R. Presence and clinical impact of human herpesvirus-6 infection in patients with moderate to critical coronavirus disease-19. *J. Med. Virol.* **2022**, *94*, 1212–1216. [CrossRef] [PubMed] [PubMed Central]
65. Lino, K.; Alves, L.S.; Trizzotti, N.; Raposo, J.V.; Souza, C.F.; da Silva, A.A.; de Paula, V.S.; Almeida, J.R. Evaluation of herpesvirus members on hospital admission in patients with systemic lupus erythematous shows higher frequency of Epstein-Barr virus and its associ-ated renal dysfunction. *J. Bras. Nefrol.* **2022**, *44*, 490–497. [CrossRef] [PubMed] [PubMed Central]
66. Raposo, J.V.; Sarmento, D.J.D.S.; Pinto, R.B.D.S.; Lopes, A.O.; Gallottini, M.; Tozetto-Mendoza, T.R.; Braz-Silva, P.H.; de Paula, V.S. Longitu-dinal study on oral shedding of human betaherpesviruses 6 and 7 in renal transplant recipients reveals active replication. *J. Oral Microbiol.* **2020**, *12*, 1785801. [CrossRef] [PubMed] [PubMed Central]
67. Guimarães, A.C.S.; Vedovi, J.V.R.; Ribeiro, C.R.d.A.; Martinelli, K.G.; Machado, M.P.; Manso, P.P.d.A.; de Oliveira, B.C.E.P.D.; Bergamini, M.L.; de Rosa, C.S.; Tozetto-Mendoza, T.R.; et al. Cytomegalovirus in Adenoma and Carcinoma Lesions: Detecting Mono-Infection and Co-Infection in Salivary Glands. *Int. J. Mol. Sci.* **2024**, *25*, 7502. [CrossRef] [PubMed] [PubMed Central]
68. Mazaheritehrani, E.; Sala, A.; Orsi, C.F.; Neglia, R.G.; Morace, G.; Blasi, E.; Cermelli, C. Human pathogenic viruses are retained in and released by Candida albicans biofilm in vitro. *Virus Res.* **2014**, *179*, 153–160. [CrossRef] [PubMed]
69. Ascione, C.; Sala, A.; Mazaheri-Tehrani, E.; Paulone, S.; Palmieri, B.; Blasi, E.; Cermelli, C. Herpes simplex virus-1 entrapped in Can-dida albicans biofilm displays decreased sensitivity to antivirals and UVA1 laser treatment. *Ann. Clin. Microbiol. Antimicrob.* **2017**, *16*, 72. [CrossRef] [PubMed] [PubMed Central]
70. Plotkin, B.J.; Sigar, I.M.; Tiwari, V.; Halkyard, S. Herpes Simplex Virus (HSV) Modulation of Staphylococcus aureus and Candida albicans Initiation of HeLa 299 Cell-Associated Biofilm. *Curr. Microbiol.* **2016**, *72*, 529–537. [CrossRef] [PubMed] [PubMed Central]
71. Plotkin, B.J.; Sigar, I.M.; Kaminski, A.; Kreamer, J.; Ito, B.; Kacmar, J. Kinetics of *Candida albicans* and *Staphylococcus aureus* Biofilm Initiation on Herpes Simplex Virus (HSV-1 and HSV-2) Infected Cells. *Adv. Microbiol.* **2020**, *10*, 583–598. [CrossRef]
72. Flynn, S.; Eisenstein, S. Inflammatory Bowel Disease Presentation and Diagnosis. *Surg. Clin. N. Am. D* **2019**, *99*, 1051–1062. [CrossRef] [PubMed]
73. Xun, Z.; Zhang, Q.; Xu, T.; Chen, N.; Chen, F. Dysbiosis and Ecotypes of the Salivary Microbiome Associated with Inflammatory Bowel Diseases and the Assistance in Diagnosis of Diseases Using Oral Bacterial Profiles. *Front. Microbiol.* **2018**, *9*, 1136. [CrossRef] [PubMed] [PubMed Central]

biomedicines

MDPI

Article

Impact of Coffee Consumption on Subjective Perception and Inflammatory Markers in Patients with Inflammatory Bowel Diseases

Lidia Neamți [1], Simona R. Gheorghe [1], Amalia Ventuneac [2,*], Tudor Drugan [3], Cristina Drugan [1], Ciprian N. Silaghi [1], Lidia Ciobanu [4] and Alexandra M. Crăciun [1]

1. Department of Medical Biochemistry, "Iuliu Hațieganu" University of Medicine and Pharmacy, 400012 Cluj-Napoca, Romania; lidia.neamti@umfcluj.ro (L.N.); gheorghe.simona@umfcluj.ro (S.R.G.); cdrugan@umfcluj.ro (C.D.); silaghi.ciprian@umfcluj.ro (C.N.S.); acraciun@umfcluj.ro (A.M.C.)
2. Department of Internal Medicine, 1 Medical Clinic, "Iuliu Hatieganu" University of Medicine and Pharmacy, 400006 Cluj-Napoca, Romania
3. Department of Medical Informatics and Biostatistics, "Iuliu Hațieganu" University of Medicine and Pharmacy, 400012 Cluj-Napoca, Romania; tdrugan@umfcluj.ro
4. Department of Internal Medicine and Gastroenterology, "Prof. Dr. Octavian Fodor", Regional Institute of Gastroenterology and Hepatology, "Iuliu Hatieganu" University of Medicine and Pharmacy, 400162 Cluj-Napoca, Romania; ciobanulidia@yahoo.com

* Correspondence: amalia.debo.ventuneac@elearn.umfcluj.ro

Abstract: Inflammatory bowel diseases (IBD), including Crohn's disease (CD) and ulcerative colitis (UC), are chronic conditions marked by persistent inflammation, impacting patients' quality of life. This study assessed differences in coffee consumption between CD and UC patients and its potential effects on the subjective perception and objective changes in inflammation markers in these two categories of patients. Using questionnaires, coffee consumption patterns, and perceived symptom effects were evaluated. Biological samples were collected to measure the following inflammatory markers: leukocytes, C-reactive protein (CRP), erythrocyte sedimentation rate (ESR), and fecal calprotectin (FC). Among 148 patients, 60% reported regular coffee consumption, with no significant difference between CD and UC patients. While 45.93% perceived no impact on symptoms, 48% of those reporting exacerbation continued their regular coffee consumption. FC values were significantly lower in coffee consumers than in non-consumers ($p < 0.05$), particularly in those consuming natural coffee ($p < 0.001$), and the case was observed for UC patients ($p < 0.05$). No significant differences were observed in other inflammatory markers, regardless of coffee type, frequency, or milk addition. This study highlights the commonality of coffee consumption among IBD patients and the association of lower FC levels with coffee consumption, especially in UC patients, suggesting that coffee may influence intestinal inflammatory responses.

Keywords: inflammatory bowel diseases; Crohn's disease; ulcerative colitis; coffee; inflammatory markers

1. Introduction

Crohn's disease (CD) and ulcerative colitis (UC) are inflammatory bowel diseases (IBD) with increasing incidence but an incompletely elucidated pathogenesis. In addition to genetic factors and aberrant immune responses, diet is believed to play a vital role in the occurrence of these diseases by inducing specific changes in the intestinal microbiome [1,2].

Research into the link between nutrition and IBD has increased in recent years [2]. Previous research has noted that certain dietary patterns are associated with the onset [3] but also the exacerbation of IBD [4] by inducing and maintaining a pro-inflammatory state in the intestine [5]. Various studies have investigated and identified connections between the pro- or anti-inflammatory effects of various dietary components and markers of inflammation, such as fecal calprotectin (FC) or C-reactive protein (CRP) and the erythrocyte sedimentation rate (ESR) [6]. FC is a marker of intestinal inflammation that significantly correlates with endoscopic disease activity in IBD, providing an essential tool for assessing endoscopic activity and remission, particularly in UC patients [7]. CRP and ESR are among the most used systemic inflammatory markers. Even if they show a modest correlation with endoscopic activity, they can be associated with therapeutic response, especially CRP [8].

Coffee is one of the main beverages consumed worldwide, which is why it has gained increased interest in analyzing its effects in various conditions. Coffee is a mixture of over a thousand different chemicals. While the effects of many coffee compounds on the body are not fully understood due to their relatively low concentrations, three are recognized for their significant bioactive effects: caffeine, diterpenic alcohols (cafestol and kahweol), and chlorogenic acid, along with other polyphenols [9]. Among the properties attributed to these compounds are antioxidant and anti-inflammatory effects [10]. Thus, the beneficial effects of regular coffee consumption have been described for various chronic diseases involving different degrees of inflammation, such as liver disease [11], type 2 diabetes [12], neurodegenerative diseases [13], constipation [14], or cancer [15]. Moreover, regular coffee consumption has been linked to a decrease in general mortality, but especially when related to diabetes or cardiovascular, respiratory, and infectious conditions [16]. Regarding the effect of coffee on the intestine, it has been observed that coffee consumption can increase the production of short-chain fatty acids at the intestinal level, thus having a probiotic effect [17]. Other observed effects include the stimulation of colonic motor activity [18] or increased rectal tone [19]. Some studies have also observed a protective effect against the development of UC [20,21]. These results were not dependent on caffeine content, suggesting that caffeine may not be responsible for the beneficial effects [22]. However, prolonged coffee consumption can also have negative effects, such as increased blood pressure values, predominantly in the elderly [23], or the alteration of sperm quality, possibly leading to infertility [24].

Due to the prokinetic effects on the digestive tract [25], coffee consumption is often not recommended for patients with IBD, especially during the active state of the disease [26]. However, despite the laxative effect of coffee, the anti-inflammatory compounds it contains may still have a positive impact in reducing the inflammation associated with these conditions. Although several studies have evaluated coffee consumption among patients with IBD [21,27–30], to date, no study has examined the relationship between this habit and various markers of inflammation used in clinical practice. In addition, the available studies on this topic are highly heterogeneous, which underlines the need for more extensive research on the effects of coffee consumption in order to evaluate its impact on quality of life and to provide evidence-based recommendations.

Considering the large number of coffee consumers among IBD patients [27], it is essential to understand the effects and consequences of this practice on these conditions. Therefore, this study aims to investigate the differences in coffee consumption between patients with CD and UC and to determine its potential influences on the subjective perception and objective changes of inflammatory markers in these two patient categories.

2. Materials and Methods

The study was conducted within the Regional Institute of Gastroenterology and Hepatology Cluj-Napoca, Romania, for a period of 6 years between 2017 and 2022. The included patients had clinically, endoscopically, and histologically confirmed diagnoses of CD or UC. The patients were selected randomly. All the patients who met the inclusion criteria and consented to undergo a colonoscopy were asked to participate in the study. Patients gave their informed consent to participate. The endoscopist only performed an intestinal biopsy in cases considered necessary.

Clinical and demographic data collected included the type of disease, age at inclusion in the study, age at diagnosis, gender, and smoking status. Patients with other conditions that could have influenced the inflammatory status, such as neoplasms, infections, and autoimmune diseases, or pregnant women were excluded. Depending on clinical, endoscopic, and histological activity status, based on internationally validated scores widely used in current practice, patients were assigned to one of the following subgroups: active disease and disease in remission [31]. Thus, to classify patients with CD, the Crohn's disease activity index (CDAI) was used to evaluate clinical activity, a simple endoscopic score (SES-CD) was used to evaluate endoscopic activity, and the Nani and Cortina score was applied for histological activity. Patients with a CDAI score of <150 points, an SES-CD score of <2 points, and a histological score of <2 points were classified in the remission subgroup. To classify patients with UC, the partial Mayo score was used to evaluate clinical activity, the Mayo endoscopic score was applied for the assessment of endoscopic activity, and the Nancy score was utilized for the evaluation of histological activity. A partial Mayo score of <2 points, an endoscopic Mayo score = 0 points, and a Nancy score < 1 point were considered suggestive of the disease in remission. The other patients were classified as having active disease.

Coffee consumption was assessed by completing a questionnaire previously validated on a similar population within the same hospital. Patients were asked to complete the questionnaire by entering data from the last month before collection. The questionnaire included questions about the type of coffee consumed, the frequency or the amount of consumption, the possible addition of/amount of milk or other similar products, and the eventual addition, amount and type of sweeteners. We proposed categorizing coffee types as follows: natural coffee, which refers to coffee that has been minimally processed and is closer to its natural state; soluble coffee, which is brewed coffee that has been freeze-dried or spray-dried into granules or powder for quick preparation; decaf coffee, which has most of its caffeine removed; cappuccino, a blend of equal parts espresso, steamed milk, and milk foam and other types. Measures commonly used in the kitchen were used to estimate quantities (e.g., cup, spoon). In addition, the patient's perception of coffee consumption ("Does coffee have a beneficial effect on health?"), and the impact of coffee consumption on symptoms (does it improve/worsen/does not influence the symptoms or the patient/does not know) were also evaluated.

Systemic inflammation was evaluated in serum, in the morning, in fasting condition, by leukocyte count (cells/μL), ESR (mm/h), and CRP (mg/dL). Intestinal inflammation was evaluated by measuring FC (μg/g). All inflammatory markers analyzed were quantified in the hospital laboratory. The intra-assay CV for each parameter was <10%. Thus, the number of leukocytes was counted by electrical impedance and light scattering using an automated analyzer Sysmex XN 1000 (Sysmex, Kobe, Japan); capillary photometry was used for ESR measurement on Alifax TEST1 (Alifax, Polverara, Italy), turbidimetric immunoassay was used for CRP determination on Cobas c503 (Roche Diagnostics, Rotkreuz, Switzerland) and an ELISA kit, calprotectin (Orgentec Diagnostika, Mainz, Germany) was used for FC determination. The assay sensitivity was 17.5 μg/g with an intra-assay precision of <6%.

Statistical analysis was performed using the SPSS program (version 25; IBM Corp., Armonk, NY, USA). Clinical and demographic data were presented as the mean ± standard deviation (SD), median, and interquartile range or as percentages (%). Testing for the normality of data distribution was performed by the Kolmogorov–Smirnov test, and differences between groups were evaluated by the Mann–Whitney U test in the case of non-normally distributed quantitative variables and by the Chi-square test or Fisher's exact test in the case of qualitative variables, respectively. Due to the low number of participants and the fact that quantitative variables were not normally distributed, we did not perform a power analysis. Values of $p < 0.05$ were considered statistically significant.

3. Results

The selection of subjects is presented in Figure 1, and the clinical and demographic characteristics of the patients are shown in Table 1. The onset of CD was at a younger age than that of UC. There were no differences in patient gender between the two diseases.

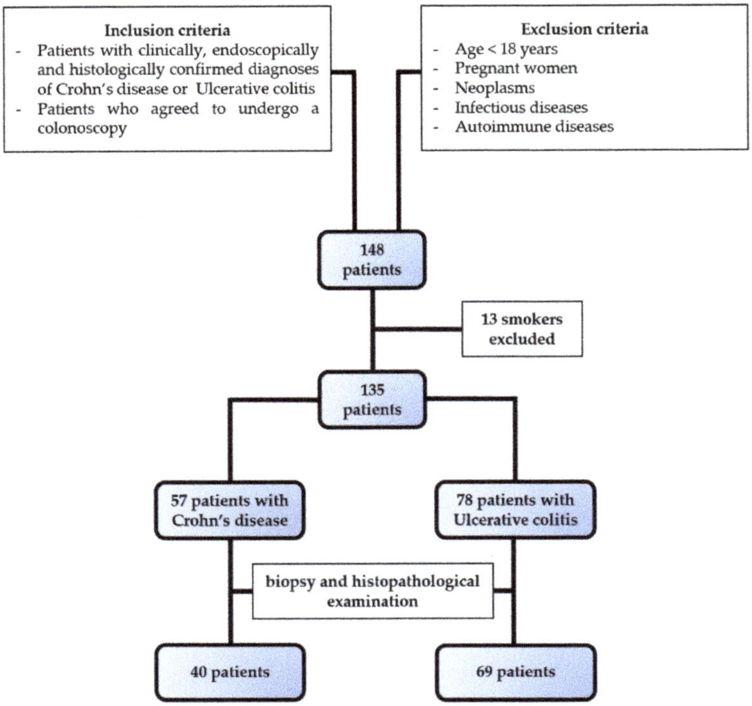

Figure 1. Selection of study population. Based on the inclusion and exclusion criteria, we selected 57 patients with Crohn's disease and 78 patients with ulcerative colitis.

Table 1. Clinical and demographic characteristics of the included subjects.

	CD $n = 57$	UC $n = 78$	p Value
Male, n (%)	28 (49.12%)	39 (50.00%)	0.92
Age at inclusion (years)	37.81 ± 13.50	44.05 ± 16.21	0.01
Age at diagnosis (years)	31.97 ± 9.92	40.38 ± 16.04	0.03
Disease activity			
Clinical, n (%)	19 (33.33%)	58 (74.36%)	<0.001
Endoscopic, n (%)	39 (78.00%)	66 (90.41%)	0.05
Histological, n (%)	36 (90.00%)	65 (94.20%)	0.46

Depending on the distribution, the data are presented as the mean ± SD or number (percentage), as appropriate. Abbreviations: CD, Crohn's disease; UC, ulcerative colitis; n, number of subjects.

Regarding disease activity, 57.04% of patients were in a state of clinical activity, 85.37% had endoscopic activity, and 92.66% had histological activity. The disease-specific activity classification is shown in Table 1. Statistically significant clinical activity differences were observed between the two diseases, without differences regarding endoscopic or histological activity.

Of the 135 patients analyzed, all completed the questionnaire in full. Of these, 60% reported regular coffee consumption. No statistically significant differences were identified regarding the proportion of patients consuming coffee between the two diseases ($p = 0.31$) or between the sexes ($p = 0.44$). Figure 2 illustrates the types of coffee consumed. Natural coffee was the predominant choice, while other types, such as soluble coffee, decaffeinated coffee, or cappuccino, were less frequently chosen. There were no significant differences in the type of coffee consumed between the sexes.

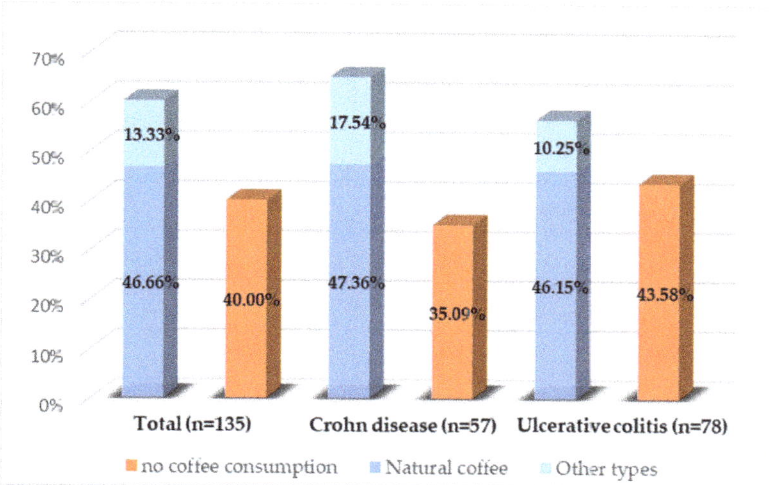

Figure 2. Coffee consumption distribution among the study population.

In terms of coffee consumption frequencies, 28.14% of all participants reported daily consumption. Additionally, 40.74% of respondents indicated adding milk to their coffee. Patients diagnosed with CD reported significantly higher rates of milk-added coffee consumption compared to those with UC ($p < 0.001$). Among all respondents, 15.15% added one spoon of milk, 63.64% added between two and four spoons, and 21.21% added more than four spoons. Regarding the use of sweeteners in coffee, 56.79% reported frequent addition, with no significant difference observed between CD and UC patients ($p = 0.07$). Within this cohort, 67.39% used white sugar, 17.39% used brown sugar, 8.70% used other types of sweeteners (e.g., stevia, saccharin, honey), and 6.52% used mixtures of sweeteners.

All patients (consumers and non-consumers of coffee) were asked about their general opinion regarding the effect of coffee on symptomatology. In total, 45.93% of patients with IBD declared that coffee consumption did not influence their symptoms; this percentage was slightly higher in CD, compared to UC (50.87% vs. 42.30%), without statistically significant differences when applying the Chi-square test ($p = 0.40$). The percentage of patients who reported the worsening of symptoms due to coffee consumption was slightly lower in CD, compared to UC (17.54% vs. 19.23%), while the proportion of patients who reported an improvement in symptoms was relatively equal between the two diseases (5.26% in CD and 5.12% in UC, respectively). However, when applying the Chi-square test, no statistically significant differences between the two diseases were found with respect to symptom aggravation ($p = 0.80$) or improvement ($p = 0.97$). A significant number of participants (30.37%) declared that they did not know if coffee consumption influenced their symptoms. Most of them belonged to the group who never consumed coffee. There were no significant differences between the sexes in the perception of coffee's effects on symptomatology.

Among the reasons why some patients avoided drinking coffee were the doctor's recommendation to avoid coffee, not feeling the need to drink coffee, or the worsening of symptoms in cases of consumption. The main symptoms associated with coffee consumption were increased stool numbers, sometimes associated with decreased consistency or worsening abdominal pain. However, 48% of the patients who reported worsening symptoms associated with coffee consumption did not give up this habit. It should be noted that five patients declared that they avoided coffee consumption only during periods of clinical activity related to the disease.

The patients were asked about their perception of the relationship between coffee consumption and its harmful effects on health. Of the total participants, 51.11% claimed that coffee consumption has no harmful effects, 17.78% claimed that coffee consumption has a negative effect on health, regardless of the amount consumed, 3.70% mentioned that this negative effect occurs only when consuming increased amounts, and 27.41% declared that they did not know whether coffee consumption influences the state of health. Among those who answered yes or did not know, 42.42% were regular coffee consumers.

Next, the connection between coffee consumption and the state of disease activity was evaluated using specific scores. No statistically significant differences were found between coffee-consuming and non-consuming patients for clinical activity ($p = 0.67$), endoscopic activity ($p = 0.22$), or histological activity ($p = 0.61$).

The influence of coffee was objectively evaluated by analyzing inflammation markers according to the type of disease and the coffee consumer/non-consumer status. The results are shown in Table 2 using the mean ± standard deviation for normally distributed variables and the median and interquartile range with the 25% and 75% percentiles for variables with a non-normal distribution. Within the whole group of patients, the FC values were significantly lower in patients who consumed coffee compared to those who did not ($p = 0.04$). However, this statistical significance was not maintained for each type of disease. No statistical significance was obtained when comparing the values of inflammatory markers according to the type of coffee, the frequency of its consumption, or the addition of milk. Regarding the addition of sweeteners, significantly lower ESR-2h values were observed in patients who consumed coffee without sweeteners compared to those who added sweeteners ($p = 0.03$).

Table 2. Inflammatory markers according to disease type and coffee consumer/non-consumer status.

	Total $n = 135$		CD $n = 57$		UC $n = 78$	
Coffee Consumption	**No**	**Yes**	**No**	**Yes**	**No**	**Yes**
Leukocyte cells/μL	7933.21 ± 2496.55	8057.28 ± 2779.64	7997.37 ± 2408.56	8501.62 ± 3194.21	7897.35 ± 2579.40	7683.64 ± 2349.46
ESR2h mm/h	44 (22–81)	40 (20–78.50)	52 (36–99)	56 (20–81)	40 (18–76)	40 (21–74)
CRP mg/dL	0.78 (0.4–3.52)	0.63 (0.39–3.12)	0.96 (0.41–6.50)	0.86 (0.41–4.84)	0.63 (0.39–3.08)	0.53 (0.39–2.13)
FC μg/g	1143 * (300–2100)	611.75 * (163.75–1754.25)	798 (175.40–2100)	548.50 (185–1247.75)	1400 (400–2100)	754.50 (126–1957)

Depending on the distribution, the data are presented as the mean ± standard deviation or median (interquartile range–25th and 75th percentile) as appropriate. Abbreviations: CD, Crohn's disease; UC, ulcerative colitis; n, number of subjects; ESR2h, two-hour erythrocyte sedimentation rate; CRP, C-reactive protein; and FC, fecal calprotectin. Statistically significant differences are marked with *.

Finally, in order to investigate whether the effect of coffee is attributable to caffeine or other compounds it contains, we analyzed whether any statistical differences in inflammatory markers can be found between patients who consumed different types of coffee. The results did not reveal statistically significant differences between instant coffee consumers and those who did not drink coffee or those who consumed other types of coffee. However, there was a significant difference between FC values in patients who exclusively consumed natural coffee and those who did not consume coffee at all, both in the overall patient sample ($p < 0.001$) and in patients with UC ($p = 0.03$), but not in CD patients ($p = 0.15$). Table 3 presents the values of inflammatory markers according to disease type and whether patients were natural coffee consumers or non-consumers. For normally distributed variables, the values are reported as the mean ± standard deviation, while for non-normally distributed variables, they are reported as median and interquartile range, including the 25th and 75th percentiles.

Table 3. Inflammatory markers according to disease type and natural coffee consumer versus non-consumer status.

	Total n = 116		CD n = 47		UC n = 70	
	No Coffee	**Natural Coffee**	**No Coffee**	**Natural Coffee**	**No Coffee**	**Natural Coffee**
Leukocyte cells/µL	7933.21 ± 2496.55	7960.95 ± 2510.66	7997.37 ± 2408.56	8354.44 ± 2908.87	7897.35 ± 2579.40	7665.83 ± 2161.32
ESR2h mm/h	44 (22–81)	40 (20–78.50)	52 (36–99)	56 (20–81)	40 (18–76)	40 (22–76)
CRP mg/dL	0.78 (0.4–3.52)	0.53 (0.4–2.14)	0.96 (0.41–6.50)	0.63 (0.41–3.26)	0.63 (0.39–3.08)	0.50 (0.39–1.48)
FC µg/g	1143 * (300–2100)	790.99 * (144–1441.50)	798 (175.40–2100)	463.50 (175–1214)	1400 * (400–2100)	623.50 * (99–1800)

Depending on the distribution, the data are presented as the mean ± standard deviation or median (interquartile range—25th and 75th percentile) as appropriate. Abbreviations: CD, Crohn's disease; UC, ulcerative colitis; n, number of subjects; ESR2h, two-hour erythrocyte sedimentation rate; CRP, C-reactive protein; and FC, fecal calprotectin. Statistically significant differences are marked with *.

4. Discussion

This study aimed to assess coffee consumption patterns among individuals with IBD by examining their subjective experiences regarding coffee's impact on their symptoms. Additionally, it aimed to objectively analyze inflammatory markers in this population in order to elucidate their potential associations with coffee consumption.

Over the years, numerous studies have investigated the influence of various environmental factors on the progression of IBD [32]. Recently, more emphasis has been placed on the role of nutrition in the pathogenesis of IBD and its potential impact on symptomatology [33]. Despite coffee being one of the most commonly consumed beverages globally and containing compounds known for its anti-inflammatory properties, its effects on IBD remain largely unexplored. To the best of our knowledge, this study represents the first attempt to investigate the impact of coffee consumption on inflammatory markers in individuals with IBD.

The decision to exclude smokers from the statistical analysis was motivated by smoking's well-known pro-inflammatory impact [34] and its paradoxical protective effect observed in patients with UC [35]. This exclusion was necessary to mitigate potential confounding effects on the study outcomes.

In our study, the number of patients exhibiting endoscopic or histological activity surpassed those reporting clinical symptoms. This observation aligns with findings from previous research, which demonstrates that intestinal lesions may not always become clinically manifest [36,37].

Coffee consumption has globally experienced a steady rise in recent decades. Europe currently leads the world in coffee consumption, averaging 5 kg per person per year [38]. Our study found that 60% of patients regularly consume coffee, with no significant variance observed between those diagnosed with CD and UC. Most patients reported daily coffee consumption, which is a pattern consistent with data from the United States, where approximately 65% of the population drinks coffee daily [39]. Preference for caffeinated coffee was predominant among participants, with only a tiny fraction opting for decaffeinated varieties, mirroring findings from a previous study on IBD patients' coffee-drinking habits [27]. This choice likely stems from individual taste preferences and the widespread belief in caffeine's potential to enhance cognitive function and mood [40]. Additionally, a notable observation was that patients with CD tended to add milk to their coffee more frequently than patients with UC. While this aspect lies beyond the scope of our study, it may be speculated that dietary preferences among IBD patients, who often avoid foods that exacerbate symptoms, could contribute to this trend [30]. Consequently, dairy consumption might have a more pronounced negative impact on UC patients compared to CD patients. However, it is crucial to acknowledge that in our study, a higher proportion of UC patients were experiencing clinical disease activity, which could further influence their dietary choices.

In contrast to the study by Barthel et al. [27], our investigation did not reveal statistically significant disparities between the two diseases in the subjective perception of coffee's effect on symptomatology. Nevertheless, a noteworthy finding was that most patients, across both conditions, who attributed coffee to an effect on symptomatology reported a negative impact. Intriguingly, this negative perception did not translate into complete abstention from coffee consumption. Such findings highlight the inconsistencies found in the existing literature regarding the relationship between coffee intake and IBD. Some studies suggest a protective role of coffee due to its anti-inflammatory [41] or anti-neoplastic properties [15]. Moreover, coffee consumption has not been linked to an increased incidence of IBD [28]; instead, it has been deemed protective [21]. Conversely, other research indicates potential pro-inflammatory effects of coffee on the healthy intestine, such as the activation of the NF-kB transcription factor [42], as well as stimulatory effects on intestinal motility, that could influence symptomatology in patients with functional bowel disorders [25]. Moreover, studies indicate that individuals with CD and UC tend to consume less coffee compared to healthy counterparts [29]. Despite negative perceptions or personal beliefs regarding coffee's harmful effects, the reason why many patients persist in its consumption remains elusive. Speculatively, perceived effects on disease progression may not be significant enough to warrant complete avoidance. Alternatively, the negative impact of coffee could be downplayed or even ignored, indicating characteristics of addiction. Additionally, some patients may be swayed by emerging evidence supporting the health benefits of coffee [11–16]. However, it is noteworthy that certain patients reported refraining from coffee consumption only during periods of clinical activity, suggesting selective avoidance of certain foods during specific disease stages, which is a finding supported by other studies [30].

Regarding the impact of coffee consumption on inflammatory markers, numerous studies have explored its influence on serum levels of CRP and various cytokines, including interleukins (ILs), such as IL-6, IL-8, and tumor necrosis factor (TNF)-alpha [43]. However, to date, no investigations have examined this relationship, specifically in patients with IBD. Consistent with previous research on serum CRP changes associated with coffee intake, our study did not reveal significant differences between coffee-consuming and non-consuming patients [44,45]. Similarly, no significant alterations were observed in other markers of systemic inflammation, such as leukocyte count or ESR-2h. Nonetheless, FC levels, a marker of intestinal inflammation, were lower among regular coffee consumers. This reduction could be attributed to the mitigating effects of coffee on acute colitis at the level of the intestinal epithelial cells, as previously demonstrated following oral caffeine administration [46]. The absence of consistent effects across different forms of IBD subgroups could be due to the relatively small sample size within each subgroup. Furthermore, our findings suggest that the association between coffee consumption and reduced FC values was significant for natural coffee drinkers rather than consumers of other coffee types. This result implies that the observed effect may be linked, at least partially, to specific compounds present in natural coffee, distinct from caffeine alone, for example, flavonoids, which are known for their fight against reactive oxygen species [47]. While no significant differences were detected between non-consumers and those preferring other types of coffee, our results underscore the importance of examining the precise composition of various coffee types and their effects on inflammatory markers in diverse conditions. Interestingly, the association between natural coffee consumption and FC levels persisted within the UC patient subgroup, hinting at the potential benefits of coffee intake for this particular condition. However, the absence of a significant similar association among CD patients underscores the necessity for further investigation to better understand coffee's impact on this subgroup.

Moreover, the addition of milk to coffee did not yield notable changes in inflammatory markers, likely due to the limited number of patients who reported this habit and possibly driven by concerns about dairy exacerbating symptoms, which is an assumption supported by other studies [30]. Nonetheless, the type of milk used goes beyond the scope of our study.

On another note, the addition of sweeteners influenced ESR-2h values, with lower levels observed in non-sweetener users. Although sugar and artificial sweeteners are generally regarded as safe, animal studies suggest that they may contribute to gastrointestinal inflammation [48]. Surveys of IBD patients indicate that between 10% and 36% perceive high-sugar foods as exacerbating their symptoms and triggering flare-ups [49].

The present study has several limitations. Firstly, the small sample size is a significant constraint, which can be attributed to the low prevalence (1.5 per 100,000 for CD and 2.4 per 100,000 for UC, respectively) and incidence rates (1.7 per 100,000 people/year for CD and 2.5 per 100,000 people/year for UC) of IBD in Romania, as well as the limited availability of patients in a single regional center [50]. Consequently, our findings may only partially represent the broader population of individuals with IBD. In addition, to ensure a robust participation rate and gather a substantial number of responses, this study focused on patients' perspectives regarding coffee consumption and its perceived effects on symptomatology. Consequently, other relevant factors, such as alcohol consumption, tea intake, or the consumption of other caffeinated beverages, were not explored. A more comprehensive approach, encompassing a broader range of dietary habits, could have provided richer insights into patients' overall eating behaviors. Additionally, it is essential to acknowledge that a questionnaire-based study has inherent limitations and cannot substitute for a clinical trial. The lack of detailed data regarding coffee processing, brewing methods, precise consumption quantities for coffee, and other additives prevented a thorough analysis of coffee's impact. More rigorous methodologies and detailed data collection would have been necessary to address these aspects, which were not feasible within the scope of this study.

The findings of our study underline the need for further research into this realm to validate and expand upon our observations regarding the influence of coffee consumption on individuals with IBD. Clinical trials play a pivotal role in furnishing robust evidence and shaping evidence-based recommendations for patient care. Moreover, it is crucial to acknowledge that some individuals may refrain from coffee consumption, either because of their own convictions or under the guidance of their healthcare provider, thus highlighting the necessity for an individualized approach to managing IBD. Continued investigation may elucidate who can benefit from coffee consumption and under what circumstances, risks, or contraindications this practice is associated with. By delving deeper into these aspects, we can refine our understanding of how coffee interacts with IBD and tailor therapeutic approaches to optimize patient outcomes.

5. Conclusions

In conclusion, while most patients reported regular coffee intake, a noteworthy proportion identified coffee as a potential influencer of intestinal symptoms. Intriguingly, despite this negative perception, many continued to consume coffee. Although systemic inflammatory markers remained largely unaffected by coffee consumption, a correlation emerged between regular coffee intake and reduced levels of FC, especially for patients who consumed natural coffee and had UC, suggesting the potential mitigating effect of coffee on intestinal inflammation. This discrepancy underlines the need for further investigation into the specific components and mechanisms regarding coffee's impact on IBD pathophysiology. Such endeavors are crucial for formulating evidence-based recommendations and guiding medical management strategies tailored to the needs of patients with IBD.

Author Contributions: Conceptualization, L.N., T.D. and A.M.C.; methodology, L.N. and T.D.; software, T.D.; formal analysis, T.D.; investigation, L.N., L.C. and A.V.; resources, L.C.; data curation, L.N.; writing—original draft preparation, L.N. and S.R.G.; writing—review and editing, A.M.C., C.N.S.,

S.R.G. and C.D.; visualization, L.N.; supervision, A.M.C., C.N.S. and C.D.; project administration, L.N. and A.V. All authors have read and agreed to the published version of the manuscript.

Funding: This research received no external funding.

Institutional Review Board Statement: This study was conducted in accordance with the Declaration of Helsinki and approved by the Ethics Committee of Iuliu Hațieganu, University of Medicine and Pharmacy, Cluj-Napoca (protocol code 93 date of approval 9 March 2020).

Informed Consent Statement: Informed consent was obtained from all subjects involved in the study.

Data Availability Statement: Data presented in this study are available upon reasonable request from the corresponding author. The data are not publicly available due to privacy regulations.

Conflicts of Interest: The authors declare no conflicts of interest.

References

1. Hansen, T.S.; Jess, T.; Vind, I.; Elkjaer, M.; Nielsen, M.F.; Gamborg, M.; Munkholm, P. Environmental factors in inflammatory bowel disease: A case-control study based on a Danish inception cohort. *J. Crohns Colitis* **2011**, *5*, 577–584. [CrossRef] [PubMed]
2. Hou, J.K.; Abraham, B.; El-Serag, H. Dietary intake and risk of developing inflammatory bowel disease: A systematic review of the literature. *Am. J. Gastroenterol.* **2011**, *106*, 563–573. [CrossRef] [PubMed]
3. Peters, V.; Bolte, L.; Schuttert, E.M.; Andreu-Sanchez, S.; Dijkstra, G.; Weersma, R.K.; Campmans-Kuijpers, M.J.E. Western and Carnivorous Dietary Patterns are Associated with Greater Likelihood of IBD Development in a Large Prospective Population-based Cohort. *J. Crohns Colitis* **2022**, *16*, 931–939. [CrossRef]
4. Peters, V.; Spooren, C.; Pierik, M.J.; Weersma, R.K.; van Dullemen, H.M.; Festen, E.A.M.; Visschedijk, M.C.; Masclee, A.A.M.; Hendrix, E.M.B.; Almeida, R.J.; et al. Dietary Intake Pattern is Associated with Occurrence of Flares in IBD Patients. *J. Crohns Colitis* **2021**, *15*, 1305–1315. [CrossRef] [PubMed]
5. Bolte, L.A.; Vich Vila, A.; Imhann, F.; Collij, V.; Gacesa, R.; Peters, V.; Wijmenga, C.; Kurilshikov, A.; Campmans-Kuijpers, M.J.E.; Fu, J.; et al. Long-term dietary patterns are associated with pro-inflammatory and anti-inflammatory features of the gut microbiome. *Gut* **2021**, *70*, 1287–1298. [CrossRef] [PubMed]
6. Naqvi, S.A.; Taylor, L.M.; Panaccione, R.; Ghosh, S.; Barkema, H.W.; Hotte, N.; Shommu, N.; Kaur, S.; Reimer, R.A.; Madsen, K.L.; et al. Dietary patterns, food groups and nutrients in Crohn's disease: Associations with gut and systemic inflammation. *Sci. Rep.* **2021**, *11*, 1674. [CrossRef] [PubMed]
7. Rokkas, T.; Portincasa, P.; Koutroubakis, I.E. Fecal calprotectin in assessing inflammatory bowel disease endoscopic activity: A diagnostic accuracy meta-analysis. *J. Gastrointest. Liver Dis.* **2018**, *27*, 299–306. [CrossRef] [PubMed]
8. Yoon, J.Y.; Park, S.J.; Hong, S.P.; Kim, T.I.; Kim, W.H.; Cheon, J.H. Correlations of C-reactive protein levels and erythrocyte sedimentation rates with endoscopic activity indices in patients with ulcerative colitis. *Dig. Dis. Sci.* **2014**, *59*, 829–837. [CrossRef] [PubMed]
9. Spiler, M.A. The chemical components of coffee. *Prog. Clin. Biol. Res.* **1984**, *158*, 91–147.
10. Gomez-Ruiz, J.A.; Leake, D.S.; Ames, J.M. In vitro antioxidant activity of coffee compounds and their metabolites. *J. Agric. Food Chem.* **2007**, *55*, 6962–6969. [CrossRef]
11. Ruhl, C.E.; Everhart, J.E. Coffee and tea consumption are associated with a lower incidence of chronic liver disease in the United States. *Gastroenterology* **2005**, *129*, 1928–1936. [CrossRef]
12. Ding, M.; Bhupathiraju, S.N.; Chen, M.; van Dam, R.M.; Hu, F.B. Caffeinated and decaffeinated coffee consumption and risk of type 2 diabetes: A systematic review and a dose-response meta-analysis. *Diabetes Care* **2014**, *37*, 569–586. [CrossRef] [PubMed]
13. Socala, K.; Szopa, A.; Serefko, A.; Poleszak, E.; Wlaz, P. Neuroprotective Effects of Coffee Bioactive Compounds: A Review. *Int. J. Mol. Sci.* **2020**, *22*, 107. [CrossRef] [PubMed]
14. Murakami, K.; Okubo, H.; Sasaki, S. Dietary intake in relation to self-reported constipation among Japanese women aged 18–20 years. *Eur. J. Clin. Nutr.* **2006**, *60*, 650–657. [CrossRef] [PubMed]
15. Arab, L. Epidemiologic evidence on coffee and cancer. *Nutr. Cancer* **2010**, *62*, 271–283. [CrossRef] [PubMed]
16. Freedman, N.D.; Park, Y.; Abnet, C.C.; Hollenbeck, A.R.; Sinha, R. Association of coffee drinking with total and cause-specific mortality. *N. Engl. J. Med.* **2012**, *366*, 1891–1904. [CrossRef] [PubMed]
17. Perez-Burillo, S.; Rajakaruna, S.; Pastoriza, S.; Paliy, O.; Angel Rufian-Henares, J. Bioactivity of food melanoidins is mediated by gut microbiota. *Food Chem.* **2020**, *316*, 126309. [CrossRef] [PubMed]
18. Rao, S.S.; Welcher, K.; Zimmerman, B.; Stumbo, P. Is coffee a colonic stimulant? *Eur. J. Gastroenterol. Hepatol.* **1998**, *10*, 113–118. [CrossRef] [PubMed]
19. Sloots, C.E.; Felt-Bersma, R.J.; West, R.L.; Kuipers, E.J. Stimulation of defecation: Effects of coffee use and nicotine on rectal tone and visceral sensitivity. *Scand. J. Gastroenterol.* **2005**, *40*, 808–813. [CrossRef]
20. Tanaka, K.; Okubo, H.; Miyake, Y.; Nagata, C.; Furukawa, S.; Andoh, A.; Yokoyama, T.; Yoshimura, N.; Mori, K.; Ninomiya, T.; et al. Coffee and caffeine intake reduces risk of ulcerative colitis: A case-control study in Japan. *J. Gastroenterol. Hepatol.* **2024**, *39*, 512–518. [CrossRef]

21. Ng, S.C.; Tang, W.; Leong, R.W.; Chen, M.; Ko, Y.; Studd, C.; Niewiadomski, O.; Bell, S.; Kamm, M.A.; de Silva, H.J.; et al. Environmental risk factors in inflammatory bowel disease: A population-based case-control study in Asia-Pacific. *Gut* **2015**, *64*, 1063–1071. [CrossRef] [PubMed]
22. Li, Q.; Liu, Y.; Sun, X.; Yin, Z.; Li, H.; Cheng, C.; Liu, L.; Zhang, R.; Liu, F.; Zhou, Q.; et al. Caffeinated and decaffeinated coffee consumption and risk of all-cause mortality: A dose-response meta-analysis of cohort studies. *J. Hum. Nutr. Diet.* **2019**, *32*, 279–287. [CrossRef] [PubMed]
23. Lopez-Garcia, E.; Orozco-Arbelaez, E.; Leon-Munoz, L.M.; Guallar-Castillon, P.; Graciani, A.; Banegas, J.R.; Rodriguez-Artalejo, F. Habitual coffee consumption and 24-h blood pressure control in older adults with hypertension. *Clin. Nutr.* **2016**, *35*, 1457–1463. [CrossRef] [PubMed]
24. Salas-Huetos, A.; Bullo, M.; Salas-Salvado, J. Dietary patterns, foods and nutrients in male fertility parameters and fecundability: A systematic review of observational studies. *Hum. Reprod. Update* **2017**, *23*, 371–389. [CrossRef] [PubMed]
25. Brown, S.R.; Cann, P.A.; Read, N.W. Effect of coffee on distal colon function. *Gut* **1990**, *31*, 450–453. [CrossRef] [PubMed]
26. Brown, A.C.; Rampertab, S.D.; Mullin, G.E. Existing dietary guidelines for Crohn's disease and ulcerative colitis. *Expert. Rev. Gastroenterol. Hepatol.* **2011**, *5*, 411–425. [CrossRef] [PubMed]
27. Barthel, C.; Wiegand, S.; Scharl, S.; Scharl, M.; Frei, P.; Vavricka, S.R.; Fried, M.; Sulz, M.C.; Wiegand, N.; Rogler, G.; et al. Patients' perceptions on the impact of coffee consumption in inflammatory bowel disease: Friend or foe?—A patient survey. *Nutr. J.* **2015**, *14*, 78. [CrossRef]
28. Georgiou, A.N.; Ntritsos, G.; Papadimitriou, N.; Dimou, N.; Evangelou, E. Cigarette Smoking, Coffee Consumption, Alcohol Intake, and Risk of Crohn's Disease and Ulcerative Colitis: A Mendelian Randomization Study. *Inflamm. Bowel Dis.* **2021**, *27*, 162–168. [CrossRef]
29. Peters, V.; Tigchelaar-Feenstra, E.F.; Imhann, F.; Dekens, J.A.M.; Swertz, M.A.: Franke, L.H.; Wijmenga, C.; Weersma, R.K.; Alizadeh, B.Z.; Dijkstra, G.; et al. Habitual dietary intake of IBD patients differs from population controls: A case-control study. *Eur. J. Nutr.* **2021**, *60*, 345–356. [CrossRef]
30. Crooks, B.; Misra, R.; Arebi, N.; Kok, K.; Brookes, M.J.; McLaughlin, J.; Limdi, J.K. The dietary practices and beliefs of British South Asian people living with inflammatory bowel disease: A multicenter study from the United Kingdom. *Intest. Res.* **2022**, *20*, 53–63. [CrossRef]
31. Sturm, A.; Maaser, C.; Calabrese, E.; Annese, V.; Fiorino, G.; Kucharzik, T.; Vavricka, S.R.; Verstockt, B.; van Rheenen, P.; Tolan, D.; et al. ECCO-ESGAR Guideline for Diagnostic Assessment in IBD Part 2: IBD scores and general principles and technical aspects. *J. Crohns Colitis* **2019**, *13*, 273–284. [CrossRef] [PubMed]
32. Singh, N.; Bernstein, C.N. Environmental risk factors for inflammatory bowel disease. *Gastroenterol. J.* **2022**, *10*, 1047–1053. [CrossRef] [PubMed]
33. Owczarek, D.; Rodacki, T.; Domagala-Rodacka, R.; Cibor, D.; Mach, T. Diet and nutritional factors in inflammatory bowel diseases. *World J. Gastroenterol.* **2016**, *22*, 895–905. [CrossRef] [PubMed]
34. Rom, O.; Avezov, K.; Aizenbud, D.; Reznick, A.Z. Cigarette smoking and inflammation revisited. *Respir. Physiol. Neurobiol.* **2013**, *187*, 5–10. [CrossRef] [PubMed]
35. Mahid, S.S.; Minor, K.S.; Soto, R.E.; Hornung, C.A.; Galandiuk, S. Smoking and inflammatory bowel disease: A meta-analysis. *Mayo Clin. Proc.* **2006**, *81*, 1462–1471. [CrossRef] [PubMed]
36. Feagins, L.A.; Melton, S.D.; Iqbal, R.; Dunbar, K.B.; Spechler, S.J. Clinical implications of histologic abnormalities in colonic biopsy specimens from patients with ulcerative colitis in clinical remission. *Inflamm. Bowel Dis.* **2013**, *19*, 1477–1482. [CrossRef] [PubMed]
37. Christensen, B.; Rubin, D.T. Understanding Endoscopic Disease Activity in IBD: How to Incorporate It into Practice. *Curr. Gastroenterol. Rep.* **2016**, *18*, 5. [CrossRef] [PubMed]
38. The International Coffee Organization. *The Coffee Report and Outlook: Coffee Consumption—Europe*; The International Coffee Organization: London, UK, 2023.
39. National Coffee Association. *National Coffee Data Trends Report*; National Coffee Association: New York, NY, USA, 2023.
40. Elliman, N.A.; Ash, J.; Green, M.W. Pre-existent expectancy effects in the relationship between caffeine and performance. *Appetite* **2010**, *55*, 355–358. [CrossRef] [PubMed]
41. Langhorst, J.; Varnhagen, I.; Schneider, S.B.; Albrecht, U.; Rueffer, A.; Stange, R.; Michalsen, A.; Dobos, G.J. Randomised clinical trial: A herbal preparation of myrrh, chamomile and coffee charcoal compared with mesalazine in maintaining remission in ulcerative colitis–A double-blind, double-dummy study. *Aliment. Pharmacol. Ther* **2013**, *38*, 490–500. [CrossRef]
42. Sauer, T.; Raithel, M.; Kressel, J.; Muscat, S.; Munch, G.; Pischetsrieder, M. Nuclear translocation of NF-kappaB in intact human gut tissue upon stimulation with coffee and roasting products. *Food Funct.* **2011**, *2*, 529–540. [CrossRef]
43. Paiva, C.; Beserra, B.; Reis, C.; Dorea, J.G.; Da Costa, T.; Amato, A.A. Consumption of coffee or caffeine and serum concentration of inflammatory markers: A systematic review. *Crit. Rev. Food Sci. Nutr.* **2019**, *59*, 652–663. [CrossRef]
44. Kempf, K.; Kolb, H.; Gartner, B.; Bytof, G.; Stiebitz, H.; Lantz, I.; Lang, R.; Hofmann, T.; Martin, S. Cardiometabolic effects of two coffee blends differing in content for major constituents in overweight adults: A randomized controlled trial. *Eur. J. Nutr.* **2015**, *54*, 845–854. [CrossRef] [PubMed]
45. Ohnaka, K.; Ikeda, M.; Maki, T.; Okada, T.; Shimazoe, T.; Adachi, M.; Nomura, M.; Takayanagi, R.; Kono, S. Effects of 16-week consumption of caffeinated and decaffeinated instant coffee on glucose metabolism in a randomized controlled trial. *J. Nutr. Metab.* **2012**, *2012*, 207426. [CrossRef] [PubMed]

46. Lee, I.A.; Low, D.; Kamba, A.; Llado, V.; Mizoguchi, E. Oral caffeine administration ameliorates acute colitis by suppressing chitinase 3-like 1 expression in intestinal epithelial cells. *J. Gastroenterol.* **2014**, *49*, 1206–1216. [CrossRef] [PubMed]
47. Steffen, Y.; Gruber, C.; Schewe, T.; Sies, H. Mono-O-methylated flavanols and other flavonoids as inhibitors of endothelial NADPH oxidase. *Arch. Biochem. Biophys.* **2008**, *469*, 209–219. [CrossRef] [PubMed]
48. Laffin, M.; Fedorak, R.; Zalasky, A.; Park, H.; Gill, A.; Agrawal, A.; Keshteli, A.; Hotte, N.; Madsen, K.L. A high-sugar diet rapidly enhances susceptibility to colitis via depletion of luminal short-chain fatty acids in mice. *Sci. Rep.* **2019**, *9*, 12294. [CrossRef] [PubMed]
49. Guida, L.; Di Giorgio, F.M.; Busacca, A.; Carrozza, L.; Ciminnisi, S.; Almasio, P.L.; Di Marco, V.; Cappello, M. Perception of the Role of Food and Dietary Modifications in Patients with Inflammatory Bowel Disease: Impact on Lifestyle. *Nutrients* **2021**, *13*, 759. [CrossRef]
50. Gheorghe, C.; Pascu, O.; Gheorghe, L.; Iacob, R.; Dumitru, E.; Tantau, M.; Vadan, R.; Goldis, A.; Balan, G.; Iacob, S.; et al. Epidemiology of inflammatory bowel disease in adults who refer to gastroenterology care in Romania: A multicentre study. *Eur. J. Gastroenterol. Hepatol.* **2004**, *16*, 1153–1159. [CrossRef]

biomedicines

MDPI

Review

Gut Microbial Targets in Inflammatory Bowel Disease: Current Position and Future Developments

Naveen Sivakumar [1,*], Ashwin Krishnamoorthy [2], Harshita Ryali [3] and Ramesh P. Arasaradnam [1,2]

1 Institute of Precision Diagnostics & Translational Medicine, University Hospitals Coventry & Warwickshire, Coventry CV2 2DX, UK; r.arasaradnam@warwick.ac.uk

2 Warwick Medical School, University of Warwick, Coventry CV4 7AL, UK; ashwin.krishnamoorthy@warwick.ac.uk

3 Southmead Hospital, North Bristol Trust, Bristol BS10 5NB, UK; harshita.ryali@nbt.nhs.uk

* Correspondence: naveen.sivakumar5@nhs.net

Abstract: Inflammatory bowel disease (IBD) is a debilitating condition in which surgery is often seen as a last resort. However, this is associated with morbidity and, in some cases, mortality. There are emerging therapies that seek to better modulate the immune response of hosts with IBD. **Aims**: The main aim of this study is to focus on novel therapies and techniques studied in the last year that are non-surgical treatments of IBD. **Methods**: We looked at all the research between March 2024 and February 2025 detailing treatment in IBD and focused on the gut microbiome and gene therapy. **Results**: Novel therapies are gaining traction in safety and popularity. The results from some animal studies show promise and, with FDA approval, some probiotic therapies show optimistic research potential for future human trials. **Conclusions**: The research into the diagnostics and novel therapies available on the horizon for humans is very promising. Animal studies have shown potentially transferrable and safe therapies that can target specific sites of inflammation. Modulating the inflammatory response is a powerful therapy with what is shown to be a reasonably safe profile to build further research on.

Keywords: inflammatory bowel disease; microbiome; microbiota; faecal transplantation; gene therapy; nanoparticle

1. Introduction

Inflammatory bowel disease (IBD) encompasses both Crohn's disease (CD) and ulcerative colitis (UC)—two functionally and histologically distinct conditions that share the element of chronic inflammation within the gastrointestinal tract and give rise to an array of sequalae, as well as increasing the risk of colorectal cancer.

IBD can be difficult to treat. Both UC and CD are heterogenous diseases, with a wide spectrum of disease activities. While UC can be cured, it requires the full surgical removal of the large bowel to achieve this, often with the result of a stoma bag for the patient, which comes with its own set of problems. CD cannot be cured; thus, the therapeutic goal is to achieve remission (Figure 1). Therefore, due to the ongoing need for medications, hospital follow-up appointments, and lost workdays for patients, IBD can present a significant financial burden to health systems and to society.

The incidence of IBD is increasing worldwide, for reasons that are not entirely certain. Some postulate that the rising IBD incidence is due to factors associated with the Western lifestyle, such as Western diet and lack of exposure to microorganisms that potentially regulate the immune system.

 https://doi.org/10.3390/biomedicines13030716

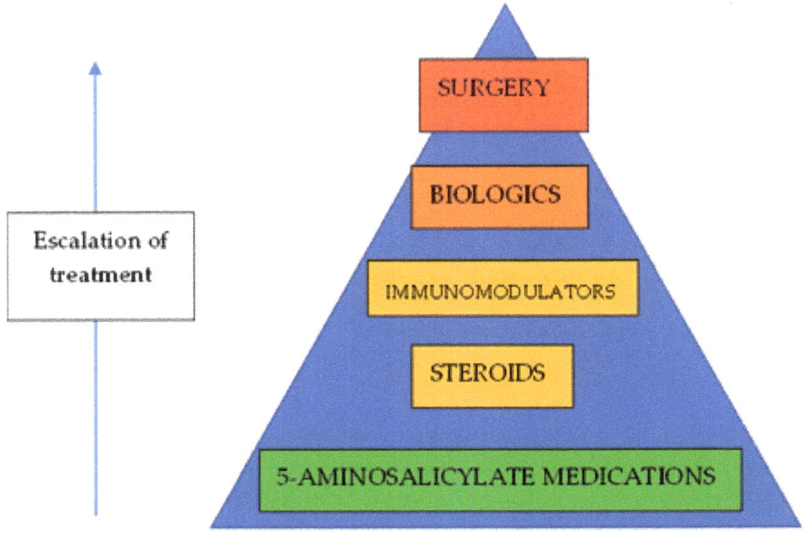

Figure 1. Treatment of IBD.

In order to focus on the treatment of IBD, we need to touch upon the aetiology of the disease. The exact cause is unknown, but it is highly likely to be a combination of genetic and environmental factors that results in altered functioning of the immune system, leading to an "attack" of the body's own gastrointestinal cells.

Therefore, the mainstay of the current medical management is related to suppressing the immune system. Various medications such as steroids, antimetabolite medication, and new "biologic" treatments (often monoclonal antibodies) that target certain biochemical pathways are used to suppress the action of the immune system. Unfortunately, this can lead to an array of unwanted side effects and toxicities. Furthermore, it is likely that there are a huge number of subsets of UC and CD, and these medications are currently not "personalised" to each individual's metabolic processes.

An evolving area of scientific interest involves the gut microbiome, which is the community of microorganisms living in the human digestive tract. Specifically, there exists a complex interplay between gut microbiome species and cells of the gastrointestinal tract, and this is implicated in both the maintenance of physiological health and the development of disease. An imbalance in the gut microbiome, in which certain deleterious species of microorganisms are increased relative to the more "favourable" species, is known as gut dysbiosis. In fact, it has been shown that IBD bacterial families that exist in abundance do not co-exist unlike in healthy individuals [1]. There are also emerging data to suggest that gut dysbiosis is associated with not just IBD but also its complications such as colorectal cancer [2,3].

Modulation of the gut microbiome could reduce inflammation and thus improve symptoms, maintain remission, and reduce relapses in IBD without dependence on medications with significant side effects. To draw a parallel, cancer treatment is evolving rapidly with the tailoring of therapies towards individual genetic mutations and "individualisation" of treatment. It is possible that the key to similar advances in IBD treatment lies within gut microbial therapeutic targets.

In this article, we aim to review the current and emerging gut microbial targets in IBD and, specifically, to elucidate the future developments most likely to impact practice.

2. Overview of the Gut Microbiome and Its Implications in IBD

In a healthy physiological state, the balance between beneficial and detrimental microorganisms in the gut is maintained, with a particular preference for certain anti-inflammatory species such as Firmicutes and Bacteroides [4,5]. Some of these beneficial bacteria were noted to be reduced in individuals with disease compared with healthy individuals, whereas the reverse seemed to be true for some potentially harmful strains. For example, certain strains of mucolytic bacteria have been found more in individuals with Crohn's and ulcerative colitis [6].

Such disruptions in the gut microbiome, dysbioses, may lead to IBD via inflammation, disruption of gut immune function, and the disruption of gut barrier function or short-chain fatty acid (SCFA) production (Figure 2). Foppa et al., 2024 [6] showed that the microbiota environment is linked to the pathogenesis of IBD via immune system change and microbiota composition. Recent reviews have even suggested that the gut microbiota can be used as a potential non-invasive biomarker for inflammatory bowel disease status and activity. This could change practice by using potentially cheaper and less invasive methods for disease surveillance. If checking the strains of bacteria in diseased individuals could accurately indicate disease activity or remission, then fewer endoscopic procedures would be required, and the potential risks to patients would be reduced.

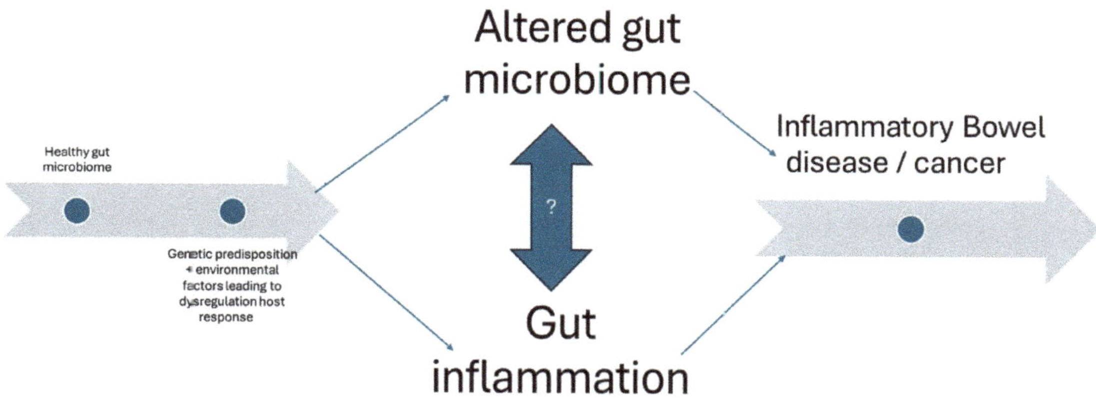

Figure 2. Overview of the relationship between altered gut microbiome and gut inflammation showing potential causative factors as well as serious sequalae.

Guo et al. [4] found that the bacteria *F. prausnitzii* is a specific marker for IBD as its prevalence was significantly lower than in IBS patients. They also found that, when considered in tandem with *E. coli*, *F. prausnitzii* could differentiate between colonic Crohn's disease and extensive colitis, implying that combinations or compositions of bacteria within a gut microbiome may be a more useful biomarker for IBD than just one strain, thus showing us potential applications for studying the gut microbiome composition as a less invasive biomarker in the diagnosis of IBD, as well as differentiating it from IBS, which can be difficult in primary care or more ambiguous presentations.

Ocansey et al., 2023 [5] found that specific bacterial clusters activate NOD2 signalling pathways. These are part of the innate immune system and are involved in the detection and initial response to pathogens. It also has a gene identified as being susceptible to IBD. These findings were linked to changes in the patients' gut microbiome, suggesting that the imbalances in the gut microbiota may contribute to the dysbiosis seen in IBD as well as to how the host's immune system responds to the disease. This would mean studying and protecting the healthy gut microbiome would be useful as a preventative measure for susceptible patients, such as those with strong family histories and genetic disposition to the disease. It may also be utilised in patients currently having IBD. There may not be enough evidence to suggest it can cure those with IBD, but the evidence seems to show that reducing dysbiosis and maintaining a healthy balance of gut bacteria will help reduce exaggerated immune responses, thus reducing flares and maintaining remission.

Haneishi et al., 2023 [7] conducted a cohort study that showed patients and mice with IBD displayed different gut microbiota composition than non-diseased individuals. Jacobs et al., 2016 [8] found the imbalance of the gut microbiota to be associated with the cause of IBD. These could imply that interventions that target the microbiota, such as probiotics or faecal microbiota transplantation (FMT), could be helpful in treating IBD symptoms.

Altered Tryptophan Metabolism in IBD as a Biomarker

Altered tryptophan (Trp) metabolism is increasingly recognised as a significant factor in the pathogenesis of IBD. Trp is an essential amino acid that has a role in gut microbiota homeostasis and is affected by many factors: probiotics, stress, ageing, and diseases including IBD [9].

Trp is a substrate for protein synthesis and is primarily metabolised via two main pathways: the kynurenine pathway (KP) and the kynurenic acid pathway (KA). Bacterial Trp metabolism differs slightly as bacteria can directly utilize Trp, but it is difficult in practice to identify which metabolites are produced, and further research would be needed to clarify this beyond the molecular level, thus making it impactful in clinical practice.

IBD is, however, associated with altered host and bacterial Trp metabolites. The plasma levels of kynurenine and KA are increased [10], whilst plasma Trp is decreased in patients with IBD [9]. It is thought the increased levels of circulating pro-inflammatory cytokines induce Trp catabolism. In animal studies, bacterial Trp metabolites are suggested to be significantly reduced in hosts with IBD, thus implying their beneficial role and potential anti-inflammatory properties. In humans with IBD, the low bacterial metabolite levels in faeces suggest that reduced Trp metabolism may be implicated in the aetiology of IBD [11]. Given the suggested relationship between Trp and its metabolites and the gut microbiome and host immune response, further research into potential therapies targeting this is warranted [9].

It could serve as a next-line treatment, broaden remission possibilities in IBD patients, and serve to potentially reduce the use of surgery to treat IBD patients.

3. Microbiota and the Role of Short-Chain Fatty Acids (SCFAs) in IBD

Certain species are responsible for the production of SCFAs. These SCFAs play an essential role with their anti-inflammatory properties and enhancement of the gut immune function. They also aid in the differentiation of regulatory T-cells into Th17 and Treg cells [12,13]. "Inflammatory reaction driven by Th cells protects the host from the detrimental pathogens"; however, "excessive activation of Th cells is associated with intestinal inflammation" [6]. The balance between pro-inflammatory Th17 and anti-inflammatory Treg cells is important in maintaining gut stability, which is directly affected by the content and diversity of the gut microbiota.

In the 1990s, a number of studies looked at a potential role for topical SCFA (butyric acid) treatment in distal ulcerative colitis through enemas or irrigation. Although trends towards beneficial effects were seen, there were no studies showing statistically significant results, and academic interest in the subject waned.

4. Prebiotics and Probiotics in IBD Treatment

Other dietary components that can affect the gut microbiome include prebiotics, postbiotics, and combinations of these known as synbiotics. Prebiotics are fermentable fibres found in foods, and probiotics are live, non-pathogenic microorganisms also implicated in the alteration of the gut microbiome for the benefit of the host. Synbiotics are a combination of the two and are thought to exert a synergistic effect [14].

Prebiotics and probiotics are thought to modulate the host immune response and improve intestinal barrier function and nutritional absorption, outcompeting pathogens for nutrition, adhesion to the gut lining, and production of antimicrobial substances [15].

Prebiotics are divided into groups based on the composition of sugars/carbohydrates. These naturally occurring compounds are found in many different foods but not in large concentrations [16]. They can be synthesised to make up for this, and, given their positive profile and therapeutic potential, it would be reasonable to assume they would be beneficial in IBD (Table 1).

Table 1. Advantages and limitations of probiotics and prebiotics.

Probiotics Pros	Prebiotics Pros	Probiotic Limitations	Prebiotic Limitations
Symptom relief	Anti-inflammatory	Strain and condition specific	Worsening of some symptoms
Enhancement of immunity	Reverses dysbiosis	Not universally effective	Limited evidence base
		Variable quality	
		Risk in immuno-compromised	

Paudel et al. [17] commented that a diet deprived of fibre would enhance mucus-eroding microbiota and, thus, leave the host susceptible to opportunistic intestinal microbes. At the very least, a lack of dietary fibre is detrimental to the healthy gut microbiome. They also commented that other studies showed that certain fibres offered protection against colitis [16]. Rau et al. [14] noted that, in some studies, prebiotics, although safe, did have some side effects such as bloating and flatulence. They also noted that caution should be exercised when recommending increased-fibre diets to patients with stricturing Crohn's disease; increased fibre is not necessarily a blanket treatment for all IBD. Whilst there is still scope for further research into prebiotic safety and efficacy, there exist some data to support the use of high-fibre diets, such as plant-based ones, to reduce symptoms in IBD [18–20].

Probiotics can also be found in fermented foods, and some have recently been marketed in the form of pills or capsules. They typically contain one or more microbial strains [12]. Rau et al. [14] noted varying outcomes of probiotics in IBD; they noted mixed reviews, with some studies showing ineffective induction of remission in UC. Some studies such as a systematic review and meta-analysis by Kaur et al. showed promising results [21], where probiotics were effective in "the induction of clinical remission in UC" and that "there were no overall differences in minor or serious adverse events when comparing probiotics with placebo". These studies, however, seemed to mainly comment on the effects of probiotics in UC. Much like prebiotics, there is more evidence required regarding the safety and efficacy of probiotics, especially in CD, in which there has been limited research thus far, before they can be applied to regular clinical practice. A Cochrane review [22] on the treatment of pouchitis following ileal pouch–anal anastomosis suggested a beneficial trend with probiotics in acute pouchitis, but robust data are still lacking.

Synbiotics in IBD also have limited research, but their potential is not to be ignored. Given the potential benefit of both prebiotics and probiotics, a synergistic combination of the two could prove useful in overcoming the current limitations in research and prove to be a safe and efficacious future treatment for IBD.

5. Faecal Microbiota Transplantation

One novel therapy that is utilised in the modulation of gut microbiome is faecal microbiota transplantation (FMT). This intervention has the potential to restore the balance in the gut microbiome between potentially pathogenic bacteria and beneficial strains. There is also the possibility of the transplantation of damaged microbiota from a healthy donor to an affected recipient [23].

FMT's exact mechanism of action is not fully understood. However, it is believed that, if successful, then the host's response to the transplant will lead to the promotion of anti-inflammatory metabolites such as SCFAs, suppressing inflammatory metabolites and reducing overall inflammation and damage to the bowel [23]. If the correct beneficial species can be identified in the donor, then FMT has the potential to become a specific treatment for an individual recipient or become a part of their personalised treatment plan.

FMT has been very successful in treating certain gastrointestinal infections, such as recurrent Clostridium difficile infection, which can cause pseudomembranous colitis.

There are many factors that determine the success of FMT in IBD. There should be careful donor and recipient screening and stringent consideration of the storage and preparation of the FMT; treatment before FMT, e.g., drug therapy or bowel preparation; route of administration; dose; and number of sessions of FMT [23,24]. Some factors identified in this systematic review of 25 studies showed these recipient factors to be associated with predictors of success when carrying out FMT: young age, less severe disease, shorter duration of disease, microbiome containing higher faecal species richness, greater abundance of *Candida*, and similarity to donor profile.

Some studies show that FMT works less well in UC than in Crohn's disease (CD). There are some reasons why it is more consistent in patients with UC than in those with CD; it seems to stem from the site of disease, as the microbial diversity of ileal and ilocolonic CD is significantly different from that of healthy controls, whilst colonic CD and UC were closer to each other [24,25].

Whilst FMT is generally safe, there have been some adverse effects reported in some trials in the younger and adolescent population with IBD. These effects include diarrhoea, abdominal cramps, bloating, and pain. These gastrointestinal symptoms are self-limiting and transient [26]. There have even been fatalities in up to 1.4% of FMT sessions [27,28].

Whilst these percentages are low, the safety of FMT is not guaranteed. These studies show that there is a need for the strict selection of patients as well as the regime they undergo as recommended by the European faecal transplant group [29].

Some upcoming advances are in the novel delivery of FMT such as colonic transendoscopic tube insertion for whole colonic treatment [30]. The tube insertions for this study were successful in all 54 patients; 98.1% of the patients were satisfied with this procedure. No discomfort or adverse events were seen. Patients were excluded if they had severe bowel lesions including stenosis, complex fistulas, or perianal lesions. This is an important consideration when selecting appropriate patients for therapy and when predicting how impactful specific therapies can be. These patients also had mesalazine delivered through their endoscopic tube, so the efficacy of FMT on its own for IBD patients is yet to be determined. Nevertheless, FMT holds promise for the future as a potential therapeutic target in IBD.

5.1. Microbiota Restoration Therapy (MRT)

FMT has, as demonstrated above, some potential side effects due to possibly unknown factors within the transplant. Another idea has focused on more defined/targeted microbial population delivery to the colon. This is known as microbiota restoration therapy (MRT). There has been promise with regards to Clostridium difficile treatment [31], although there is still more research to be carried out to solidify its therapeutic efficacy. The aim of MRT is to restore healthy gut microbiota to counter the dysbiosis in IBD. In the U.S., there has been Food and Drug administration (FDA) approval for the use of microbiome treatment containing live bacteria of qualified donor stool. This is a potentially huge step forward in the research on MRT. With this approval, its use can be studied with more reassurance and fewer administrative issues when setting up the research protocol.

5.2. Modification of Host–Microbe Interactions

The host–microbe chemical interactions in normal, healthy subjects contribute to normal gut health. They are responsible for the maintenance of gut barrier function, mucosal integrity, and clearance of pathogens. While FMT is one approach to restoring healthy gut microbiota interactions, another potential method is to modulate or modify host–microbe metabolic interactions.

Various biotechnological companies have examined these interactions and developed certain therapeutic targets and are studying their utility in IBD patients.

An experimental drug, EB8018, has been developed with the aim of blocking invasive *E. Coli* species' adherence onto intestinal epithelial cells and is currently in phase 1b trials. Other compounds still in their preclinical phase of study include SG-2-0776, which is being researched in a preclinical model of IBD [17,32].

The compounds SYMB-104 and SYMB-202 show promise in increasing the levels of Treg cells and reducing overall levels of intestinal inflammation. This shows promise for a system-targeted approach in personalising treatment for IBD patients. If it can specifically target colonic inflammation whilst maintaining low immunogenicity, then we may see a more effective and lasting treatment on the horizon. And, for patients, this translates to effective medical treatment, greater variety of treatment, more room for escalation without surgery, and ultimately living with their disease symptom free in remission [32].

6. Nanoparticle Gene Delivery

One other novel advancement for the delivery of treatment in IBD is the development of oral nanomedicines, which have been shown to directly affect and restore damaged intestinal epithelium. Nanoparticles are defined as particles between 1 and 100 nanometres in size. There are 1,000,000 nanometres in 1 millimetre. Some of these studies have shown promising therapeutic benefit in mouse large and small bowel samples. These 3-D tissue culture models served as a safe predictive base for disease sequalae and response to novel therapies such as nanomedicines [33].

These 3-d models showed strong anti-inflammatory responses and the ability to target very specific parts of the inflammatory process, in recent years, even being able to modulate mRNA expression selectively [34].

Research shows problems with gene expression in many pathologies including inflammatory bowel disease. Veiga et al. [34] has shown ways to overcome some of the technological challenges when using modified messenger RNA (mmRNA), such as the ability to successfully transcribe large amounts of mRNA in vitro, instability of the mRNA in vivo, the amount of immune response the host has in response to the therapy, and the ability to target specific cells.

This shows exciting promise for the future of disease therapy and the application of mRNA-related therapies. There is potential to introduce IL-10, a predominantly anti-inflammatory cytokine associated with the regulation of IBD, mRNA as a novel therapy. The potential benefit of mRNA therapies also lies in their lower risk for genomic integration compared with their DNA-based treatment counterparts.

Veiga et al. [34] designed lipid nanoparticles (LNPs) to overcome potential shortcomings and to avoid using other vectors such as viruses, which may have hindered long-term therapy options. LNPs would prevent the degradation of RNA molecules and reduce the host immune response to them, which is ideal. It is also a feasible and replicable preparation method that allows a more standardised approach in its adoption as a novel treatment [35]. They used transmission electron microscopy to ascertain the efficiency of LNP encapsulation, which was ~100% [36,37].

They were also able to add targeting antibodies for the cell-specific delivery of mmRNA, and this method did not hamper mRNA encapsulation. Therefore, the therapy should be specific and only target the colon.

Safety and sustainability often go hand in hand when describing therapies. So, in order to check that the novel therapies are not just novel and are of potential use to humans, we must look at how specific such therapy is and whether there are any potential areas for development especially with systemic inflammatory reactions.

To assess the immunogenicity of their LNPs, splenic inflammatory cytokines were analysed via ELISA as a marker of systemic inflammation, and these were found to be in lower amounts than IL-10 levels in the colon and in control groups. This shows us that they targeted the specific expression of IL-10 in colonic mice models, with induced inflammatory bowel disease, without the systemic involvement of other organs. Pathological disease signs were also used as a marker including weight loss, erythema, and inflammatory infiltration of the colon. These were also found to be significantly reduced in the treated mice, and the control groups showed minimal reduction in these signs; thus, proving its therapeutic potential and safety to trial in human studies. The pro-inflammatory markers they looked at originated from the spleen, and the mice were sacrificed to look at their colonic histology after day 10. So, whilst there are very promising human implications for this treatment, there is scope for further analysis on the long-term safety and other systemic markers.

7. Conclusions

The research into the diagnostics and novel therapies available on the horizon for humans is very promising. Animal studies have shown potentially transferrable and safe therapies that can target specific sites of inflammation. Modulating the inflammatory response is a powerful therapy with what is shown to be a reasonably safe profile to build further research on. If properly and successfully developed, it would have life changing potential for refractory disease and provide patients with therapies associated with fewer side effects as compared to surgery. There is also potential for those with other inflammatory conditions to benefit from these innovative modes of treatment. The implications mentioned in this review for targeted gene therapy, effective treatment with low immunogenicity, and a safe side effect profile can be adapted to other conditions [38].

Author Contributions: Conceptualisation, N.S., H.R., A.K. and R.P.A.; review of the literature: N.S., H.R., A.K. and R.P.A.; writing—original draft preparation: N.S., H.R. and A.K.; writing—review and editing: N.S., H.R., A.K. and R.P.A.; supervision: A.K. and R.P.A. All authors have read and agreed to the published version of the manuscript.

Funding: This research received no external funding.

Institutional Review Board Statement: This study did not require ethical approval.

Data Availability Statement: No new data were created.

Conflicts of Interest: The authors declare no conflicts of interest.

Abbreviations

The following abbreviations are used in this manuscript:

IBD	Inflammatory bowel disease
UC	Ulcerative colitis
SCFAs	Short-chain fatty acids
FMT	Faecal microbiota transplantation
MRT	Microbiota restoration therapy
mRNA	Messenger ribonucleic acid
mmRNA	Modified messenger ribonucleic acid
ELISA	Enzyme-linked immunosorbent assay

References

1. Cao, Z.; Sugimura, N.; Burgermeister, E.; Ebert, M.P.; Zuo, T.; Lan, P. The gut virome: A new microbiome component in health and disease. *eBioMedicine* **2022**, *81*, 104113. [CrossRef]
2. Zhang, F.; Aschenbrenner, D.; Yoo, J.Y.; Zuo, T. The gut mycobiome in health, disease, and clinical applications in association with the gut bacterial microbiome assembly. *Lancet Microbe* **2022**, *3*, E969–E983. [CrossRef]
3. Boppana, K.; E Almansouri, N.; Bakkannavar, S.; Faheem, Y.; Jaiswal, A.; Shergill, K.; Nath, T.S. Alterations in Gut Microbiota as Early Biomarkers for Predicting Inflammatory Bowel Disease Onset and Progression: A Systematic Review. *Cureus* **2024**, *16*, e58080. [CrossRef] [PubMed]
4. Guo, X.; Huang, C.; Xu, J.; Xu, H.; Liu, L.; Zhao, H.; Wang, J.; Huang, W.; Peng, W.; Chen, Y.; et al. Gut Microbiota Is a Potential Biomarker in Inflammatory Bowel Disease. *Front. Nutr.* **2022**, *8*, 818902. [CrossRef] [PubMed]
5. Ocansey, D.K.W.; Fang, S.; Yuan, X.; Qian, H.; Zhou, M.; Olovo, C.V.; Zhang, X.; Mao, F. The diagnostic and prognostic potential of gut bacteria in inflammatory bowel disease. *Gut Microbes* **2023**, *15*, 2176118. [CrossRef]
6. Foppa, C.; Rizkala, T.; Repici, A.; Hassan, C.; Spinelli, A. Microbiota and IBD: Current knowledge and future perspectives. *Dig. Liver Dis.* **2024**, *56*, 911–922. [CrossRef] [PubMed]
7. Haneishi, Y.; Furuya, Y.; Hasegawa, M.; Picarelli, A.; Rossi, M.; Miyamoto, J. Inflammatory Bowel Diseases and Gut Microbiota. *Int. J. Mol. Sci.* **2023**, *24*, 3817. [CrossRef]
8. Jacobs, J.P.; Goudarzi, M.; Singh, N.; Tong, M.; McHardy, I.H.; Ruegger, P.; Asadourian, M.; Moon, B.H.; Ayson, A.; Borneman, J.; et al. A Disease-Associated Microbial and Metabolomics State in Relatives of Pediatric Inflammatory Bowel Disease Patients. *Cell. Mol. Gastroenterol. Hepatol.* **2016**, *2*, 750–766. [CrossRef]
9. Forrest, C.M.; Gould, S.R.; Darlington, L.G.; Stone, T.W. Levels of purine, kynurenine and lipid peroxidation products in patients with inflammatory bowel disease. *Adv. Exp. Med. Biol.* **2003**, *527*, 395–400.
10. Lamas, B.; Richard, M.L.; Leducq, V.; Pham, H.-P.; Michel, M.-L.; Da Costa, G.; Bridonneau, C.; Jegou, S.; Hoffmann, T.W.; Natividad, J.M.; et al. CARD9 impacts colitis by altering gut microbiota metabolism of tryptophan into aryl hydrocarbon receptor ligands. *Nat. Med.* **2016**, *22*, 598–605. [CrossRef]
11. Khan, I.; Ullah, N.; Zha, L.; Bai, Y.; Khan, A.; Zhao, T.; Che, T.; Zhang, C. Alteration of Gut Microbiota in Inflammatory Bowel Disease (IBD): Cause or Consequence? IBD Treatment Targeting the Gut Microbiome. *Pathogens* **2019**, *8*, 126. [CrossRef] [PubMed]
12. Caparrós, E.; Wiest, R.; Scharl, M.; Rogler, G.; Casbas, A.G.; Yilmaz, B.; Wawrzyniak, M.; Francés, R. Dysbiotic microbiota interactions in Crohn's disease. *Gut Microbes* **2021**, *13*, 1949096. [CrossRef] [PubMed]
13. Gao, J.; Xu, K.; Liu, H.; Liu, G.; Bai, M.; Peng, C.; Li, T.; Yin, Y. Impact of the Gut Microbiota on Intestinal Immunity Mediated by Tryptophan Metabolism. *Front. Cell. Infect. Microbiol.* **2018**, *8*, 13. [CrossRef]
14. Rau, S.; Gregg, A.; Yaceczko, S.; Berkeley, L.i.m.k.e.t.k.a.i. Prebiotics and Probiotics for Gastrointestinal Disorders. *Nutrients* **2024**, *16*, 778. [CrossRef]
15. Markowiak, P.; Śliżewska, K. Effects of Probiotics, Prebiotics, and Synbiotics on Human Health. *Nutrients* **2017**, *9*, 1021. [CrossRef]
16. Qin, Y.-Q.; Wang, L.-Y.; Yang, X.-Y.; Xu, Y.-J.; Fan, G.; Fan, Y.-G.; Ren, J.-N.; An, Q.; Li, X. Inulin: Properties and health benefits. *Food Funct.* **2023**, *14*, 2948–2968. [CrossRef]

17. Paudel, D.; Nair, D.V.T.; Joseph, G.; Castro, R.; Tiwari, A.K.; Singh, V. Gastrointestinal microbiota-directed nutritional and therapeutic interventions for inflammatory bowel disease: Opportunities and challenges. *Gastroenterol. Rep.* **2023**, *12*, goae033. [CrossRef]
18. Bretin, A.; Zou, J.; Yeoh, B.S.; Ngo, V.L.; Winer, S.; Winer, D.A.; Reddivari, L.; Pellizzon, M.; Walters, W.A.; Patterson, A.D.; et al. Psyllium Fiber Protects Against Colitis Via Activation of Bile Acid Sensor Farnesoid X Receptor. *Cell. Mol. Gastroenterol. Hepatol.* **2023**, *15*, 1421–1442. [CrossRef] [PubMed]
19. Limketkai, B.N.; Hamideh, M.; Shah, R.; Sauk, J.S.; Jaffe, N. Dietary Patterns and Their Association with Symptoms Activity in Inflammatory Bowel Diseases. *Inflamm. Bowel Dis.* **2022**, *28*, 1627–1636. [CrossRef]
20. Limketkai, B.N.; Godoy-Brewer, G.; Parian, A.M.; Noorian, S.; Krishna, M.; Shah, N.D.; White, J.; Mullin, G.E. Dietary Interventions for the Treatment of Inflammatory Bowel Diseases: An Updated Systematic Review and Meta-analysis. *Clin. Gastroenterol. Hepatol. Off. Clin. Pract. J. Am. Gastroenterol. Assoc.* **2022**, *21*, 2508–2525. [CrossRef]
21. Kaur, L.; Gordon, M.; Baines, P.A.; Iheozor-Ejiofor, Z.; Sinopoulou, V.; Akobeng, A.K. Probiotics for induction of remission in ulcerative colitis. *Cochrane Database Syst. Rev.* **2020**, *3*, CD005573. [PubMed]
22. Nguyen, N.; Zhang, B.; Holubar, S.D.; Pardi, D.S.; Singh, S. Treatment and prevention of pouchitis after ileal pouch-anal anastomosis for chronic ulcerative colitis. *Cochrane Database Syst. Rev.* **2019**, *5*, CD001176. [PubMed]
23. Arora, U.; Kedia, S.; Ahuja, V. The practice of fecal microbiota transplantation in inflammatory bowel disease. *Intest. Res.* **2023**, *22*, 44–64. [CrossRef]
24. Imhann, F.; Vila, A.V.; Bonder, M.J.; Fu, J.; Gevers, D.; Visschedijk, M.C.; Spekhorst, L.M.; Alberts, R.; Franke, L.; van Dullemen, H.M.; et al. Systematic review of donor and recipient predictive biomarkers of response to faecal microbiota transplantation in patients with ulcerative colitis. *eBioMedicine* **2022**, *81*, 104088.
25. Marcella, C.; Cui, B.; Kelly, C.R.; Ianiro, G.; Cammarota, G.; Zhang, F. Interplay of host genetics and gut microbiota underlying the onset and clinical presentation of inflammatory bowel disease. *Gut* **2016**, *67*, 108–119.
26. Marcella, C.; Cui, B.; Kelly, C.R.; Ianiro, G.; Cammarota, G.; Zhang, F. Systematic review: The global incidence of faecal microbiota transplantation-related adverse events from 2000 to 2020. *Aliment. Pharmacol. Ther.* **2020**, *53*, 33–42. [CrossRef]
27. Quera, R.; Espinoza, R.; Estay, C.; Rivera, D. Bacteremia as an adverse event of fecal microbiota transplantation in a patient with Crohn's disease and recurrent Clostridium difficile infection. *J. Crohn's Colitis* **2014**, *8*, 252–253. [CrossRef]
28. Kao, D.; Roach, B.; Silva, M.; Beck, P.; Rioux, K.; Kaplan, G.G.; Chang, H.-J.; Coward, S.; Goodman, K.J.; Xu, H.; et al. Effect of Oral Capsule– vs Colonoscopy-Delivered Fecal Microbiota Transplantation on Recurrent Clostridium difficile Infection. *JAMA* **2017**, *318*, 1985. [CrossRef]
29. Keller, J.J.; Ooijevaar, R.E.; Hvas, C.L.; Terveer, E.M.; Lieberknecht, S.C.; Högenauer, C.; Arkkila, P.; Sokol, H.; Gridnyev, O.; Mégraud, F.; et al. A standardised model for stool banking for faecal microbiota transplantation: A consensus report from a multidisciplinary UEG working group. *United Eur. Gastroenterol. J.* **2021**, *9*, 229–247. [CrossRef]
30. Peng, Z.; Xiang, J.; He, Z.; Zhang, T.; Xu, L.; Cui, B.; Li, P.; Huang, G.; Ji, G.; Nie, Y.; et al. Colonic transendoscopic enteral tubing: A novel way of transplanting fecal microbiota. *Endosc. Int. Open* **2016**, *4*, E610–E613. [CrossRef]
31. Reinisch, W. Fecal Microbiota Transplantation in Inflammatory Bowel Disease. *Dig. Dis.* **2017**, *35*, 123. [CrossRef] [PubMed]
32. Cully, M. Microbiome therapeutics go small molecule. *Nat. Rev. Drug Discov.* **2019**, *18*, 569–572. [CrossRef] [PubMed]
33. Sadman Sakib Zou, S. Attenuation of Chronic Inflammation in Intestinal Organoids with Graphene Oxide-Mediated Tumor Necrosis Factor-α_Small Interfering RNA Delivery. *Langmuir* **2024**, *40*, 3402–3413.
34. Veiga, N.; Goldsmith, M.; Granot, Y.; Rosenblum, D.; Dammes, N.; Kedmi, R.; Ramishetti, S.; Peer, D. Cell specific delivery of modified mRNA expressing therapeutic proteins to leukocytes. *Nat. Commun.* **2018**, *9*, 4493. [CrossRef]
35. Karp, J.M.; Peer, D. Focus on RNA interference: From nanoformulations to in vivo delivery. *Nanotechnology* **2017**, *29*, 010201. [CrossRef] [PubMed]
36. Cohen, Z.R.; Ramishetti, S.; Peshes-Yaloz, N.; Goldsmith, M.; Wohl, A.; Zibly, Z.; Peer, D. Localized RNAi Therapeutics of Chemoresistant Grade IV Glioma Using Hyaluronan-Grafted Lipid-Based Nanoparticles. *ACS Nano* **2015**, *9*, 1581–1591. [CrossRef]
37. Mizrahy, S.; Hazan-Halevy, I.; Dammes, N.; Landesman-Milo, D.; Peer, D. Current Progress in Non-viral RNAi-Based Delivery Strategies to Lymphocytes. *Mol. Ther.* **2017**, *25*, 1491–1500. [CrossRef]
38. Romano, A.; Mortellaro, A. The New Frontiers of Gene Therapy and Gene Editing in Inflammatory Diseases. *Hum. Gene Ther.* **2024**, *35*, 219–231. [CrossRef]

biomedicines

MDPI

Article

Infliximab in Inflammatory Bowel Disease: Leveraging Physiologically Based Pharmacokinetic Modeling in the Clinical Context

Zvonimir Petric [1,*], João Gonçalves [2] and Paulo Paixão [1]

1 Department of Pharmacological Sciences, Research Institute for Medicines, Faculty of Pharmacy, University of Lisbon, 1649-004 Lisbon, Portugal

2 Biopharmaceutical and Molecular Biotechnology Unit, Research Institute for Medicines, Faculty of Pharmacy, University of Lisbon, 1649-004 Lisbon, Portugal

* Correspondence: petric.zvonimir@gmail.com

Abstract: In this study, a physiologically based pharmacokinetic (PBPK) modeling framework was employed to explore infliximab exposure following intravenous (5 mg/kg) and subcutaneous administration (encompassing the approved 120 mg flat-fixed dose as a switching option) in virtual adult and pediatric patients with inflammatory bowel disease (IBD). The PBPK model and corresponding simulations were conducted using the PK-Sim® software platform. The PBPK simulation indicated that a 120 mg subcutaneous flat-fixed dose might not be optimal for heavier adults with IBD, suggesting the need for infliximab dose escalation. For an older virtual pediatric patient (14 years old), subcutaneous administration of a 120 mg flat-fixed dose appears to be a feasible IBD treatment option. In the final exploration scenario, the model was extended to predict hypothetical subcutaneous infliximab doses in a virtual pediatric population (6–18 years old), stratified into three weight bands (20–30 kg, 30–45 kg, and 45–70 kg), that would yield post-switch trough concentrations of infliximab comparable to those seen in adults with the 120 mg flat-fixed subcutaneous dose. The PBPK-model-informed dose suggestions were 40 mg for the 20–30 kg band, 80 mg for the 30–45 kg band, and 120 mg for the 45–70 kg band. As demonstrated in this paper, the PBPK modeling framework can serve as a versatile tool in clinical pharmacology to investigate various clinical scenarios, such as exploring alternative dosing regimens and routes of administration, ultimately advancing IBD treatment across diverse (sub)populations of clinical interest.

Keywords: physiologically based pharmacokinetic (PBPK) modeling; infliximab; inflammatory bowel disease (IBD); clinical pharmacology

1. Introduction

Inflammatory bowel disease (IBD) encompasses two closely related yet distinct intestinal disorders: Crohn's disease and ulcerative colitis. The etiology and pathophysiology of IBD remain complex and multifaceted. While the exact mechanisms are still being elucidated, it is believed that a combination of genetic predisposition, environmental factors, lifestyle choices, mucosal immunity mediated by the intestinal barrier, and alterations in the gut microbiome contribute to the development of the disease and its inflammation. Infliximab, initially approved for medical use by the U.S. Food and Drug Administration agency in 1998, stands out as one of the blockbuster monoclonal antibodies (MAbs) that has reshaped the pharmacological landscape in the treatment of IBD. Specifically, infliximab binds to and neutralizes (i.e., blocks) the pleiotropic cytokine tumor necrosis factor-alpha (TNF-α), a pivotal player in the pathogenesis of IBD. Over time, or following the initiation of pharmacological treatment with infliximab, the complex interactions among (patho)physiology, immunology, and pharmacology frequently lead to a diminished clinical response. From a clinical standpoint, it has been observed that the clearance of infliximab tends to increase with the severity of the disease. Infliximab clearance is influenced by the individual's pharmacokinetic, pharmacodynamic, and immune context. Specifically, there is a positive correlation between infliximab clearance and the extent of gut inflammation, which, in combination with immunogenicity, may lead to reduced effective drug concentrations in patients [1]. This is exemplified by the notably lower trough concentrations observed in non-responders compared to responders [2]. As a result, this exposure metric is widely employed in concentration-guided dosing approaches, encompassing dose escalation or de-escalation [1,2].

In Europe, infliximab is approved for use in both adult and pediatric populations with IBD, starting from six years of age [3]. Typically, the administration of monoclonal antibodies in pediatric patients is adapted from adult protocols. Infliximab, administered intravenously in children, follows a dosing regimen based on body weight (5 mg/kg) during both the induction and maintenance phases at designated time intervals, which is the same as in adults. However, depending on the clinical response, dose escalation or shortening the dosing intervals to less than 8 weeks might be necessary [3].

Just recently, infliximab has gained approval for subcutaneous administration as maintenance therapy in adults. This involves switching to a flat-fixed dose of 120 mg solution for injection (available in a pre-filled syringe and pre-filled pen) at week 6 following the intravenous induction phase (5 mg/kg) [4]. This innovative, subcutaneous, biosimilar infliximab can also be referred to as a biobetter, owing to its clinical novelty and improved pharmacokinetic profile compared to the intravenous originator. From a patient's standpoint, subcutaneous administration is anticipated to enhance adherence and offer overall benefits to adult patients, resulting in better treatment effectiveness [4]. However, clinical data supporting the feasibility of switching to subcutaneous infliximab in the pediatric population is lacking at the moment [5].

Quantitative Clinical Pharmacology Tools

Pharmacokinetic (PK) modeling, a cornerstone of pharmacometrics (the science of quantitative pharmacology) and often hailed as a state-of-the-art pharmacological tool, plays a pivotal role in clinical pharmacology. It assists in understanding drug behavior within the body, optimizing dosing regimens, and predicting drug exposure across diverse scenarios. A PK model can be conceived as a simplified empirical representation of biological processes, including drug input, distribution, and elimination, which are the fundamental aspects of pharmacokinetics within the human body [6]. However, when such an empirical model describing the fate of a drug in the body is enriched with the physical, (patho)physiological, and biochemical context of a living system, mechanistic physiological models are obtained. These models can depict physiological and biochemical processes within a virtual human. In addition to describing the pharmacokinetics of a drug, these models aid in understanding the drug's fate within the body. Such models also have the capability to describe virtual human characteristics by utilizing known or extrapolated physiological parameters [7–9]. In some cases, if certain physiological parameters are not known, their values can be determined by fitting the simulation predictions to experimental data, such as the drug concentration–time profile. Namely, because of the physiological foundation, most parameters in such models are not reliant on specific drug knowledge or pharmacokinetic measurements [9].

Drug-specific properties, encompassing physicochemical and biochemical characteristics, are pivotal in determining how the body processes a drug. Factors such as molecular weight, solubility, lipophilicity, and interactions with transporters—both influx and efflux—can significantly influence drug absorption. Furthermore, the disposition of small molecules may be impacted by their affinity for binding to proteins in plasma or tissue components, as well as to cytochrome P-450 (CYP) enzymes and target receptors [8]. In contrast, the disposition of large protein molecules (e.g., MAbs) is independent of CYPs, and they are mainly eliminated through catabolism. The physicochemical complexity, structural differences, and greater target selectivity and specificity of MAbs, compared to small molecule drugs, consequently affect the choice of administration route and dosing regimen. These properties ultimately manifest as clinically meaningful aspects within the realm of pharmacokinetics, such as bioavailability, volume of distribution, clearance, half-life, and various exposure metrics including the area under the concentration–time curve, maximum concentration, and trough concentration. Consequently, the framework that integrates anatomical and physiological features of a virtual individual (or population) of interest with drug-specific physicochemical and biochemical properties, utilized to characterize the pharmacokinetics of a drug, is known as physiologically based pharmacokinetic (PBPK) modeling (Figure 1). Finally, the PBPK simulation prediction, based on the corresponding model, encompasses not only the (patho)physiology of a virtual human and drug-specific properties but also the pharmacokinetic profile of the drug, its formulation, and its dosing regimen.

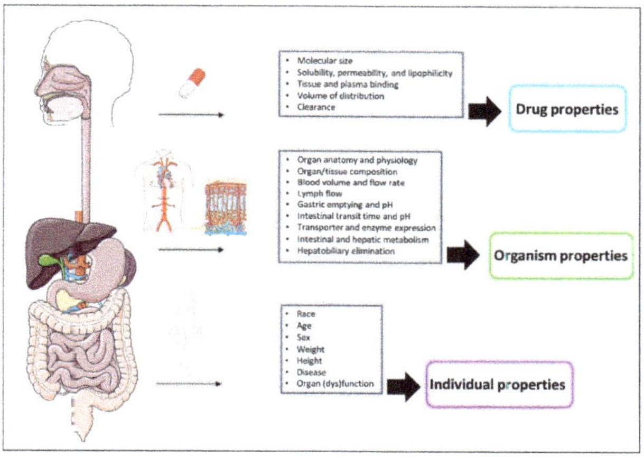

Figure 1. Example of integrated components of the PBPK modeling framework (graphics are with permission from Servier Medical Art by Servier, licensed under CC BY 4.0 [10]). Note that the selection of drug properties depends on the classification of the drug as either a small molecule or large molecule (e.g., MAb).

The fundamental assumption underlying any PBPK model is the division of the body into multiple networks of compartments, each representing organs, or part of organs, and tissues interconnected via the blood system (venous and arterial blood pool) (Figure 2) [8]. From a mathematical standpoint, the PBPK model describes the input and transfer of a drug throughout the system using mass balance differential equations. However, despite its mathematical underpinnings, PBPK modeling can offer advantages in comprehending complex clinical contexts [11], supporting drug labeling recommendations [12], or guiding dosing decisions [13], i.e., aiding in addressing questions within the realm of clinical pharmacology.

One of the primary advantages of PBPK modeling is its ability to allow users to adjust, as needed, the variability (i.e., differences) in physiological and biochemical parameters in the virtual human(s). This enables the virtual patient (or population) to reflect the characteristics of its real-life counterpart [7,8]. The versatility of the PBPK framework allows for the customization of PBPK models to accommodate various conditions such as hepatic impairment.

For instance, parameters like organ blood flow rate, liver volume, albumin and hematocrit values, and the expression profiles of CYP enzymes can be modified to mirror the pathophysiological context associated with the severity of hepatic impairment. This capability enables drawing inferences about the drug of interest, i.e., its disposition, and exposure, all of which is influenced by the impairment.

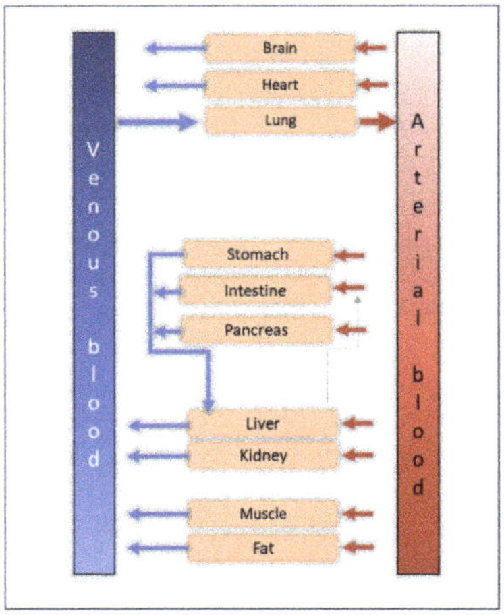

Figure 2. Graphical conceptualization of a PBPK model for a hypothetical drug with enterohepatic circulation. Drug input can be, for example, via the intravenous route, directly into the venous blood pool. Compartments in a PBPK model represent the actual anatomy and physiology relevant to drug input and disposition.

In cases where the nature of the disease is too complex to be straightforwardly set up in the software (e.g., gut inflammation in IBD), users can explore alternative methods to mimic the real-life impact of the disease on drug disposition [14]. In this paper, the versatility of the PBPK framework is demonstrated in virtual patients, including both adults and children, treated with infliximab via intravenous and subcutaneous administration. Additionally, the PBPK framework is utilized for model-informed dose suggestions in target (sub)populations of clinical interest.

2. Materials and Methods

The PBPK modeling exercise was performed using the modeling platform PK-Sim® (version 11.2, Open Systems Pharmacology Suite, Bayer Technology Services, Leverkusen, Germany). This modeling platform offers a model specifically tailored to explain the pharmacokinetics of protein drugs and large molecules (e.g., MAbs), which is developed as an extension of a standard model for small molecules (please see the Supplementary Materials for additional information on methodology, including Figure S1) [9,15].

For large molecules and proteins, hydrodynamic radius (solute radius) is estimated from the molecular weight set in the "Basic physico-chemistry" tab. Additionally, the infliximab PBPK model included the expression profile of TNF-α (already built into the software database), with its relative expression in plasma set to 1. TNF-α half-lives in the liver and intestine were left unchanged, but its reference concentration was set to 0.20 pM [16].

PKSim® does not include a subcutaneous administration building block. To compensate for this, the fat compartment was designated as the target organ for the subcutaneous delivery of infliximab, with the plasma as the target compartment. A first-order absorption process, based on the literature data [17], was assumed for modeling the absorption. The dosage modification was implemented to accurately represent the true concentration of infliximab in the biophase, taking into consideration the bioavailability (F) of subcutaneous infliximab. The bioavailability value was taken from the population PK model of the subcutaneous infliximab formulation [17]. Lastly, bioavailability (F) and the absorption rate constant (Ka) were kept consistent across all exploration scenarios involving the subcutaneous administration of infliximab.

The PBPK model of infliximab was initially developed to represent a virtual human (i.e., a virtual twin) corresponding to the average (typical), i.e., mean, pharmacokinetic, and biometric profile of the population in a real-world trial—specifically, healthy adults receiving intravenous infliximab (5 mg/kg) [18,19] (Table 1). The baseline model incorporated inputs obtained from the software, built-in parameter identification, as well as from the literature (Table 2).

Table 1. Published clinical trial data on infliximab used for fitting [18] and model validation [14,17,20–22].

1. Clinical trial in healthy adults, single intravenous dose 5 mg/kg [18]
2. Clinical trial in adult patients with IBD [20] intravenous dose 5 mg/kg induction + maintenance up to week 54 subcutaneous switch, dose: 120 mg (skin of abdomen or upper thigh) subcutaneous switch, dose: 240 mg (skin of abdomen or upper thigh)
3. Clinical trial in adult patients with IBD, population pharmacokinetic study (subcutaneous switch to 120 mg in adults with IBD) and simulations on smaller, average, and heavier adult patients [17]
4. Clinical trial in pediatric population with IBD (intravenous route 5 mg/kg, ulcerative colitis) [14,21]
5. Clinical trial in older pediatric population with IBD (post-switch to subcutaneous 120 mg, skin of abdomen or upper thigh) [22]

Table 2. Input parameters for a baseline PBPK model in virtual healthy adults.

TNF-α
Reference concentration: 0.2 pm [16]
Localization: plasma and interstitial space; relative expression: 1 [14]
Infliximab
Molecular weight: 149.9 kDa [1]
Radius (solute): 5.18 nm [23]
Kd (FcRn) in endosomal space: 0.73 μmol/L [24]
Kd (FcRn) plasma/interstitial *: 4.54 mmol/L (i.e., negligible binding affinity [25])Kd (TNF-α) *: 120.17 pmol/L (100 pmol/L [26])
Koff (TNF-α) *: 1.331/ms (111/ms [27])
Kass (FcRn)*: 0.72 L/μmol/min (0.80 L/μmol/min [28])
Anatomy and physiology of a virtual healthy adult
Fraction endosomal: 0.20 [28]
Specific clearance in endosome *: 0.911/min
Fraction recycled to plasma: 1 [28]
Fraction of endosomal uptake from plasma *: 0.53
Rate constant for endosomal uptake: 0.291/min [28]
Rate constant for recycling from endosomal space *: 0.301/min
Kd (FcRn, endogenous IgG) in plasma/interstitial space: 10,000 μmol/L [28]
Kd (FcRn, endogenous IgG) in endosome: 0.63 μmol/L [28]
Kass (FcRn, endogenous IgG): 0.87 L/ μmol/min [28]

Fitted values are denoted by an asterisk (*), while values reported in the literature are shown in brackets. Kd (FcRn)—dissociation constant of infliximab for FcRn (neonatal fragment crystallizable receptor) in the endosomal space, or in the plasma/interstitial space (in neutral very weak affinity); Kd (TNF-α)—dissociation constant of infliximab for TNF-α (tumor necrosis factor alpha); Koff (TNF-α)—dissociation rate constant of infliximab for TNF-α; Kass (FcRn)—association constant of infliximab for FcRn; endogenous IgG—endogenous immunoglobulin G with its dissociation (Kd) and association (Kass) constant for FcRn.

The clinical trial dataset [18] in Table 1 was used for fitting this baseline model, while other trials were utilized for model validation across various clinical scenarios of interest, such as exploration of the subcutaneous administration route, different doses, or different target (sub)populations. Pharmacokinetic data on infliximab were digitized using WebPlot Digitizer® (version 4.5, Pacifica, Carpinteria, CA, USA). Illustrations were made by Servier Medical Art tools under the free CC BY 4.0 license [10].

An overview of the PBPK modeling exploration of infliximab in this paper is provided in Figure 3.

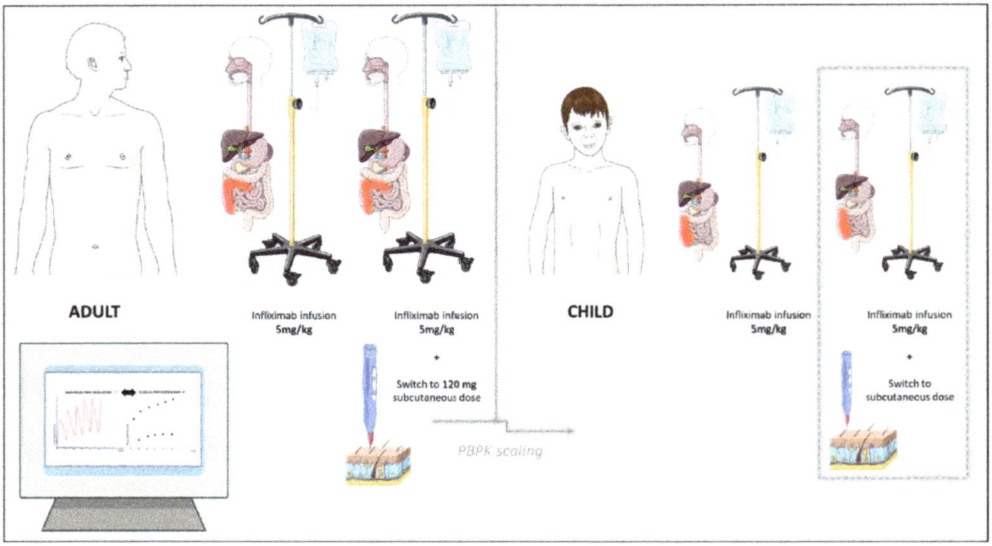

Figure 3. General overview of the PBPK modeling exploration of infliximab in this paper (graphics with permission from Servier Medical Art by Servier, licensed under CC BY 4.0 [10]). Pharmacokinetic profiles of a typical (mean) virtual healthy individual (70 kg), virtual adult patient (70 kg), virtual heavy adult (120 kg), and virtual pediatric patient (14-year-old child) with IBD were compared with the mean concentration–time profile derived from real-world clinical trials. The dashed line represents a hypothetical "what-if" scenario involving a switch to subcutaneous infliximab and exploration of the PBPK-model-informed dose suggestion in a typical virtual pediatric patient (14 years of age) and virtual pediatric populations (6–18 years of age) stratified by weight.

3. Results and Discussion

This paper showcases the adaptability of the PBPK framework in patients with IBD, encompassing both adults and children, who are undergoing infliximab treatment via intravenous (5 mg/kg) and subcutaneous routes (encompassing the flat-fixed 120 mg dose). Furthermore, the PBPK model is utilized to propose model-informed dose suggestions post-switch to subcutaneous infliximab in a typical heavy adult (120 kg), a pediatric patient (14-year-old child, 60 kg), and a pediatric population (6–18 years of age stratified by weight). In essence, the PBPK simulations are employed to examine dosing strategies and to explore hypothetical clinical scenarios in target (sub)populations pertinent to infliximab dosing in the context of IBD.

3.1. PBPK Model Development for a Virtual Healthy Adult after Single Intravenous Administration of Infliximab (5 mg/kg)

A baseline PBPK model was constructed for a virtual healthy adult (representing a typical adult individual, 70 kg) receiving a single-dose intravenous infusion of infliximab (5 mg/kg over a duration of 2 h). The endosomal clearance rate for the typical adult healthy individual was determined by fitting the PK profiles from the trial [18] (via built-in parameter identification) to 0.91 per minute. Relevant input parameters of the baseline PBPK model are outlined in Table 2, while the fitted profile is shown in Figure 4. Trial data for a healthy individual were digitized from [18].

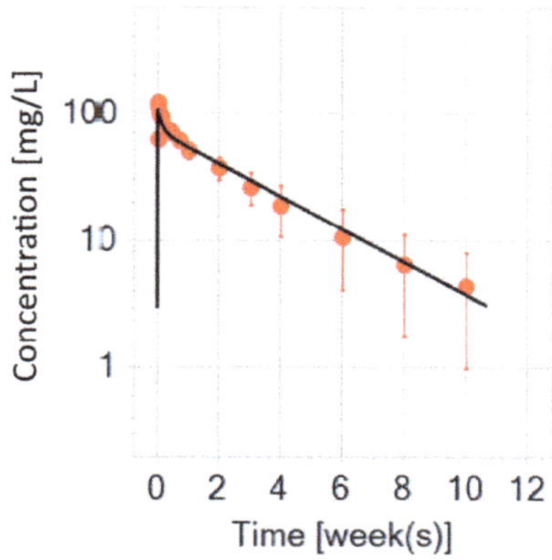

Figure 4. Fitted baseline PBPK model of infliximab on a semi-logarithmic scale for a typical healthy adult (black curve) after a single intravenous treatment (5 mg/kg), corresponding to a typical healthy adult from a trial. The red dots represent the average pharmacokinetic profile digitized from the trial data in healthy adult individuals.

3.2. PBPK Model Development for a Virtual Adult with IBD after Intravenous Administrations of Infliximab (5 mg/kg)

As previously noted, the severity of IBD can vary widely among patients, with both immune- and non-immune-mediated factors negatively impacting drug exposure. To address all the factors contributing to increased infliximab clearance, a process in the physiological compartment (i.e., endosome) was manually adjusted (as a lumped proxy for those factors) to fit an average infliximab pharmacokinetic profile in patients with IBD. Consequently, virtual adult patients with moderate to severe IBD were assigned a specific endosomal clearance rate of 1.6 per minute, which resulted in the simulation prediction shown in Figure 5. Trial data from an adult patient was digitized from [20].

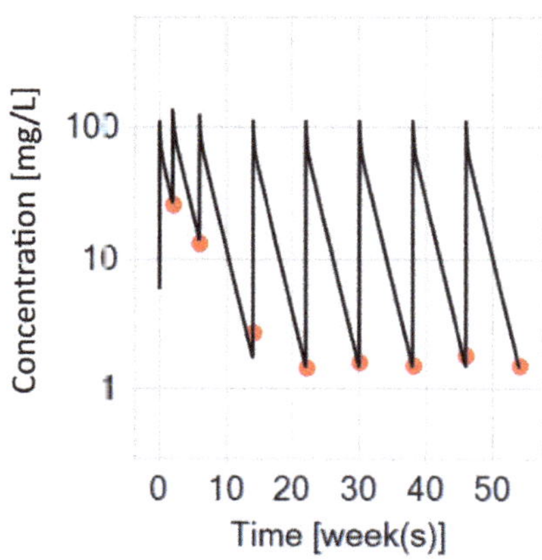

Figure 5. Infliximab PBPK simulation on a semi-logarithmic scale for a typical adult patient with IBD (black curve) after intravenous treatments (5 mg/kg), representing the mean adult patient from a trial. The red dots represent the mean trough concentrations digitized from the trial data in adult patients with IBD.

3.3. PBPK Modeling Exploration for Virtual Adults with IBD (Typical and Heavy) after Switching to Subcutaneous Infliximab

Given the recent introduction of a biobetter of infliximab, the PBPK model was assessed to determine its capability in describing the exposure profile following the switch (at week 6) to subcutaneous infliximab at a flat-fixed dose of 120 mg in adult patients with IBD.

As stated earlier, to ensure that the actual concentration of infliximab in the biophase is properly represented in the PBPK-simulated prediction, the infliximab subcutaneous input was modeled as a first-order absorption with an estimated absorption rate constant (Ka) of 0.0114 1/h. Additionally, the dose was corrected for the estimated bioavailability (F) of 0.79. Both values were taken from the population PK study of subcutaneous infliximab [17].

The PBPK simulation prediction for a typical virtual adult (70 kg) was compared to clinical data and contextualized with predicted intervals (5th and 95th percentile) derived from the population PK study [17] (Figure 6A). To evaluate the model's predictive performance after infliximab switching (120 mg) in a typical heavy patient (120 kg), a second simulation was conducted (Figure 6B). Since there is also a clinical trial [20] which tested the subcutaneous dose of 240 mg, simulation prediction was extended to test the model performance in the typical heavy patient (120 kg) receiving 240 mg of subcutaneous infliximab (Figure 6C). It is important to mention that the subcutaneous dose of 240 mg is not approved by the regulating authority. Trial data for adult patients was digitized from [20] while the prediction interval from the population PK study was digitized from [17].

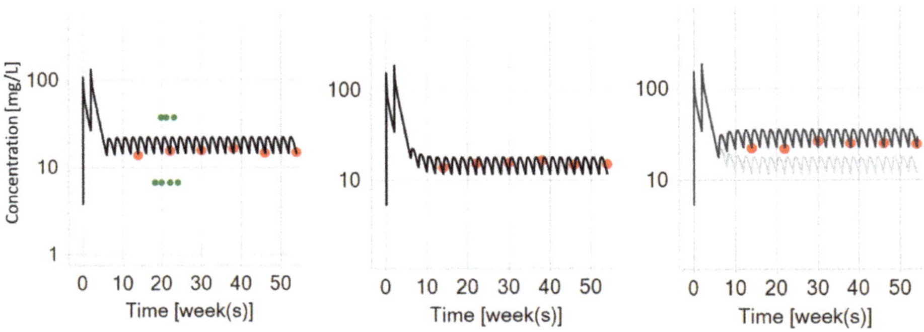

A B C

Figure 6. Infliximab PBPK simulation on a semi-logarithmic scale for a typical adult patient with IBD following the switch to subcutaneous infliximab (black curve) at week 6. (**A**) The image displays the prediction after a flat-fixed dose of 120 mg in a typical adult (70 kg). (**B**) The image displays the prediction after a flat-fixed dose of 120 mg in a typical heavy adult (120 kg). (**C**) The image displays the prediction after a dose of 240 mg in a typical heavy adult (120 kg). The gray curve is the prediction with a flat-fixed dose of 120 mg for the same individual (i.e., prediction (**B**)) for better visual comparison. Notice how the simulation prediction in a heavier patient (prediction (**B**)) indicates underexposure in the trough concentrations with flat-fixed (120 mg) subcutaneous infliximab dosing, while dose escalation to 240 mg (prediction (**C**)) shows a better fit to the trial data. The red dots represent digitized trough concentrations in adult patients post-switching to 120 mg subcutaneous infliximab at week 6, while the green dots represent the digitized prediction interval (5th and 95th percentile).

3.4. PBPK Modeling Exploration for an Older Virtual Child (14-Year-Old, 60 kg) with IBD after Intravenous Administrations of Infliximab (5 mg/kg)

To assess model prediction in the pediatric population, a virtual pediatric patient (14-year-old, 60 kg) was scaled from the adult patient with IBD. The simulation results are presented in Figure 7. Trial data from pediatric patients were sourced from [14] (originally digitized from [21]).

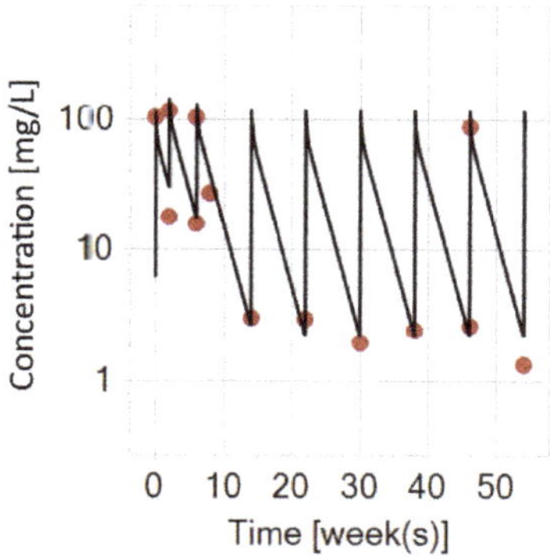

Figure 7. Infliximab PBPK simulation on a semi-logarithmic scale for a typical older pediatric patient (14-year-old child, 60 kg) after intravenous (5 mg/kg) administrations (black curve). The red dots represent the mean trough concentrations and maximal concentrations digitized from the trial data in pediatric patients.

3.5. PBPK Modeling Exploration for an Older Virtual Child (14-Year-Old, 60 kg) with IBD after Switching to a Flat-Fixed Dose of Subcutaneous Infliximab (120 mg)

Currently there is no approved subcutaneous formulation of infliximab for pediatric patients. However, older and heavier pediatric patients could have benefit from such a formulation [22]. Therefore, the infliximab PBPK model was extended to explore this route of administration in such a patient. In the absence of real-world clinical data for pediatric patients in this scenario, trough concentrations from a typical adult patient (post-switch to 120 mg) were digitized from [20] and used for comparison (Figure 8). In adult patients, median trough concentrations of infliximab post-switch to 120 mg were shown to vary between 11 and 20 mg/L, contingent on the study (see the discussion).

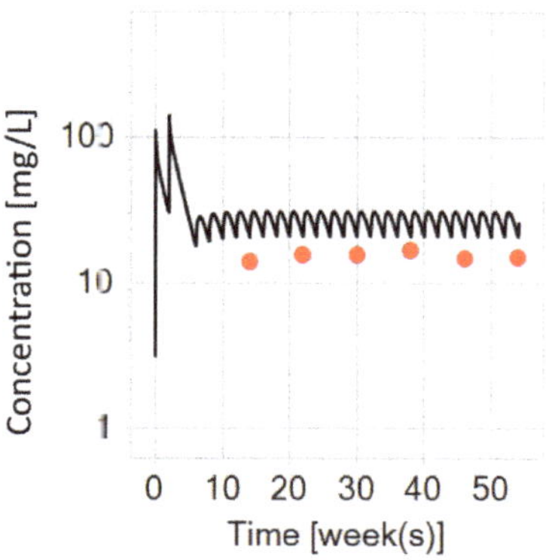

Figure 8. Infliximab PBPK simulation on a semi-logarithmic scale for a typical older child with IBD (14-year-old, 60 kg) after switching to a subcutaneous dose of 120 mg (black curve) at week 6. The red dots represent trough concentrations digitized from the trial data in adult patients post-switching to 120 mg subcutaneous infliximab.

3.6. PBPK Modeling Exploration for a Virtual Pediatric Population Stratified by Weight Bands after Switching to Subcutaneous Infliximab: A PBPK-Model-Informed Dose Suggestion

In the final exploration scenario, the goal was to utilize PBPK simulations for proposing the suitable subcutaneous dose (post-switching) in the pediatric population across the approved age range for the intravenous route (6–18 years), stratified into three weight bands based on estimated weight by age [29]: 20–30 kg, 30–45 kg, and 45–70 kg (Figure 9, top, middle, and bottom image, respectively). Each weight band contained 50 simulated pediatric patients (i.e., 150 in total across the simulated age ranges). As already mentioned, given the absence of real-world clinical data for pediatric patients, trough concentrations from a typical adult patient after switching to 120 mg were used as the target exposure metric that would guide the choice of a corresponding subcutaneous dose for each weight band (if such administration were to exist). Figure 9 shows the median concentration and simulated prediction interval (5th–95th percentile) for each weight band along with the corresponding PBPK-model-informed dose suggestion: 40 mg (top prediction), 80 mg (middle prediction), and 120 mg (bottom prediction).

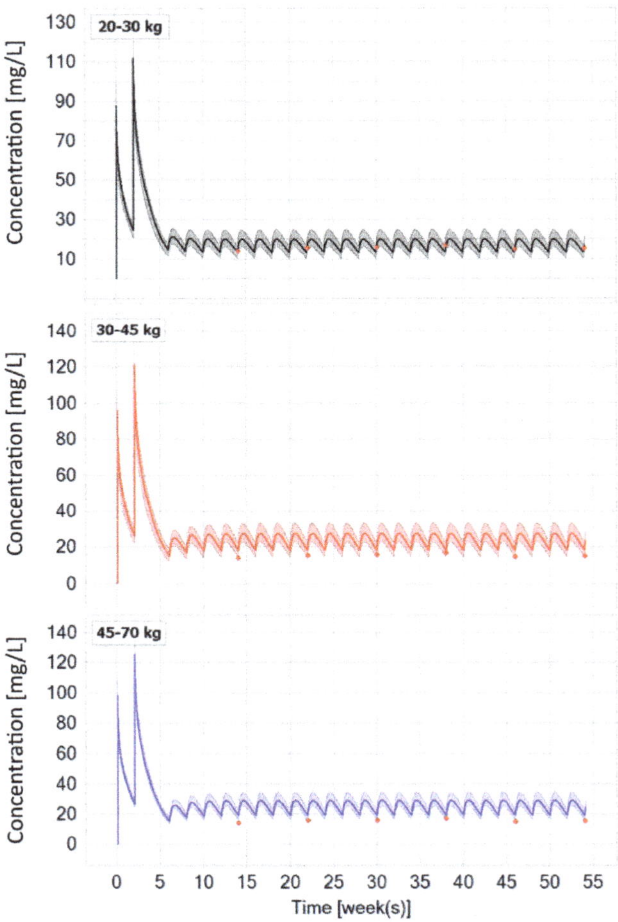

Figure 9. Infliximab PBPK simulations for a pediatric population stratified into three weight bands post-switch to subcutaneous infliximab at week 6. The PBPK-model-informed dose suggestion indicates that, to achieve comparable infliximab exposure metrics as in adults receiving 120 mg, pediatric patients weighing 20–30 kg would require a dose of at least 40 mg (typical pediatric patient), with a slightly higher dose needed to cover the entire prediction interval ((**top**) prediction). For patients weighing 30–45 kg, the suggested dose is 80 mg ((**middle**) prediction), while those weighing 45–70 kg would require 120 mg ((**bottom**) prediction). The red dots represent digitized trough concentrations in adult patients after switching to 120 mg subcutaneous infliximab.

For the virtual healthy individual (Figure 4), overlaying the mean pharmacokinetic profile from trial [18] demonstrates that the PBPK model is able to capture the average exposure of infliximab after a single intravenous administration (5 mg/kg). This was further confirmed through a comparison of exposure metrics and pharmacokinetic parameters between a typical virtual heathy individual and real-life healthy trial participant. Namely, the area under the concentration–time curve (after a single 5 mg/kg dose) was quite comparable, totaling 40,311 mg × h/L in the simulation, compared to 38,000 mg × h/L observed in the clinical trial. Similarly, the simulated maximum concentration reached 110 mg/L, while in the trial it peaked at 121 mg/L. Additionally, the simulated infliximab clearance and apparent volume of distribution (0.009 L/h and 0.07 L/kg, respectively) were also comparable with the average dataset-derived PK parameters (0.01 L/h and 0.09 L/kg, respectively). The exposure metrics and PK parameters derived from the simulation prediction also closely match those from other publications [30]. Lastly, the baseline prediction was also plotted against trial observations, demonstrating an even distribution around the line of identity.

Pharmacological treatments with MAbs (and some small molecules) often exhibit a phenomenon where the drug's pharmacodynamics influences its pharmacokinetics. This contrasts with the more common situation where pharmacokinetics governs pharmacodynamics, i.e., drug effect [1]. This intricate bidirectional interplay can stem from dose-dependent nonlinear elimination, termed target-mediated drug disposition, wherein drug–target complexes may impact drug effectiveness. Furthermore, the high inflammatory burden in the context of IBD triggers other elimination mechanisms, further contributing to underexposure and loss of effect, such as drug degradation via metalloproteinases [31] or excessive protein loss (which includes the elimination of MAbs) due to the leaky gut [1]. Finally, the formation of neutralizing and non-neutralizing anti-drug antibodies (i.e., immunogenicity) further contributes to underexposure (or vice versa), affecting both pharmacokinetics and pharmacodynamics. Hence, when these processes converge, they can result in unpredictable clinical outcomes and varying treatment success rates, due to faster drug elimination than expected. Therefore, adjusting the endosomal clearance rate in virtual patients with IBD to mimic the observed clinical scenario (i.e., increased infliximab clearance and underexposure when compared to healthy adults), served as a proxy accounting for the multitude of immune-mediated and non-immune-mediated pathways.

In the pharmacokinetic profile, the adult virtual IBD patient exhibited 1.5 times faster infliximab clearance compared to the clinically observed clearance in a healthy individual (0.015 L/h vs. 0.01 L/h, respectively), which aligns well with the true clinical IBD scenario after intravenous administration (5 mg/kg) (Figure 5).

The PBPK simulation of the virtual adult with IBD, after intravenous administration of infliximab, indicated a half-life of infliximab of 9.93 days, which is consistent with the clinically reported infliximab half-life of 9.5 days (with 5 mg/kg dosing) [32]. The maximal predicted concentration reached 115.5 mg/L in the maintenance phase, compared to a median of 120 mg/L in the trial dataset. Additionally, the simulation predicted a trough concentration of 1.5 mg/L (week 22), while the real-word data [33] reported a mean trough concentration of 2.9 mg/L (±2.6), i.e., adjusted geometric least squares mean of 1.8 mg/L. At week 30, Schreiber et al. [34] reported a median trough concentration of 2.3 mg/L (with the predicted interval 5th–95th percentile: 0.1–8.6). Finally, examining three larger study comparisons (C0168T72, REACH, and ACT) [35], the reported median maximal concentrations during the induction phase (with 5 mg/kg) were 115 mg/L, 109 mg/L, and 132 mg/L. In the same report [35], the median trough concentrations at week 30 were reported as 1.9 mg/L, 1.8 mg/L, and 2.5 mg/L. Since the simulated prediction of the virtual adult with IBD represents a mean virtual human, reflecting the mean of all adult real-world patients from the trial, the general conclusion, based on previously discussed exposure metrics and PK parameters, is that the PBPK model prediction in Figure 5 can effectively capture the overall trend of data in a typical adult patient with IBD after intravenous (5 mg/kg) administrations of infliximab.

PKSim® lacks the subcutaneous administration option in the administration building block. As a simplification, the fat compartment was chosen as the target organ for subcutaneous input with the plasma as the target compartment. In modeling the input from the subcutaneous formulation, a first-order process was assumed according to the literature data [36], while the half-life of absorption was derived from the estimated absorption rate constant [17]. The PBPK simulation following the switch to 120 mg subcutaneous infliximab at week 6 (Figure 6, prediction A) indicates that the model effectively captured trough concentrations in a virtual adult patient (70 kg) with IBD. Moreover, simulation for a virtual heavier adult patient (120 kg) with IBD also indicates underexposure trends in trough concentrations with a 120 mg flat-fixed dose (Figure 6B). This suggests that heavier individuals with IBD could benefit from dose escalation. To test this, a typical heavy patient weighing 120 kg was compared with the real-word trial [20] encompassing a subcutaneous dose of 240 mg, which resulted in better overlapping of the mean trend of trough concentrations (Figure 6C).

These indications of a possible need for dose escalation in heavier subjects align with the conclusions drawn from the population PK study conducted by Hanzel et al. [17]. However, as subcutaneous infliximab is currently only approved in a flat-fixed dose of 120 mg, dose adjustments after switching are not expected to occur (for now).

When examining the reported trough concentrations of infliximab from various clinical trials after switching, slight variations can be expected. For instance, at week 8, Roblin et al. [37] (taken from [38]) report a median trough of 11 mg/L (with an interquartile range: 7.5–15.1), while Falquina et al. [39] report 14.1 mg/L (with an interquartile range: 12.2–22.7). In the simulation in Figure 6, prediction A, the typical adult patient had a trough concentration around 14 mg/L (at week 8), which indicates that the model is able to capture the general trend. Schreiber et al. [34] at week 30 reported a median trough concentration of 13.27 mg/L (with a predicted interval 5th–95th percentile: 5.6–26.8) for 120 mg dosing, while for 240 mg dosing, the reported median was 26.54 mg/L (with a predicted interval 5th–95th percentile: 11.2–53.2). In the prediction for the 240 mg regimen (Figure 6, prediction C), a typical heavy patient had a trough concentration of 23 mg/L. The same study [34] reported the steady state median maximum concentration (at weeks 22–30) for the 120 mg regimen to be 18.24 mg/L (with a predicted interval 5th–95th percentile: 10.14–32.63). This also aligns well with model prediction in Figure 6A, where the maximum concentration for a typical adult patient was 22.8 mg/L for the same regimen. For the 240 mg regimen (Figure 6, prediction C), the same exposure metric was around 36 mg/L for the heavy adult, while the reported value from the trial was 36.48 mg/L (with a predicted interval 5th–95th percentile: 20.3–65.15). Additionally, the PBPK model estimated half-life as 10.97 days and a clearance of 0.013 L/h (for a 120 mg flat-fixed dose). These values are comparable to those estimated by population PK modeling in a typical adult IBD patient by Hanzel et al. [17] of 10.8 days and 0.015 L/h, respectively. Hence, it can be inferred that the PBPK simulation was able to capture the general trend of the data in adult patients with IBD after switching to 120 mg flat-fixed subcutaneous infliximab dose (Figure 6A).

It is also worth reiterating that the PBPK model indicated underexposure in heavier patients with 120 mg flat-fixed dosing (Figure 6B). Therefore, additional clinical trials are warranted to validate this simulation finding and ascertain the necessity of dose adjustments for heavier adults.

When determining the dose of MAbs in pediatric patients, it is common to employ weight-based dosing (i.e., mg/kg) extrapolated from adult dosing protocols. However, this method fails to consider the maturation process, as well as the (patho)physiological and biochemical differences between these two populations, relying solely on changes in size [14,19,40]. Therefore, in cases of such extrapolation, younger pediatric patients (infants) are often underdosed.

PBPK modeling, with its mechanistic approach, provides an additional opportunity, especially when combined with allometric scaling, to refine pediatric trial design and determine better dosing strategies for pediatric patients.

In Figure 7, it seems that the PBPK simulation for the intravenous administration (5 mg/kg) slightly better captured the maximum concentrations of the induction phase in the typical pediatric patient (14-year-old child, 60 kg) which was also noted by other researchers [14]. However, variable disease-mediated influences on drug elimination over time must be also taken into account when interpreting trough concentrations in the context of PBPK modeling. In the same virtual pediatric patient, the infliximab half-life was 10.96 days which is in accordance with the reported values of 10.5 days [41] and 10.9 days [42]. The simulated trough concentration was 2.1 mg/L, while Adedokun et al. [43] reported a median of 1.9 (at week 30) for the 5 mg/kg intravenous dosing. Hence, it can be concluded that the PBPK simulation for a typical pediatric patent (14 years old, 60 kg) in Figure 7 was able to capture the general trend of the data, after the intravenous administration (5 mg/kg) of infliximab.

It is interesting to mention that in the trial by Adedokun et al. [43], there was no observed difference in infliximab pharmacokinetics between the stratified pediatric groups (6–12 vs. 12–17 years) with ulcerative colitis. Additionally, it was inferred that infliximab pharmacokinetics in pediatric patients were consistent with adult data, despite observing that the median serum infliximab concentrations were approximately 20% lower in children at various time points. However, it has been concluded that younger pediatric patients (median age 8) are underexposed with weight-based (mg/kg) intravenous dosing of infliximab compared to older pediatric patients (median age 14) [44]. In addition to this complex narrative, another study (C0168T72) [35] reported a higher percentage of participants in the younger age group discontinuing infliximab treatment (5 mg/kg) by week 8 due to non-response compared to those in the older age group. Nonetheless, the rates of discontinuation were similar after stratification in the maintenance phase [35]. Conclusively, these uncertainties underscore the complexity of treatment and disease dynamics and the need for further investigation to optimize the therapeutic and clinical outcomes with infliximab in pediatric (sub)populations with IBD.

The power of PBPK modeling can be leveraged also as a tool for model-informed dose suggestions in various clinical contexts. Hence, in the final two explorations, the PBPK framework was extended to these "what-if" scenarios in pediatric patients with IBD.

As already mentioned, there is no subcutaneous biobetter of infliximab intended for the pediatric population (the currently approved dose remains for adults only at a flat-fixed dose of 120 mg). Until now, there has been only one pediatric study [22] performed on seven individuals, that examined switching to the 120 mg infliximab dose in older (15–18 years) and heavier children (>50 kg, median 61 kg). In this trial, the median trough infliximab concentrations after switching were approximated to 14 mg/L (at 40 weeks post-switch). This concentration was also the upper limit of quantification, so it was not possible to accurately measure values above this threshold in four out of six children, clearly indicating that the true trough concentrations were higher with a flat-fixed 120 mg dosing [22].

The PBPK simulation of a typical older pediatric patient (14-year-old, 60 kg) (Figure 8) resulted in a trough infliximab concentration of 21 mg/L post-switching to 120 mg, which suggests that the PBPK model would be able to capture the higher true trend of the pediatric clinical trial data. Since there is no data for comparison at the moment, trough concentrations from the adult trial were used for visual inspection and for comparability. Namely, in Figure 8, a slightly higher trough concentration can be seen when compared to adults. However, this was not (for now) shown to be concerning in terms of safety [22]. Hence, it seems that the flat-fixed subcutaneous dose of 120 mg may be suitable (in terms of both effectiveness and safety) for older and heavier pediatric patients. Nonetheless, further clinical trials are necessary to comprehensively evaluate the advantages of subcutaneous administration and determine appropriate dose adjustments of infliximab in the pediatric population.

In the final exploration scenario (Figure 9), the developed PBPK model was applied to the virtual population. Similar to the approach for a typical virtual patient (adult or child with IBD), this approach provided insights into PBPK-model-informed dose suggestions for the target (sub)populations of interest.

Since infliximab is approved for treating IBD from the age of 6 and above, the target population (i.e., 150 pediatric individuals, 6–18 years of age) was stratified by weight [29] into three groups: 20–30 kg, 30–45 kg, and 45–70 kg. The choice of post-switch subcutaneous infliximab dose was guided by achieving comparable trough concentrations to those observed with the flat-fixed 120 mg dose in adults (Figure 9).

The PBPK-model-informed suggestion for pediatric patients weighing between 20 and 35 kg was 40 mg, with a slightly higher dose required to cover the entire prediction interval in this weight group (Figure 9, top). For patients weighing 35–45 kg, the suggested dose to cover the entire prediction was 80 mg (Figure 9, middle image), and for those weighing 45–70 kg, it was 120 mg (Figure 9, bottom image). The corresponding PBPK simulations show post-switch median trough concentrations around 14 mg/L, 18 mg/L, and 18.5 mg/L, respectively (with 5th–95th percentile intervals of 11.5–17 mg/L, 14.5–22 mg/L, and 16–23 mg/L).

Due to the slight differences in the reported trough concentrations after switching to subcutaneous infliximab, it is challenging to set a typical value for this exposure metric. Namely, the reported median trough concentrations, depending on the real-world trial in adults, ranged from 11 to 20 mg/L [37,39,45]. Based on that, it can be inferred that the PBPK predictions for the tested weight bands with the corresponding model-informed dose suggestions yielded exposure metrics comparable to those in adults receiving a flat-fixed 120 mg dose of subcutaneous infliximab. In addition, for the heaviest pediatric band (>45 kg) which corresponds to children older than 14 years of age, the prediction again confirms the suitability of administering a flat-fixed dose of 120 mg that is registered for adults.

It is also worth mentioning that the modeling assumption of the same bioavailability after subcutaneous administration of MAbs in younger children may also be debated, given the general anatomical differences in injection sites between children and adults [46]. These differences would imply, for example, variations in monoclonal antibody uptake, lymph flow, local degradation (catabolism), immunogenicity, and target-mediated drug disposition, which could be clinically relevant for the rate and extent of absorption among pediatric patients with IBD and contribute to a further increase in between-patient variability in pharmacokinetics, pharmacodynamics, and consequently, clinical outcomes [47]. One must also take into account the possible variability between pediatric patients and consequently modify the subcutaneous dose of infliximab to accommodate such variability if shown to be clinically relevant. Therefore, future clinical trials are anticipated to provide insights that can address the current uncertainties and further refine modeling approaches.

3.7. Limitations and Future Perspectives of the Study

In clinical settings, modeling and simulation approaches still face fragmentation and limited uptake. Nonetheless, there is a growing recognition of their significance, particularly in the realm of population pharmacokinetic and pharmacodynamic modeling.

PBPK modeling, while powerful, is inherently complex and demands expertise across multiple domains, including clinical pharmacology, pharmacokinetics, pharmacodynamics, physiology, and software proficiency. Due to its reliance on input parameters, the lack of comprehensive knowledge about them can undermine the reliability of predictions. PBPK models heavily rely on assumptions and approximations, posing challenges for model validation. This introduces uncertainty (error) into simulation predictions, further complicating the assessment of model reliability and its extrapolation abilities. In other words, the virtual human is as good as the real counterpart if the totality of accurate information is supported and undoubtedly confirmed by a fair amount of clinical evidence [8,13,48,49].

In this study, a more simplistic PBPK approach was employed, with some of the input parameters identified by an in-built software algorithm to match the observed clinical data. However, this common practice in modeling can introduce the likelihood of model/parameter identifiability issues, as the fitted values may not represent the true or experimentally determined values [48,49]. In other words, various parameter sets can generally yield similar fitting results. Additionally, apart from relying on robust clinical data, adjustments made to one parameter can cascade to others, ultimately affecting the overall parameter values of the model. However, in this study, the input parameters were very closely similar (or within the same order of magnitude) as the reported values in the literature, and as such, they enabled the PBPK model to capture general trends in the explored clinical scenarios.

Tailoring treatments with proper dosing options for individual patients is crucial for therapeutic success and personalized care. Extending the application of PBPK modeling beyond drug discovery and development into clinical settings could offer relevant information for clinicians. The future perspectives of the study involve comparing simulated scenarios with real-life clinical studies, while also encouraging drug manufacturers to assess their products' effectiveness across all patient (sub)groups and advance the field of personalized medicine.

4. Conclusions

Utilizing state-of-the-art quantitative pharmacology tools represents the future approach for advancing pharmacological treatments in IBD. Hence, PBPK modeling, as a mechanistic framework, holds the capability to comprehensively incorporate both known and unknown disease mechanisms, as well as drug-specific characteristics. Leveraging this approach enables the exploration of novel strategies for more effective disease management.

PBPK modeling is commonly utilized in the drug development process. However, this study demonstrates its versatility in exploring diverse clinical scenarios related to infliximab use in the context of IBD. This includes investigating alternative dosing regimens and routes of administration across individuals and (sub)populations of clinical interest.

Finally, while simulations involving virtual individuals and populations must be complemented with real-life studies, the PBPK framework can also prompt drug manufacturers to reconsider the versatility of their products in effectively covering all patient groups.

Supplementary Materials: The following supporting information on methodology can be downloaded at: https://www.mdpi.com/article/10.3390/biomedicines12091974/s1, Figure S1: Graphical representation of fold errors.

Author Contributions: Conceptualization: Z.P. and P.P.; methodology and formal software analysis: Z.P.; writing—original draft preparation: Z.P.; writing—review and editing: Z.P., P.P. and J.G. All authors have read and agreed to the published version of the manuscript.

Funding: This research received no external funding.

Institutional Review Board Statement: Not applicable.

Informed Consent Statement: Not applicable.

Data Availability Statement: The original contributions presented in the study are included in the article/Supplementary Materials. Further inquiries can be directed to the corresponding authors.

Acknowledgments: Z.P. would like to thank Senior Scientist Priyata Kalra, from Simulations Plus, for fruitful discussions and broadening horizons relevant to PBPK modeling.

Conflicts of Interest: Z.P. and P.P. declare no conflicts of interest. J.G. has received research grants and has been an invited speaker and advisor for Biogen, AstraZeneca, Pfizer, Sandoz, Novartis, and Hikma. The funders had no role in the design of the study; in the collection, analyses, or interpretation of the data; in the writing of the manuscript, or in the decision to publish the results.

References

1. Petric, Z.; Goncalves, J.; Paixao, P. Under the Umbrella of Clinical Pharmacology: Inflammatory Bowel Disease, Infliximab and Adalimumab, and a Bridge to an Era of Biosimilars. *Pharmaceutics* **2022**, *14*, 1766. [CrossRef]
2. Ungar, B.; Mazor, Y.; Weisshof, R.; Yanai, H.; Ron, Y.; Goren, I.; Waizbard, A.; Yavzori, M.; Fudim, E.; Picard, O.; et al. Induction infliximab levels among patients with acute severe ulcerative colitis compared with patients with moderately severe ulcerative colitis. *Aliment. Pharmacol. Ther.* **2016**, *43*, 1293–1299. [CrossRef] [PubMed]
3. European Medicines Agency (EMA). Remicade (Infliximab) Assessment Report. Available online: https://www.ema.europa.eu/en/medicines/human/EPAR/remicade (accessed on 26 June 2024).
4. Smith, P.J.; Fumery, M.; Leong, R.W.; Novak, K.; Dignass, A. Real-world experience with subcutaneous infliximab: Broadening treatment strategies for inflammatory bowel disease. *Expert. Rev. Clin. Immunol.* **2023**, *19*, 1143–1156. [CrossRef] [PubMed]
5. Vandenplas, Y.; Broekaert, I.; Domellöf, M.; Indrio, F.; Lapillonne, A.; Pienar, C.; Ribes-Koninckx, C.; Shamir, R.; Szajewska, H.; Thapar, N.; et al. An ESPGHAN position paper on the diagnosis, management and prevention of cow's milk allergy. *J. Pediatr. Gastroenterol. Nutr.* **2024**, *78*, 386–413. [CrossRef] [PubMed]
6. Mould, D.R.; Upton, R.N. Basic concepts in population modeling, simulation, and model-based drug development. *CPT Pharmacomet. Syst. Pharmacol.* **2012**, *1*, 1–14. [CrossRef]
7. Jones, H.; Rowland-Yeo, K. Basic concepts in physiologically based pharmacokinetic modeling in drug discovery and development. *CPT Pharmacomet. Syst. Pharmacol.* **2013**, *2*, 1–12. [CrossRef] [PubMed]
8. Peters, S.A. *Physiologically Based Pharmacokinetic (PBPK) Modeling and Simulations: Principles, Methods, and Applications in the Pharmaceutical Industry*; John Wiley & Sons: Hoboken, NJ, USA, 2022.
9. Open Systems Pharmacology Suite, Manual. Available online: https://docs.open-systems-pharmacology.org/ (accessed on 26 June 2024).
10. Servier—Servier Medical Art licensed under CC BY 4.0. Available online: https://smart.servier.com/ (accessed on 26 June 2024).
11. Perry, C.; Davis, G.; Conner, T.M.; Zhang, T. Utilization of Physiologically Based Pharmacokinetic Modeling in Clinical Pharmacology and Therapeutics: An Overview. *Curr. Pharmacol. Rep.* **2020**, *6*, 71–84. [CrossRef]
12. Luzon, E.; Blake, K.; Cole, S.; Nordmark, A.; Versantvoort, C.; Berglund, E.G. Physiologically based pharmacokinetic modeling in regulatory decision-making at the European Medicines Agency. *Clin. Pharmacol. Ther.* **2017**, *102*, 98–105. [CrossRef]
13. Rowland Yeo, K.; Gil Bergland, E.; Chen, Y. Dose Optimization Informed by PBPK Modeling: State-of-the Art and Future. *Clin. Pharmacol. Ther.* **2024**, *116*, 563–576. [CrossRef]
14. Malik, P.R.V.; Edginton, A.N. Physiologically-Based Pharmacokinetic Modeling vs. Allometric Scaling for the Prediction of Infliximab Pharmacokinetics in Pediatric Patients. *CPT Pharmacomet. Syst. Pharmacol.* **2019**, *8*, 835–844. [CrossRef]
15. Rippe, B.; Haraldsson, B. Transport of macromolecules across microvascular walls: The two-pore theory. *Physiol. Rev.* **1994**, *74*, 163–219. [CrossRef] [PubMed]
16. Pedersen, M.E.; Haegebaert, R.M.S.; Østergaard, J.; Jensen, H. Size-based characterization of adalimumab and TNF-α interactions using flow induced dispersion analysis: Assessment of avidity-stabilized multiple bound species. *Sci. Rep.* **2021**, *11*, 4754. [CrossRef] [PubMed]
17. Hanzel, J.; Bukkems, L.H.; Gecse, K.B.; D'Haens, G.R.; Mathôt, R.A.A. Population pharmacokinetics of subcutaneous infliximab CT-P13 in Crohn's disease and ulcerative colitis. *Aliment. Pharmacol. Ther.* **2021**, *54*, 1309–1319. [CrossRef]
18. EMA, Clinical Trial Register. Available online: https://clinicaldata.ema.europa.eu/web/cdp (accessed on 25 June 2024).
19. Zunino, C.; Perrier, J.; Gualano, V.; Zhou, H.; Lukacova, V.; Le Merdy, M. Validation of PBPK-Based Translation to Predict Monoclonal Antibody Pharmacokinetics in Pediatric Populations. In Proceedings of the 2023 AAPS National Biotechnology Conference, Philadelphia, PA, USA, 23–26 April 2023.
20. Reinisch, W.; Jang, B.I.; Borzan, V.; Lahat, A.; Pukitis, A.; Osipenko, M.; Mostovoy, Y.; Schreiber, S.; Ben-Horin, S.; Lee, S.J.; et al. DOP62 A novel formulation of CT-P13 (infliximab biosimilar) for subcutaneous administration: 1-year result from a Phase I open-label randomised controlled trial in patients with active Crohn's disease. *J. Crohns Colitis* **2019**, *13*, S066–S067. [CrossRef]
21. Adedokun, O.J.; Sandborn, W.J.; Feagan, B.G.; Rutgeerts, P.; Xu, Z.; Marano, C.W.; Johanns, J.; Zhou, H.; Davis, H.M.; Cornillie, F.; et al. Association Between Serum Concentration of Infliximab and Efficacy in Adult Patients with Ulcerative Colitis. *Gastroenterology* **2014**, *147*, 1296–1307.e5. [CrossRef]
22. Gianolio, L.; Armstrong, K.; Swann, E.; Shepherd, R.; Henderson, P.; Wilson, D.C.; Russell, R.K. Effectiveness of Switching to Subcutaneous Infliximab in Pediatric Inflammatory Bowel Disease Patients on Intravenous Maintenance Therapy. *J. Pediatr. Gastroenterol. Nutr.* **2023**, *77*, 235–239. [CrossRef]
23. McInnes, S.J.P.; Turner, C.T.; Al-Bataineh, S.A.; Airaghi Leccardi, M.J.I.; Irani, Y.; Williams, K.A.; Cowin, A.J.; Voelcker, N.H. Surface engineering of porous silicon to optimise therapeutic antibody loading and release. *J. Mater. Chem. B* **2015**, *3*, 4123–4133. [CrossRef] [PubMed]
24. Suzuki, T.; Ishii-Watabe, A.; Tada, M.; Kobayashi, T.; Kanayasu-Toyoda, T.; Kawanishi, T.; Yamaguchi, T. Importance of neonatal FcR in regulating the serum half-life of therapeutic proteins containing the Fc domain of human IgG1: A comparative study of the affinity of monoclonal antibodies and Fc-fusion proteins to human neonatal FcR. *J. Immunol.* **2010**, *184*, 1968–1976. [CrossRef]

25. Grevys, A.; Frick, R.; Mester, S.; Flem-Karlsen, K.; Nilsen, J.; Foss, S.; Sand, K.M.K.; Emrich, T.; Fischer, J.A.A.; Greiff, V.; et al. Antibody variable sequences have a pronounced effect on cellular transport and plasma half-life. *iScience* **2022**, *25*, 103746. [CrossRef]
26. Scallon, B.J.; Moore, M.A.; Trinh, H.; Knight, D.M.; Ghrayeb, J. Chimeric anti-TNF-α monoclonal antibody cA2 binds recombinant transmembrane TNF-α and activates immune effector functions. *Cytokine* **1995**, *7*, 251–259. [CrossRef]
27. Li, X.; Jusko, W.; Cao, Y. Role of interstitial fluid turnover on target suppression by therapeutic biologics using a minimal physiologically-based pharmacokinetic (mPBPK) model. *J. Pharmacol. Exp. Ther.* **2018**, *367*, 1–8. [CrossRef]
28. Niederalt, C.; Kuepfer, L.; Solodenko, J.; Eissing, T.; Siegmund, H.U.; Block, M.; Willmann, S.; Lippert, J. A generic whole body physiologically based pharmacokinetic model for therapeutic proteins in PK-Sim. *J. Pharmacokinet. Pharmacodyn.* **2018**, *45*, 235–257. [CrossRef]
29. Children's Health Queensland: Estimated Weight Based on Age. Available online: https://www.childrens.health.qld.gov.au/ (accessed on 26 June 2024).
30. Lambert, J.; Wyand, M.; Lassen, C.; Shneyer, L.; Thomson, E.; Knight, A.; Willers, J.; Kay, J. Bioavailability, safety and immunogenicity of biosimilar infliximab (BOW015) compared to reference infliximab. *Int. J. Clin. Pharmacol. Ther.* **2016**, *54*, 315–322. [CrossRef]
31. Marônek, M.; Marafini, I.; Gardlík, R.; Link, R.; Troncone, E.; Monteleone, G. Metalloproteinases in Inflammatory Bowel Diseases. *J. Inflamm. Res.* **2021**, *14*, 1029–1041. [CrossRef]
32. Klotz, U.; Teml, A.; Schwab, M. Clinical Pharmacokinetics and Use of Infliximab. *Clin. Pharmacokinet.* **2007**, *46*, 645–660. [CrossRef]
33. Schreiber, S.; Ben-Horin, S.; Leszczyszyn, J.; Dudkowiak, R.; Lahat, A.; Gawdis-Wojnarska, B.; Pukitis, A.; Horynski, M.; Farkas, K.; Kierkus, J.; et al. Randomized Controlled Trial: Subcutaneous vs Intravenous Infliximab CT-P13 Maintenance in Inflammatory Bowel Disease. *Gastroenterology* **2021**, *160*, 2340–2353. [CrossRef]
34. Schreiber, S.; Jang, B.; Borzan, V.; Lahat, A.; Pukitis, A.; Osipenko, M.; Mostovoy, Y.; Ben-Horin, S.; Ye, B.D.; Lee, S.J.; et al. Tu2018—Novel Formulation of CT-P13 (Infliximab Biosimilar) for Subcutaneous Administration: Initial Results from a Phase I Open-Label Randomized Controlled Trial in Patients with Active Crohn's Disease. *Gastroenterology* **2018**, *6*, S-1371. [CrossRef]
35. European Medicines Agency (EMA). Assessment Report on Remsima (Infliximab). Available online: https://www.ema.europa.eu/en/documents/assessment-report/remsima-epar-public-assessment-report_en.pdf (accessed on 26 June 2024).
36. Pan, X.; Stader, F.; Abduljalil, K.; Gill, K.L.; Johnson, T.N.; Gardner, I.; Jamei, M. Development and Application of a Physiologically-Based Pharmacokinetic Model to Predict the Pharmacokinetics of Therapeutic Proteins from Full-term Neonates to Adolescents. *AAPS J.* **2020**, *22*, 76. [CrossRef]
37. Roblin, X.; Veyrard, P.; Bastide, L.; Berger, A.E.; Barrau, M.; Paucelle, A.-S.; Waeckel, L.; Kwiatek, S.; Flourie, B.; Nancey, S.; et al. Subcutaneous injection of infliximab CT-P13 results in stable drug levels within 14-day treatment cycle in Crohn's disease. *Aliment. Pharmacol. Ther.* **2022**, *56*, 77–83. [CrossRef]
38. Little, R.D.; Ward, M.G.; Wright, E.; Jois, A.J.; Boussioutas, A.; Hold, G.L.; Gibson, P.R.; Sparrow, M.P. Therapeutic Drug Monitoring of Subcutaneous Infliximab in Inflammatory Bowel Disease—Understanding Pharmacokinetics and Exposure Response Relationships in a New Era of Subcutaneous Biologics. *J. Clin. Med.* **2022**, *11*, 6173. [CrossRef]
39. Falquina, I.C.M.; Chumillas, R.M.S.; Garcia, L.A.; González, B.V.; Cuesta, N.R.; Hernández, L.A.; Pascual, L.A.; Aladrén, B.S. P617 Switching from an intensified regimen of infliximab to a subcutaneous standard dose in adults with Inflammatory Bowel Disease: Our experience in a tertiary hospital. *J. Crohns. Colitis.* **2022**, *16*, i544–i545. [CrossRef]
40. Malik, P.; Edginton, A. Pediatric physiology in relation to the pharmacokinetics of monoclonal antibodies. *Expert. Opin. Drug. Metab. Toxicol.* **2018**, *14*, 585–599. [CrossRef]
41. Cornillie, F.; Shealy, D.; D'Haens, G.; Geboes, K.; Van Assche, G.; Ceuppens, J.; Wagner, C.; Schaible, T.; Plevy, S.E.; Targan, S.R.; et al. Infliximab induces potent anti-inflammatory and local immunomodulatory activity but no systemic immune suppression in patients with Crohn's disease. *Aliment. Pharmacol. Ther.* **2001**, *15*, 463–473. [CrossRef]
42. Ternant, D.; Mulleman, D.; Degenne, D.; Willot, S.; Guillaumin, J.M.; Watier, H.; Goupille, P.; Paintaud, G. An enzyme-linked immunosorbent assay for therapeutic drug monitoring of infliximab. *Ther. Drug. Monit.* **2006**, *28*, 169–174. [CrossRef]
43. Adedokun, O.J.; Xu, Z.; Padgett, L.; Blank, M.; Johanns, J.; Griffiths, A.; Ford, J.; Zhou, H.; Guzzo, C.; Davis, H.M.; et al. Pharmacokinetics of infliximab in children with moderate-to-severe ulcerative colitis: Results from a randomized, multicenter, open-label, phase 3 study. *Inflamm. Bowel Dis.* **2013**, *19*, 2753–2762. [CrossRef]
44. Jongsma, M.M.E.; Winter, D.A.; Huynh, H.Q.; Norsa, L.; Hussey, S.; Kolho, K.L.; Bronsky, J.; Assa, A.; Cohen, S.; Lev-Tzion, R.; et al. Infliximab in young paediatric IBD patients: It is all about the dosing. *Eur. J. Pediatr.* **2020**, *179*, 1935–1944. [CrossRef]
45. Argüelles-Arias, F.; Fernández Álvarez, P.; Castro Laria, L.; Maldonado Pérez, B.; Belvis Jiménez, M.; Merino-Bohórquez, V.; Caunedo Álvarez, A.; Calleja Hernández, M. Switch to subcutaneous infliximab during the SARS-CoV-2 pandemic: Preliminary results. *Rev. Esp. Enferm. Dig.* **2022**, *114*, 118–119. [CrossRef]
46. Derraik, J.G.; Rademaker, M.; Cutfield, W.S.; Pinto, T.E.; Tregurtha, S.; Faherty, A.; Peart, J.M.; Drury, P.L.; Hofman, P.L. Effects of age, gender, BMI, and anatomical site on skin thickness in children and adults with diabetes. *PLoS ONE* **2014**, *9*, e86637. [CrossRef]
47. Davis, J.D.; Bravo Padros, M.; Conrado, D.J.; Ganguly, S.; Guan, X.; Hassan, H.E.; Hazra, A.; Irvin, S.C.; Jayachandran, P.; Kosloski, M.P.; et al. Subcutaneous Administration of Monoclonal Antibodies: Pharmacology, Delivery, Immunogenicity, and Learnings from Applications to Clinical Development. *Clin. Pharmacol. Ther.* **2024**, *115*, 422–439. [CrossRef]

48. Shebley, M.; Sandhu, P.; Emami Riedmaier, A.; Jamei, M.; Narayanan, R.; Patel, A.; Peters, S.A.; Reddy, V.P.; Zheng, M.; de Zwart, L.; et al. Physiologically Based Pharmacokinetic Model Qualification and Reporting Procedures for Regulatory Submissions: A Consortium Perspective. *Clin. Pharmacol. Ther.* **2018**, *104*, 88–110. [CrossRef]
49. Basu, S.; Lien, Y.T.K.; Vozmediano, V.; Schlender, J.F.; Eissing, T.; Schmidt, S.; Niederalt, C. Physiologically Based Pharmacokinetic Modeling of Monoclonal Antibodies in Pediatric Populations Using PK-Sim. *Front. Pharmacol.* **2020**, *11*, 868. [CrossRef] [PubMed]

biomedicines

MDPI

Article

Review and External Evaluation of Population Pharmacokinetic Models for Vedolizumab in Patients with Inflammatory Bowel Disease: Assessing Predictive Performance and Clinical Applicability

Marija Jovanović [1], Ana Homšek [1], Srđan Marković [2,3], Đorđe Kralj [2], Petar Svorcan [2,3], Tamara Knežević Ivanovski [2], Olga Odanović [2] and Katarina Vučićević [1,*]

1 Department of Pharmacokinetics and Clinical Pharmacy, Faculty of Pharmacy, University of Belgrade, 11221 Belgrade, Serbia
2 Department of Gastroenterology and Hepatology, University Hospital Medical Center "Zvezdara", 11000 Belgrade, Serbia
3 Faculty of Medicine, University of Belgrade, 11000 Belgrade, Serbia
* Correspondence: katarina.vucicevic@pharmacy.bg.ac.rs

Abstract: Background/Objectives: Several population pharmacokinetic models of vedolizumab (VDZ) are available for inflammatory bowel disease (IBD) patients. However, their predictive performance in real-world clinical settings remains unknown. This study aims to externally evaluate the published VDZ pharmacokinetic models, focusing on their predictive performance and simulation-based clinical applicability. Methods: A literature search was conducted through PubMed to identify VDZ population pharmacokinetic models. A total of 114 VDZ concentrations from 106 IBD patients treated at the University Medical Center "Zvezdara", Republic of Serbia, served as the external evaluation cohort. The predictive performance of the models was assessed using prediction- and simulation-based diagnostics. Furthermore, the models were utilized for Monte Carlo simulations to generate concentration–time profiles based on 24 covariate combinations specified within the models. Results: Four published pharmacokinetic models of VDZ were included in the evaluation. Using the external dataset, the median prediction error (MDPE) ranged from 13.82% to 25.57%, while the median absolute prediction error (MAPE) varied between 41.64% and 47.56%. None of the models fully met the combined criteria in the prediction-based diagnostics. However, in simulation-based diagnostics, pvcVPC showed satisfactory results, despite wide prediction intervals. Analysis of NPDE revealed that only the models by Rosario et al. and Okamoto et al. fulfilled the evaluation criteria. Simulation analysis further demonstrated that the median VDZ concentration remains above 12 μg/mL at week 22 during maintenance treatment for approximately 45–60% of patients with the best-case covariate combinations and an 8-week dosing frequency. Conclusions: None of the published models satisfied the combined criteria (MDPE, MAPE, percentages of prediction error within ±20% and ±30%), rendering them unsuitable for a priori predictions. However, two models demonstrated better suitability for simulation-based applications.

Keywords: predictive performance; simulations; prediction error; NONMEM; vedolizumab; pharmacokinetics

1. Introduction

Vedolizumab (VDZ) is a humanized monoclonal antibody (mAb) that blocks the interaction of α4β7 integrin and mucosal addressin cell adhesion molecule-1 (MAdCAM-1), thereby inhibiting the migration of memory T cells into inflamed intestinal tissue [1]. According to the European Summary of Product Characteristics, this drug is indicated for the treatment of adults with moderately to severely active ulcerative colitis (UC) or Crohn's disease (CD). It is reserved for patients who have not responded to, have responded inadequately to, or cannot tolerate conventional therapy (glucocorticosteroids, immunosuppressants) or the tumor necrosis factor-alpha (TNFα) antagonist. The recommended dosing regimen of VDZ is 300 mg administered as an intravenous infusion at 0, 2, and 6 weeks, and every 8 weeks thereafter (Q8W) [2]. In certain cases, an increased dosing frequency of every 4 weeks (Q4W) may be considered for patients who no longer respond to the Q8W regimen [3].

Given the limited number of biologic agents approved for the treatment of UC and CD, therapy optimization becomes paramount. Various factors, such as sex, body size, immunogenicity, albumin levels, and the use of immunosuppressants, have been associated with the accelerated clearance (CL) of mAb, implying wide variability between patients [4]. Thus, therapeutic drug monitoring (TDM) stands out as a crucial tool for the individualization of biologic therapy, whether using a reactive or proactive approach [5]. Reactive TDM of infliximab has become an essential part of managing patients with inflammatory bowel disease (IBD), with growing evidence highlighting the benefits of proactive approach as well [6,7]. For VDZ, TDM is typically recommended at the end of the induction phase in non-responders, and in patients when secondary loss of response is confirmed [5]. However, evidence supporting the routine monitoring of VDZ trough concentrations remains limited, and specific time-dependent and exposure-response targets are still unclear [8,9]. Nevertheless, TDM of VDZ is being utilized more frequently in various clinical settings, even in the absence of robust supporting evidence. Addressing the challenges posed by VDZ pharmacokinetic variability and standardizing TDM practices could provide the basis for establishing universally accepted TDM protocols [9]. In this context, model-informed precision dosing (MIPD) could serve as a valuable tool for personalized biologic therapy. MIPD typically uses a Bayesian approach and population pharmacokinetic models to predict the optimal dosing for achieving a target drug concentration [4]. The method can be used a priori (based on patient covariates) to determine the starting dose, or a posteriori (based on covariates and one or more observed concentrations) to generate a Bayesian posterior parameter distribution, allowing prediction of the next dose [10].

A population pharmacokinetic analysis of VDZ was previously performed in patients with UC or CD using extensively collected data from phase 1 and 2 studies, as well as sparsely collected data from the phase 3 GEMINI studies, in a predominantly Western population. According to this model, only extreme albumin and body weight values were identified as potentially clinically relevant predictors for the linear clearance (CL_L) of VDZ [11]. Subsequently, other authors have usually adapted this model to specific populations and study conditions [3,12–14]. However, the potential use of the developed models in real-world clinical settings remains unknown and requires validation in an independent cohort. Therefore, this study aims to assess the predictive performance of published population pharmacokinetic models of VDZ in patients with IBD to determine their applicability for our population and to subsequently use them in the clinical setting within MIPD. Specifically, the study sought to assess the models' capacity for a priori predictions using patient covariates only, as well as their utility in simulation-based application. Moreover, the models were utilized for Monte Carlo simulations to generate and compare concentration–time profiles based on clinically important covariate combinations specified within the models.

2. Methods

2.1. Literature Search

A systematic literature search for published original articles on population pharmacokinetic models for VDZ in patients with IBD until November 2024 was conducted in PubMed, with the language being limited to English. The population studies were searched for using the following terms: (Vedolizumab) AND (pharmacokinetic model OR population pharmacokinetics OR population pharmacokinetic model* OR nonlinear mixed effects model* OR NONMEM OR pharmacometric) AND (Inflammatory Bowel Diseases OR Crohn Disease OR Crohn's Disease OR ulcerative colitis OR IBD). Moreover, the reference lists of the relevant articles were searched for additional literature. The models were excluded if (1) the study was not a population pharmacokinetic analysis (nonlinear mixed effects modeling analysis) of VDZ in patients with IBD; (2) model parameters were not available for external evaluation; (3) the publications were conference abstracts or review articles; or (4) models were constructed on a population unrepresentative for our population (e.g., pediatric population). The following information was extracted from the articles: patient characteristics, software, pharmacokinetic model structure, typical value of pharmacokinetic parameters, inter-individual variability (IIV), inter-occasion variability (IOV), residual variability (RV), and covariates significantly influencing CL_L with potential clinical relevance.

2.2. External Evaluation Cohort

We enrolled 106 adult patients diagnosed with UC or CD from the University Medical Center "Zvezdara", Belgrade, Republic of Serbia, who were treated with VDZ and underwent TDM during the induction or maintenance phase. The study protocol was approved by the institutional Ethics Committee (No. IRB00009457, on 5 October 2022). The design and conduct of this clinical study adhered to the ethical standards outlined in the Declaration of Helsinki. During the induction phase, VDZ (Entyvio®, 300 mg vial solution for infusion, Takeda Italia S.P.A., Rome, Italy) was administered as a 30 min intravenous infusion at a standard dose of 300 mg at weeks 0, 2, and 6. Maintenance dosing intervals were 4, 6, or 8 weeks, depending on clinical assessment and the individual patient's response to treatment.

The required data were extracted from the patients' medical records, and included VDZ therapy and TDM data (date of therapy initiation, dosing regimen, exact time and date of blood sampling for TDM, and measured concentration), co-therapy (prior and current), demographic (age, sex, body weight), clinical (disease type), and laboratory characteristics including serum albumin concentrations. Patients were excluded from the analysis if data about VDZ dosing and TDM were missing.

VDZ concentration measurements were performed using commercially available R-Biopharm® ELISA tests on a Dynex DS2 analyzer (Dynex Technologies, Chantilly, VA, USA) in the biochemical laboratory of University Hospital Medical Center "Zvezdara", Belgrade, Republic of Serbia.

2.3. External Predictability Evaluation

The external evaluation was conducted using NONMEM version 7.5 (ICON Development Solutions, Ellicott City, MD, USA). The programs R and RStudio were used for the pre- and post-processing of input/output. Published population pharmacokinetic models were coded by inputting the equations and parameter values into the control file and executing with an iteration of 0 (MAXEVAL = 0). Only covariates with potential clinical relevance were considered. Covariates with missing data were assigned the reference values from the selected model. Because no data on anti-drug antibodies (ADAs) were available in the validation dataset, this variable was not considered. Prediction- and simulation-based diagnostics were used to assess the predictive performances of the selected models.

External validation of a model was based on comparison between predictions obtained with the models and VDZ measurements in the external dataset. The predictions represent a priori predictions based on the patients' covariates with potential clinical relevance. Several metrics used for model evaluation have been previously described [10,15]. The bias and precision of prediction were evaluated using the mean prediction error (MPE, Equation (1)) and root mean square error (RMSE, Equation (2)).

$$\mathrm{MPE} = \frac{\Sigma(\hat{\mathrm{Y}} - \mathrm{Y})}{\mathrm{n}} \tag{1}$$

$$\mathrm{RMSE} = \sqrt{\frac{\Sigma(\hat{\mathrm{Y}} - \mathrm{Y})^2}{\mathrm{n}}} \tag{2}$$

in which $\hat{Y}$ represents the population-predicted VDZ concentration, Y represents the observed VDZ concentration, and n is the number of observations [16]. Relative prediction errors were expressed as a percentage of the measured value (PE (%)) using Equation (3).

$$\mathrm{PE}(\%) = \frac{\hat{\mathrm{Y}} - \mathrm{Y}}{\mathrm{Y}} \cdot 100 \tag{3}$$

The median prediction error (MDPE (%)), median absolute prediction error (MAPE (%)), and PE (%) values that fell within the range of ±20% (F20) and ±30% (F30) were applied to further evaluate the accuracy and precision of the models, as previously described [17]. To enable a more comprehensive comparison of the models, the results were presented as an overall comparison and as a group comparison. Predictive performance was evaluated across subgroups defined by specific covariates. Moreover, to assess the overall model fit, measured values were plotted against population predictions.

Simulation-based diagnostics were performed using prediction- and variability-corrected visual predictive checks (pvcVPCs). The model of interest was used to generate 1000 simulations of the observed data. The 95% confidence intervals (CI) for the 5th, 50th, and 95th percentiles of the simulations were compared with the prediction- and variability-corrected observations, binning automatically, and plotted against an independent variable. In addition, the normalized prediction distribution error (NPDE) was determined using an add-on R package (NPDE, version 3.5, www.npde.biostat.fr, accessed on 1 October 2024). A total of 1000 datasets were simulated based on the reported final model parameters. A normal distribution N(0, 1) of NPDEs was tested using the Wilcoxon signed-rank test to assess whether the mean value significantly differed from zero and the Fisher variance test to compare the variance to one. Additionally, the Shapiro–Wilk test was conducted to compare the distribution of the NPDE to a normal distribution. Finally, a global test with an adjusted *p*-value of all the three tests was used to identify the best model. To visualize the distribution, quantile–quantile (QQ) plots and histograms of NPDE were presented by the NPDE package in R.

2.4. Monte Carlo Simulations Using Selected Models

Finally, the models were utilized for Monte Carlo simulations to generate concentration–time profiles based on covariate combinations specified within the models and the Q8W dosing regimen. VDZ trough levels in week 22 were compared among subgroups. Specifically, different albumin levels (30 g/L and 40 g/L), body weight (50 kg, 70 kg, and 100 kg), prior biologic therapy, and ADA status were considered, resulting in 24 unique covariate combinations that defined the subgroups. Additionally, VDZ concentrations were simulated (n = 1000) to assess Q8W and Q4W regimens for the best-case (no previous biologic exposure, body weight = 70 kg, no ADA, albumin = 40 g/L) and worst-case (previous biologic exposure, body weight = 100 kg, ADA, albumin = 30 g/L) covariate combinations. For the selected models, the proportion of concentrations in the maintenance phase (week 22) exceeding 12 μg/mL was calculated.

3. Results

3.1. Review of Selected Population Pharmacokinetic Models

A total of 31 results were found and collected in the PubMed search using the keywords mentioned in Section 2. An independent literature review revealed only one additional result. Following the application of inclusion and exclusion criteria, four population pharmacokinetic models [3,11,13,14] of VDZ in IBD patients were finally selected (Figure 1). The model by Rosario et al. characterized the pharmacokinetics of VDZ using a two-compartment model with parallel linear and nonlinear elimination [11], which served as a reference model. Subsequent studies updated this model to fit their specific datasets. All selected models were developed/updated using NONMEM® software (version 7.5). More detailed information about the selected studies and models can be found in Table 1. In all studies, VDZ was intravenously administered.

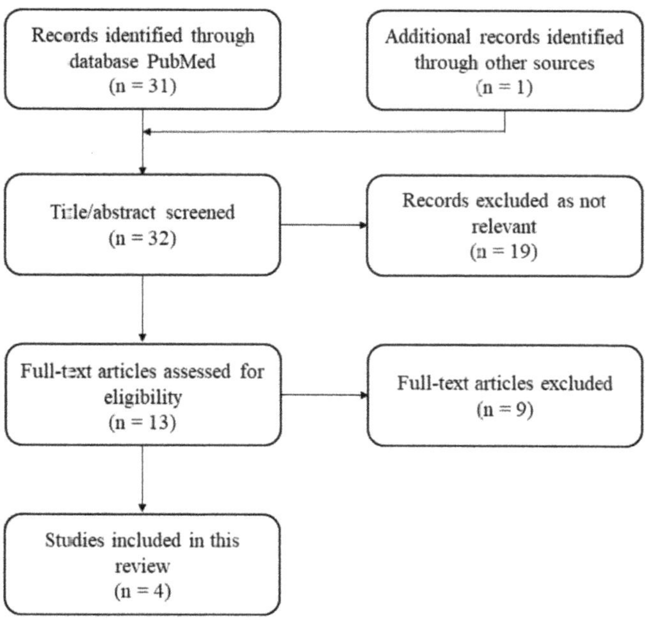

Figure 1. Flow chart of the article selection.

Table 1. Summary of selected (developed/updated) population pharmacokinetic studies of vedolizumab (VDZ) and identified factors of variability in linear clearance with potential clinical relevance.

Reference	Population Number of Subjects (Disease Type); Age	Software/Model	Typical Value of Pharmacokinetic Parameters, IIV, IOV and RV	Covariates Significantly Influenced CL_L with Potential Clinical Relevance
Developed population pharmacokinetic models				
Rosario et al., 2015 [11]	2554 individuals: 87 healthy volunteers from phase 1 study, 46 patients from phase 2 study (UC), and 891, 1115, and 415 patients from phase 3 GEMINI 1 (UC), GEMINI 2 (CD), and GEMINI 3 (CD) studies; age median (range): 36 (18–78) years	NONMEM/ 2-COMP model with parallel linear and nonlinear elimination	CL_L: 0.159 L/day (UC) CL_L: 0.155 L/day (CD) K_m: 0.964 μg/mL V_{max}: 0.265 mg/day Q: 0.12 L/day V_1: 3.19 L V_2: 1.65 L IIV CL_L: 34.6%, corrCL_L–V_1: 0.566, IIV V_1: 19.1%, corrCL_L–V_{max}: −0.192, corrV_1–V_{max}: −0.267, IIV V_{max}: 105% Proportional error: 0.0554 (23.5%)	ALB, WT
Population pharmacokinetic model reanalysis/update of previous model				
Okamoto et al., 2020 [3]	1933 individuals: 9 patients from phase 1 study (CPH-001, UC), 743, 966, 152, and 63 patients from phase 3 GEMINI 1 (UC), GEMINI 2 (CD), CCT-101 (UC), and CCT-001 (CD) studies; age median (range): 36 (17–79) years	NONMEM/ 2-COMP model with parallel linear and nonlinear elimination	CL_L: 0.165 L/day (ADA−) 0.246 L/day (ADA+) K_m: 0.851 μg/mL V_{max}: 0.238 mg/day Q: 0.161 L/day V_1: 3.16 L V_2: 1.84 L IIV CL_L: 30.8% corr CL_L–V_1: 0.581 IIV V_1: 20.2% corr CL_L–V_2: 0.0188 corr V_1-V_2: 0.371 IIV V_2: 70.2% IOV CL_L: 20.3% Proportional error: 0.0318 (17.8%)	WT, ALB, ADA status and titer

Table 1. *Cont.*

Reference	Population Number of Subjects (Disease Type); Age	Software/Model	Typical Value of Pharmacokinetic Parameters, IIV, IOV and RV	Covariates Significantly Influenced CL_L with Potential Clinical Relevance
Pauwels et al., 2021 [13]	37 patients: 12 (UC), 3 (IBD-U), 22 (CD); age median (IQR): 39 (26–50) years	NONMEM/ Serum PK model: 2-COMP model with parallel linear and nonlinear elimination Serum-tissue PK model: 3-comp model	Serum PK model: CL_L: 0.159 L/day (UC), 0.155 L/day (CD) K_m: 0.964 mg/L V_{max}: 0.265 mg/day Q: 0.12 L/day V_1: 3.19 L V_2: 1.65 L Serum—tissue PK model: Q_2: 0.07 L/day V_3: 1.31 L	ALB
Hanzel et al., 2022 [14]	108 patients from LOVE-CD trial; age median (IQR): 36 (28–46) years	NONMEM/ 2-COMP model with parallel linear and nonlinear elimination	CL_L: 0.215 L/day K_m: 0.964 mg/L fixed V_{max}: 0.265 mg/day fixed Q: 0.12 L/day fixed V_1: 4.92 L V_2: 1.65 L fixed IIV CL_L: 26.2% IOV CL_L: 15.2% Additive error: 0.469 mg/L Proportional error: 18.9%	ALB, ADA status, no previous biologic exposure

IIV—inter-individual variability in %; IOV—inter-occasional variability in %; RV—residual variability; 2-COMP—2-compartment model; IQR—interquartile range; COMP—compartment; PK—pharmacokinetic; CL_L—clearance of linear elimination pathway; K_m—concentration at half-maximum elimination rate; V_{max}—maximum elimination rate; V_1—apparent volume of the central compartment; V_2—apparent volume of the peripheral compartment; V_3—apparent volume of the third compartment; Q—apparent intercompartmental clearance between first and second compartment; Q_2—apparent intercompartmental clearance between second and third compartment; corr—correlation coefficient; ALB—albumin; ADA—anti-drug antibody; WT—body weight.

Typical values for CL_L in the studies ranged from 0.155 to 0.215 L/day, regardless of the disease type [3,11,13,14]. CL_L in ADA positive patients was 0.246 L/day in the study by Okamoto et al. [3]. The typical values of V_1 and V_2 ranged from 3.16 to 4.92 L, and from 1.65 to 1.84 L, respectively. The reported typical value of K_m was 0.851–0.964 μg/mL, while the typical value of V_{max} was 0.238–0.265 mg/day. Three models reported the IIV (percent coefficient of variation) associated with CL_L [3,11,14], with values ranging from 26.2% to 34.6%, and two models reported IIV associated with V_1 of 19.1% [11] and 20.2% [3]. IOV was accounted for by Okamoto et al. (an occasion was defined as a dosing interval with at least one associated pharmacokinetic measurement) with an effect on the CL_L of 20.3% [3], and Hanzel et al. (occasion was defined as induction—up to the week 14 dose, or maintenance—from week 14 onward) with an effect on the CL_L of 15.2% [14]. The residual variation was described with a proportional model [3,11] or a combined proportional and additive model [14]. Random effects were not reported for the model by Pauwels et al. [13].

Identified covariates with potential clinical relevance for CL_L were ADA, serum albumin, body weight, and previous biologic exposure (Table 1). Rosario et al. described several covariates in the population model, but only the effects of albumin and body weight at extreme values on CL_L had the potential to be clinically meaningful (effect sizes greater than ±25%) [11]. Thus, only these two covariates were accounted in the external evaluation analysis. On the other hand, the effects of fecal calprotectin (FCP), Crohn's Disease Activity Index (CDAI) score, partial Mayo score, age, prior TNF-α antagonist therapy status, ADA status (ELISA assay), and concomitant therapy use on VDZ CL_L were not considered clinically important in the Rosario et al. model [11], and Bayesian 95% credible intervals 95% (CDIs) for most effects contained the null effect. In the subsequent analysis, the remaining effects of sex and CRP were not clinically important. Only graphical evaluation implied that at week 6, UC patients with a Mayo endoscopic sub-score of 3 had, on average, 25% higher CL_L than patients with a sub-score of 0 [11].

Okamoto et al. updated the reference model in order to assess the impact of covariates on its pharmacokinetics in Asian and non-Asian UC and CD patients. This analysis had updated electrochemiluminescence (ECL) assay data and time-varying ADA in the dataset, so continuous titer data could be used for modeling the ADA effect. Albumin, body weight, and ADA were assigned as clinically meaningful predictors of VDZ CL_L, while the effect of race and diagnosis on CL_L was negligible [3]. The external evaluation analysis included albumin and body weight as covariates, as ADA values were not available for this analysis.

Pauwels et al. reanalyzed the reference model with two compartments, incorporating a third compartment to account for intestinal tissue concentrations, thereby developing a serum–tissue pharmacokinetic model. In the serum pharmacokinetic model, the negative impact of albumin on CL_L was incorporated, while body weight data were not available and therefore not considered [13].

Hanzel et al. developed a new VDZ model, building upon a previously published two-compartment model with parallel linear and nonlinear elimination. Their results demonstrated that CL_L was higher in patients with lower serum albumin concentrations, in the presence of ADA, and in patients with prior exposure to other biologic therapy [14]. Consequently, these covariates were considered in the external evaluation analysis.

3.2. Characteristics of External Cohort

Our cohort for external evaluation included data from 62 patients with UC and 44 patients with CD. The characteristics of patients and therapy are given in Table 2. A total of 114 VDZ trough concentration measurements were obtained during the follow-up period.

Table 2. Patient and therapy characteristics of the external evaluation dataset.

Characteristic (Units)	n (%)/Mean ± SD (Range)
Diagnosis	
UC	62 (58.49%)
CD	44 (41.51%)
Age (years)	49.76 ± 17.43 (21–78)
Sex (male)	55 (51.9%)
Body weight (kg)	71.94 ± 12.76 (44–110)
Albumin (g/L) *	42.93 ± 4.63 (30–55)
Immunomodulatory drug	86 (81.1%)
Prior anti-TNFα therapy	44 (41.5%)
Vedolizumab concentrations (μg/mL)	
TAD 4 weeks	26.09 ± 14.30 (5.309–62.79)
TAD 6 weeks	23.43 ± 8.53 (9.119–43.08)
TAD 8 weeks	15.39 ± 11.40 (3.02–47.22)

n—number; SD—standard deviation; UC—ulcerative colitis; CD—Crohn's disease; TAD—time after dose; * Missing data in 62 patients (54.4%).

3.3. Prediction-Based Diagnostics

The prediction-based diagnostic results are summarized in Table 3, while the population-predicted values vs. measured values are presented in Figure 2 and relative PE (%) in the boxplot in Figure 3. Although none of the models met the combined criteria of MDPE $\leq \pm 20\%$, MAPE $\leq 30\%$, F20 $\geq 35\%$, and F30 $\geq 50\%$ (Table 3), the models proposed by Pauwels et al. and Hanzel et al. exhibited lower MDPE ($\leq 20\%$) compared to the other two models, demonstrating superior accuracy. However, the CI of MPE included 0 only for the model by Pauwels et al. [13]. In terms of precision, the model of Hanzel et al. [14] showed the lowest MAPE of 41.64%, but, in general, all models exceeded the acceptable limit of 30%.

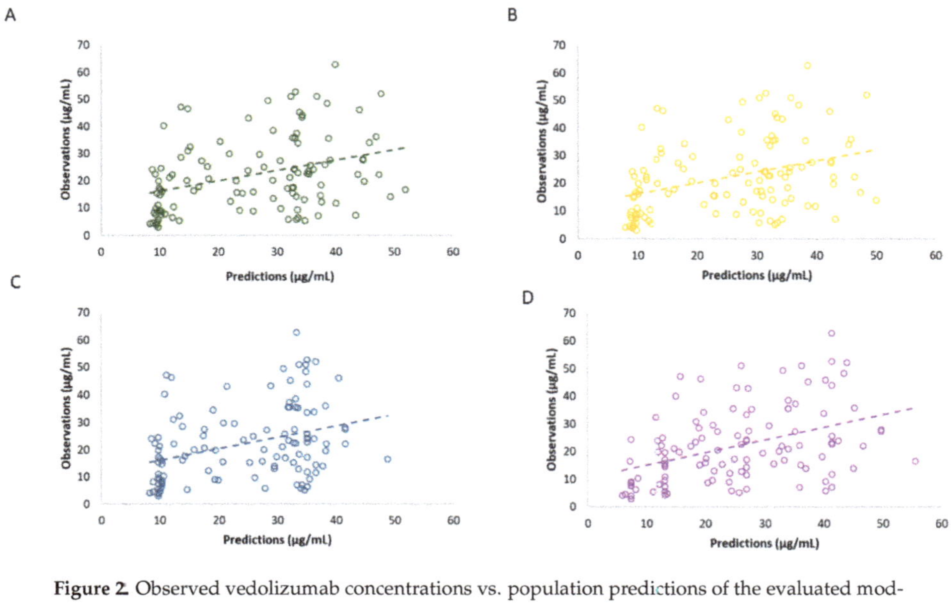

Figure 2. Observed vedolizumab concentrations vs. population predictions of the evaluated models: (**A**) Rosario et al., 2015 [11], (**B**) Okamoto et al., 2021 [3], (**C**) Pauwels et al., 2021 [13], and (**D**) Hanzel et al., 2022 [14]. Values are shown as points with a dashed regression line through the data.

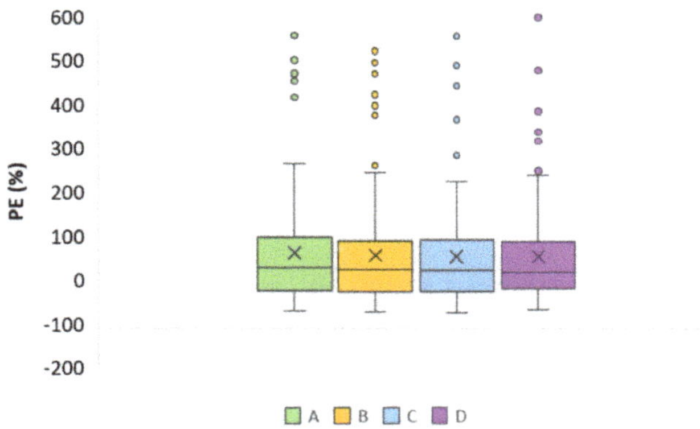

Figure 3. Boxplot for prediction error (PE (%)) of the evaluated models: (A) Rosario et al., 2015 [11], (B) Okamoto et al., 2021 [3], (C) Pauwels et al., 2021 [13], and (D) Hanzel et al., 2022 [14]. The × represents the mean value, the central line within each box represents the median, while the edges of the box denote the interquartile range (IQR); the vertical lines are whiskers and individual points are outliers.

Table 3. Comparison of population (PRED) predictions to observations for the evaluated population models of vedolizumab (VDZ).

Population PK Model	MPE (µg/mL) 95% CI	MDPE (%)	RMSPE (µg/mL)	F20 (%)	F30 (%)	MAPE (%)
Rosario et al., 2015 [11]	3.77 1.05–6.50	25.57	15.25	20.18	29.82	47.56
Okamoto et al., 2021 [3]	2.84 0.156–5.53	20.75	14.85	21.05	28.95	44.58
Pauwels et al., 2021 [13]	2.06 −0.567–4.68	18.63	14.38	21.93	28.07	45.96
Hanzel et al., 2022 [14]	2.91 0.331–5.49	13.82	14.30	25.44	38.60	41.64

MPE—mean prediction error, CI—confidence interval, MDPE—median prediction error, RMSPE—root mean square prediction error; F20—percentages of PE% within ±20%, F30—percentages of PE% within ±30%, MAPE—median absolute prediction error.

The prediction-based performance was evaluated across subgroups defined by specific covariate. All of the models performed better in terms of accuracy and precision for the subgroup with low–normal albumin levels, while subgroups with different body weights (≤70 kg and >70 kg) showed variable results. The Hanzel et al. [14] model showed superior characteristics for the subgroup of patients with prior biologic exposure. However, none of the models showed compliance with the combined criteria.

3.4. Simulation-Based Diagnostics

In the simulation-based diagnostics, the pvcVPC was used for diagnosis if the model accurately predicted both the central trend and the variability of the data (Figure 4). The results showed that the 5th and 95th (90%) percentile PIs covered most of the observations for each model. Although performance of the models was similar, slight deviations may be observed between observed and simulated data for each model, with the most obvious deviation at the 5th percentiles of the Hanzel et al. model [14].

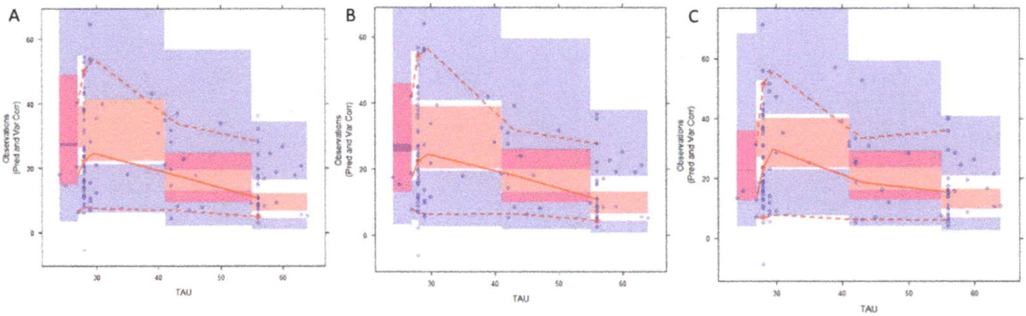

Figure 4. Prediction- and variability-corrected visual predictive check (pvcVPC) of the evaluated models: (**A**) Rosario et al., 2015 [11], (**B**) Okamoto et al., 2021 [3], and (**C**) Hanzel et al., 2022 [14]; prediction- and variability-corrected concentrations (μg/mL) vs. time after dose (days). The open black circles represent the observed vedolizumab (VDZ) concentrations. Solid and dashed red lines represent the median, 5th, and 95th percentiles of the observed data. The semi-transparent red shaded area represents the simulation-based 95% confidence interval (CI) for the median, while the semi-transparent blue fields represent the 95% CI around the 5th and 95th percentiles of the simulation-based prediction intervals.

Plots illustrating the NPDE of the evaluated models are presented on Figure 5, and results of statistical analysis are presented in Table 4. Statistical analysis confirmed normal distribution of NPDE N(0,1) for the Rosario et al. [11] and Okamoto et al. [3] models (Table 4). Even though the majority of NPDE values for the Hanzel et al. [14] model were within the range of plus or minus 1.96, variance was significantly different from one ($p < 0.01$).

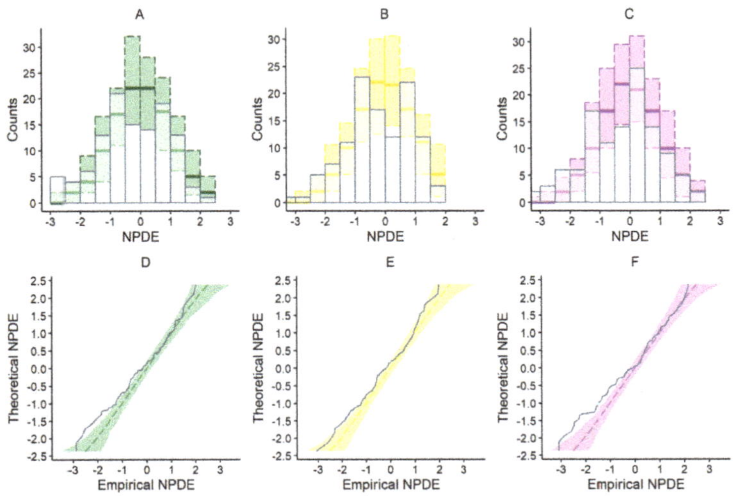

Figure 5. Plots illustrating normalized prediction distribution errors (NPDEs) of the evaluated models; histogram of NPDE of models: (**A**) Rosario et al., 2015 [11], (**B**) Okamoto et al., 2021 [3], and (**C**) Hanzel et al., 2022 [14]; QQ plot of theoretical NPDE vs. empirical NPDE of models (**D**) Rosario et al., 2015 [11], (**E**) Okamoto et al., 2021 [3], and (**F**) Hanzel et al., 2022 [14].

Table 4. Statistical tests for evaluating the normality of the normalized prediction distribution errors (NPDEs).

Population PK Model	Wilcoxon *	Fisher *	Shapiro–Wilks *	Global *
Rosario et al., 2015 [11]	0.0958	0.155	0.381	0.0958
Okamoto et al., 2021 [3]	0.132	1	0.578	0.132
Hanzel et al., 2022 [14]	0.0802	0.00894	0.394	0.00894

* data are expressed as *p*-values.

3.5. Simulated VDZ Concentration-Time Profiles

Simulated VDZ concentration–time profiles for 24 distinct subgroups, defined by combinations of covariates, following the recommended dosing regimen, are presented in Figures S1–S3 for the three evaluated models. Median concentrations based on 1000 simulations for 8-week and 4-week dosing frequencies in the maintenance phase are shown in Figure 6, comparing the best-case (no previous biologic therapy, body weight = 70 kg, no ADA, albumin = 40 g/L) and the worst-case (previous biologic therapy, body weight = 100 kg, ADA, albumin = 30 g/L) scenarios. Table 5 displays median simulated VDZ trough concentrations at week 22 after 300 mg Q8W in the maintenance phase for different covariate combinations across various models. Additionally, Table 6 summarizes the percentage of virtual patients whose VDZ troughs exceeded 12 μg/mL in week 22 for different dosing scenarios.

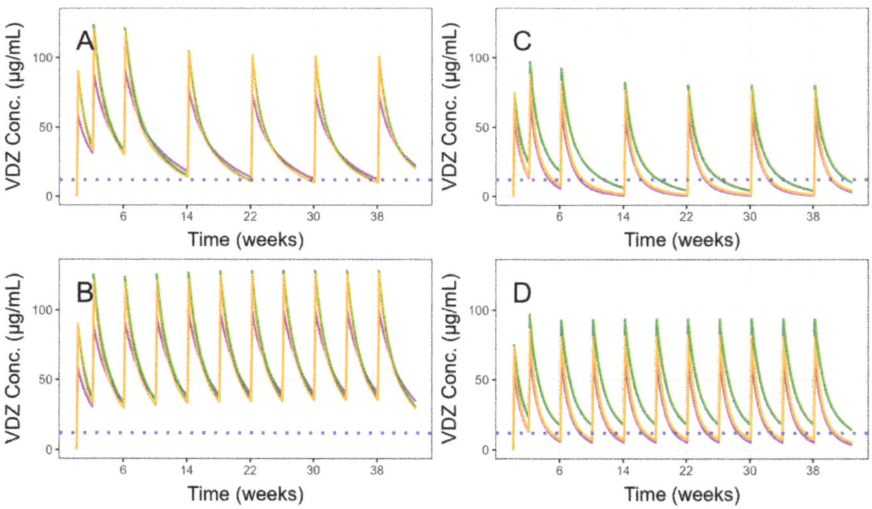

Figure 6. Simulated median vedolizumab (VDZ) pharmacokinetic profiles for the best-case: no previous biologic exposure, body weight = 70 kg, no ADA, albumin = 40 g/L (**A**,**B**) and the worst-case: previous biologic exposure, body weight = 100 kg, ADA, albumin = 30 g/L combination of covariates (**C**,**D**) following dosing frequency of 8 weeks (**A**,**C**) and 4 weeks (**B**,**D**) in the maintenance phase using three population pharmacokinetic models. Purple—Hanzel et al., 2022 [14], yellow—Okamoto et al. [3], green—Rosario et al. [11]. Blue dotted line represents y = 12 μg/mL.

Table 5. Simulated vedolizumab trough concentration in week 22 after 300 mg every 8 weeks in the maintenance treatment based on a combination of covariates using different population pharmacokinetic models.

Population PK Model	Median Trough Concentration (IQR) of Vedolizumab (VDZ) in Week 22 [μg/mL]	
	Best-Case Combination of Covariates [1]	Worst-Case Combination of Covariates [2]
Hanzel et al. [14]	13.83 (3.62–34.46)	0.77 (0.12–4.61)
Okamoto et al. [3]	10.86 (1.54–35.89)	1.32 (0.03–8.20)
Rosario et al. [11] *	10.98 (1.74–37.19)	4.31 (0.36–18.86)

[1] no previous biologic exposure = 70 kg, no ADA, albumin = 40 g/L; [2] previous biologic exposure, body weight = 100 kg, ADA, albumin = 30 g/L; * for Crohn's disease indication.

Table 6. Percent of simulated patients with vedolizumab (VDZ) trough concentration above 12 μg/mL in week 22 using different population pharmacokinetic (PK) models.

Population PK Model	Patients with Trough Concentration of Vedolizumab (VDZ) >12 μg/mL in Week 22 [%]	
	Best-Case Combination of Covariates [1] and 300 mg Every 8 Weeks During Maintenance	Worst-Case Combination of Covariates [2] and 300 mg Every 4 Weeks During Maintenance
Hanzel et al. [14]	60.8	9.5
Okamoto et al. [3]	44.1	22.6
Rosario et al. [11] *	45.5	77.3

[1] no previous biologic exposure, body weight = 70 kg, no ADA, albumin = 40 g/L; [2] previous biologic exposure, body weight = 100 kg, ADA, albumin = 30 g/L; * for Crohn's disease indication.

4. Discussion

The individualization of biologic exposure is challenging due to the substantial within- and between-subject variability in CL, which may be better predicted using population pharmacokinetic models. Although several population pharmacokinetic studies of VDZ are available for adult IBD patients, the predictability of models has not been assessed on an independent population. To the best of our knowledge, this study is the first to evaluate the published population models using an external dataset. In our study, a validation dataset consisting of 114 VDZ concentrations obtained from 106 IBD patients was used to explore the predictive performance of four population models for VDZ in adults. The evaluation was performed using prediction-based and simulation-based diagnostics.

Previous population analyses characterized the pharmacokinetics of VDZ by a two-compartment model with a nonlinear elimination mechanism at low concentrations and a linear pathway at higher, therapeutic concentrations (Table 1). The nonlinear elimination is related to saturable, target-mediated mechanisms such as receptor-mediated endocytosis, while the linear pathway involves non-saturable components such as Fc-mediated elimination [1,11]. According to the selected models, clinically relevant change in CL_L can be expected with extreme values of (low) albumin and (high) body weight, ADA, and previous biologic therapy. However, a portion of the variability in CL_L (26.2–34.6%) remains unexplained, suggesting that factors influencing VDZ pharmacokinetics have not yet been definitively established.

In our external evaluation analysis, none of the models met the combined criteria of MDPE $\leq \pm 20\%$, MAPE $\leq 30\%$, F20 $\geq 35\%$, and F30 $\geq 50\%$ (Table 3). Among the evaluated models, the MDPE (%) results indicated that the predictions from the models by Pauwels et al. and Hanzel et al. demonstrated acceptable accuracy. However, based on MPE results, only the CI for the Pauwels et al. model included 0. Due to the significant skewness and variability observed in the MPE data for each model, MDPE likely provides a more reliable representation of the overall trend. Regarding the precision, the Hanzel et al. model showed the best MAPE of 41.64%, but in general all models exceeded the acceptable limit of 30%. Consistently, the evaluated models displayed similar results in overall model fit, with notable dispersion of population predictions (Figure 2). Interestingly, all models provided better accuracy and precision for the subgroup of patients for whom albumin levels were low–normal (approximately below 40 g/L), but in general none fulfilled the combined criteria. Perhaps a more heterogenous dataset is required to assess predictive performance in covariate-defined subgroups. Overall, all models exhibited bias in population predictions, indicating limited utility for a priori dose adjustments based solely on population parameters and identified covariates. Significant bias in population predictions has also been reported for other monoclonal antibodies used in IBD treatment, such as infliximab [18]. Nevertheless, Bayesian forecasting is expected to improve the precision and accuracy of predictions by incorporating prior concentration data, warranting further evaluation of population models combined with Bayesian estimation. Indeed, for drugs with fixed initial dosing regimens, a posteriori predictions are generally more valuable for optimizing dosing strategies. However, in the absence of TDM data for a posteriori MIPD, predictions based solely on patient covariates may still serve as a useful tool to identify individuals at higher risk of inadequate response. Despite their poor performance in population-based predictions, three tested models showed better results in simulation-based diagnostics performed by pvcVPC (Figure 4). While slight deviations were noted between observed and simulated data for each model, the results suggest that these models are better suited for exploring "what if" scenarios through simulations than prediction-based applications [19]. This divergence between prediction-based and simulation-based evaluations has also been noted in studies involving other therapeutic agents [20,21]. However, additional analysis of NPDE (Figure 5, Table 4) revealed that only the models by Rosario et al. [11] and Okamoto et al. [3] completely fulfilled the criteria. While the majority of NPDEs were within the range of plus or minus 1.96, the variance was significantly different from one ($p < 0.01$) for the model of Hanzel et al [14].

In general, the selected models showed poor population prediction, likely influenced by multiple factors. The extrapolation may have been limited by missing some clinically relevant covariates in the evaluation dataset, such as ADA or albumin values in some patients. This limitation may be a potential reason for the detection of several outliers presented in Figure 3. Furthermore, the variables contributing to VDZ pharmacokinetic variability have not been definitively established. Although several covariates were described previously, only albumin, body weight, ADA, and previous biologic therapy showed a clinically relevant change in CL_L in selected population models. Consequently, the external validation of these models may have been hindered by their inability to account for all covariates relevant to the external population.

Albumin levels were consistently found to be negatively associated with CL_L across all evaluated VDZ models, aligning with previous findings [4]. While the exact mechanism underlying this effect is not fully understood, it has been proposed that reduced expression or activity of the neonatal Fc receptor (FcRn) in IBD patients impairs salvage of albumin and IgG, reflecting increased antibody CL. Another possible mechanism is that inflammation of the gastrointestinal tract in IBD patients may lead to an atypical elimination route [11]. Both Rosario et al. [11] and Okamoto et al. [3] emphasized that only the extremely low albumin levels were identified as potentially clinically important predictors of CL_L. Although none of the patients in the study by Pauwels et al. [13] had low albumin levels (<32 g/L), this covariate was incorporated into the model to confirm previous findings [13]. Hanzel et al. [14] calculated that CL_L increased at lower albumin levels (28 g/L) for 26% compared to a typical patient [14]. Indeed, the clinical relevance of this covariate for VDZ pharmacokinetics was confirmed in other studies as well [12].

The disposition of monoclonal antibodies, including VDZ, is often described as a function of body size [4,22]. The models by Rosario et al. [11] and Okamoto et al. [3] incorporated body weight using allometric scaling. Allometric power coefficients were fixed to 0.75 for V_{max} and Q, and to 1.0 for V_2, while the weight effect was estimated for V_1 and CL_L. Both studies found that only extreme body weight values were identified as potentially clinically important predictors of CL_L [3,11]. Rosario et al. [11] noted that a typical individual weighing 120 kg had a 19% probability of having a CL_L value more than 25% higher than in a patient weighing 70 kg [11]. In contrast, Hanzel et al. [14] did not find an effect of body weight on VDZ pharmacokinetics, likely due to the narrower body weight range in their cohort [14]. In addition to body size, other demographic variables, such as age, sex, and race, were also evaluated as potential covariates. Okamoto et al. [3] studied the pharmacokinetics of VDZ in Asian and non-Asian patients, finding only a small clinically insignificant effect of race [3]. Similarly, age and sex were determined not to be a significant or clinically relevant covariates for VDZ CL_L in selected studies [3,11,14].

As exogenous proteins, therapeutic monoclonal antibodies can provoke an immune response, leading to the production of ADA, which can accelerate the elimination of biologics [4]. In the study by Rosario et al., the presence of ADAs (either persistently or transiently) was found to increase VDZ CL_L by only 12%, a statistically significant but clinically insignificant effect [11]. In contrast, Okamoto et al. [3] identified a positive ADA titer as a potentially clinically important predictor of CL_L. Specifically, CL_L increased from 0.165 in ADA-negative patients (<10 titers) to 0.246 L/day in ADA-positive patients (titer 250) [3]. Moreover, Hanzel et al. [14] observed a marked increase in CL_L by 89% in the presence of ADAs [14]. Simulated concentration–time profiles across various covariate subgroups revealed a dominant effect of ADA on CL_L, particularly for the models developed by Hanzel et al. [14] and Okamoto et al. [3] (Figures S1 and S2). These findings highlight the significance of ADA as a covariate affecting VDZ pharmacokinetics and underscore the potential for immunogenicity to influence therapeutic outcomes in clinical settings.

Monoclonal antibody interactions with small-molecule drugs are generally not anticipated [22]. However, prior biologic therapy has occasionally been associated with higher CL of monoclonal antibodies in IBD patients [4]. Hanzel et al. found that CL_L increased by 25% in patients who had prior exposure to biologics compared to those with no prior exposure [14]. This impact of prior biologic therapy on clearance was reflected in the simulated concentrations (Figure S1). On the other hand, Rosario et al. [11] detected a minor 4% increase in CL_L in patients who had been treated with and failed prior TNF-α antagonist therapy, although this effect was not deemed clinically meaningful. Moreover, immunomodulatory therapies, or amino-salicylate or corticosteroid therapy, were not detected as being important for the pharmacokinetic variability of VDZ [11,14].

There was no clinically meaningful effect of IBD diagnosis on CL_L in the model by Okamoto et al. [3]. Likewise, typical estimates of CL_L were similar between UC and CD patients within the Rosario et al. model [11]. The effect of the partial Mayo score and the CDAI score at baseline had no effect on VDZ CL_L in Rosario et al. model [11]. However, a trend toward lower CL_L, and therefore higher concentrations, in UC patients with a lower Mayo endoscopic sub-score was noted. As additional measures of disease severity, the effects of FCP and CRP concentrations on VDZ CL_L were evaluated. While the effect of FCP was statistically significant, it was small and not considered to be clinically relevant. Similarly, subsequent post hoc analysis suggested that the effect of CRP on VDZ CL_L was also not clinically relevant [11]. Hanzel et al. tested CDAI, CRP, and Simple Endoscopic Score for Crohn's Disease (SES-CD) at baseline as covariates, but no effect was detected [14].

During the standard induction phase, VDZ trough levels are typically around 27 µg/mL. In the maintenance phase, mean steady-state trough levels are approximately

12 μg/mL for a dosing frequency of Q8W and 36 μg/mL for a dosing frequency of Q4W [2,23–25]. In general, VDZ trough concentration >20 μg/mL at week 6 and >12 μg/mL during maintenance are proposed thresholds [26–28]. Our simulation analysis reveals that the median concentration is above 12 μg/mL in week 22 during maintenance for approximately 45–60% patients with best-case combinations of covariates and the dosing frequency Q8W (Table 6). Simulated concentrations are notably lower for worst-case combinations of covariates (Table 5, Figure 6), which implies that alternative dosing could be more appropriate. However, simulation analysis with intensified dosing showed variable results. While simulation based on the model by Rosario et al. [11] predicts approximately 77% of the concentration above the threshold, the two other models with an incorporated ADA influence predict notably lower percentages (Table 6, Figure 6). Thus, in patients with ADA-negative status, the Q4W dosing regimen might be appropriate. On the other hand, sub-therapeutic concentrations are likely in ADA-positive patients, especially when additional significant covariates are present (Figures S1 and S2). Moreover, at low VDZ concentrations, nonlinear elimination becomes predominant, further contributing to an increase in CL. Thus, alternative biologic therapy, rather than a pharmacokinetic-guided dosing regimen, might be more suitable for these patients. Yet, it should be noted that VDZ is a humanized monoclonal antibody and its immunogenicity is generally low [12].

Our study has several limitations. As previously mentioned, due to the retrospective nature of data collection from routine TDM, albumin levels were not available for every patient, and ADAs are not part of routine monitoring as VDZ immunogenicity is generally low. Consequently, in subgroup analysis, missing data on albumin were categorized as a low–normal level. On the other hand, it is expected that Bayesian forecasting could enhance predictions by utilizing previous concentration points. Unfortunately, this approach could not be applied in our analysis as most patients had only a single VDZ concentration measurement available. Lastly, due to the small number of published VDZ population pharmacokinetic models, we included articles with overlapping datasets but excluded those that were missing key pharmacokinetic parameters. These limitations may have impacted the generalizability and accuracy of the results, and future studies with more comprehensive datasets are necessary to validate and improve model predictions.

5. Conclusions

We evaluated four published VDZ population pharmacokinetic models for patients with IBD using an independent dataset from our center. The external predictive performance of these models was not satisfactory in prediction-based diagnostics, which indicates that a priori predictions based solely on covariates remains challenging. However, combining model-based dosing with therapeutic drug monitoring (TDM) could offer a more reliable approach for a posteriori predictions, and this should be further explored in future studies. When drug concentration measurements are available, Bayesian estimation enables the derivation of individual pharmacokinetic parameters, allowing the optimization of dosing strategies tailored to each patient. Our findings suggest that two of the tested models may, in particular, be more suitable for simulation-based applications. The simulations conducted using these models contribute valuable insights into optimizing the VDZ dosing regimen for patients with varying characteristics. These results emphasize the potential utility of simulation-based approaches in tailoring treatment for individual patients, although further validation is required to fully assess their clinical applicability.

Supplementary Materials: The following supporting information can be downloaded at: https://www.mdpi.com/article/10.3390/biomedicines13010043/s1, Figure S1: Simulated vedolizumab (VDZ) concentrations with various combinations of covariates (ALB = albumin level, ADA = anti-drug antibody status, BW = body weight, ATNF naive = no previous biologic therapy) for dosing regimen

(300 mg, dosing frequency Q8W) for the model by Hanzel et al., 2022 [14]; Figure S2: Simulated vedolizumab (VDZ) concentrations with various combinations of covariates (ALB = albumin level, ADA = anti-drug antibody status, BW = body weight, ATNF naive = no previous biologic therapy) for dosing regimen (300 mg, dosing frequency Q8W) for the model by Okamoto et al., 2020 [3]; Figure S3: Simulated vedolizumab (VDZ) concentrations with various combinations of covariates (ALB = albumin level, ADA = anti-drug antibody status, BW = body weight, ATNF naive = no previous biologic therapy) for dosing regimen (300 mg, dosing frequency Q8W) for the model by Rosario et al., 2015 [11].

Author Contributions: S.M., P.S. and K.V. conceptualized and designed the research. S.M., Đ.K., T.K.I. and O.O. performed the research and patient recruitment. Đ.K., T.K.I., O.O. and A.H. performed data curation. M.J. and K.V. analyzed the data. M.J., A.H., S.M. and K.V. wrote the first draft of the paper. P.S., Đ.K., T.K.I. and O.O. revised the paper. All authors have read and agreed to the published version of the manuscript.

Funding: This research was supported by the Science Fund of the Republic of Serbia, through grant agreement No. 6777, Improving Clinical Outcomes with Precision Dosing in Patients with Inflammatory Bowel Disease Through Investigating Variability of Monoclonal Antibodies Based on Population Pharmacokinetic-Pharmacodynamic Modeling—optYmAb.

Institutional Review Board Statement: The study followed the principles of the Declaration of Helsinki and was approved by the local ethical committee of University Clinical Hospital Centre "Zvezdara" (approval code n. IRB00009457).

Informed Consent Statement: Informed consent was obtained from all subjects involved in the study.

Data Availability Statement: The data presented in this study are available on request from the corresponding author due to privacy and ethical reasons.

Conflicts of Interest: The authors declare no competing interests for this work.

References

1. Rosario, M.; Dirks, N.L.; Milch, C.; Parikh, A.; Bargfrede, M.; Wyant, T.; Fedyk, E.; Fox, I. A review of the clinical pharmacokinetics, pharmacodynamics, and immunogenicity of vedolizumab. *Clin. Pharmacokinet.* **2017**, *56*, 1287–1301. [CrossRef] [PubMed]
2. SmPC Entyvio. Summary of Product Characteristics for Entyvio 300 mg Powder for Concentrate for Solution for Infusion. Available online: https://www.medicines.org.uk/emc/product/5442/smpc#gref (accessed on 1 October 2024).
3. Okamoto, H.; Dirks, N.L.; Rosario, M.; Hori, T.; Hibi, T. Population pharmacokinetics of vedolizumab in Asian and non-Asian patients with ulcerative colitis and Crohn's disease. *Intest. Res.* **2021**, *19*, 95–105. [CrossRef] [PubMed]
4. Deyhim, T.; Cheifetz, A.S.; Papamichael, K. Drug clearance in patients with inflammatory bowel disease treated with biologics. *J. Clin. Med.* **2023**, *12*, 7132. [CrossRef]
5. Papamichael, K.; Cheifetz, A.S.; Melmed, G.Y.; Irving, P.M.; Vande Casteele, N.; Kozuch, P.L.; Raffals, L.E.; Baidoo, L.; Bressler, B.; Devlin, S.M.; et al. Appropriate therapeutic drug monitoring of biologic agents for patients with inflammatory bowel diseases. *Clin. Gastroenterol. Hepatol.* **2019**, *17*, 1655–1668.e3. [CrossRef] [PubMed]
6. Sethi, S.; Dias, S.; Kumar, A.; Blackwell, J.; Brookes, M.J.; Segal, J.P. Meta-analysis: The efficacy of therapeutic drug monitoring of anti-TNF-therapy in inflammatory bowel disease. *Aliment. Pharmacol. Ther.* **2023**, *57*, 1362–1374. [CrossRef]
7. Cheifetz, A.S.; Abreu, M.T.; Afif, W.; Cross, R.K.; Dubinsky, M.C.; Loftus, E.V., Jr.; Osterman, M.T.; Saroufim, A.; Siegel, C.A.; Yarur, A.J.; et al. A comprehensive literature review and expert consensus statement on therapeutic drug monitoring of biologics in inflammatory bowel disease. *Am. J. Gastroenterol.* **2021**, *116*, 2014–2025. [CrossRef]
8. Dreesen, E.; Verstockt, B.; Bian, S.; de Bruyn, M.; Compernolle, G.; Tops, S.; Noman, M.; Van Assche, G.; Ferrante, M.; Gils, A.; et al. Evidence to support monitoring of vedolizumab trough concentrations in patients with inflammatory bowel diseases. *Clin. Gastroenterol. Hepatol.* **2018**, *16*, 1937–1946.e8. [CrossRef]
9. Di Paolo, A.; Luci, G. Personalized medicine of monoclonal antibodies in inflammatory bowel disease: Pharmacogenetics, therapeutic drug monitoring, and beyond. *Front. Pharmacol.* **2020**, *11*, 610806. [CrossRef]
10. El Hassani, M.; Marsot, A. External evaluation of population pharmacokinetic models for precision dosing: Current state and knowledge gaps. *Clin. Pharmacokinet.* **2023**, *62*, 533–540. [CrossRef]

11. Rosario, M.; Dirks, N.L.; Gastonguay, M.R.; Fasanmade, A.A.; Wyant, T.; Parikh, A.; Sandborn, W.J.; Feagan, B.G.; Reinisch, W.; Fox, I. Population pharmacokinetics-pharmacodynamics of vedolizumab in patients with ulcerative colitis and Crohn's disease. *Aliment. Pharmacol. Ther.* **2015**, *42*, 188–202. [CrossRef]
12. Wyant, T.; Yang, L.; Rosario, M. Comparison of the ELISA and ECL assay for vedolizumab anti-drug antibodies: Assessing the impact on pharmacokinetics and safety outcomes of the phase 3 GEMINI trials. *AAPS J.* **2020**, *23*, 3. [CrossRef] [PubMed]
13. Pauwels, R.W.M.; Proietti, E.; van der Woude, C.J.; Oudijk, L.; Crombag, M.B.S.; Peppelenbosch, M.P.; Grohmann, U.; Fuhler, G.M.; de Vries, A.C. Vedolizumab tissue concentration correlates to mucosal inflammation and objective treatment response in inflammatory bowel disease. *Inflamm. Bowel Dis.* **2021**, *27*, 1813–1820. [CrossRef] [PubMed]
14. Hanzel, J.; Dreesen, E.; Vermeire, S.; Lowenberg, M.; Hoentjen, F.; Bossuyt, P.; Clasquin, E.; Baert, F.J.; D'Haens, G.R.; Mathot, R. Pharmacokinetic-pharmacodynamic model of vedolizumab for targeting endoscopic remission in patients with Crohn disease: Posthoc analysis of the LOVE-CD study. *Inflamm. Bowel Dis.* **2022**, *28*, 689–699. [CrossRef]
15. Brendel, K.; Dartois, C.; Comets, E.; Lemenuel-Diot, A.; Laveille, C.; Tranchand, B.; Girard, P.; Laffont, C.M.; Mentre, F. Are population pharmacokinetic and/or pharmacodynamic models adequately evaluated? A survey of the literature from 2002 to 2004. *Clin. Pharmacokinet.* **2007**, *46*, 221–234. [CrossRef]
16. Sheiner, L.B.; Beal, S.L. Some suggestions for measuring predictive performance. *J. Pharmacokinet. Biopharm.* **1981**, *9*, 503–512. [CrossRef]
17. Chen, S.; Huang, L.; Huang, W.; Zheng, Y.; Shen, L.; Liu, M.; Chen, W.; Wu, X. External evaluation of population pharmacokinetic models for high-dose methotrexate in adult patients with hematological tumors. *J. Clin. Pharmacol.* **2024**, *64*, 437–448. [CrossRef]
18. Konecki, C.; Feliu, C.; Cazaubon, Y.; Giusti, D.; Tonye-Libyh, M.; Brixi, H.; Cadiot, G.; Biron, A.; Djerada, Z. External evaluation of population pharmacokinetic models and bayes-based dosing of infliximab. *Pharmaceutics* **2021**, *13*, 1191. [CrossRef]
19. Cheng, Y.; Wang, C.Y.; Li, Z.R.; Pan, Y.; Liu, M.B.; Jiao, Z. Can population pharmacokinetics of antibiotics be extrapolated? Implications of external evaluations. *Clin. Pharmacokinet.* **2021**, *60*, 53–68. [CrossRef]
20. Ryu, S.; Jung, W.J.; Jiao, Z.; Chae, J.W.; Yun, H.Y. External evaluation of the predictive performance of seven population pharmacokinetic models for phenobarbital in neonates. *Br. J. Clin. Pharmacol.* **2021**, *87*, 3878–3889. [CrossRef]
21. Zhao, C.Y.; Jiao, Z.; Mao, J.J.; Qiu, X.Y. External evaluation of published population pharmacokinetic models of tacrolimus in adult renal transplant recipients. *Br. J. Clin. Pharmacol.* **2016**, *81*, 891–907. [CrossRef]
22. Dirks, N.L.; Meibohm, B. Population pharmacokinetics of therapeutic monoclonal antibodies. *Clin. Pharmacokinet.* **2010**, *49*, 633–659. [CrossRef] [PubMed]
23. Feagan, B.G.; Rutgeerts, P.; Sands, B.E.; Hanauer, S.; Colombel, J.F.; Sandborn, W.J.; Van Assche, G.; Axler, J.; Kim, H.J.; Danese, S.; et al. Vedolizumab as induction and maintenance therapy for ulcerative colitis. *N. Engl. J. Med.* **2013**, *369*, 699–710. [CrossRef] [PubMed]
24. Sandborn, W.J.; Feagan, B.G.; Rutgeerts, P.; Hanauer, S.; Colombel, J.F.; Sands, B.E.; Lukas, M.; Fedorak, R.N.; Lee, S.; Bressler, B.; et al. Vedolizumab as induction and maintenance therapy for Crohn's disease. *N. Engl. J. Med.* **2013**, *369*, 711–721. [CrossRef] [PubMed]
25. Sands, B.E.; Feagan, B.G.; Rutgeerts, P.; Colombel, J.F.; Sandborn, W.J.; Sy, R.; D'Haens, G.; Ben-Horin, S.; Xu, J.; Rosario, M.; et al. Effects of vedolizumab induction therapy for patients with Crohn's disease in whom tumor necrosis factor antagonist treatment failed. *Gastroenterology* **2014**, *147*, 618–627.e3. [CrossRef]
26. Singh, S.; Dulai, P.S.; Vande Casteele, N.; Battat, R.; Fumery, M.; Boland, B.S.; Sandborn, W.J. Systematic review with meta-analysis: Association between vedolizumab trough concentration and clinical outcomes in patients with inflammatory bowel diseases. *Aliment. Pharmacol. Ther.* **2019**, *50*, 848–857. [CrossRef]
27. Steenholdt, C.; Lorentsen, R.D.; Petersen, P.N.; Widigson, E.S.; Kloft, C.; Klaasen, R.A.; Brynskov, J. Therapeutic drug monitoring of vedolizumab therapy in inflammatory bowel disease. *J. Gastroenterol. Hepatol.* **2024**, *39*, 1088–1098. [CrossRef]
28. Alsoud, D.; Vermeire, S.; Verstockt, B. Monitoring vedolizumab and ustekinumab drug levels in patients with inflammatory bowel disease: Hype or hope? *Curr. Opin. Pharmacol.* **2020**, *55*, 17–30. [CrossRef]

biomedicines

MDPI

Systematic Review

Comparative Efficacy of Subcutaneous Versus Intravenous Interleukin 12/23 Inhibitors for the Remission of Moderate to Severe Crohn's Disease: A Systematic Review and Meta-Analysis

Nouran Alwisi [1], Rana Ismail [1], Hissa Al-Kuwari [1], Khalifa H. Al-Ansari [1], Mohammed A. Al-Matwi [1], Noor A. Aweer [1], Wejdan N. Al-Marri [1], Yousif Al-Kubaisi [1], Muneera Al-Mohannadi [2], Shahd Hamran [1], Suhail A. R. Doi [1], Habib H. Farooqui [1,*] and Tawanda Chivese [1,*]

[1] College of Medicine, QU Health, Qatar University, Doha P.O. Box 2713, Qatar; na2104730@qu.edu.qa (N.A.); ri2108210@qu.edu.qa (R.I.); ha2104524@qu.edu.qa (H.A.-K.); ka1801508@qu.edu.qa (K.H.A.-A.); ma2104272@qu.edu.qa (M.A.A.-M.); na2003836@qu.edu.qa (N.A.A.); wa1903516@qu.edu.qa (W.N.A.-M.); ya1808493@qu.edu.qa (Y.A.-K.); sh2004556@qu.edu.qa (S.H.); sdoi@qu.edu.qa (S.A.R.D.)

[2] Department of Gastroenterology and Hepatology, Hamad Medical Corporation, Doha P.O. Box 3050, Qatar; ma.mohannadi@hamad.qa

* Correspondence: hfarooqui@qu.edu.qa (H.H.F.); tchivese@uw.edu (T.C.); Tel.: +974-4403-7833 (H.H.F.); +974-4403-7831 (T.C.)

Abstract: Background/Objectives: Interleukin 12/23 inhibitors are a newer class of monoclonal antibodies used to induce and maintain remission for Crohn's disease (CD), a chronic inflammatory bowel disease, when patients do not respond to conventional immunomodulatory drugs or first-line monoclonal antibody therapies. Although biologics are best administered intravenously, subcutaneous administration has been trialed, with mixed results. This research synthesized evidence on the efficacy and safety of subcutaneous compared to intravenous administration of interleukin 12/23 inhibitors for moderate to severe CD. **Methods**: In this systematic review and meta-analysis, we searched Cochrane, PubMed, SCOPUS, CINHAL, and preprint archives for randomized controlled trials (RCTs) that compared the efficacy and safety of subcutaneous to intravenous interleukin 12/23 inhibitors for the remission of CD. After study quality assessment, a meta-analysis was carried out using a bias-adjusted inverse variance heterogeneity model, heterogeneity was assessed using I^2, and publication bias was performed using Doi plots. Evidence certainty was assessed using Grading of Recommendations, Assessment, Development, and Evaluations (GRADE). **Results**: Seven RCTs, with 2179 participants, all with moderate to severe CD, were included. After meta-analysis, subcutaneous compared to intravenous administration showed similar efficacy for the induction of remission (OR 0.77, 95%CI 0.53–1.12), with no-to-low heterogeneity ($I^2 = 0\%$, $p = 0.97$). For the maintenance of remission, only two studies had analyzable data, and they showed that subcutaneous interleukin 12/23 inhibitors were equal or better compared to intravenous administration. Further syntheses showed that subcutaneous compared to intravenous administration of interleukin 12/23 inhibitors had almost similar odds of adverse events (OR 0.91, 95%CI 0.63–1.32, $I^2 = 39\%$), serious adverse events (OR 0.97, 95%CI 0.61–1.53, $I^2 = 0\%$), and treatment discontinuation (OR 1.06, 95%CI 0.67–1.68, $I^2 = 0\%$). **Conclusions**: In individuals with moderate to severe CD, subcutaneous administration has similar efficacy for inducing remission with comparable safety. More RCTs are needed to confirm these findings.

Keywords: Crohn's disease (CD); interleukin inhibitors; monoclonal antibodies (mAbs); subcutaneous (SC); intravenous (IV); meta-analysis

1. Introduction

Crohn's disease (CD) is a chronic, disabling, and progressive inflammatory bowel disease (IBD) of the gastrointestinal tract [1]. Once classified as rare, the prevalence of IBD, which CD belongs to, is increasing in step with the rapid epidemiological transitions occurring in low- and middle-income countries (LMIC) [2–4]. Between 1990 and 2019, the number of people affected by IBD increased from 3.3 to 4.9 million, highlighting the growing disease burden of IBD globally [5]. Chronic inflammation is associated with the accumulation of tissue damage that can lead to disease complications such as strictures, fistulae, and surgical resections [1]. CD has a significant negative impact on the health-related and social quality of life of diagnosed individuals, and this includes recurring disease activity, extra-intestinal manifestations, and decreased social functioning and productivity, and has been linked to colonic cancer [6–8]. Up to half of individuals with CD will experience a disease complication requiring surgery within 10 years of diagnosis [1]. The Montreal Classification categorizes CD into phenotypes based on age at diagnosis, disease location, and aggressiveness of the disease [3,9,10]. Evidence suggests that some of the CD phenotypes that initially present as mild disease tend to evolve into complicated moderate to severe phenotypes which require more aggressive pharmacotherapy and surgical interventions, over time [11]. The health and social impact of CD is worse for individuals with severe phenotypes [12]. These phenotypes contribute a large proportion of difficult-to-treat CD, a subtype of CD that has limited treatment options [13].

Since 1975, biologic therapies have evolved through the decades and have become part of treatment protocols for several diseases such as IBD, rheumatoid arthritis, and some cancers [14,15]. Available treatment modalities for CD target the resolution of clinical symptoms, such as diarrhea and extraintestinal manifestations, and endoscopic remission, which includes lack of inflammation, ulceration, and bleeding in the affected areas [9,10]. According to recent guidelines, people with moderate-to-severe CD are started on either Tumor Necrosis Factor alpha (TNF-α) inhibitor monotherapy, such as infliximab and adalimumab, or combined therapy consisting of TNF-α inhibitors and immunomodulators (thiopurines, 5-aminosalicylic acid (5-ASA), methotrexate) for the induction and maintenance of remission, with the use of corticosteroids for short-term management of flare-ups [16]. However, around one-third of individuals on TNF-α inhibitors do not achieve induction of remission, and of those who achieve initial remission, around one-half fail to maintain remission subsequently [17]. For these individuals with refractory CD, treatment options are limited as surgical approaches generally do not result in long-term remission, while the repeated use of corticosteroids comes with significant risks [17].

The lack of treatment options has led to the development of interleukin 12 and 23 (IL-12/IL-23) inhibitors, another group of monoclonal antibodies, the most common being Ustekinamab [18]. IL-12/IL-23 are pro-inflammatory cytokines, sharing a similar p40 subunit, which are produced by immune cells in response to antigens [18]. The first generation of IL-12/IL-23 monoclonal antibodies, primarily the drug Ustekinamb, blocks the shared p40 subunits of the two cytokines, but increased understanding of the pathophysiology of CD has led to the development of selective anti-IL-23 monoclonal antibodies, which inhibit the p19 subunit of IL-23 while preserving IL-12 functionality [17,18]. Examples of the selective anti-IL-23 monoclonal antibodies include Mirikizumab, Risankizumab, and Guselkumab [11].

IL-12/IL-23 inhibitors are active proteins and therefore have been traditionally administered using the intravenous route [19,20]. For the treatment of CD, IL-12/IL-23 inhibitors are administered through a series of intravenous infusions [21]. Advantages of the intravenous administration of IL-12/IL-23 inhibitors include a quicker drug effect, better control of dosages, continuous drug administration, and larger dose infusion and allows drug administration in people who are unable to take drugs via oral and other routes [22]. Recent advances have resulted in formulations of IL-12/IL-23 inhibitors that can be delivered via subcutaneous injections [20]. This route enhances adherence and lowers treatment costs, as it allows self-administration, improves individual mobility, reduces hospital stay, reduces overall costs, and enables the administration of biologics in people with poor venous access [22]. Additionally, subcutaneous injections typically take minutes compared to the hours needed for intravenous infusions, which makes it a compelling and efficient alternative, favored by both individuals and healthcare providers [23,24].

Results from randomized controlled trials that have compared the efficacy of subcutaneous and intravenous administration of IL-12/IL-23 inhibitors have been inconsistent [25–31]. Generally, subcutaneous IL-12/IL-23 inhibitors were found to be inferior in efficacy when compared to intravenous infusion for the induction of remission [28–30]. One study, however, demonstrated the superiority of the subcutaneous route for the induction of CD remission [25]. For the maintenance of remission, there are only a few studies, and their findings suggest that subcutaneous administration of IL-12/IL-23 inhibitors may match or supersede the efficacy of intravenous infusions [30,31]. Given the disparity in the results of existing clinical trials, there is a need to synthesize existing evidence on the comparative efficacy of subcutaneous and intravenous routes of IL-12/IL-23 inhibitors, to enable clinicians to make informed choices with their patients. In this meta-analysis, we synthesized the evidence from existing randomized controlled trials on the efficacy and safety of the subcutaneous route of administration of IL-12/IL-23 inhibitors compared to the intravenous infusion, for CD remission.

2. Methods

2.1. Study Design

This is a systematic review and meta-analysis which was conducted according to the Preferred Reporting Items for Systematic Reviews and Meta-Analyses (PRISMA) guidelines [32]. The protocol for this study is registered in the International Prospective Register of Systematic Reviews (PROSPERO) (CRD42024484820).

2.2. Data Sources

A search was conducted of Cochrane Central Register of Controlled Trials (CENTRAL), Scopus, PubMed, Cumulated Index to Nursing and Allied Health Literature (CINAHL), the databases of preprints (medRXIV), Google Scholar, ClinicalTrials.gov, and references. This search covered databases up to the 20th of September 2024, with no language restrictions. The search strategy is shown in the Supplementary Materials.

2.3. Search Terms

2.3.1. Search Terms for Interleukin 12/23 Inhibitors

"Monoclonal antibody" OR "Monoclonal antibodies" OR "Biologics" OR "Ustekinumab" OR "Stelara" OR "Wezlana" OR "CNTO-1275" OR "CNTO1275" OR "anti-IL-12" OR "anti-IL-23" OR "Anti-IL-12/23 Therapy" OR "IL-12/23 Blocker" OR "IL-12/23 Inhibitor" OR "Guselkumab" OR "Tremfya" OR "Risankizumab" OR "Skyrizi" OR "Brazikumab" OR "Mirikizumab" OR "Omvoh".

2.3.2. Search Terms for Crohn's Disease

"Crohn's Disease" OR "Crohns Disease" OR "Crohn Disease" OR "CD" OR "Crohn's Enteritis" OR "Regional Enteritis" OR "Ileocolitis" OR "Ileitis, Terminal" OR "Terminal

Ileitis" OR "Ileitis, Regional" OR "Regional Ileitides" OR "Regional Ileitis" OR "Enteritis, Granulomatous" OR "Granulomatous Enteritis" OR "Refractory Crohn's Disease" OR "Severe Crohn's Disease" OR "Mild-to-Moderate Crohn's Disease".

2.3.3. Search Terms for Route of Administration

"Subcutaneous" OR "SC" OR "SQ" OR "SubQ" OR "Sub-Q" OR "Subcut" OR "SubC" OR "Subcu" OR "Hypodermic" OR "Hypodermal" OR "Intracutaneous" OR "Intravenous" OR "Drip" OR "Endovenous" OR "IV" OR "Venous" OR "Infusion"

2.4. Procedure for the Selection of Studies

The study records obtained from the literature search were imported into EndNote 20 software for de-duplication. Subsequently, the records were uploaded to the Rayyan systematic review management website (https://www.rayyan.ai/ (accessed on 17 August 2024)) for screening based on the title and abstract. Preliminarily included study records were then retrieved in full text and manually assessed for eligibility by two independent investigators. In cases of disagreement, a third investigator was consulted to make the final decision.

2.5. Eligibility

Studies were eligible for inclusion if they were RCTs evaluating the efficacy and safety of subcutaneous compared to intravenous IL-12/IL-23 inhibitors in participants with CD. We excluded observational studies and trials where the comparator was placebo. This approach was adopted to ensure that only studies with a direct, head-to-head comparison between subcutaneous and intravenous administration of IL-12/IL-23 inhibitors in CD were included.

2.6. Outcomes

The primary efficacy outcomes were the induction and maintenance of remission, which were defined by the Crohn's Disease Activity Index (CDAI) as asymptomatic remission <150 or a Harvey Bradshaw Index (HBI) of $\leq$4 points [33]. The secondary efficacy outcomes were endoscopic remission, defined as a Simple Endoscopic Score for Crohn's Disease (SES-CD) of 0–2, and endoscopic response, defined as a $\geq$50% reduction from baseline in SES-CD [34]. The primary safety outcome was any adverse events. The secondary safety outcomes were all-cause mortality, treatment discontinuation, and serious adverse events.

2.7. Data Extraction

Data were extracted from the included studies on Microsoft Excel. Eight authors (NA, RI, HA, K-HA, M-AA, N-AA, W-NA, YA) independently extracted data on the characteristics such as study design, date, location, number of participants, and selected demographic characteristics (e.g., age, gender, comorbidities, type, and severity of CD). Data regarding the treatment regimen included the drugs used, the dosages, and the duration of treatment. Data related to the study outcome included the number of individuals in both the subcutaneous and intravenous groups who achieved induced remission, the number of participants in these groups who maintained remission, the number of individuals who developed at least one adverse event, and the number of individuals that developed at least one serious adverse event, death, or treatment discontinuation.

2.8. Assessing the Quality of Included Studies

The quality of the included studies was evaluated using the Methodological Standard for Epidemiological Research (MASTER) scale, comprising seven domains subdivided into 36 safeguards [35]. These domains are to assess the internal validity of included studies including selection bias, information bias, confounding, and bias in the study design and in the analysis and interpretation of results.

2.9. Data Synthesis

Characteristics of included studies are displayed in tables and narratively described. For outcomes (maintenance of remission and endoscopic remission) where there were insufficient studies for meta-analysis, results are described narratively. A meta-analysis was carried out for induction, endoscopic response, mortality, and safety outcomes using a bias-adjusted meta-analysis model—the quality-effects model [36]—which is a model under the common parameters assumption. The study level unadjusted odds ratios (ORs) and their 95% CIs were recalculated for each of the binary outcomes and then synthesized to compute overall effects as this is considered the optimal binary measure in meta-analysis [37]. The quality-effects model modifies variance weights using the quality ranking of the studies, thereby decreasing bias in the synthesized results [38]. Sensitivity analysis was conducted using leave-one-out analysis. We used the I^2 statistic, Cochran's Q p-value, and tau^2 to quantify heterogeneity, and I^2 values of 25%, 50%, and 75% were assigned into low, moderate, and high inconsistency categories, respectively [39,40]. We investigated publication bias using Doi plots and the LFK index [41]. GRADE was used to report the evidence for each outcome. We used Stata version 18 (College Station, TX, USA) with the *metan* module in Stata.

2.10. Ethics

This systematic review utilized published data; therefore, there was no need for ethical approval.

3. Results

3.1. Search Results

A total of 3287 studies were identified through the search. After eliminating duplicates and a manual screening process based on the title and abstract, 37 studies underwent full-text screening. Out of these, 30 studies were excluded for the reasons indicated in Figure 1. After the full-text screening, most of the studies were excluded because they did not compare the administration routes (n = 12). Ultimately, seven trials were included [25–31], four of them were included in the induction analysis [25,28–30], two studies were included in the maintenance analysis [30,31], and two trials did not provide data on either induction or maintenance [26,27]. Further, seven RCTs [25–31] were included in the analysis of adverse events and serious adverse events [25–31], five trials in the treatment discontinuation analysis [25,28–31], and six trials in the mortality analysis [25–29,31].

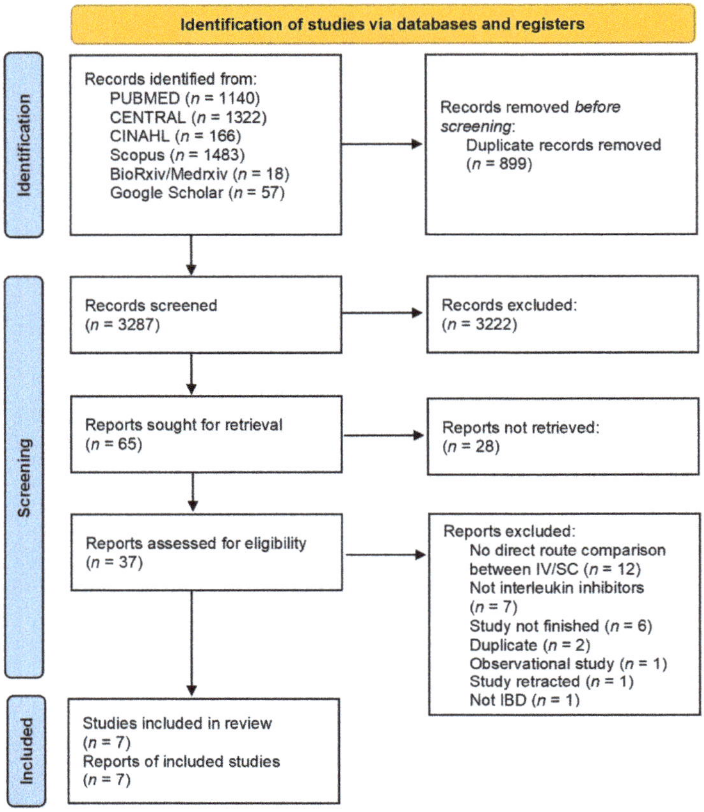

Figure 1. PRISMA flow diagram.

3.2. Characteristics of Included Studies

The seven selected studies [25–31] involved 2179 participants from more than 40 countries with most studies from the United States, Canada, and Germany. All seven trials included participants with moderate to severe CD [25–31]. Three of the studies [28–30] investigated subcutaneous Ustekinumab, two investigated Risankizumab [26,27], one investigated subcutaneous Mirikizumab [31], and one investigated Brazikumab [25]. However, the two studies [26,27] that compared subcutaneous to intravenous Risankizumab only reported data on adverse events. The characteristics of the included studies are shown in Table 1.

Table 1. Characteristics of included studies.

Author, Year	Type of IBD	Specific Biologic	SC/IV Sample Size	Phase of Remission	Follow-Up Period (Months)	Mechanism of Action
Schreiber, 2023 [28] (NCT,03782376)	Crohn's Disease	SC: Ustekinumab: 90 mg IV: Ustekinumab: 6 mg/kg	SC:107 IV:108	Induction	8	IL-12/IL-23 Inhibitor
Sandborn, 2008 [30] (NCT,00265122)	Crohn's Disease	SC: Ustekinumab: 90 mg IV: Ustekinumab: 4.5 mg/kg	SC:65 IV:66	Induction and Maintenance	5.22	IL-12/IL-23 Inhibitor
Sandborn, 2022 [29] (NCT,03466411)	Crohn's Disease	SC: Ustekinumab: 90 mg IV: Guselkumab: 200 mg, 600 mg, 1200 mg	SC:63 IV:185	Induction	2.78	IL-12/IL-23 Inhibitor
Sands, 2021 [31] (NCT,02891226)	Crohn's Disease	SC: Mirikizumab: 300 mg IV: Mirikizumab: 1000 mg	SC:46 IV:41	Maintenance	12	IL-23 Inhibitor
NCT,02574637 [25]	Crohn's Disease	SC: Brazikumab: 35, 70, 105, 210 mg IV: Brazikumab: 700 mg	SC:10 IV:5	Induction	6.4	IL-23 Inhibitor
NCT,03104413 [26]	Crohn's Disease	SC: Risankizumab: 180, 360 mg IV: Risankizumab: 1200 mg	SC: 83 IV: 453	Adverse events	10.1	IL-23 Inhibitor
NCT,03105128 [27]	Crohn's Disease	SC: Risankizumab: 180, 360 mg IV: Risankizumab: 1200 mg	SC:135 IV:812	Adverse events	10.1	IL-23 Inhibitor

3.3. Assessment of the Quality of Included Studies

Most of the included trials obtained MASTER scale scores ranging from 32 to 35 out of 36, with an average of 33.5, signifying an overall high quality of evidence (Supplementary Figure S1 and Supplementary Table S1). The temporal precedence domains were met by all the studies except one [28] because of the possible presence of carry-over effects. All the trials were multicenter trials and therefore the safeguard of equal care delivery was not met.

3.4. Induction of Remission

Four RCTs [25,28–30] compared subcutaneous to intravenous IL-12/IL-23 inhibitors for the induction of remission in CD. Three of these trials [28–30] investigated subcutaneous Ustekinumab and the remaining one studied Brazikumab [25]. In the overall synthesis, the odds of inducing remission were reduced by almost 23% in the subcutaneous group compared to the intravenous group (OR 0.77, 95%CI 0.53–1.12), with the confidence interval suggesting that the treatments could be similar, with no-to-low heterogeneity (I^2 = 0%) (Figure 2) and major asymmetry (Supplementary Figure S2), suggesting concerns with publication bias. The Galbraith plot (Supplementary Figure S3) showed an effect near the null, represented by an almost horizontal line. The results were consistent after sensitivity analysis using leave-one-out (Supplementary Figure S4), and after restricting the analysis to Ustekinumab only. The summary GRADE rating for this outcome was of moderate-certainty evidence (Supplementary Table S2).

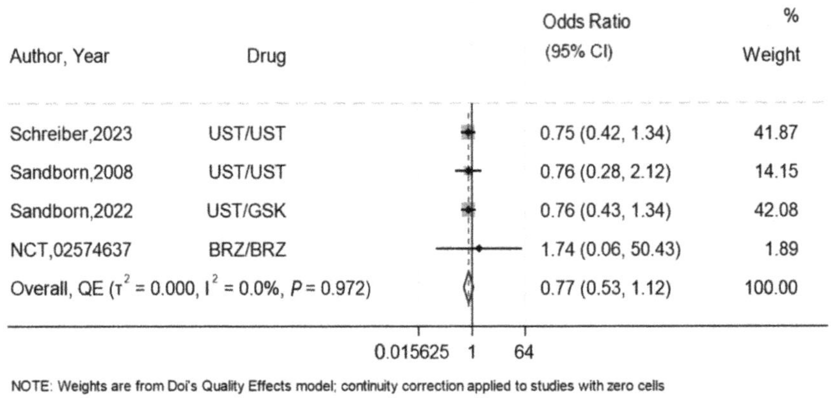

Figure 2. Forest plot showing efficacy of subcutaneous compared to intravenous interleukin 12/23 inhibitors for induction of remission. NB: This forest plot shows the overall analysis for the odds of inducing remission using the subcutaneous compared to the intravenous route in four RCTs [25,28–30]. The figure includes a line of no effect (vertical black line), meta-analytical estimates with confidence intervals (blue diamonds), study weights (gray boxes), study effect sizes (black dots), confidence intervals for study effect sizes (horizontal black lines), and a line representing the overall odds ratio (red dotted line). Abbreviations: Ustekinumab (UST), Guselkumab (GSK), and Brazikumab (BRZ).

3.5. *Maintenance of Remission*

Two RCTs [30,31] compared subcutaneous to intravenous IL-12/IL-23 inhibitors for maintaining CD remission. The first trial [30] showed nearly 40% higher odds in achieving remission with subcutaneous compared to intravenous Ustekinumab in weeks 12 and 16, while week 14 showed nearly the same odds of maintaining remission in both routes. The second trial [31] showed higher odds of maintaining remission when subcutaneous Mirikizumab was used compared to the intravenous route (Supplementary Figure S5).

3.6. *Endoscopic Response and Remission*

Three RCTs [28,29,31] reported endoscopic response, and the overall odds ratio and its 95%CI suggested no difference in the odds of achieving an endoscopic response with the subcutaneous administration compared to the intravenous administration, with no-to-low heterogeneity (OR 0.73, 95%CI 0.46–1.15, I^2 = 0%) and no asymmetry in the Doi plots, suggesting no publication bias (Supplementary Figures S6 and S7). The summary GRADE rating for endoscopic response was of high-certainty evidence (Supplementary Table S2). Two RCTs [28,31] reported endoscopic remission (Supplementary Figure S8). The first trial [28] showed a 76% decrease in the odds of achieving endoscopic remission using subcutaneous compared to intravenous Ustekinumab (OR 0.24, 95%CI 0.06–0.90). The second trial [31] showed two-fold higher odds of achieving endoscopic remission using subcutaneous compared to intravenous Mirikizumab (OR 2.00, 95%CI 0.74–5.36).

3.7. *Any Adverse Events and Serious Adverse Events*

A total of seven RCTs reported adverse events [25–31], and the overall effect estimate showed similar odds of adverse events with subcutaneous administration compared to intravenous, with low heterogeneity (OR 0.91, 95%CI 0.63–1.32, I^2 = 39%) and no asymmetry in the Doi plot, suggesting no publication bias (Figure 3A, Supplementary Figure S9). Data from the same seven RCTs [25–31] reported the serious adverse events, with the overall effect showing nearly the same odds of serious adverse events, with no-to-low heterogeneity (OR 0.97, 95%CI 0.61–1.53, I^2 = 0%) and minor asymmetry in the Doi plot suggesting little-to-no publication bias (Figure 3B, Supplementary Figure S10). The summary GRADE rating for both outcomes was of high-certainty evidence (Supplementary Table S2).

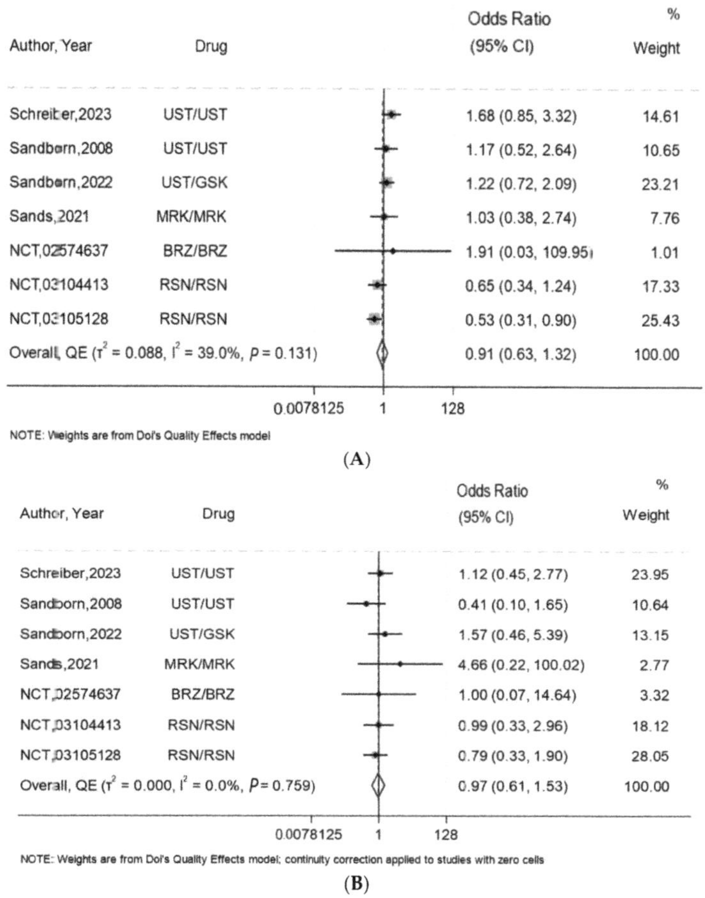

Figure 3. Forest plots showing adverse events and serious adverse events of subcutaneous compared to intravenous interleukin 12/23 inhibitors. NB: This forest plot shows the analysis of the safety outcomes of (**A**) the development of adverse events and (**B**) serious adverse events in individuals with CD using subcutaneous compared to the intravenous interleukin 12/23 inhibitors in seven RCTs [25–31]. The figure includes a line of no effect (vertical black line), meta-analytical estimates with confidence intervals (blue diamonds), study weights (gray boxes), study effect sizes (black dots), confidence intervals for study effect sizes (horizontal black lines), and a line representing the overall odds ratio (red dotted line). Abbreviations: Ustekinumab (UST), Guselkumab (GSK), Brazikumab (BRZ), Mirikizumab (MRK), and Risankizumab (RSN).

3.7.1. Treatment Discontinuation

Overall, five RCTs [25,28–31] reported data on treatment discontinuation, and the overall effect estimate showed almost similar odds of treatment discontinuation with subcutaneous compared to intravenous administration, with no-to-low heterogeneity (OR 1.06, 95%CI 0.67–1.68, $I^2 = 0\%$) (Figure 4, Supplementary Figure S11). The summary GRADE rating for this outcome was of moderate-certainty evidence due to possible publication bias (Supplementary Table S2). The most common reasons for discontinuation across both groups were due to lack of efficacy and voluntary withdrawal (Supplementary Table S3).

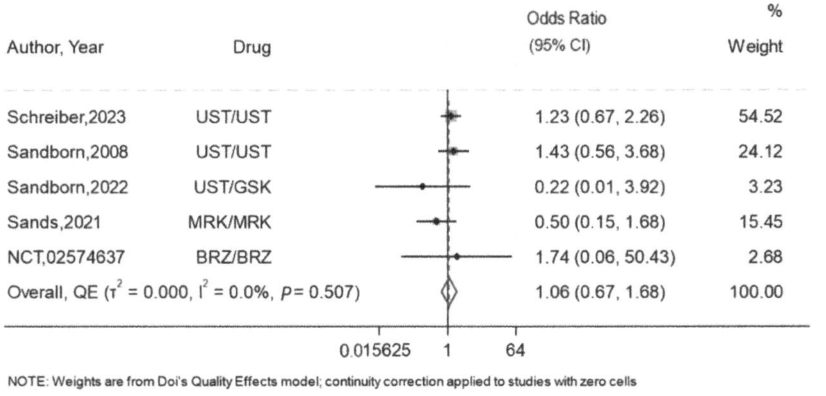

Figure 4. Forest plot for the effect of subcutaneous compared to intravenous interleukin 12/23 inhibitors on treatment discontinuation. NB: This forest plot shows the overall analysis for the odds of treatment discontinuation with the subcutaneous compared to the intravenous route using IL12/23 inhibitors in five RCTs [25,28–31]. The figure includes a line of no effect (vertical black line), meta-analytical estimates with confidence intervals (blue diamonds), study weights (gray boxes), study effect sizes (black dots), confidence intervals for study effect sizes (horizontal black lines), and a line representing the overall odds ratio (red dotted line). Abbreviations: Ustekinumab (UST), Guselkumab (GSK), Brazikumab (BRZ), and Mirikizumab (MRK).

3.7.2. Hospitalization

One RCT [29] reported the number of hospitalizations, and the results suggested similar odds of hospitalization in the subcutaneous arm compared to the intravenous arm (OR 0.97, 95%CI 0.04–24.08).

3.7.3. Mortality

Out of the included RCTs, six reported the mortality outcome [25–29,31]. The overall synthesis showed almost similar odds of mortality in the subcutaneous compared to the intravenous route, with no-to-low heterogeneity (OR 1.17, 95%CI 0.27–5.20, $I^2 = 0\%$) (Figure 5) and no evidence of publication bias (Supplementary Figure S12). The summary GRADE rating for this outcome was of high-certainty evidence (Supplementary Table S2).

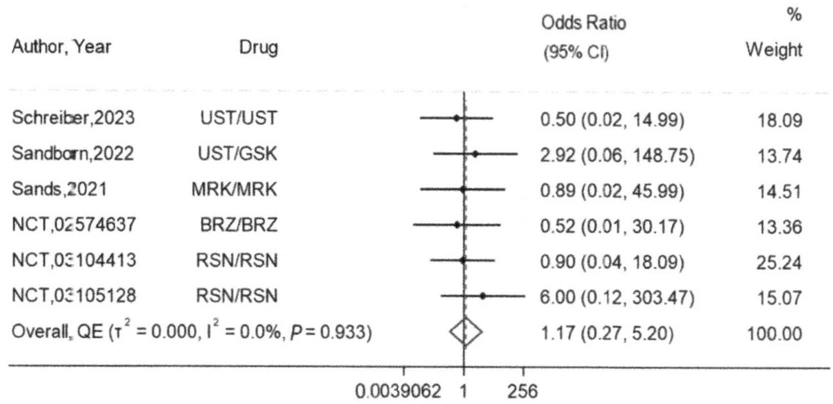

Figure 5 Forest plot for the effect of subcutaneous compared to intravenous interleukin 12/23 inhibitors on mortality. NB: This forest plot shows the overall analysis for the odds of mortality using the subcutaneous compared to the intravenous route in six RCTs [25–29,31]. The figure includes a line of no effect (vertical black line), meta-analytical estimates with confidence intervals (blue diamonds), study weights (gray boxes), study effect sizes (black dots), confidence intervals for study effect sizes (horizontal black lines), and a line representing the overall odds ratio (red dotted line). Abbreviations: Ustekinumab (UST), Guselkumab (GSK), Brazikumab (BRZ), and Mirikizumab (MRK).

4. Discussion

In this meta-analysis of seven RCTs, we found that subcutaneous administration of IL-12/IL-23 inhibitors, compared to intravenous administration, was associated with a small non-significant decrease in efficacy when used for induction of remission in individuals with CD. As for the safety of subcutaneous IL-12/IL-23 inhibitors, similar odds of adverse events were observed compared to intravenous IL-12/IL-23 inhibitors. However, for the maintenance of remission, data from two trials suggested that the subcutaneous route was similar to the intravenous in efficacy. Additionally, the subcutaneous route showed almost similar odds of mortality compared to the intravenous route.

We found that subcutaneous administration showed no difference in the odds of induction of remission in individuals with CD, with low-certainty GRADE evidence. The one existing meta-analysis comparing the subcutaneous and intravenous administration of IL-12/IL-23 inhibitors for the induction of CD remission used observational studies, which is associated with key methodological limitations [42], including an indirect comparison of the two administration routes across studies that were performed separately for each of the routes. This lacks the rigor of a head-to-head trial, as the study populations were different. While the analysis concluded that subcutaneous Ustekinumab was superior in inducing a clinical response, the conclusions are not based on high-quality data and analysis. Notably, current guidelines do not provide explicit recommendations regarding the subcutaneous route for the induction phase, due to the lack of robust evidence regarding the efficacy of subcutaneous interleukin inhibitors compared to the intravenous route, which this meta-analysis now addresses.

Our findings suggest that subcutaneous administration of IL-12/IL-23 inhibitors had similar odds of maintaining remission compared to the intravenous route. However, our findings are limited as only two RCTs have so far been conducted and have provided data for maintaining remission. One of the two RCTs [30] showed that subcutaneous Ustekinumab increased the odds of maintaining remission by 40% and 44% in weeks 12 and 16, respectively. The second included RCT [31] and showed a two-fold increase in the odds of maintaining remission in subcutaneous compared to intravenous Mirikizumab at 52 weeks.

In both trials, the 95%CIs include the null, suggesting that the two routes could be similar. There are no existing meta-analyses that compare the two routes of administration of IL-12/IL-23 inhibitors in maintaining remission. Nonetheless, some meta-analyses have shown that subcutaneous administration of anti-TNF-α monoclonal antibodies, which are another class of biologics commonly prescribed to individuals with CD, may result in similar efficacy to intravenous infusions. Subcutaneous adalimumab showed similar efficacy in maintaining remission in individuals with CD compared to intravenous Infliximab in one published meta-analysis [43]. The same has been observed for subcutaneous infliximab when compared to intravenous infliximab or subcutaneous/intravenous Vedolizumab in another meta-analysis of 13 RCTs, although this study had limitations of indirect comparisons [44]. Despite the different mechanism of action between these drugs and IL 12/23 inhibitors, the findings support the results of subcutaneous IL 12/23 inhibitors in maintaining remission in the tow studies in this current meta-analysis. Although there are multiple available IL-12/IL-23 inhibitors, the current European Crohn's and Colitis Organization (ECCO) guidelines recommend the use of subcutaneous Ustekinumab to maintain clinical remission in individuals with CD who achieved remission with Ustekinumab [45]. This might be due to the lack of data on subcutaneous formulations of other monoclonal antibodies. For example, there are two RCTs, the ADVANCE and MOTIVATE trials, which initially set out to compare subcutaneous to intravenous Risankizumab, in addition to intravenous vs. placebo [46]. However, the two trials have not reported the efficacy findings of the comparison for subcutaneous and intravenous administration of this selective IL-23 blocker and data on safety comparisons used in our meta-analysis were only available on ClinicalTrials.gov [46].

Our current meta-analysis found that adverse events and treatment discontinuation were almost similar between subcutaneous and intravenous IL-12/IL-23 inhibitors. Again, there are no previous meta-analyses that compare either adverse events or drug discontinuation between the two routes of administration, both of which are key factors in influencing outcomes, especially in individuals who are refractory to other therapies. Although there was a slight increase in the odds of mortality in the subcutaneous group, the confidence interval suggested that there was no clinically important difference in mortality between the two routes of administration. Our findings suggest that it is equally safe to administer IL-12/IL-23 inhibitors via the subcutaneous route as compared to intravenous administration, although more trials are still required. A similar safety profile is important for individuals on biologic treatment, as many report preferring intravenous over subcutaneous administration because they feel safer in a hospital setting [47]. Thus, with a similar safety profile, providers can reassure individuals that the subcutaneous formulation is as safe as the intravenous one, and that they can return to the hospital if they feel any side-effects.

The strength of this meta-analysis includes the comprehensive search and rigorous analysis that was carried out, and the use of GRADE evidence of certainty makes the results easier for translation into practice guidelines and clinical practice. To the best of our knowledge, this study provides the only direct comparison between subcutaneous and intravenous IL-12/IL-23 inhibitors administration using data from RCTs, both of which are available for induction and maintenance of remission. A limitation of this study is that there were insufficient data on the maintenance of remission in CD, limiting our ability to draw reliable conclusions. Limitations of the included studies include the lack of consistent and objective measures of remission, the variable induction timing between the studies, the lack of classification of disease severity, and the lack of data on the use of rescue steroids during the trial period in most studies. Additionally, two trials, the ADVANCE [46] and the MOTIVATE [46], have published data on just the intravenous versus placebo comparisons and therefore could not be included in the efficacy outcomes. More trials that compared the subcutaneous and intravenous routes for IL-12/IL-23 inhibitors are needed to improve evidence certainty.

5. Conclusions

In individuals with moderate to severe CD, subcutaneous administration of IL-12/IL-23 inhibitors has similar efficacy to intravenous administration for the induction and maintenance of CD remission and safety. However, for robust conclusions about the use of this route for IL12/23 inhibitors for the maintenance of CD remission, more studies are needed.

Supplementary Materials: The following supporting information can be downloaded at https://www.mdpi.com/article/10.3390/biomedicines13030702/s1. Figure S1: Quality assessment of included studies using the MASTER scale/Equal Recruitment (brown) has 4 safeguards, Equal Retention (dark green) has 5 safeguards, Equal Ascertainment (sky blue) has 7 safeguards, Equal Implantation (purple) has 6 safeguards, Equal Prognosis (light green) has 6 safeguards, Sufficient Analysis (blue) has 3 safeguards, Temporal Precedence has 5 safeguards (yellow); Figure S2: DOI plot for induction of remission/The Doi plot shows major asymmetry, confirmed by the LFK index = 4.20, indicating asymmetry and that publication bias is more likely to be present; Figure S3: Galbraith plot for induction of remission/The Galbraith plot shows the four studies that reported the induction of remission at the highest timepoint of the study, one study is overlapping with another study. The regression line showed an effect near the null. All studies, fall within the 95% CIs (the dashed lines) suggesting no heterogeneity; Figure S4: Sensitivity analysis for the induction/The forest plot shows the Sensitivity analysis for (A) the induction of remission to examine the influence of each study on the meta-analytic outcome estimate(A). (B) shows the induction of remission with Ustekinumab only. The results support those of the main outcome analysis of inducing and maintaining remission. Abbreviations: Ustekinumab (UST), Guselkumab (GSK), Brazikumab (BRZ); Figure S5: Descriptive Forest plot for maintenance of CD remission/This forest plot shows the results of two trials that compared maintenance of CD remission between subcutaneous and intravenous routes. The first trial measured outcomes at three time-points (12, 14 and 16 weeks). The study results were not meta-analysed because data from the different weeks for Sandborn 2008 came from the same participants. Abbreviations: Ustekinumab (UST), Mirikizumab (MRK); Figure S6: Forest plot for endoscopic response/The forest plot shows the results of trials that compared the subcutaneous to the intravenous routes in achieving endoscopic response. Abbreviations: Ustekinumab (UST), Guselkumab (GSK), Mirikizumab (MRK); Figure S7: Doi plot for endoscopic response/The Doi plot shows no asymmetry, confirmed by the LFK index = −0.65 indicating no publication bias; Figure S8: Descriptive Forest plot for endoscopic remission/This forest plot shows the results of two trials that compared endoscopic remission of CD between subcutaneous and intravenous routes. Mirikizumab shows two-fold increase in the odds, while Ustekinumab shows 76% decrease in the odds of endoscopic remission; Figure S9: Doi plot for developing adverse events/The Doi plot shows no asymmetry, confirmed by the LFK index = 0.47 indicating no publication bias; Figure S10: Doi plot for developing serious adverse events/The Doi plot shows minor asymmetry, confirmed by the LFK index =1.28 suggesting publication bias is less likely; Figure S11: Doi plot for drug discontinuation/The Doi plot shows major asymmetry, confirmed by the LFK index =-2.44 suggesting presence of publication bias; Figure S12: Doi plot for mortality/The Doi plot shows no asymmetry, confirmed by the LFK index =1.00 suggesting absence of publication bias; Table S1: MASTER scale; Table S2: GRADE Rating for main outcomes; Table S3: Reasons for treatment discontinuation.

Author Contributions: N.A.—Conceptualization, Investigation, Formal Analysis, Validation, Visualization, Data Curation, Resources, Software, Methodology, Writing—Original Draft Preparation, Writing—Review and Editing, and Project Administration. R.I.—Conceptualization, Investigation, Formal Analysis, Validation, Visualization, Data Curation, Resources, Software, Methodology, Writing—Original Draft Preparation, and Writing—Review and Editing. H.A.-K.—Conceptualization, Investigation, Validation, Visualization, Data Curation, Resources, Software, Methodology, Writing—

Original Draft Preparation, and Writing—Review and Editing. K.H.A.-A.—Conceptualization, Investigation, Validation, Visualization, Data Curation, Resources, Software, Methodology, Writing—Original Draft Preparation, and Writing—Review and Editing. M.A.A.-M.—Conceptualization, Investigation, Validation, Visualization, Data Curation, Resources, Software, Methodology, Writing—Original Draft Preparation, and Writing—Review and Editing. N.A.A.—Conceptualization, Investigation, Validation, Visualization, Data Curation, Resources, Software, Methodology, Writing—Original Draft Preparation, and Writing—Review and Editing. W.N.A.-M.—Conceptualization, Investigation, Validation, Visualization, Data Curation, Resources, Software, Methodology, Writing—Original Draft Preparation, and Writing—Review and Editing. Y.A.-K.—Conceptualization, Investigation, Validation, Visualization, Data Curation, Resources, Software, Methodology, Writing—Original Draft Preparation, and Writing—Review and Editing. M.A.-M.—Methodology, Investigation, and Writing—Review and Editing. S.H.—Investigation, Validation, Visualization, Data Curation, Resources, Software, Methodology, and Writing—Review and Editing. S.A.R.D.—Formal Analysis, Methodology, Writing—Review and Editing. H.H.F.—Investigation, Validation, Visualization, Data Curation, Resources, Software, Methodology, Writing—Review and Editing, and Supervision. T.C.—Conceptualization, Investigation, Formal Analysis, Validation, Visualization, Resources, Software, Methodology, Writing—Review and Editing, Supervision, and Guarantor of Review. All authors have read and agreed to the published version of the manuscript.

Funding: This work was supported by the Qatar National Research Fund, Undergraduate Research Experience Program (UREP) (Grant ID: UREP31-179-3-047). Open Access Funding was provided by the Qatar National Library.

Institutional Review Board Statement: Not applicable.

Informed Consent Statement: Not applicable.

Data Availability Statement: This is a meta-analysis. Data are included in primary studies according to policies of parent journals.

Acknowledgments: We would like to express our deepest appreciation to the Department of Population Medicine at Qatar University for their continuous help throughout the research process.

Conflicts of Interest: The authors have no conflicts of interest to declare. All co-authors have seen and agree with the contents of the manuscript and there is no financial interest to report. We certify that the submission is original work and is not under review at any other publication. This manuscript has no conflicts of interest with Hamad Medical Corporation.

References

1. Ungaro, R.C.; Aggarwal, S.; Topaloglu, O.; Lee, W.J.; Clark, R.; Colombel, J.F. Systematic review and meta-analysis: Efficacy and safety of early biologic treatment in adult and paediatric patients with Crohn's disease. *Aliment. Pharmacol. Ther.* **2020**, *51*, 831–842. [CrossRef] [PubMed]
2. Abdallah, B.; Arif, M.; Al-Malki, M.; Hourani, R.; Al-Maadeed, T.; Khodr, N.; Al-Kuwari, G.; Al-Siddiqi, M.; Kane, T.; Chivese, T. The Association Between Inflammatory Bowel Disease and Exposure to Tobacco Smoking: A Case-Control Study in Qatar. *Int. J. Gen. Med.* **2023**, *16*, 233–242. [CrossRef] [PubMed]
3. Chivese, T.; Esterhuizen, T.M.; Basson, A.R.; Watermeyer, G. Correction: The Influence of Second-Hand Cigarette Smoke Exposure during Childhood and Active Cigarette Smoking on Crohn's Disease Phenotype Defined by the Montreal Classification Scheme in a Western Cape Population, South Africa. *PLoS ONE* **2018**, *13*, e0190822. [CrossRef] [PubMed]
4. Ng, S.C.; Shi, H.Y.; Hamidi, N.; Underwood, F.E.; Tang, W.; Benchimol, E.I.; Panaccione, R.; Ghosh, S.; Wu, J.C.Y.; Chan, F.K.L.; et al. Worldwide incidence and prevalence of inflammatory bowel disease in the 21st century: A systematic review of population-based studies. *Lancet* **2017**, *390*, 2769–2778. [CrossRef]
5. Wang, R.; Li, Z.; Liu, S.; Zhang, D. Global, regional and national burden of inflammatory bowel disease in 204 countries and territories from 1990 to 2019: A systematic analysis based on the Global Burden of Disease Study 2019. *BMJ Open* **2023**, *13*, e065186. [CrossRef]
6. Radford, S.J.; McGing, J.; Czuber-Dochan, W.; Moran, G. Systematic review: The impact of inflammatory bowel disease-related fatigue on health-related quality of life. *Frontline Gastroenterol.* **2021**, *12*, 11–21. [CrossRef]

7. Rogler, G.; Singh, A.; Kavanaugh, A.; Rubin, D.T. Extraintestinal Manifestations of Inflammatory Bowel Disease: Current Concepts, Treatment, and Implications for Disease Management. *Gastroenterology* **2021**, *161*, 1118–1132. [CrossRef]
8. Wan, Q.; Zhao, R.; Xia, L.; Wu, Y.; Zhou, Y.; Wang, Y.; Cui, Y.; Shen, X.; Wu, X.T. Inflammatory bowel disease and risk of gastric, small bowel and colorectal cancer: A meta-analysis of 26 observational studies. *J. Cancer Res. Clin. Oncol.* **2021**, *147*, 1077–1087. [CrossRef]
9. Cai, Z.; Wang, S.; Li, J. Treatment of Inflammatory Bowel Disease: A Comprehensive Review. *Front. Med.* **2021**, *8*, 765474. [CrossRef]
10. Hazel, K.; O'Connor, A. Emerging treatments for inflammatory bowel disease. *Ther. Adv. Chronic Dis.* **2020**, *11*, 2040622319899297. [CrossRef]
11. Cosnes, J.; Cattan, S.; Blain, A.; Beaugerie, L.; Carbonnel, F.; Parc, R.; Gendre, J.P. Long-term evolution of disease behavior of Crohn's disease. *Inflamm. Bowel Dis.* **2002**, *8*, 244–250. [CrossRef] [PubMed]
12. Ananthakrishnan, A.N.; Shi, H.Y.; Tang, W.; Law, C.C.; Sung, J.J.; Chan, F.K.; Ng, S.C. Systematic Review and Meta-analysis: Phenotype and Clinical Outcomes of Older-onset Inflammatory Bowel Disease. *J. Crohn's Colitis* **2016**, *10*, 1224–1236. [CrossRef]
13. Parigi, T.L.; D'Amico, F.; Abreu, M.T.; Dignass, A.; Dotan, I.; Magro, F.; Griffiths, A.M.; Jairath, V.; Iacucci, M.; Mantzaris, G.J.; et al. Difficult-to-treat inflammatory bowel disease: Results from an international consensus meeting. *Lancet Gastroenterol. Hepatol.* **2023**, *8*, 853–859. [CrossRef]
14. Breedveld, F.C. Therapeutic monoclonal antibodies. *Lancet* **2000**, *355*, 735–740. [CrossRef] [PubMed]
15. Lamb, C.A.; Kennedy, N.A.; Raine, T.; Hendy, P.A.; Smith, P.J.; Limdi, J.K.; Hayee, B.; Lomer, M.C.E.; Parkes, G.C.; Selinger, C.; et al. British Society of Gastroenterology consensus guidelines on the management of inflammatory bowel disease in adults. *Gut* **2019**, *68* (Suppl. S3), s1–s106. [CrossRef]
16. Feuerstein, J.D.; Ho, E.Y.; Shmidt, E.; Singh, H.; Falck-Ytter, Y.; Sultan, S.; Terdiman, J.P. AGA Clinical Practice Guidelines on the Medical Management of Moderate to Severe Luminal and Perianal Fistulizing Crohn's Disease. *Gastroenterology* **2021**, *160*, 2496–2508. [CrossRef]
17. Gisbert, J.P.; Chaparro, M. Predictors of Primary Response to Biologic Treatment [Anti-TNF, Vedolizumab, and Ustekinumab] in Patients with Inflammatory Bowel Disease: From Basic Science to Clinical Practice. *J. Crohn's Colitis* **2020**, *14*, 694–709. [CrossRef]
18. Fanizza, J.; D'Amico, F.; Lusetti, F.; Fasulo, E.; Allocca, M.; Furfaro, F.; Zilli, A.; Parigi, T.L.; Radice, S.; Peyrin-Biroulet, L.; et al. The Role of IL-23 Inhibitors in Crohn's Disease. *J. Clin. Med.* **2023**, *13*, 224. [CrossRef] [PubMed]
19. Jin, J.F.; Zhu, L.L.; Chen, M.; Xu, H.M.; Wang, H.F.; Feng, X.Q.; Zhu, X.P.; Zhou, Q. The optimal choice of medication administration route regarding intravenous, intramuscular, and subcutaneous injection. *Patient Prefer. Adherence* **2015**, *9*, 923–942. [CrossRef]
20. Xu, Z.; Leu, J.H.; Xu, Y.; Nnane, I.; Liva, S.G.; Wang-Lin, S.X.; Kudgus-Lokken, R.; Vermeulen, A.; Ouellet, D. Development of Therapeutic Proteins for a New Subcutaneous Route of Administration After the Establishment of Intravenous Dosages: A Systematic Review. *Clin. Pharmacol. Ther.* **2023**, *113*, 1011–1029. [CrossRef]
21. Ordás, I.; Mould, D.R.; Feagan, B.G.; Sandborn, W.J. Anti-TNF monoclonal antibodies in inflammatory bowel disease: Pharmacokinetics-based dosing paradigms. *Clin. Pharmacol. Ther.* **2012**, *91*, 635–646. [CrossRef] [PubMed]
22. Stoner, K.L.; Harder, H.; Fallowfield, L.J.; Jenkins, V.A. Intravenous versus Subcutaneous Drug Administration. Which Do Patients Prefer? A Systematic Review. *Patient* **2014**, *8*, 145–153. [CrossRef] [PubMed]
23. De Cock, E.; Pivot, X.; Hauser, N.; Verma, S.; Kritikou, P.; Millar, D.; Knoop, A. A time and motion study of subcutaneous versus intravenous trastuzumab in patients with HER2-positive early breast cancer. *Cancer Med.* **2016**, *5*, 389–397. [CrossRef] [PubMed]
24. Schreiber, S.; Ben-Horin, S.; Leszczyszyn, J.; Dudkowiak, R.; Lahat, A.; Gawdis-Wojnarska, B.; Pukitis, A.; Horynski, M.; Farkas, K.; Kierkus, J.; et al. Randomized Controlled Trial: Subcutaneous vs Intravenous Infliximab CT-P13 Maintenance in Inflammatory Bowel Disease. *Gastroenterology* **2021**, *160*, 2340–2353. [CrossRef] [PubMed]
25. NCT02574637. Evaluation of Efficacy and Safety of Brazikumab (MEDI2070) in Participants with Active, Moderate to Severe Crohn's Disease. 2021. Available online: https://clinicaltrials.gov/study/NCT02574637 (accessed on 3 February 2024).
26. NCT03104413. A Study to Assess the Efficacy and Safety of Risankizumab in Participants with Moderately to Severely Active Crohn's Disease Who Failed Prior Biologic Treatment. 2022. Available online: https://clinicaltrials.gov/study/NCT03104413 (accessed on 28 February 2024).
27. NCT03105128. A Study of the Efficacy and Safety of Risankizumab in Participants with Moderately to Severely Active Crohn's Disease. 2022. Available online: https://clinicaltrials.gov/study/NCT03105128 (accessed on 28 February 2024).
28. Schreiber, S.W.; Lee, S.; van der Woude, C.J.; Marín-Jiménez, I.; Wolf, D.; Schnoy, E.; Salzberg, B.; Busse, C.; Nazar, M.; Langholff, W.; et al. P436 Efficacy and safety of intravenous ustekinumab re-induction therapy in Crohn's disease patients with secondary loss of response to ustekinumab maintenance therapy: Week 16 results from the POWER trial. *J. Crohn's Colitis* **2023**, *17* (Suppl. S1), i564–i566. [CrossRef]
29. Sandborn, W.J.; D'Haens, G.R.; Reinisch, W.; Panés, J.; Chan, D.; Gonzalez, S.; Weisel, K.; Germinaro, M.; Frustaci, M.E.; Yang, Z.; et al. Guselkumab for the Treatment of Crohn's Disease: Induction Results From the Phase 2 GALAXI-1 Study. *Gastroenterology* **2022**, *162*, 1650–1664.e8. [CrossRef]

30. Sandborn, W.J.; Feagan, B.G.; Fedorak, R.N.; Scherl, E.; Fleisher, M.R.; Katz, S.; Johanns, J.; Blank, M.; Rutgeerts, P. A randomized trial of Ustekinumab, a human interleukin-12/23 monoclonal antibody, in patients with moderate-to-severe Crohn's disease. *Gastroenterology* **2008**, *135*, 1130–1141. [CrossRef]
31. Sands, B.E.; Peyrin-Biroulet, L.; Kierkus, J.; Higgins, P.D.R.; Fischer, M.; Jairath, V.; Hirai, F.; D'Haens, G.; Belin, R.M.; Miller, D.; et al. Efficacy and Safety of Mirikizumab in a Randomized Phase 2 Study of Patients with Crohn's Disease. *Gastroenterology* **2021**, *162*, 495–508. [CrossRef]
32. Page, M.J.; McKenzie, J.E.; Bossuyt, P.M.; Boutron, I.; Hoffmann, T.C.; Mulrow, C.D.; Shamseer, L.; Tetzlaff, J.M.; Akl, E.A.; Brennan, S.E.; et al. The PRISMA 2020 statement: An updated guideline for reporting systematic reviews. *BMJ* **2021**, *372*, n71. [CrossRef]
33. Harvey, R.F.; Bradshaw, J.M. A simple index of Crohn's-disease activity. *Lancet* **1980**, *1*, 514. [CrossRef]
34. Vuitton, L.; Marteau, P.; Sandborn, W.J.; Levesque, B.G.; Feagan, B.; Vermeire, S.; Danese, S.; D'Haens, G.; Lowenberg, M.; Khanna, R.; et al. IOIBD technical review on endoscopic indices for Crohn's disease clinical trials. *Gut* **2016**, *65*, 1447–1455. [CrossRef] [PubMed]
35. Stone, J.C.; Glass, K.; Clark, J.; Ritskes-Hoitinga, M.; Munn, Z.; Tugwell, P.; Doi, S.A.R. The MethodologicAl STandards for Epidemiological Research (MASTER) scale demonstrated a unified framework for bias assessment. *J. Clin. Epidemiol.* **2021**, *134*, 52–64. [CrossRef]
36. Doi, S.A.; Thalib, L. A quality-effects model for meta-analysis. *Epidemiology* **2008**, *19*, 94–100. [CrossRef]
37. Doi, S.A.; Furuya-Kanamori, L.; Xu, C.; Lin, L.; Chivese, T.; Thalib, L. Controversy and Debate: Questionable utility of the relative risk in clinical research: Paper 1: A call for change to practice. *J. Clin. Epidemiol.* **2022**, *142*, 271–279. [CrossRef] [PubMed]
38. Stone, J.C.; Glass, K.; Munn, Z.; Tugwell, P.; Doi, S.A.R. Comparison of bias adjustment methods in meta-analysis suggests that quality effects modeling may have less limitations than other approaches. *J. Clin. Epidemiol.* **2020**, *117*, 36–45. [CrossRef] [PubMed]
39. Higgins, J.P.T.; Thomas, J.; Chandler, J.; Cumpston, M.; Li, T.; Page, M.J.; Welch, V.A. (Eds.) *Cochrane Handbook for Systematic Reviews of Interventions Version 6.3 (Updated February 2022)*; John Wiley & Sons: Chichester, UK, 2019. Available online: www.training.cochrane.org/handbook (accessed on 18 June 2023).
40. Thompson, S.G. Systematic Review: Why sources of heterogeneity in meta-analysis should be investigated. *BMJ* **1994**, *309*, 1351. [CrossRef]
41. Furuya-Kanamori, L.; Barendregt, J.J.; Doi, S.A.R. A new improved graphical and quantitative method for detecting bias in meta-analysis. *Int. J. Evid. Based Healthc.* **2018**, *16*, 195–203. [CrossRef]
42. Macaluso, F.S.; Maida, M.; Ventimiglia, M.; Cottone, M.; Orlando, A. Effectiveness and safety of Ustekinumab for the treatment of Crohn's disease in real-life experiences: A meta-analysis of observational studies. *Expert. Opin. Biol. Ther.* **2020**, *20*, 193–203. [CrossRef]
43. Yang, H.H.; Huang, Y.; Zhou, X.C.; Wang, R.N. Efficacy and safety of adalimumab in comparison to infliximab for Crohn's disease: A systematic review and meta-analysis. *World J. Clin. Cases* **2022**, *10*, 6091–6104. [CrossRef]
44. Peyrin-Biroulet, L.; Bossuyt, P.; Bettenworth, D.; Loftus, E.V., Jr.; Anjie, S.I.; D'Haens, G.; Saruta, M.; Arkkila, P.; Park, H.; Choi, D.; et al. Comparative Efficacy of Subcutaneous and Intravenous Infliximab and Vedolizumab for Maintenance Treatment of TNF-naive Adult Patients with Inflammatory Bowel Disease: A Systematic Literature Review and Network Meta-analysis. *Dig. Dis. Sci.* **2024**, *69*, 1808–1825. [CrossRef]
45. Gordon, H.; Minozzi, S.; Kopylov, U.; Verstockt, B.; Chaparro, M.; Buskens, C.; Warusavitarne, J.; Agrawal, M.; Allocca, M.; Atreya, R.; et al. ECCO Guidelines on Therapeutics in Crohn's Disease: Medical Treatment. *J. Crohn's Colitis* **2024**, *18*, 1531–1555. [CrossRef] [PubMed]
46. D'Haens, G.; Panaccione, R.; Baert, F.; Bossuyt, P.; Colombel, J.F.; Danese, S.; Dubinsky, M.; Feagan, B.G.; Hisamatsu, T.; Lim, A.; et al. Risankizumab as induction therapy for Crohn's disease: Results from the phase 3 ADVANCE and MOTIVATE induction trials. *Lancet* **2022**, *399*, 2015–2030. [CrossRef] [PubMed]
47. Overton, P.M.; Shalet, N.; Somers, F.; Allen, J.A. Patient Preferences for Subcutaneous versus Intravenous Administration of Treatment for Chronic Immune System Disorders: A Systematic Review. *Patient Prefer. Adherence* **2021**, *15*, 811–834. [CrossRef] [PubMed]

biomedicines

MDPI

Article

High-Throughput Whole-Exome Sequencing and Large-Scale Computational Analysis to Identify the Genetic Biomarkers to Predict the Vedolizumab Response Status in Inflammatory Bowel Disease Patients from Saudi Arabia

Hanin Aljohani [1], Doaa Anbarserry [1], Mahmoud Mosli [2,3,4], Amani Ujaimi [5,6], Duaa Bakhshwin [1], Ramu Elango [5,6,*] and Sameer Alharthi [1,3,*]

1 Department of Clinical Pharmacology, Faculty of Medicine, King Abdulaziz University, Jeddah 22252, Saudi Arabia; hsaleamaljohani@stu.kau.edu sa (H.A.); dserri@kau.edu.sa (D.A.); dbakhshwin@kau.edu.sa (D.B.)
2 Department of Medicine, Faculty of Medicine, King Abdulaziz University, Jeddah 22252, Saudi Arabia; mmosli@kau.edu.sa
3 Inflammatory Bowel Disease Research Group, King Abdulaziz University, Jeddah 22252, Saudi Arabia
4 Inflammatory Bowel Disease Unit, King Abdulaziz University Hospital, King Abdulaziz University, Jeddah 22252, Saudi Arabia
5 Princess Al-Jawahara Cernter of Excellence in Research of Hereditary Disorders (PACER-HD), King Abdulaziz University, Jeddah 22252, Saudi Arabia; aaujaimi@gmail.com
6 Department of Genetic Medicine, Faculty of Medicine, King Abdulaziz University, Jeddah 22252, Saudi Arabia
* Correspondence: relango305@gmail.com (R.E.); salharthe@kau.edu.sa (S.A.)

Abstract: Background/Objectives: Vedolizumab (VDZ) is the new monoclonal drug targeting $\alpha4\beta7$ integrin for patients with moderate/severe IBD. Between 30 and 45% of patients fail to respond to VDZ after 14–16 weeks of treatment. The aim of the study was to explore the genetic profile of vedolizumab-treated Arab IBD patients in Saudi Arabia to identify the potential biomarkers to differentiate the responders from non-responders. **Methods**: A cohort of 16 patients with IBD, including 4 with Crohn's disease and 12 with ulcerative colitis, were recruited. Following 16 weeks of VDZ treatment, nine were found to be responders and seven non-responders. Blood samples were collected for the whole exome sequencing of DNA from all patients. The variants in the whole-exome sequencing data were analyzed with a variety of bioinformatics tools and databases, such as Polyphen2, Mutation Taster, CADD, FATHMM, Open Target Platform, TOPPFun, STRING, and GTEx. **Results**: More than 1.6 million variants from 16 samples were analyzed. The rare variant analysis prioritized NOD2, IL23, IL10, IL27, and TRAF1 genes in non-responders. NOD2, IL23, IL10, IL27, and TRAF1 were found to be the significant IBD risk factors in multiple genome-wide association studies, and their pro-inflammatory activity might contribute to the inherent resistance to VDZ. Rare variants of CARD9, TYK2, IL4, and NLRP1 genes present in VDZ responders enhance the anti-inflammatory/immune modulation effects. **Conclusions**: This investigation is the first to apply whole-exome sequencing to identify the potential drug response biomarkers for the IBD drug VDZ in Saudi Arabia.

Keywords: vedolizumab; genetic biomarkers; ulcerative colitis; Crohn's disease; drug response; whole-exome sequencing; rare variants

1. Introduction

Inflammatory bowel disease (IBD) is a persistent and progressive disease of the digestive tract, caused by an inappropriate immune system response to microorganisms [1].

IBD is a broad term that is classified into two major forms, Crohn's disease (CD) and ulcerative colitis (UC), depending on their specific anatomical sites [2]. It is estimated that there are approximately 1.5 million IBD patients in the United States, 2.2 million in Europe, and a substantial number worldwide [3]. In Saudi Arabia, the epidemiology of IBD remains unknown; however, several studies in various regions suggest an increase in incidence over the years, ranging from 0.32 per 100,000 to 1.66 per 100,000 per year [4–6].

Over the last two decades, different highly promising therapies have emerged for autoimmune and inflammatory conditions such as IBD. However, a major challenge is that not all patients respond to these treatments [7]. Approximately 30% of IBD patients do not respond to anti-TNF therapy (PNR: primary non-response), and nearly half of patients who respond to anti-TNF therapy lose clinical benefit within the first year, requiring dose escalation or treatment modification (LOS: secondary loss of response) [8,9]. PNR and LOS result in unsuccessful disease control and the exacerbation of symptoms [10]. Between 10 and 40 percent of patients exhibited PNR to anti-TNF medications after the initial treatment period of 14 weeks, while an additional 24 to 46 percent suffered LOS after one year of anti-TNF medication [11–13]. A new monoclonal antibody that blocks the activity of integrin alpha 4 beta 7 was developed in 2014. Vedolizumab (VDZ) is a monoclonal antibody that prevents the movement of white blood cells in the intestine by disrupting the connection between a protein called integrin alpha 4 beta 7 and mucosal vascular addressin cell adhesion molecule 1 (MADCAM-1). A significant association between clinical remission at week 14 and median VDZ value at week 6 (25.1 μg/mL 95% confidence interval: 16.5–42.9), compared to non-responders, was reported from Saudi Arabia [14].

A combination of multiple factors, including environmental, genetic, immune, and gut microbiota factors, leads to an abnormal immune system. This defect triggers the production of inflammatory cytokines and adhesion molecules, which initiate the inflammatory process [15]. A few reports indicated a connection between immune cell phenotype and the effectiveness of VDZ. The pathogenesis of IBD involves the participation of both innate and adaptive immune cells, including CD4+ helper T cells and macrophages in the patient's colonic mucosa.

A lack of biomarkers to predict the non-responders to various drugs early leads to the persistence and severity of symptoms in IBD patients. Next-generation sequencing (whole-exome and whole-genome sequencing) and the large-scale generation of variants in populations are used to identify the causal or contributing genes and variants for IBD [16–18]. The same technologies can be used to identify biomarkers at the molecular level (rare variants with minor allele frequency <0.05) for drug response status. Multiple studies have documented pharmacological parameters, such as peak and trough level, predicting the effectiveness of VDZ [14,19]. The GWASs (genome-wide association studies) were mainly used to identify 100s of disease susceptibility loci but not the drug response biomarkers in IBD so far. The current study is the first to apply whole-exome sequencing to study the complex disease drug response in the Saudi Arabian population, marking a unique ethnic-specific contribution. It assesses the exomes, bringing to light rare but significant genetic variations relevant to IBD drug response. The discovery and validation of these biomarkers could optimize treatment effectiveness and pave the way for more personalized treatment plans for IBD patients.

The aim of the study was to explore the genetic profile of the vedolizumab-treated IBD patients to identify the potential biomarkers for responders among Arabs of Saudi Arabia.

2. Materials and Methods

This study is one part of research for which Institutional Research Ethics Board approval was obtained prior to participant recruitment and sample collection (KAUH-REC

No. 480-20) [14]. Patients were diagnosed with IBD by gastroenterologists at King AbdulAziz University Hospital in Jeddah, Saudi Arabia. Informed consent was obtained from all participants prior to collecting clinical data and blood samples during the study phase. Blood samples were collected in EDTA vials for DNA analysis and stored at −80 °C till they were used.

1. Participant profile:

The following Table 1 presents the inclusion/exclusion criteria used to identify and recruit the participants for the study.

Table 1. Inclusion/exclusion criteria to identify and to recruit the participants.

Inclusion Criteria	Exclusion Criteria
Aged between 18 and 80 years; male or female Saudi patients; capable of giving voluntary informed consent; diagnosis of moderate-to-severe active UC/CD (Mayo endoscopic sub-score > 1 for UC OR presence of frank ulcerations for CD); and patients naïve to VDZ.	Signs of abdominal abscess; any colonic resection; either total or subtotal colectomy; known fixed stenosis of the intestine, ileostomy, or colostomy; use of non-permitted IBD therapies within 30 or 60 days; active or dormant TB infection; hepatitis C or B chronic infection; malignancy; small or large bowel malignancy; being incapable of complying with study protocols or attending study visits.

The data collection form in Supplementary Materials: Research information comprises several items, including clinical and family history and physical examination with the clinical scoring. All patients who started vedolizumab treatment between October 2020 and September 2021 were identified and offered the option to join the research project. Of the 25 patients who fulfilled the criteria as VDZ-naïve IBD patients, only 16 joined and signed the informed consent form for data and sample collection. At weeks 0, 2, and 6, patients received vedolizumab intravenous infusion (300 mg) for the induction phase and underwent a follow-up assessment at week 14. After 14 weeks of VDZ treatment, the clinical outcome was evaluated with partial Mayo score for UC and CD activity and Harvey Bradshaw scores for CD, which was confirmed by the significant VDZ trough level differences (25.1 µg/mL 95% CI: 16.5–42.9 for responders and 7.7 µg/mL, 95% CI: 4.6–10.6 for non-responders; $p = 0.002$).The general study workflow is presented in Figure 1.

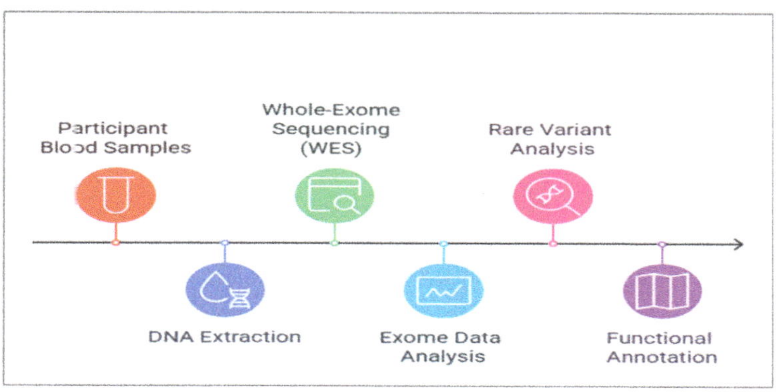

Figure 1. General workflow of the study.

2. Exome sequence generation:

WES: DNA extraction: About 2–4 mL of venous blood samples were collected once during the study period for DNA isolation and extractions using the standard DNA extraction procedures of the lab. Quality control of DNA: The quantity of DNA was measured by the picogreen method using Victor 3 fluorometry, and again by fluorescence-based quantification for WES library preparation. Assessing the nature of the DNA: The assessment was carried out by the agarose gel electrophoresis method. DNA fragments <1 kb: A 2100 Bioanalyzer was used to check the size, and the Femto-Pulse method was used to fragment the high-molecular DNA. The Exome Capture Library from Agilent (version 7) was used to capture the targeted exome fragments, amplified by PCR. After the purification of captured fragments, extensive QC checks were carried out. Once the samples passed the QC check, the samples were loaded into the NGS machine for sequence generation for downstream analysis, as illustrated in Figure 2.

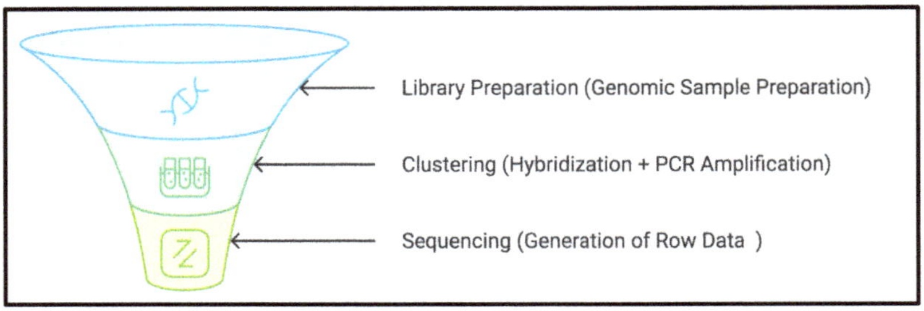

Figure 2. WES general workflow.

3. The following chart provides the exome variant analysis workflow from Raw Data generated by the NGS machine to the annotated variants, (Figures 2 and 3). Tables 2 and 3 lists the various tools and databases (with versions) used for WES data analysis and variant annotations.

Table 2. Databases used (including version) for the variant identification and annotation.

Software	Version
Mapping Reference	Hg38 (original GRCh38-NCBI, Dec.2013).
dbSNP	154
1000Genome	Phase3
Clinvar	07/2021
ESP	ESP6500SI_V2
dbNSFP	dbNSFPv4.2c

Table 3. Computational tools used to curate the exome sequence and annotate the variants.

Software	Version
BWA	Bwa-0.7.17
Picard	Picard-tools-2.18.2-SNAPSHOT
GATK	GATKv4.0.5.1
SnpEff	SnpEff 5.0e 9 March 2021

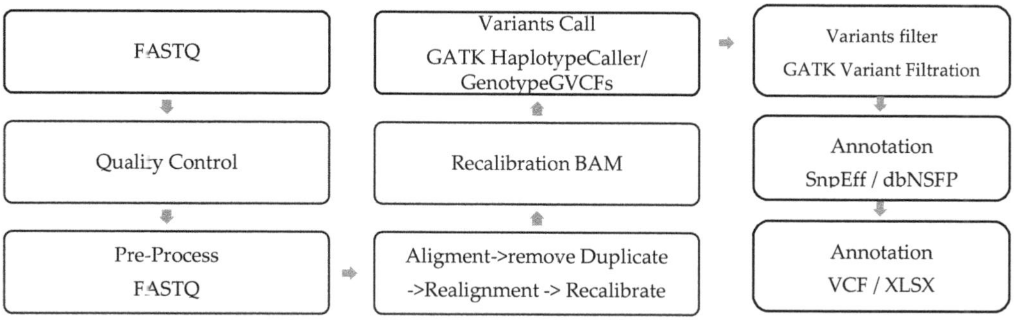

Figure 3. Exome sequence data analysis process and workflow.

For variant analysis and selection, pathogenicity prediction, sequence conservation, and variant location with reference to genes, many tools were used: Poyphen2, Mutation Taster, CADD, FATHMM, etc. Only variants located in the coding region were selected for downstream analysis. Population frequency data of variants in 1K genome, ExAC, gnomAD, and RGC Million Exome variants databases were extensively used to select the rare variants with MAF <0.05 in different ethnic groups. The filtered variants from responder and non-responder groups were classified with three d levels of rare minor allele frequency (MAF) categories in all ethnic populations of the 1K, ExAC, and gnomAD databases. The minor allele frequency categories selected are (a) rare: 3 to 5% (0.03–0.05), (b) very rare: 1 to 2.99% (0.01–0.0299), and (c) extremely rare: less than 1% (<0.01).

In order to prioritize the genes and variants and to explore the Molecular Functions, Biological Processes, Cellular Components, pathways, drug targets, and the causal natures of the genes, multiple bioinformatic tools and databases were extensively used. For biological functional and pathway analysis, some of the tools and databases used are TOPPFun, Open Target Platform, KEGG, Reactome, STRING db, GTEX, etc. (Table 4).

Table 4. Examples of some of the complex biological databases with extensive bioinformatic output for complex queries used.

Evidence Tool	Outcomes
Open Target Platform	This website provides access to multiple computational tools and databases that aid in identifying the causal or functional annotations between the clinical phenotype and drug target genes [20].
TOPPFun	The ToppGene platform is used to enrich a group of genes based on function and cellular localization, pathways, etc., to prioritize candidate genes by extensively using an array of protein interaction and functional annotations network datasets [21].
STRING database	This protein–protein interaction database encompass both physical and functional connections of all genes [22].
Genotype-Tissue Expression (GTEx)	Human gene expression data resource from various tissues and organs used to correlate their relationships to genetic variation [23].
RGC	New whole-exome/genome database from more than a million people of different ethnicities in the public domain for minor allele frequency of variants to identify the rare variants in the world population [24].

3. Results

3.1. Participant Profile

Sixteen (sixteen out of twenty-five) IBD participants fulfilled the inclusion and exclusion criteria, including four with CD and twelve with UC. Others did not agree to join the research project and were not included in the study. The average age of the nine male and seven female patients in this study was 30 years. After 14 weeks of VDZ treatment, the clinical outcome was assessed by partial Mayo score for UC and CD activity and Harvey Bradshaw scores for CD, which was confirmed, but with significant differences in VDZ trough levels (25.1 µg/mL, 95% confidence interval: 16.5–42.9 for responders and 7.7 µg/mL, 95% confidence interval: 4.6–10.6, p = 0.002). Nine were classified as responders (R group), and seven were non-responders (NR group), for VDZ based on the above-mentioned internationally accepted standards by the clinical team.

3.2. WES Analysis

On average, 99.99% of the exome library fragments passed the quality score of Phred 30 from the target regions. Sequences that passed the Phred Q score were processed for downstream analysis. An average of 60,447,882 reads for each sample of DNA was generated, with an average sequence size of 140 bp and an average throughput depth of 198.5; the mean depth of the target regions was 96.7. A total of 1.7 million variants were identified in 16 samples with ~120 K variants per exome.

3.3. Stringent Variant Prioritization

The pooled responder group (nine participants) had 2590, 3308, and 9276 extremely rare, very rare, and rare variants, respectively. For the NR group (seven participants), 1808, 2421, and 5839 extremely rare, very rare, and rare variants were identified and pooled, respectively (Table 5).

Table 5. Total rare variants in responder and non-responder groups based on MAF. (Range: extremely rare <0.01; very rare 0.01–0.0299; and rare 0.03–0.05).

	Variant Prioritizations		
Group	**Extreme Rare**	**Very Rare**	**Rare**
R	2590	3308	9276
NR	1808	2421	5839

Prioritized variants were mapped to genes for R and NR groups, and the overlapped ones were excluded from the downstream analysis (Figure 4). The IBD GWAS data from the GWAS catalogue were compared with R and NR unique genes to find the interesting potential candidate genes.

3.3.1. Prioritization Candidate Genes for R (Responder) and NR (Non-Responder) Groups

Figure 3 shows 123 and 68 genes in responder and non-responder groups' overlaps with IBD loci. A search for functional annotation support for both sets of genes for their role in IBD development and/or autoimmunity from Open Target Platform (OTP) and TOPPFun was performed. Finally, 25 and 18 from R (from 6526) and NR (from 4365 genes) groups, respectively, were prioritized using various stringent genetic, genomic, and functional criteria as strong potential candidate biomarkers. Gene ontology: Of the prioritized 25 responder genes, 4 could affect the immune aspect through positive regulation of the adaptive immune response and NF-kb transcription factor activity as biological processes, whereas, of the 18 NR genes, 5 were enriched with the positive regulation of cytokine secretion and response and mediated IL-12 production.

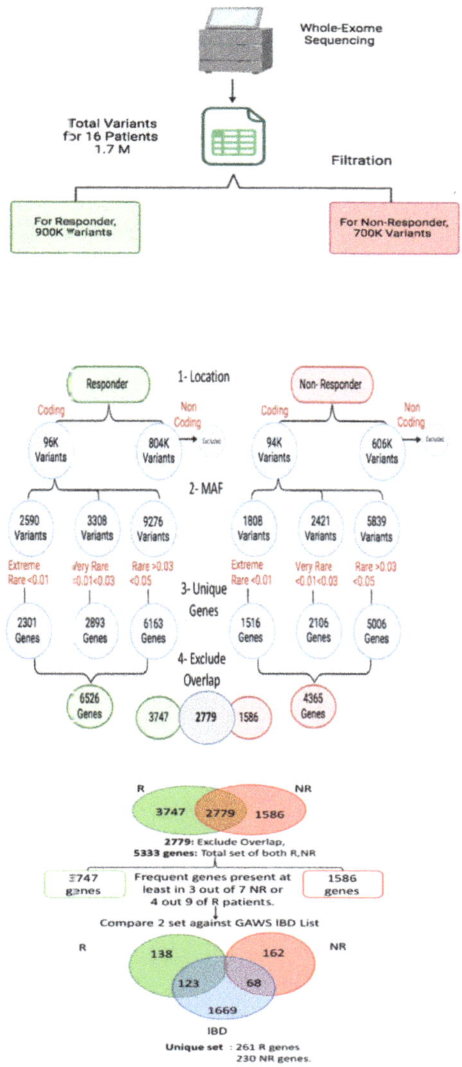

Figure 4. WES data workflow of variants to prioritized genes from responders and non-responders to VDZ in Saudi Arabian patients.

Functional Enrichment

- Biological pathways: Four responder candidate genes (CARD9, NLRP1, IL-4, and TYK2) may enhance the action of VDZ. These genes play an important role in one or multiple functions and pathways. These include the anti-inflammatory effect, impairment of the activation of NFkB by decreased secretion of cytokines by innate immune cells, induction of Th-2 cells to produce anti-inflammatory and immunomodulatory factors, and activation of the JAK/STAT pathway. These are involved in the following pathways: (a) immune system, (b) NLRP1 inflammasome signaling, (c) nucleotide-binding domain leucine-rich repeat-containing receptor NLR signaling, and (d) interleukin-10 signaling. Table 6 lists the key biological functions of these key genes, which potentially enhance the response to VDZ.

- The five non-responder (NR) candidate genes (NOD2, TRAF1, IL10RA, IL-23R, and IL27) enhance the activation of pro-inflammatory cytokines through MAPK and NFkB pathways, modulate innate and acquired immunity, and activate Th-17 cells, leading to the production of pro-inflammatory cytokines. These functions might contribute to the poor response to VDZ in IBD patients through the following pathways: (a) NOD-NFkB signaling, (b) ulcerative colitis signaling, and (c) the PID-NFkB canonical pathway. Those genes were also found to be associated with the development of the other common autoimmune disease, rheumatoid arthritis. Table 7 highlights the main biological functions of NR genes possibly contributing to poor or non-responder status to VDZ. The activation of pro-inflammatory cytokines through NFκB pathways by NOD2 and TRAF and modulation of immunity by IL10RA and IL27 genes was found.
- Protein–protein Interaction: The STRING protein–protein interaction database search resulted in findings of critical gene networks for both R and NR sets of genes, Figures 5 and 6. The R group gene network was enriched with the cytokine processes and pathways, which include IL13RA1 and IL-12RB2. They play a crucial role with IL-4 in the anti-inflammatory process. The strong interaction between the four responder group genes highlights their potential contribution to the positive response to VDZ.
- Figure 7 explains the role of CARD9 in inhibiting the NFkB pathway, which leads to the suppression of the Th-1 cell, which is responsible for producing pro-inflammatory cytokines. They inhibit cytokine secretion. Moreover, Th-1 cells inhibited by IL-4 and TYK2 suppress the production of cytokines.

Table 6. Major biological role of the potential candidate gene in the VDZ responders group.

Gene Name	Function
CARD9	Impairs the activation of RelB, a subunit of non-canonical NFkB, ↓cytokines and chemokines production by innate immune cells.
IL4	Anti-inflammatory and immunomodulatory factor, induces Th2 cell differentiation and expression.
NLRP1	Innate immune sensor to attenuate IL18, IL-1β levels.
TYK2	Activation of the Janus kinase/transcriptional signaling and activation factor (JAK/STAT) pathway.

Table 7. Major biological roles of the potential candidate genes in VDZ non-responders.

Gene Name	Function
NOD2	Activation of pro-inflammatory cytokines and regulation of inflammation and cell apoptosis via the MAPK and NF-κB pathways.
IL10RA	Regulates both innate and acquired immunity.
IL23R	Activation and development of the Th17 lineage and its effect on dendritic cells and macrophages results in the production of a variety of pro-inflammatory molecules.
IL27	Th17 differentiation and immune regulation.
TRAF1	Canonical and non-canonical NFκB pathways activating MAP kinases.

Gene Prioritization

Gene ontology

R

261 to 25 genes

Immune aspect through positive regulation of adaptive immune response and NF-kb transcription factor activity as biological process.

NR

320 to 18 genes

Positive regulation of cytokine secretion and response and mediation of IL-12 production.

Functional Enrichment -Biological Pathway

4 out of 25 genes

Immune System

Nlrp1 inflammasome Signaling Pathway

Nucleotide-Binding Domain Leucine-Rich Repeat-Containing Receptor Nlr Signaling Pathways

5 out of 18 genes

1- NOD-NFkB Signaling Pathway
2- Ulcerative Colitis Signaling
3- PID-NFkB Canonical Pathway
4- Associated With Rheumatoid Arthritis

- Protein–Protein Interaction

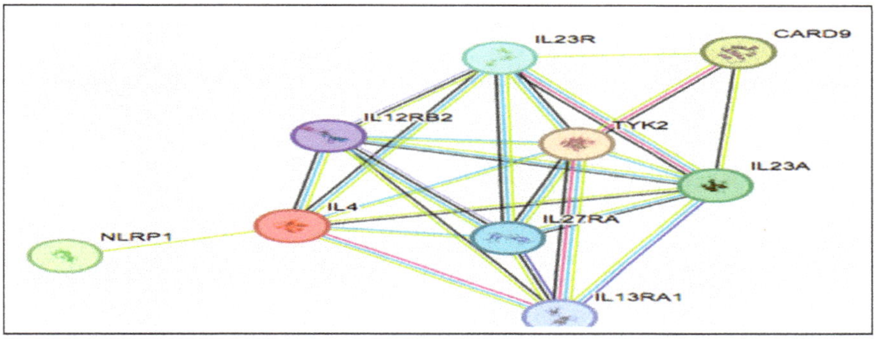

Figure 5. Network of responder genes (STRING protein–protein interaction dataset).

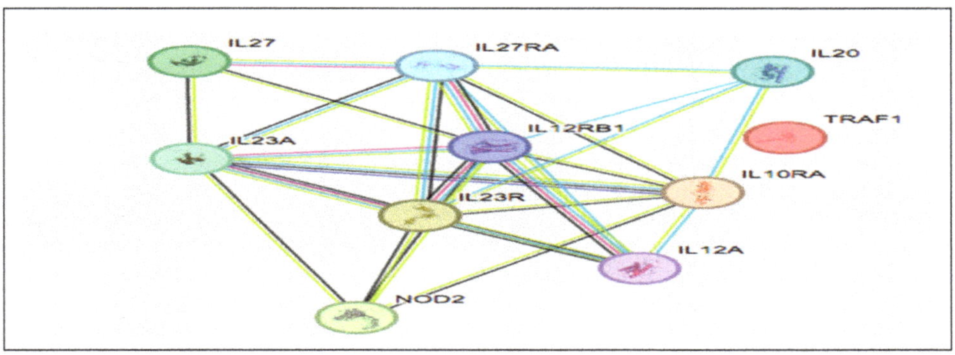

Figure 6. Network of genes from non-responders (STRING protein–protein interaction database).

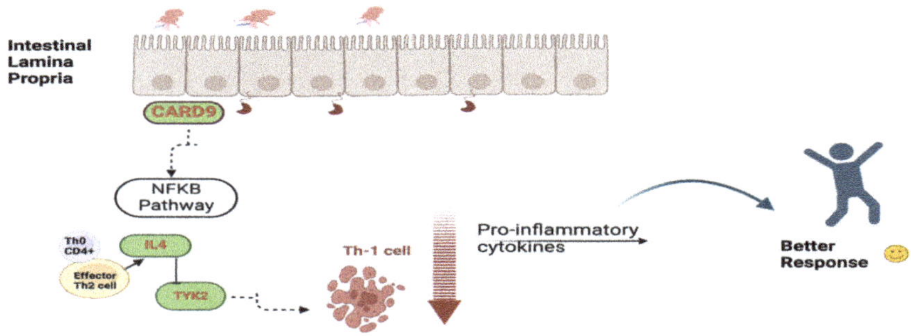

Figure 7. Biological functional roles of candidate genes in VDZ responder group.

To further validate the biological pathways of the listed genes in the responder group, the GTEx database was explored regarding different tissues for changes in the expression of samples with variants and normal alleles. The GTEx analysis revealed a significant change in the expression of the rare variant of the IL-4R gene (rs2234895) in the esophagus; $p = 3.07^{-2}$. Additionally, the TYK2 gene variant (rs2304255) showed significant expression in both the esophagus and small intestine ($p = 4.5^{-4}$ and 1.29^{-2}, respectively) when compared to the normal allele carriers. Furthermore, the NLRP1 gene variant (rs12150220) demonstrated highly significant expression changes ($p = 6.17^{-3}$) in the esophagus (Figure 8).

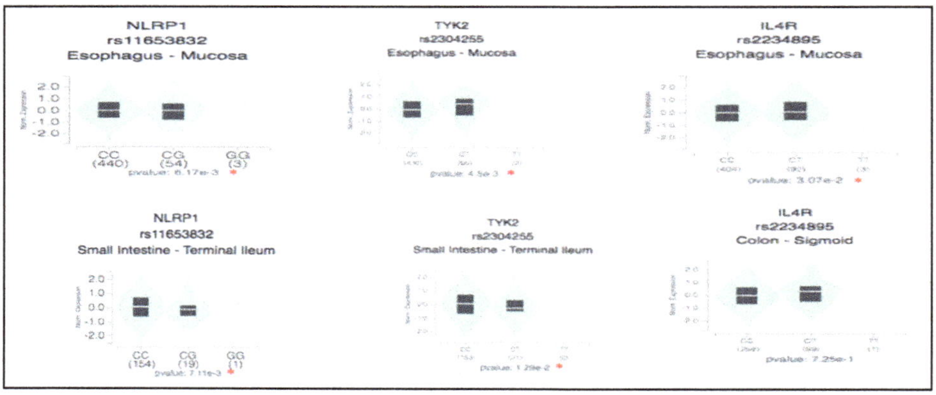

Figure 8. Genotype-Tissue Expression (GTEx) of genes in the responder group in different tissues. * denotes statistically significantly different gene expression recorded in specific tissue between the carriers of the rare variant and common alleles.

For NR candidate genes, Figure 5 shows the protein interaction gene network from the STRING. Enrichment analysis of the biological functions and pathways indicates their role in cytokine processes and pathways, which include IL-20 and IL-12. They play a key role in the non-response status by triggering inflammation in the target tissues through their aberrant expressions. The non-responder groups' genes, by interacting with the key partners, may contribute to hindering the response to VDZ, leading to the severity of the disease symptoms.

The biological functions and processes of the non-responder genes' network are shown in Figure 9. Functional and pathway enrichment of these genes reveals that the IL23R and IL10RA activate the dendritic cells, triggering the MAPK signaling activity. This activation stimulates the Th-1 cell to produce pro-inflammatory cytokines, which upregulate the cytokine secretion. At the same time, NOD2 and TRAF1 enhance the NFkB singling cascade through the activation of macrophages; this will induce the Th-1 cells to produce more pro-inflammatory cytokines. The non-responsive status, in this case, is due to the aggregation of pro-inflammatory cytokines that counteract the inhibitory action of VDZ.

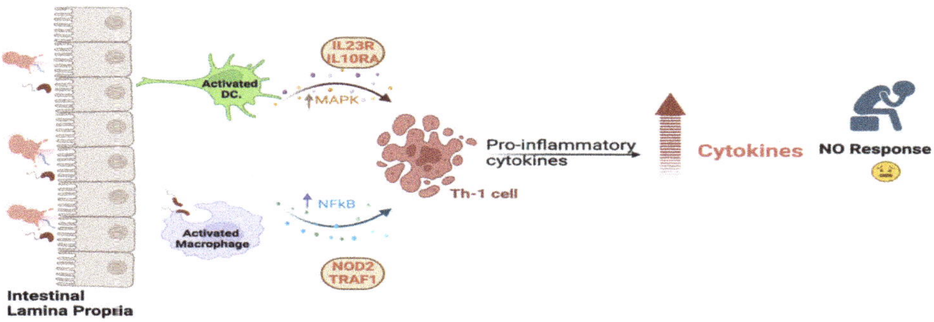

Figure 9. Biological functional roles of candidate genes in VDZ non-responder group.

To further validate the biological pathways of the candidate genes in the non-responder group, GTEx profiles in a variety of tissues were searched for in the gene variants. We observed a significant change in the expression of the TRAF1 gene with the rare variant (rs34119250) in the esophagus and sigmoid colon ($p = 7.16^{-9}$ and 2.88^{-5}, respectively). Additionally, with the NOD2 gene variant (rs5743291), a significant change in expression was observed in the sigmoid colon ($p = 1.09^{-2}$) and skin $p = 2.36^{-3}$) (see Figure 10). IL23R and IL10RA did not show any significant changes in their expression between rare and common variant carriers in any tissues analyzed.

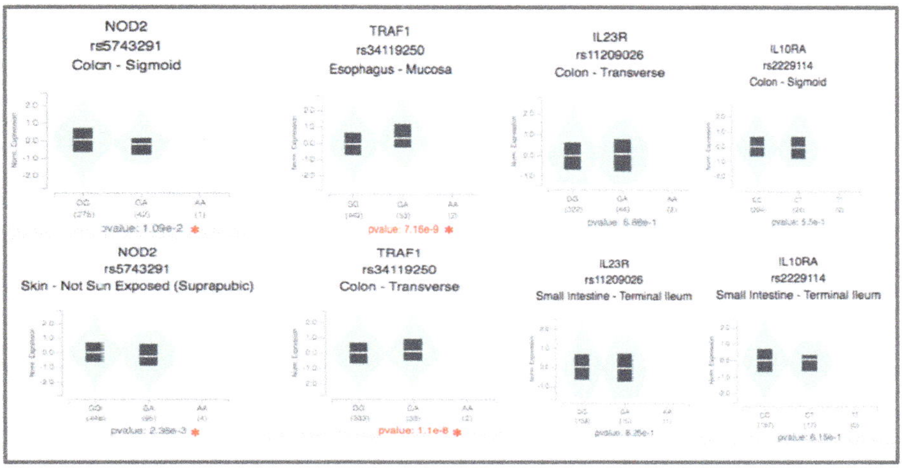

Figure 10. Genotype-Tissue Expression (GTEx) of non-responder genes. * denotes statistically significantly different gene expression recorded in specific tissues between the carriers of the rare variant and common alleles.

The global population's MAF is changing rapidly due to the increasing number of samples from various ethnic groups that have been added to the variant databases, such as the RGC Million Exome db, the largest genomic database. All candidate gene rare variants were searched for in the pooled Middle Eastern Arab data along with global MAF data and are presented in Table 8. This reveals differences in variant frequencies in Arabs when compared to other ethnic groups; for example, in the IL27 variant—low, the IL4 variant—high, and the NLRP1 variant—very high (approximately 9 out of 100 Arabs have this variant, when compared to approximately 2.4 in 1 million from RGC).

Table 8. Alleles' frequency in Middle Eastern Arabs compared to other populations in non-responder and responder variants.

Gene/SNP	MAF	1000 G	GnomAD	RGC—All	RGC—Arab	Saudi MAF
Non-Responder						
NOD2	rs5743291	0.0332	0.063	0.077	0.114	0.0694
IL-23R	rs11209026	0.023	0.042	0.055	0.057	0.0486
IL-10RA	rs2229114	0.017	0.032	0.040	0.040	0.0312
IL-27	rs147413292	0.020	0.050	0.053	0.058	0.0347
TRAF1	rs34119250	0.034	0.051	0.060	0.062	0.0694
Responder						
CARD9	rs114895119	0.002	0.004	0.004	0.009	0.0035
TYK2	rs2304255	0.044	0.062	0.066	0.071	0.0417
IL-4	rs2234895	0.047	0.069	0.077	0.112	0.1146
NLRP1	rs11653832	-	0.00000119	0.000002433	0	0.0938

4. Discussion

Most genetic studies on IBD have largely concentrated on identifying the common disease susceptibility variants with small effect sizes through GWASs in Caucasians [25]. However, rare and highly penetrant variations identified through population-specific cohorts or family-focused research have immense potential to catch the variants with high effect sizes on complex diseases such as IBD [17,26]. Many large-scale sporadic case-control studies on WES-based rare variant burden analysis (RVB) have previously identified several strong risk loci for complex diseases, such as schizophrenia [27], Alzheimer's disease [28], autism [29], and CD [30]. According to a recent systemic review and meta-analysis of IBD in the Arab world, the consanguinity rate in Saudi Arabian IBD patients is high, 57.6%, which is similar to that in the general population as well [4,31]. The present study, by a novel approach, utilized the exome data from highly consanguineous Saudi Arabian ABD patients with biological functional enrichment with a range of bioinformatic tools and databases to identify the unique genetic signature for VDZ drug response.

This study utilized the power of large-scale multi-domain computational biological databases and tools to prioritize the rare coding variants in genes and key disease pathways, aiming to facilitate personalized genomic analysis of patients. This study prioritized NOD2, IL23, IL10, IL27, TRAF1, CARD9, TYK2, IL4, and NLRP1 genes with rare variants from non-responders and responders, respectively, as potential candidate biomarkers for VDZ drug response. A stringent filtration for allele frequency, biological functions, and genetic evidence resulted in 261 and 230 genes in responders and non-responders, respectively. Genes prioritized by GWASs that overlap in both responder and non-responder groups play a crucial role in the etiology of IBD through the inflammatory pathway [32,33] and cytokine interaction process [34–36]. The network interaction of non-responder potential candidate genes showed many cytokines that play a role in IBD pathogenesis. IL-20 and IL-12RB1 with the co-expression of IL-12 is a key regulator of the inflammatory cascade of non-responder genes, confirming a previous study [37]. This demonstrates a clear role for *IL-12* in the initiation of intestinal inflammation, disrupting the epithelial barrier. IL23, on the other hand, is important in chronic intestinal inflammation [38]. Moreover, most of the identified non-responder potential predictive markers are related to pro-inflammatory cytokines/chemokines or their receptors (NOD2, IL23R, TRAF1, IL10RA, and IL27) [32]. The majority of these genes interact with IL12A. The activity of IL23 is dependent on

IL12RB1, a type 1 transmembrane receptor that physically associates with the p40 domain common to both IL12 and IL23 and promotes their respective signaling pathways [39]. All the previous studies identified the critical role of NOD2, IL23, IL10RA, and TRAF1 as risk factors for IBD in GW studies and in animal models for UC or CD [40–42].

Most NR genes act on pro-inflammatory cytokine secretion; for example, *NOD2* activates NFκB and MAPK, and, thus, the transcription of pro-inflammatory molecules such as IL6, IL8, IL1β, and TNF-α, which alter Paneth cells' ability to recognize and eliminate invading pathogens that cause the development of inflammatory bowel lesions [43,44]. Also, TRAF1 regulates both canonical and non-canonical *NFκB* pathways as well as MAP kinase activation, and influences pro-inflammatory cytokine production and inflammatory responses [42,45]. This upregulation of pro-inflammatory cytokines may potentially hinder the VDZ in inhibiting the alpha 4 beta 7 integrin. Two prior meta-analyses have examined NOD2/CARD15 polymorphisms in CD to confirm the non-responder role of NOD2 in IBD therapy [41,46]. Moreover, a few animal models support the role of *NOD2* and TRAF1 in the development of CD [47,48]. In addition, interleukin-23 (*IL23*) is a pro-inflammatory cytokine, produced primarily by macrophages and antigen-presenting cells (APCs) after antigen stimulation. Studies conducted in both mice and humans have shown that IL23 acts as a major pathogenic pro-inflammatory factor in IBD [49,50]. Targeting the IL23 pathway is an important opportunity for drug development. Multiple lines of evidence support the IL23 blockade as a therapeutic strategy for IBD [51]. In a mouse model, an IL23 blockade suppressed T cell-mediated colitis and reduced inflammation to a greater extent than an IL12 blockade alone. Ustekinumab is a monoclonal antibody that targets the shared p40 subunit of IL-12/23 and is approved for the treatment of moderate-to-severe CD and UC [51].

The responder genes enhance the drug action of VDZ by its anti-inflammatory/immune-modulatory effect [43,52,53]. Moreover, most of the key interactors of responder genes through IL13RA1 act as pleiotropic cytokines in the activation of IL4 to induce inhibitory responses, which contribute to inflammatory diseases [54]. Anti-inflammatory cytokines play a crucial role in controlling pro-inflammatory cytokine production. This investigation identified rare variants in IL-4 in more responders than in non-responders. A possible explanation for this might be that it is contributing to the enhanced production/action of anti-inflammatory cytokines in IBD by VDZ [55]. Previous studies confirm that IL-4 acts as an anti-inflammatory and immunomodulatory factor by suppressing the pro-inflammatory IL1, IL6, IL12, and TNF-alpha secretion [56]. IL4 promotes the healing processes accomplished by macrophages and has an alleviating effect upon patients with colitis [57]. TYK2 is involved in the signaling pathway of various cytokines, including IL4, which are responsible for transmitting signals from cytokine receptors to the nucleus. Therefore, TYK2 is necessary for IL4 to exert its effects on immune cells. In an animal model, the administration of the antagonist of IL4 receptorα for the treatment of atopic dermatitis has caused enteritis as a side effect [58]. These findings lead to the assumption that the immune response mediated by Th2 cells may act as a protective factor against VDZ IBD. In addition, CARD9 (Caspase Recruitment Domain 9) plays a role in the response to bacteria by interacting with NOD2 [59]. The previous studies reported the protective role of *CARD9* S12NΔ11 (with the deletion of exon 11) as a protective variant. This allele truncates the CARD9 C-terminus of the protein to provide strong protection against IBD. Those individuals with CARD9 S12NΔ11 have decreased TNF-α and IL-6 production [60]. Rare variants of NLRP1 in the responders may attenuate gastrointestinal inflammation. Knock-out *Nlrp1b(−/−)* mice demonstrated significant increases in morbidity, inflammation, and tumorigenesis [53]. Taken together, these data identify NLRP1 as an essential mediator of the host immune response during IBD and cancer. These findings are consistent with a model whereby multiple NLR inflammasomes attenuate disease pathobiology through modulating IL-1β and IL18 levels in the colon [53]. In the current study, rare variants of these genes among the responders highlight potential biomarkers for better VDZ response. The current study results emphasize the importance of the early prediction of drug response, which is essential to prevent disease resistance and damage to the intestines in drug-resistant and poorly responding patients.

We acknowledge some limitations of this study. First, this study involved a small sample size, which limits the robustness of the findings. The recruitment of more patients could help in validating the potential candidate genes identified in this study. The main reasons for the small sample size in this study are (a) the poor response of patients in joining as participants in this research project in general, especially during and after the pandemic, due to the restricted movement of the population; (b) the cost of the WES processing is high; and (c) a limited number of patients were allowed to be treated with this drug due to limited hospital funds and stringent patient selection for this costly treatment regimen in Saudi Arabia. Second, a lack of large-scale population-specific genomic variant databases in the Arab world in the public domain restricted us in confirming the minor allele frequency in the local Arab population, which is genetically unique. Last, a lack of large-scale GWASs in the genetically unique Arab populations has also contributed to the sparse knowledge of the genetic susceptibility to complex diseases, including IBD. The lack of laboratory-based validation in many IBD patients treated with VDZ is also a limitation of this study.

5. Conclusions

This is the first study to explore WES data for IBD drug response in the Middle Eastern Arab region. More than a million variants across the exomes of the 16 IBD patients were searched for and analyzed with a variety of advanced bioinformatic tools for pathogenicity prediction, population frequencies, protein–protein interaction networks, pathways, functional enrichment, etc., and animal models were also analyzed. This study highlights the potential critical genetic signature of Saudi Arabian IBD patient response/non-response status to VDZ. The present investigation lays the foundation to integrate WES with extensive integrated multi-omics data analysis to identify drug response candidate genes for chronic complex diseases in Saudi Arabia. Future research should look for rare variant burdens in the target genes and other critical pathway genes in large sample sizes for more validation. This will have the positive downstream effect of improving drug adherence. Moreover, this will help clinical management teams and the government cover more IBD patients nationwide who are predicted to be responders to the drug and reduce the economic burden of patient care. Predicting responders early will spur the rapid introduction of an efficient personalized medical management program for IBD across the country.

Supplementary Materials: The supporting information can be downloaded at https://www.mdpi.com/article/10.3390/biomedicines13020459/s1. Informed consent, and Data capture Sheets.

Author Contributions: Conceptualization, M.M., S.A. and R.E.; Participant recruitment and clinical data capture: M.M., D.A. and D.B.; methodology, software: H.A., A.U. and R.E.; validation, H.A., D.A., M.M. and R.E.; Data analysis: H.A. and R.E.; data curation, H.A., D.A., S.A. and R.E.; writing—original draft preparation, H.A., D.A., D.B., R.E. and S.A.; review and editing of the manuscript: H.A., D.A., R.E. and S.A.; supervision: D.B., R.E. and S.A. All authors have read and agreed to the published version of the manuscript.

Funding: There were no external funding sources or sponsoring societies for this study.

Institutional Review Board Statement: This study was approved by the Institutional Ethical Committee of King Abdulaziz University Hospital (480-20, 2020). The study design conforms to the 1975 Declaration of Helsinki.

Informed Consent Statement: Informed consent was obtained from all subjects involved in the study.

Data Availability Statement: Data that support the findings of this study are available from the corresponding author upon request.

Conflicts of Interest: The authors declare no competing interests.

Abbreviations

The following abbreviations are used in this manuscript:

IBD	inflammatory bowel disease
MACAM-1	mucosal vascular addressin cell adhesion molecule
KSA	Kingdom of Saudi Arabia
VDZ	vedolizumab

References

1. Ghouri, Y.A.; Tahan, V.; Shen, B. Secondary causes of inflammatory bowel diseases. *World J. Gastroenterol.* **2020**, *26*, 3998–4017. [CrossRef] [PubMed]
2. Malik, T.A. Inflammatory bowel disease: Historical perspective, epidemiology, and risk factors. *Surg. Clin.* **2015**, *95*, 1105–1122.
3. Ananthakrishnan, A.N. Epidemiology and risk factors for IBD. *Nat. Rev. Gastroenterol. Hepatol.* **2015**, *12*, 205–217. [CrossRef] [PubMed]
4. Mosli, M.; Alawadhi, S.; Hasan, F.; Abou Rached, A.; Sanai, F.; Danese, S. Incidence, prevalence, and clinical epidemiology of inflammatory bowel disease in the Arab world: A systematic review and meta-analysis. *Inflamm. Intest. Dis.* **2021**, *6*, 123–131. [CrossRef]
5. Al-Ghamdi, A.S.; A Al-Mofleh, I.; Al-Rashed, R.S.; Al-Amri, S.M.; Aljebreen, A.M.; Isnani, A.C.; El-Badawi, R. Epidemiology and outcome of Crohn's disease in a teaching hospital in Riyadh. *World J. Gastroenterol.* **2004**, *10*, 1341. [CrossRef] [PubMed]
6. Windsor, J.W.; Kaplan, G.G. Evolving epidemiology of IBD. *Curr. Gastroenterol. Rep.* **2019**, *21*, 40. [CrossRef]
7. Kopylov, U.; Seidman, E. Predicting durable response or resistance to antitumor necrosis factor therapy in inflammatory bowel disease. *Ther. Adv. Gastroenterol.* **2016**, *9*, 513–526. [CrossRef]
8. Adegbola, S.O.; Sahnan, K.; Warusavitarne, J.; Hart, A.; Tozer, P. Anti-TNF therapy in Crohn's disease. *Int. J. Mol. Sci.* **2018**, *19*, 2244. [CrossRef]
9. Billioud, V.; Sandborn, W.J.; Peyrin-Biroulet, L. Loss of response and need for adalimumab dose intensification in Crohn's disease: A systematic review. *Off. J. Am. Coll. Gastroenterol.* **2011**, *106*, 674–684. [CrossRef]
10. Rutgeerts, P.; D'Haens, G.; Targan, S.; Vasiliauskas, E.; Hanauer, S.B.; Present, D.H.; Mayer, L.; Van Hogezand, R.A.; Braakman, T.; DeWoody, K.L. Efficacy and safety of retreatment with anti–tumor necrosis factor antibody (infliximab) to maintain remission in Crohn's disease. *Gastroenterology* **1999**, *117*, 761–769. [CrossRef]
11. Sprakes, M.B.; Ford, A.C.; Warren, L.; Greer, D.; Hamlin, J. Efficacy, tolerability, and predictors of response to infliximab therapy for Crohn's disease: A large single centre experience. *J. Crohn's Colitis* **2012**, *6*, 143–153. [CrossRef] [PubMed]
12. Peyrin-Biroulet, L.; Danese, S.; Argollo, M.; Pouillon, L.; Peppas, S.; Gonzalez-Lorenzo, M.; Lytras, T.; Bonovas, S. Loss of response to vedolizumab and ability of dose intensification to restore response in patients with Crohn's disease or ulcerative colitis: A systematic review and meta-analysis. *Clin. Gastroenterol. Hepatol.* **2019**, *17*, 838–846.e2. [CrossRef] [PubMed]
13. Ungar, B.; Malickova, K.; Hanžel, J.; Abu Arisha, M.; Paul, S.; Rocha, C.; Ben Shatach, Z.; Abitbol, C.M.; Haj Natour, O.; Selinger, L. Dose optimisation for loss of response to Vedolizumab—Pharmacokinetics and immune mechanisms. *J. Crohn's Colitis* **2021**, *15*, 1707–1719. [CrossRef] [PubMed]
14. Anbarserry, D.; Mosli, M.; Qari, Y.; Saadah, O.; Bokhary, R.; Esmat, A.; Alsieni, M.; Shaker, A.; Elango, R.; Alharthi, S. The use of therapeutic drug monitoring for early identification of vedolizumab response in Saudi Arabian patients with inflammatory bowel disease. *Sci. Rep.* **2023**, *13*, 1771. [CrossRef]
15. McDowell, C.; Farooq, U.; Haseeb, M. *Inflammatory Bowel Disease*; StatPearls: Treasure Island, FL, USA, 2023.
16. Yang, S.-K.; Hong, M.; Choi, H.; Zhao, W.; Jung, Y.; Haritunians, T.; Ye, B.D.; Kim, K.-J.; Park, S.H.; Lee, I. Immunochip analysis identification of 6 additional susceptibility loci for Crohn's disease in Koreans. *Inflamm. Bowel Dis.* **2015**, *21*, 1–7. [CrossRef]
17. Jan, R.M.; Al-Numan, H.H.; Al-Twaty, N.H.; Alrayes, N.; Alsufyani, H.A.; Alaifan, M.A.; Alhussaini, B.H.; Shaik, N.A.; Awan, Z.; Qari, Y.; et al. Rare variant burden analysis from exomes of three consanguineous families reveals LILRB1 and PRSS3 as potential key proteins in inflammatory bowel disease pathogenesis. *Front. Med.* **2023**, *10*, 1164305. [CrossRef]

18. Al-Numan, H.H.; Jan, R.M.; Al-Saud, N.b.S.; Rashidi, O.M.; Alrayes, N.M.; Alsufyani, H.A.; Mujalli, A.; Shaik, N.A.; Mosli, M.H.; Elango, R. Exome sequencing identifies the extremely rare ITGAV and FN1 variants in early onset inflammatory bowel disease patients. *Front. Pediatr.* **2022**, *10*, 895074. [CrossRef]
19. Yacoub, W.; Williet, N.; Pouillon, L.; Di-Bernado, T.; De Carvalho Bittencourt, M.; Nancey, S.; Lopez, A.; Paul, S.; Zallot, C.; Roblin, X. Early vedolizumab trough levels predict mucosal healing in inflammatory bowel disease: A multicentre prospective observational study. *Aliment. Pharmacol. Ther.* **2018**, *47*, 906–912. [CrossRef]
20. Ochoa, D.; Hercules, A.; Carmona, M.; Suveges, D.; Baker, J.; Malangone, C.; Lopez, I.; Miranda, A.; Cruz-Castillo, C.; Fumis, L.; et al. The next-generation Open Targets Platform: Reimagined, redesigned, rebuilt. *Nucleic Acids Res.* **2022**, *51*, D1353–D1359. [CrossRef]
21. ToppGene. 2023. Available online: http://toppgene.cchmc.org (accessed on 1 January 2023).
22. Szklarczyk, D.; Kirsch, R.; Koutrouli, M.; Nastou, K.; Mehryary, F.; Hachilif, R.; Gable, A.L.; Fang, T.; Doncheva, N.T.; Pyysalo, S. The STRING database in 2023: Protein–protein association networks and functional enrichment analyses for any sequenced genome of interest. *Nucleic Acids Res.* **2023**, *51*, D638–D646. [CrossRef]
23. Westra, H.-J.; Peters, M.J.; Esko, T.; Yaghootkar, H.; Schurmann, C.; Kettunen, J.; Christiansen, M.W.; Fairfax, B.P.; Schramm, K.; Powell, J.E. Systematic identification of trans eQTLs as putative drivers of known disease associations. *Nat. Genet.* **2013**, *45*, 1238–1243. [CrossRef] [PubMed]
24. Regeneron Pharmaceuticals, Inc. Global Terms of Use. 2024. Available online: https://www.regeneron.com/terms (accessed on 20 December 2024).
25. Lee, J.C.; Biasci, D.; Roberts, R.; Gearry, R.B.; Mansfield, J.C.; Ahmad, T.; Prescott, N.J.; Satsangi, J.; Wilson, D.C.; Jostins, L. Genome-wide association study identifies distinct genetic contributions to prognosis and susceptibility in Crohn's disease. *Nat. Genet.* **2017**, *49*, 262–268. [CrossRef] [PubMed]
26. Cordero, R.Y.; Cordero, J.B.; Stiemke, A.B.; Datta, L.W; Buyske, S.; Kugathasan, S.; McGovern, D.P.; Brant, S.R.; Simpson, C.L. Trans-ancestry, Bayesian meta-analysis discovers 20 novel risk loci for inflammatory bowel disease in an African American, East Asian and European cohort. *Hum. Mol. Genet.* **2023**, *32*, 873–882. [CrossRef] [PubMed]
27. Singh, T.; Poterba, T.; Curtis, D.; Akil, H.; Al Eissa, M.; Barchas, J.D.; Bass, N.; Bigdeli, T.B.; Breen, G.; Bromet, E.J. Rare coding variants in ten genes confer substantial risk for schizophrenia. *Nature* **2022**, *604*, 509–516. [CrossRef]
28. Sims, R.; Van Der Lee, S.J.; Naj, A.C.; Bellenguez, C.; Badarinarayan, N.; Jakobsdottir, J.; Kunkle, B.W.; Boland, A.; Raybould, R.; Bis, J.C. Rare coding variants in PLCG2, ABI3, and TREM2 implicate microglial-mediated innate immunity in Alzheimer's disease. *Nat. Genet.* **2017**, *49*, 1373–1384. [CrossRef]
29. Balicza, P.; Varga, N.Á.; Bolgár, B.; Pentelényi, K.; Bencsik, R.; Gál, A.; Gézsi, A.; Prekop, C.; Molnár, V.; Molnár, M.J. Comprehensive analysis of rare variants of 101 autism-linked genes in a Hungarian cohort of autism spectrum disorder patients. *Front. Genet.* **2019**, *10*, 434. [CrossRef]
30. Sazonovs, A.; Stevens, C.R.; Venkataraman, G.R.; Yuan, K.; Avila, B.; Abreu, M.T.; Ahmad, T.; Allez, M.; Ananthakrishnan, A.N.; Atzmon, G. Large-scale sequencing identifies multiple genes and rare variants associated with Crohn's disease susceptibility. *Nat. Genet.* **2022**, *54*, 1275–1283. [CrossRef]
31. Yousef, N.A.; ElHarouni, A.A.; Shaik, N.A.; Banaganapalli, B.; Al Ghamdi, A.F.; Galal, A.H.; Alahmadi, T.S.; Shuaib, T.; Aljeaid, D.; Alshaer, D.S. Nationwide survey on awareness of consanguinity and genetic diseases in Saudi Arabia: Challenges and potential solutions to reduce the national healthcare burden. *Hum. Genom.* **2024**, *18*, 138. [CrossRef]
32. Gajendran, M.; Loganathan, P.; Catinella, A.P.; Hashash, J.G. A comprehensive review and update on Crohn's disease. *Disease-a-Month* **2018**, *64*, 20–57. [CrossRef]
33. Michail, S.; Bultron, G.; DePaolo, R.W. Genetic variants associated with Crohn's disease. *Appl. Clin. Genet.* **2013**, *6*, 25–32. [CrossRef]
34. Kopitar-Jerala, N. The role of interferons in inflammation and inflammasome activation. *Front. Immunol.* **2017**, *8*, 873. [CrossRef] [PubMed]
35. Gurung, P.; Malireddi, R.S.; Anand, P.K.; Demon, D.; Walle, L.V.; Liu, Z.; Vogel, P.; Lamkanfi, M.; Kanneganti, T.-D. Toll or interleukin-1 receptor (TIR) domain-containing adaptor inducing interferon-β (TRIF)-mediated caspase-11 protease production integrates Toll-like receptor 4 (TLR4) protein-and Nlrp3 inflammasome-mediated host defense against enteropathogens. *J. Biol. Chem.* **2012**, *287*, 34474–34483. [CrossRef] [PubMed]
36. Glas, J.; Seiderer, J.; Wagner, J.; Olszak, T.; Fries, C.; Tillack, C.; Friedrich, M.; Beigel, F.; Stallhofer, J.; Steib, C. Analysis of IL12B gene variants in inflammatory bowel disease. *PLoS ONE* **2012**, *7*, e34349. [CrossRef]
37. Robinson, R.T. IL12Rβ1: The cytokine receptor that we used to know. *Cytokine* **2015**, *71*, 348–359. [CrossRef]
38. Greving, C.N.A.; Towne, J.E. A role for IL-12 in IBD after all? *Immunity* **2019**, *51*, 209–211. [CrossRef]
39. Vignali, D.A.; Kuchroo, V.K. IL-12 family cytokines: Immunological playmakers. *Nat. Immunol.* **2012**, *13*, 722–728. [CrossRef]
40. Hugot, J.-P.; Chamaillard, M.; Zouali, H.; Lesage, S.; Cézard, J.-P.; Belaiche, J.; Almer, S.; Tysk, C.; O'Morain, C.A.; Gassull, M. Association of NOD2 leucine-rich repeat variants with susceptibility to Crohn's disease. *Nature* **2001**, *411*, 599–603. [CrossRef]

41. Solon, J.G.; Burke, J.P.; Walsh, S.R.; Coffey, J.C. The effect of NOD2 polymorphism on postsurgical recurrence in Crohn's disease: A systematic review and meta-analysis of available literature. *Inflamm. Bowel Dis.* **2013**, *19*, 1099–1105. [CrossRef]
42. Sughra, K.; Birbach, A.; de Martin, R.; Schmid, J.A. Interaction of the TNFR-receptor associated factor TRAF1 with I-kappa B kinase-2 and TRAF2 indicates a regulatory function for NF-kappa B signaling. *PLoS ONE* **2010**, *5*, e12683. [CrossRef]
43. Rückert, Y.; Schindler, U.; Heinig, T.; Nikolaus, S.; Raedler, A.; Schreiber, S. IL-4 signaling mechanisms in inflammatory bowel disease mononuclear phagocytes. *Inflamm. Bowel Dis.* **1996**, *2*, 244–252. [CrossRef]
44. Jarmakiewicz-Czaja, S.; Zielińska, M.; Sokal, A.; Filip, R. Genetic and epigenetic etiology of inflammatory bowel disease: An update. *Genes* **2022**, *13*, 2388. [CrossRef]
45. Cy, W. NF-kappaB antiapoptosis: Induction of TRAF1 and TRAF2 and c-IAP1 and c-IAP2 to suppress caspase-8 activation. *Science* **1998**, *281*, 1680–1683.
46. Adler, J.; Rangwalla, S.C.; Dwamena, B.A.; Higgins, P.D. The prognostic power of the NOD2 genotype for complicated Crohn's disease: A meta-analysis. *Off. J. Am. Coll. Gastroenterol.* **2011**, *106*, 699–712. [CrossRef] [PubMed]
47. Kobayashi, K.S.; Chamaillard, M.; Ogura, Y.; Henegariu, O.; Inohara, N.; Nuñez, G.; Flavell, R.A. Nod2-dependent regulation of innate and adaptive immunity in the intestinal tract. *Science* **2005**, *307*, 731–734. [CrossRef]
48. Leo, E.; Deveraux, Q.L.; Buchholtz, C.; Welsh, K.; Matsuzawa, S.-I.; Stennicke, H.R.; Salvesen, G.S.; Reed, J.C. TRAF1 is a substrate of caspases activated during tumor necrosis factor receptor-α-induced apoptosis. *J. Biol. Chem.* **2001**, *276*, 8087–8093. [CrossRef]
49. Trinchieri, G.; Pflanz, S.; Kastelein, R.A. The IL-12 family of heterodimeric cytokines: New players in the regulation of T cell responses. *Immunity* **2003**, *19*, 641–644. [CrossRef]
50. Gheita, T.A.; El Gazzar, I.I.; El-Fishawy, H.S.; Aboul-Ezz, M.A.; Kenawy, S.A. Involvement of IL-23 in enteropathic arthritis patients with inflammatory bowel disease: Preliminary results. *Clin. Rheumatol.* **2014**, *33*, 713–717. [CrossRef]
51. Engel, T.; Yung, D.E.; Ma, C.; Pariente, B.; WIls, P.; Eliakim, R.; Ungar, B.; Ben-Horin, S.; Kopylov, U. Effectiveness and safety of Ustekinumab for Crohn's disease; systematic review and pooled analysis of real-world evidence. *Dig. Liver Dis.* **2019**, *51*, 1232–1240. [CrossRef]
52. Drummond, R.A.; Franco, L.M.; Lionakis, M.S. Human CARD9: A critical molecule of fungal immune surveillance. *Front. Immunol.* **2018**, *9*, 1836. [CrossRef]
53. Williams, T.M.; Leeth, R.A.; Rothschild, D.E.; Coutermarsh-Ott, S.L.; McDaniel, D.K.; Simmons, A.E.; Heid, B.; Cecere, T.E.; Allen, I.C. The NLRP1 inflammasome attenuates colitis and colitis-associated tumorigenesis. *J. Immunol.* **2015**, *194*, 3369–3380. [CrossRef]
54. Seyfizadeh, N.; Seyfizadeh, N.; Gharibi, T.; Babaloo, Z. Interleukin-13 as an important cytokine: A review on its roles in some human diseases. *Acta Microbiol. Immunol. Hung.* **2015**, *62*, 341–378. [CrossRef] [PubMed]
55. Vebr, M.; Pomahačová, R.; Sýkora, J.; Schwarz, J. A Narrative Review of Cytokine Networks: Pathophysiological and Therapeutic Implications for Inflammatory Bowel Disease Pathogenesis. *Biomedicines* **2023**, *11*, 3229. [CrossRef] [PubMed]
56. Opal, S.M.; DePalo, V.A. Anti-inflammatory cytokines. *Chest* **2000**, *117*, 1162–1172. [CrossRef] [PubMed]
57. Emam, A.A.; Shehab, M.M.; Allah, M.A.; Elkoumi, M.A.; Abdelaal, N.M.; Mosabah, A.A.; Zakaria, M.T.; Sherif, A.M.; Soliman, M.M.; El-Kaffas, R.M. Interleukin-4-590C/T gene polymorphism in Egyptian children with acute lower respiratory infection: A multicenter study. *Pediatr. Pulmonol.* **2019**, *54*, 297–302. [CrossRef]
58. Luo, X.; Villablanca, E.J. Type 2 immunity in intestinal homeostasis and inflammatory bowel disease. *Biochem. Soc. Trans.* **2021**, *49*, 2371–2380. [CrossRef]
59. Cao, Z.; Conway, K.L.; Heath, R.J.; Rush, J.S.; Leshchiner, E.S.; Ramirez-Ortiz, Z.G.; Nedelsky, N.B.; Huang, H.; Ng, A.; Gardet, A. Ubiquitin ligase TRIM62 regulates CARD9-mediated anti-fungal immunity and intestinal inflammation. *Immunity* **2015**, *43*, 715–726. [CrossRef]
60. Winer, D.A.; Luck, H.; Tsai, S.; Winer, S. The intestinal immune system in obesity and insulin resistance. *Cell Metab.* **2016**, *23*, 413–426. [CrossRef]

biomedicines

MDPI

Article

Identifying Common Genetic Etiologies Between Inflammatory Bowel Disease and Related Immune-Mediated Diseases

Xianqiang Liu [1,2,†], Dingchang Li [1,2,†], Yue Zhang [1], Hao Liu [2,3], Peng Chen [1,2], Yingjie Zhao [1,2], Piero Ruscitti [4], Wen Zhao [2,3,*] and Guanglong Dong [2,*]

[1] Medical School of Chinese PLA, Beijing 100853, China; dr_liuxianqiang@163.com (X.L.)
[2] Department of General Surgery, The First Medical Center, Chinese PLA General Hospital, No. 28 Fuxing Road, Haidian District, Beijing 100853, China
[3] School of Medicine, Nankai University, Tianjin 300071, China
[4] Rheumatology Unit, Department of Biotechnological and Applied Clinical Sciences, University of L'Aquila, 67100 L'Aquila, Italy
* Correspondence: zhaowen2021@163.com (W.Z.); dongguanglong@301hospital.com.cn (G.D.)
† These authors contributed equally to this work.

Abstract: Background: Patients with inflammatory bowel disease (IBD) have an increased risk of developing immune-mediated diseases. However, the genetic basis of IBD is complex, and an integrated approach should be used to elucidate the complex genetic relationship between IBD and immune-mediated diseases. Methods: The genetic relationship between IBD and 16 immune-mediated diseases was examined using linkage disequilibrium score regression. GWAS data were synthesized from two IBD databases using the METAL, and multi-trait analysis of genome-wide association studies was performed to enhance statistical robustness and identify novel genetic associations. Independent risk loci were meticulously examined using conditional and joint genome-wide multi-trait analysis, multi-marker analysis of genomic annotation, and functional mapping and annotation of significant genetic loci, integrating the information of quantitative trait loci and different methodologies to identify risk-related genes and proteins. Results: The results revealed four immune-mediated diseases (AS, psoriasis, iridocyclitis, and PsA) with a significant relationship with IBD. The multi-trait analysis revealed 909 gene loci of statistical significance. Of these loci, 28 genetic variants were closely related to IBD, and 7 single-nucleotide polymorphisms represented novel independent risk loci. In addition, 14 genes and 514 proteins were found to be associated with susceptibility to immune-mediated diseases. Notably, IL1RL1 emerged as a key player, present within pleiotropic genes across multiple protein databases, highlighting its potential as a therapeutic target. Conclusions: This study suggests that the common polygenic determinants between IBD and immune-mediated diseases are widely distributed across the genome. The findings not only support a shared genetic relationship between IBD and immune-mediated diseases but also provide novel therapeutic targets for these diseases.

Keywords: inflammatory bowel disease; GWAS; genetics; MTAG; immune-mediated diseases; IL-1; autoinflammation

1. Introduction

Inflammatory bowel disease (IBD), which includes both Crohn's disease and ulcerative colitis, is a chronic inflammatory disorder. It arises from an abnormal immune reaction to intestinal bacteria in individuals with a genetic predisposition, leading to recurring and damaging inflammation of the gastrointestinal tract [1]. Millions of individuals have IBD worldwide, with approximately 2.2 million diagnosed cases in Europe alone [2]. Immune-mediated diseases frequently co-occur within families, with individuals with one condition having an increased risk of other conditions [3,4]. Common susceptibility loci identified in various immune-mediated diseases suggest a shared genetic basis involving polygenic susceptibility genes [5,6]. Comorbidities and associations between inflammatory bowel disease and immune-mediated diseases have been widely reported. Genome-wide association studies (GWASs) have validated a genetic relationship between IBD and several immune-mediated diseases, including celiac disease [7], rheumatoid arthritis (RA) [8], ankylosing spondylitis (AS) [9], and primary sclerosing cholangitis [10]. Numerous signaling pathways are involved in this relationship, with tumor necrosis factor (TNF) and nuclear factor kappa-light-chain-enhancer of activated B cells (NF-κB) playing a crucial role in inflammation and other immune responses [11,12].

Despite significant advancements in understanding these relationships, studies focusing on single diseases may overlook key genetic loci and regulatory mechanisms. Therefore, multi-trait analysis is important for expanding the phenotypic spectrum of research, identifying risk loci, and investigating the shared genetic etiological factors between diseases [13]. The shared genetic causes may indicate potential pleiotropy, acting as genetic confounding factors between traits [14,15]. Therefore, cross-trait analysis based on GWAS data has been proposed to identify pleiotropic genes or loci across multiple traits [16,17]. These pleiotropic loci may serve as valuable targets for preventing or treating multiple diseases simultaneously.

In this pleiotropic GWAS, summary data from large-scale GWASs on IBD (International Inflammatory Bowel Disease Consortium and FinnGen database) and 16 immune-mediated diseases were utilized. Various statistical methods (PLACO, MAGMA, POPS, SMR, and BLISS) were used to assess pleiotropic associations between IBD and immune-mediated diseases based on single-nucleotide variants (SNVs), gene levels, protein levels, and biological pathways to identify shared genetic etiological factors. Furthermore, gene set variation analysis (GSVA) was performed based on the transcriptomic profiles of patients with IBD to establish a pleiotropic gene score, and the relationship between this score and immune cell infiltration was subsequently analyzed to subtype IBD patients. We hope that this study will contribute to a better understanding of the genetic structure and potential therapeutic mechanisms of IBD. Figure 1 depicts the comprehensive design of this study.

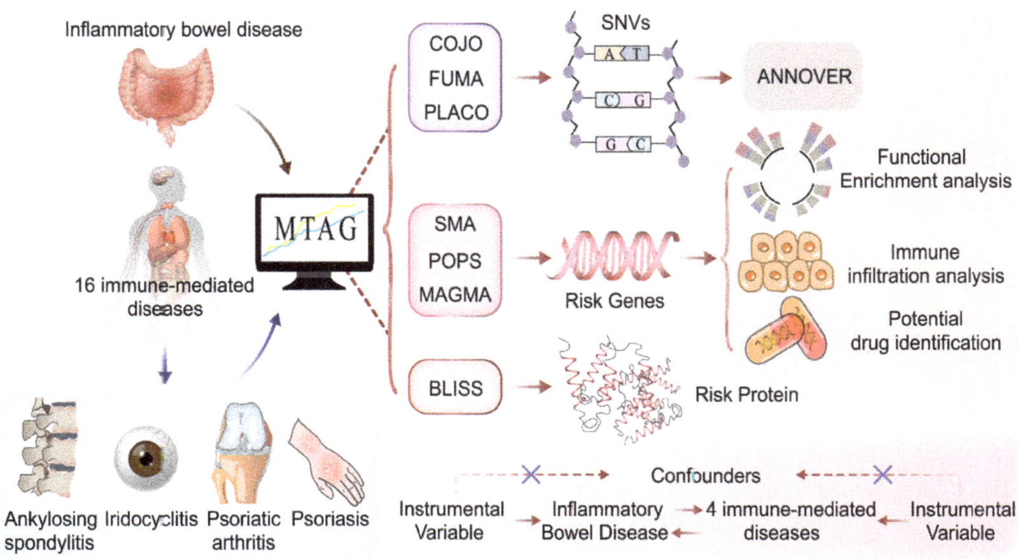

Figure 1. The overall study design. LDSC analysis was first conducted on IBD and 16 immune-mediated diseases, revealing a genetic correlation between IBD and conditions such as AS, psoriasis, iridocyclitis, and PsA. Following this, MTAG analysis was performed, and the indings were elaborated

at the levels of single-nucleotide variants (SNVs), genes, and proteins. The figure was created using Adobe Illustrator. AS, ankylosing spondylitis; PsA, psoriatic arthritis; LDSC, linkage disequilibrium score regression; POPS, polygenic priority score; MAGMA, multi-marker analysis of genomic annotation; COJO, conditional and joint analysis; BLISS, Biomarker Imputation from Summary Statistics; SMR, Summary-based Mendelian randomization; MR, Mendelian randomization.

2. Materials and Methods

2.1. Collection of GWAS Summary Data

GWAS summary statistics were obtained from publicly available datasets of European ancestry. GWAS summary data on IBD were extracted from the International IBD Genetics Consortium [18], which includes 12,882 patients and 21,770 control individuals, and a FinnGen database (Finn-IBD), which includes 9083 patients and 392,974 control individuals. Additionally, data on 16 prevalent immune-mediated diseases were obtained from the FinnGen database [19], including AS, psoriasis, iridocyclitis, psoriatic arthritis (PsA), celiac disease, sarcoidosis, primary sclerosing cholangitis, multiple sclerosis, immune-mediated hyperthyroidism, RA, type 1 diabetes mellitus, hypothyroidism, adult-onset Still's disease, hidradenitis suppurativa, gout, and systemic lupus erythematosus. Based on data availability, these 16 diseases were chosen across an inflammatory spectrum from autoinflammatory to autoimmune diseases as two-end stages and "intermediate" phenotypes according to a continuum of different pathologic conditions associated with a deregulated and aberrant immune response [20]. Data aligning with the GRCh38 reference were converted to GRCh37 using the liftOver tool to ensure consistency [21].

The characteristics of the study population are outlined in Supplementary Table S1. To investigate the genetic composition of patients with IBD, quantitative trait loci (QTL) data were integrated, including plasma protein QTLs (pQTLs) and expression QTLs (eQTLs) from 54 specific samples (such as small intestine terminal ileum and Colon Sigmoid). Blood eQTL data were extracted from the expansive eQTLGen Consortium database, documenting single-nucleotide polymorphisms (SNPs) associated with various traits in 31,684 individuals [22]. Plasma pQTL data were extracted from the deCODE [23], ARIC, and UKBPP [24] database.

2.2. Assessment of Genetic Correlations Between IBD and Immune-Mediated Diseases

Linkage disequilibrium score regression (LDSC) was used to assess the genetic relationship between IBD and 16 immune-mediated diseases based on GWAS summary data from two IBD datasets. In particular, the 1000 Genomes Project data for European ancestry was harnessed for LD scores within these analyses [25]. In LDSC, no constraints were imposed on the intercept, as sample overlap influences only the intercept, leaving the regression slope and genetic correlation unaffected. The Benjamini and Hochberg (BH) correction was applied to mitigate the impact of multiple testing, with an FDR-p value < 0.05 confirming significant genetic associations. Immune-mediated diseases that showed positive results in both dataset (The International Inflammatory Bowel Disease Genetics Consortium and Finngen database) analyses were included in the subsequent analysis.

2.3. Meta-Analysis of GWASs

A meta-analysis was conducted to combine data from two sources of IBD. Using Metasoft, the heterogeneity index (I^2) and p-value based on Cochran's Q test (P_het) were calculated. In cases of heterogeneity ($I^2 \geq 50$ or $P\_het < 0.05$), p-values from the random-effects model were prioritized [26,27].

2.4. Integrated Analysis of Traits of IBD and Associated Immune-Mediated Diseases

Based on the results of the abovementioned analyses, the multi-trait analysis of GWASs (MTAG) method was used to assess the phenotypes of immune-mediated diseases that exhibited a significant genetic correlation with META-IBD. The MTAG involves the use of the generalized inverse-variance weighted (IVW) approach to enhance statistical power and facilitate the identification of genetic relationships for each trait. Essentially, the MTAG processes the GWAS summary data of individual traits to produce trait-specific effects for shared SNPs while integrating LDSC to adjust for sample overlap between related traits [28]. In this process, the GWAS data of immune-related disease phenotypes with confirmed genetic correlations to IBD were integrated to generate MTAG-IBD.

2.5. Identification of Genetic Risk Factors for IBD

2.5.1. Identification of Independent Risk Loci

To further elucidate the genomic risks associated with IBD, distinct independent signals within genomic loci linked to MTAG-IBD were examined. This was achieved through conditional and joint association analyses using the stepwise model selection framework provided by GCTA–conditional and joint analysis (COJO) [29]. The analysis focused on multi-allelic variants displaying significant associations (P.mtag $< 5 \times 10^{-8}$) within recognized genomic risk loci, with additional signals being validated based on a joint p-value threshold of $<5 \times 10^{-8}$. This investigation utilized the European ancestry reference cohort dataset from the third phase of the 1000 Genomes Project [25]. For pairs of traits showing significant genetic correlation or overlap, pleiotropic analysis under the composite null hypothesis (PLACO) was employed to detect potential pleiotropic SNVs. This analysis computed squared Z scores for each variant, and SNPs with exceedingly high Z values (>80) were excluded. Subsequently, the hypothesis of no pleiotropy was assessed using the intersection–union test method with a horizontal α, leading to determining the final pleiotropic p-values. Significant pleiotropic variants were identified as SNVs with p-values $< 5 \times 10^{-8}$. Following the PLACO results, the identified loci were mapped to neighboring genes to investigate the shared biological mechanisms underlying these pleiotropic loci. Additional annotation was performed using the Functional Mapping and Annotation (FUMA) platform [30]. Strict criteria were applied, setting the maximum p-value for lead SNVs at $<5 \times 10^{-8}$ while adopting a more inclusive significance threshold of $p < 0.05$. Independent SNV identification was based on an r^2 threshold of less than 0.6, with lead SNVs requiring an r^2 of less than 0.1 within a 1 Mb radius. The criteria for defining genomic risk loci included merging regions with lead SNVs less than 250 kb apart. SNVs validated through COJO and FUMA analyses were classified as risk variants for COPD. These variants were annotated using ANNOVAR [31], and their potential deleterious impact was evaluated through combined annotation-dependent depletion (CADD) scores, with values exceeding 12.37 suggesting a higher likelihood of harmful effects [32]. RegulomeDB (RDB) [33] provides a classification score ranging from 1a to 7, indicating the regulatory function of SNPs based on eQTLs and chromatin marks. A score of 1a represents the strongest biological evidence for the SNP as a regulatory element.

2.5.2. Genetic Insights into IBD

In a comprehensive analysis targeting the genetic underpinnings of IBD, three distinct strategies were implemented. For each approach, p-values were corrected for the false discovery rate (FDR) using the BH method, with genes displaying an FDR < 0.05 and those consistently identified by three approaches being deemed significantly associated risk genes. The multi-marker analysis of genomic annotation (MAGMA) and polygenic priority score (POPS) were applied to identify and prioritize relevant genes [34,35]. The gene-centric analysis conducted in the MAGMA was derived from an extensive catalog of protein-coding genes, and when combined with the POPS, it enabled a more refined gene prioritization strategy. This methodology integrated summary GWAS data with comprehensive expression datasets and biological pathways, establishing a POPS threshold greater than 1 for gene selection.

The Summary-based Mendelian randomization (SMR) approach was simultaneously applied, utilizing the MTAG-IBD and eQTL dataset summary statistics to identify genes whose expression levels are associated with complex traits driven by pleiotropy. SMR uses SNPs as instrumental variables to test the causal effect of the exposure on the outcome [36]. The accompanying Heterogeneity in Dependent Instruments (HEIDI) test was also employed to assess whether the causal effect detected by SMR was due to linkage disequilibrium (p-HEIDI < 0.01). Consequently, genes with an FDR < 0.05 and p-HEIDI > 0.01 were considered potential susceptibility genes associated with the genetic risk underlying MTAG-IBD.

Phenotypic and genomic enrichment analyses were performed to assess the biological relevance of genes associated with IBD. Phenotypic enrichment analysis was performed using the Mammalian Phenotype Ontology from Mouse Genome Informatics (MGI) [37], and the specificity of mammalian phenotype (MP)-related genes was compared with that of non-MP-related genes. The genomic enrichment analysis was performed using data from the Kyoto Encyclopedia of Genes and Genomes (KEGG) pathways and Gene Ontology (GO) pathway databases [38,39].

2.5.3. Proteomic Insights into IBD

To unravel the complex proteomic profiles linked with IBD and immune-mediated diseases, this study utilized the "Biomarker Imputation from Summary Statistics (BLISS)" technique [40]. BLISS introduces a novel approach for developing protein interpolation models directly from summary-level pQTL data, thereby enabling the creation of comprehensive European PWAS models. This was accomplished by employing extensive pQTL information from large repositories, including the UKB, deCODE, and ARIC studies. In this research segment, the BH procedure continued to be applied to ascertain the FDR of p-values. Proteins exhibiting an FDR of less than 0.05 were recognized as significant risk proteins, highlighting their potential role in the pathophysiology of IBD and related immune-mediated diseases.

2.6. *Construction of Drug–Gene Interaction Networks*

The Drug–Gene Interaction Database (DGIdb, http://www.dgidb.org/, accessed on 28 May 2024) [41] was used to predict FDA-approved drugs interacting with pleiotropic genes. Subsequently, Cytoscape software (version 3.9.1) was used to construct a drug–gene interaction network based on the predictions.

2.7. *Two-Sample MR*

The widely recognized instrumental variable technique, MR analysis, was employed to discern causal relationships between IBD and four immune-related diseases. SNPs associated with exposure served as instruments [42,43], while data derived from GWAS summaries were utilized to pinpoint variants correlated with IBD and four immune-related diseases, adhering to a p-value threshold of $<5.0 \times 10^{-8}$. Additionally, to account for linkage disequilibrium, a clumping procedure was employed on these SNPs using specific parameters (kb = 10,000, $r^2 = 0.001$). To ensure the robustness of the instrumental variables, the coefficient of determination (r^2) and F-statistic were computed, incorporating only those SNPs with F-values exceeding 10. Furthermore, the MR-PRESSO method, employing 1000 iterations, was utilized to identify outliers [14]. LDlink facilitated the exclusion of confounding SNPs, and the identified outliers were subsequently removed for reassessment.

2.8. *GSVA and Immune Cell Infiltration Analysis*

To assess the role of pleiotropic genes in the immunophenotyping of IBD patients, GSVA analysis was performed to evaluate immune cell infiltration; mRNA expression data were extracted from three datasets (GSE75214, GSE3365, and GSE87466) from the Gene Expression Omnibus (GEO) database [44], including 344 patients with IBD and 85 healthy individuals. Risk-related genes were quantified using the single-sample gene set enrichment analysis (ssGSEA) algorithm. Based on the ssGSEA outcomes, patients in the IBD cohort were classified with high or low immune infiltration [45].

3. Results

3.1. Genetic Relationship Between IBD and Multiple Immune-Mediated Diseases

In investigating genetic correlations, we conducted LDSC analyses on IBD from two sources and 16 immune-mediated diseases. After applying BH correction, we identified significant genetic correlations between IBD from both sources and four immune-mediated diseases (AS, psoriasis, iridocyclitis, and PsA) (Supplementary Table S2). Subsequently, we integrated the GWAS summary statistics from both IBD sources to create a consolidated dataset (META-IBD), which included 9,749,028 SNPs. After excluding the complex MHC region, we identified 8033 statistically significant genetic loci.

3.2. Genetic Landscape of IBD Identified Through Multi-Trait Analysis

To further investigate the complex genetic architecture of IBD, we performed a multi-trait analysis using the META-IBD dataset and four immune-mediated diseases. Using the MTAG method, we generated an enhanced IBD dataset (MTAG-IBD) that included 8,247,243 SNPs. From this MTAG-IBD dataset, we identified 8657 significant SNPs. Notably, this analysis revealed 909 novel SNPs that had not been previously detected in individual IBD GWAS summaries or the META-IBD dataset.

3.3. Genetic Markers Associated with IBD

Using the advanced GCTA-COJO tool, we conducted conditional and joint association analyses on the MTAG-IBD dataset. Through this rigorous process, we identified 363 SNPs (Supplementary Table S3). Subsequently, the PLACO analysis identified 9344 SNPs as potential pleiotropic variants across four IBD–immune-mediated disease pairs (Figure 2A–D). Further analysis using the FUMA platform revealed 159 lead SNPs (Supplementary Table S4). Notably, 38 SNPs (28 unique) were consistently identified in both the COJO and PLACO analyses, establishing them as independent genetic risk loci for IBD–immune-mediated diseases. Utilizing the ANNOVAR tool for further detailed gene annotation, we identified two variants—rs11209026 (IL23R) and rs1990760 (IFIH1)—located within the exonic regions. Notably, both of these variants have CADD scores exceeding 12.37. This suggests the potential pathogenic effects of these single-nucleotide variants (SNPs).

3.4. Genes Associated with the Risk of IBD

The MAGMA revealed 1426 genes associated with immune-mediated disease risk SNPs (Supplementary Table S5). Subsequently, POPSs revealed 137 (104 unique) genes (POPSs > 1) potentially associated with the risk of IBD (Supplementary Table S6). SMR analysis showed that 14 of the 104 genes were associated with immune-mediated diseases (Figure 3A) (Supplementary Table S7). The analysis of tissue-specific gene expression revealed that disease–gene associations for pleiotropic genes were predominantly concentrated in the spleen and small intestine terminal ileum compartments (Figure 3D). Genomic enrichment analysis indicated that the risk-related genes were significantly enriched in biological processes related to the active regulation of inflammatory responses and immune effects, including positive regulation of leukocyte adhesion. In addition, the genes were enriched in Th17 cell differentiation, cytokine–cytokine receptor interactions, and the c TNF signaling pathway (Supplementary Table S8) (Figure 3B,C). These results suggest that the risk-related genes contributed to the pathogenesis of IBD and associated immune-mediated diseases. Phenotypic enrichment analysis showed that the genes were significantly enriched in two biological processes, including the immune system and hematopoietic system, demonstrating the complex nature of IBD and its systemic impacts (Supplementary Table S9).

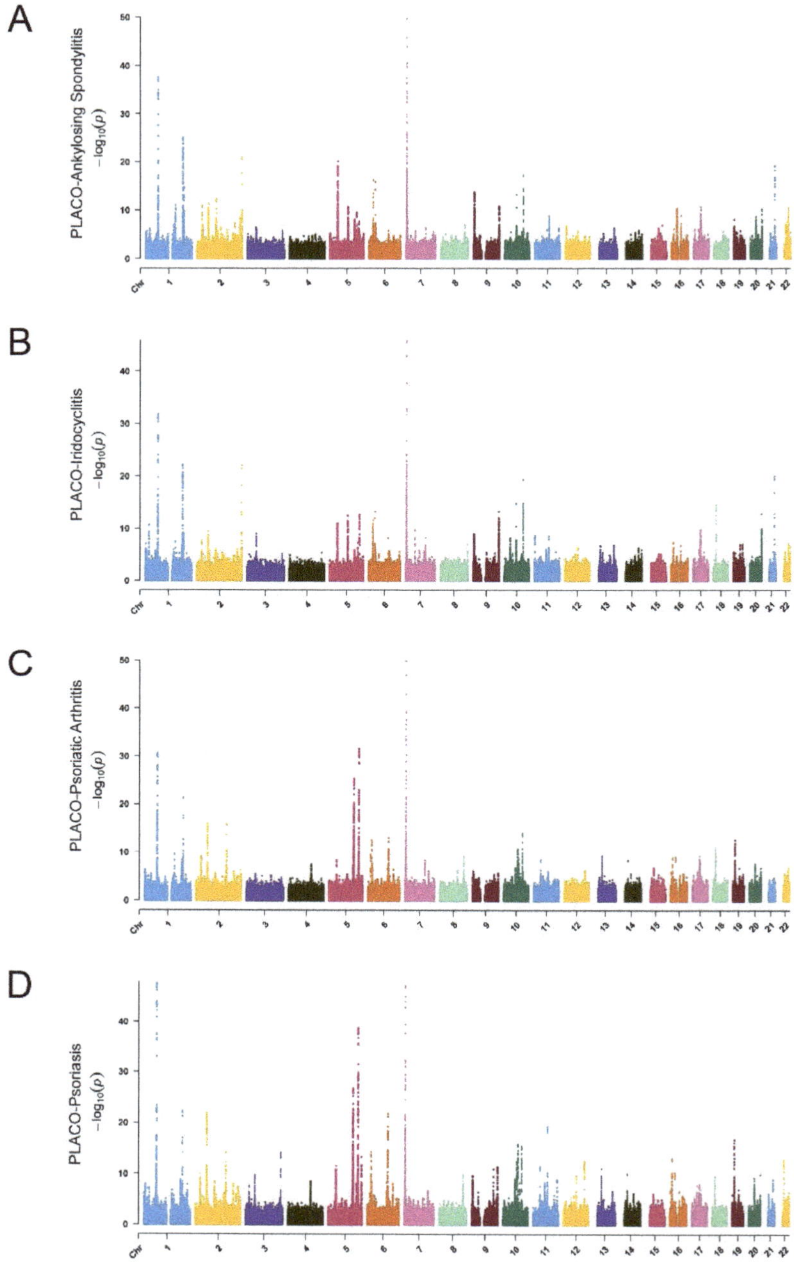

Figure 2. Manhattan plots of gene-based enrichments of PLACO associations with (**A**) ankylosing spondylitis, (**B**) iridocyclitis, (**C**) psoriatic arthritis, and (**D**) psoriasis. The x-axis shows chromosomal position, and the y-axis shows association p-values on a $-\log_{10}$ scale.

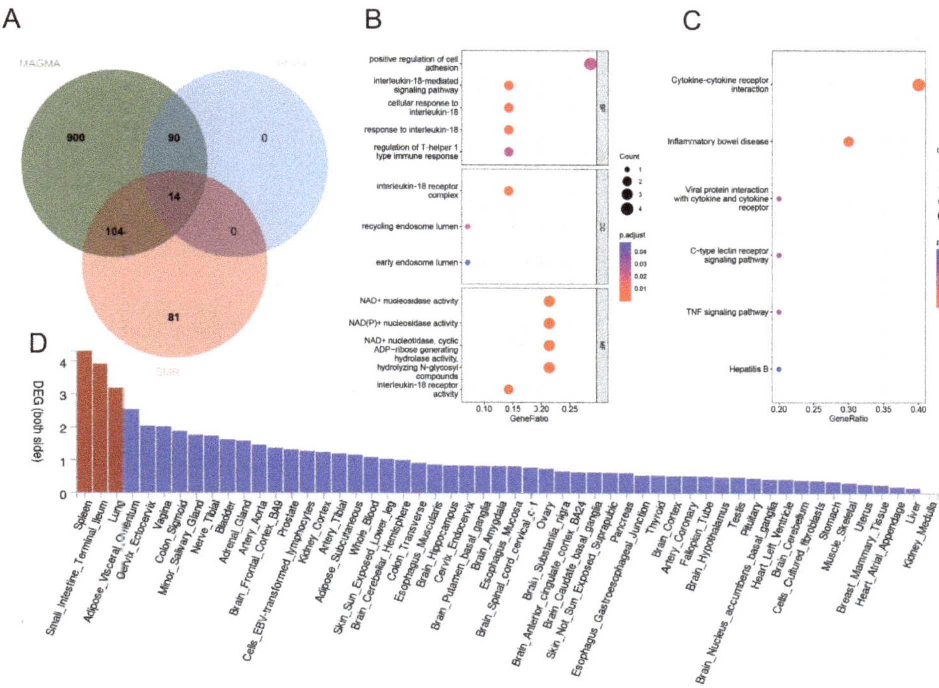

Figure 3. Enrichment analysis for identified pleiotropic genes. (**A**) The Wayne diagram showing POPS, MAGMA, and SMR pleiotropic gene screening. Significant types of pathways based on GO (**B**) and KEGG enrichment analyses (**C**). BP, biological process; CC, cellular component; MF, molecular function; KEGG, Kyoto encyclopedia of genes and genomes pathway. (**D**) Enrichment of differentially expressed genes among all identified pleiotropic genes across 54 GTEx tissues. The *y*-axis shows the *p*-values with a scale of $-\log_{10}$. The bars in red represent significant enrichment with Bonferroni adjustment for multiple-hypothesis testing.

3.5. Proteins Associated with the Risk of IBD and Associated Immune-Mediated Diseases

Based on the BLISS method combined with MTAG-IBD data, we evaluated 2923, 4953, and 4428 plasma proteins in the UKB, ARIC, and deCODE cohorts, respectively. The results revealed 514 proteins associated with the risk of IBD and associated immune-mediated diseases (Supplementary Table S10). KEGG enrichment analysis of these risk-associated proteins revealed significant enrichment in pathways such as cytokine–cytokine receptor interaction, JAK-STAT signaling, and TNF signaling (Supplementary Table S11). In particular, IL1RL1 was found to be present both within the pleiotropic genes and across the aforementioned three protein databases, suggesting a possible common thread and a potential therapeutic target.

3.6. Predicted Drug–Gene Interactions

Cytoscape was used to construct a drug–gene interaction network (Figure 4 and Supplementary Table S12). A total of 32 interactions were observed between 32 small-molecule drugs and 4 pleiotropic genes (MAP3K8, EGR2, PIM3, and SMAD3), which may represent novel therapeutic targets for IBD.

3.7. Results of Two-Sample MR

Bidirectional MR was performed to investigate the potential causal relationship between IBD and immune-mediated diseases. The results indicate a potential causal relationship between META-IBD and iridocyclitis [OR: 1.19; 95% CI: 1.13–1.24], AS [OR: 1.34; 95% CI: 1.25–1.44], and PsA [OR: 1.15; 95% CI: 1.07–1.22], with increased incidence rates.

Reverse MR demonstrates that iridocyclitis [OR: 1.10; 95% CI: 1.02–1.20] and AS [OR: 1.07; 95% CI: 1.04–1.11] have an inverse causal relationship with the incidence of META-IBD (Figure 5). Scatter plots, funnel plots, and leave-one-out sensitivity analysis are represented in Figure 6 (Supplementary Tables S13 and S14).

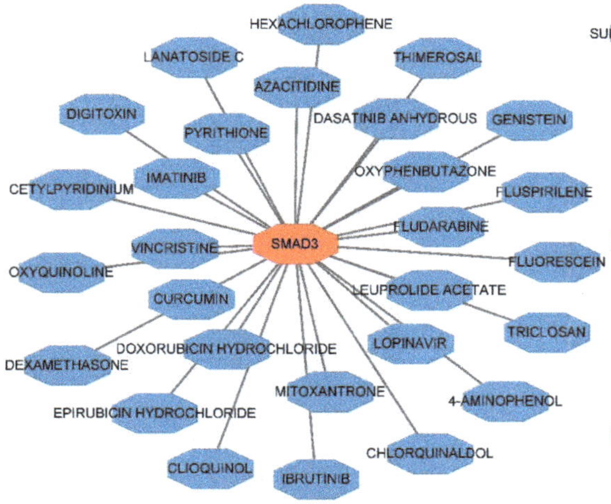

Figure 4. The drug–gene interaction network of the annotated genes through DGIdb. The genes are highlighted in red, whereas the drugs are highlighted in blue.

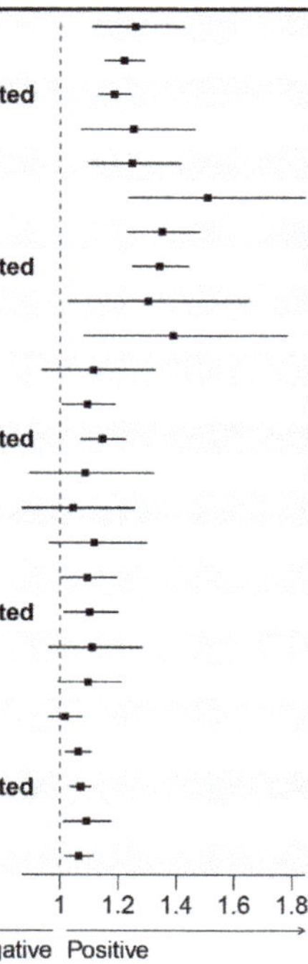

exposure	outcome	method	nsnp	pval	OR (95% CI)
IBD	Iridocyclitis	MR Egger	91	0.000	1.259 (1.111 to 1.426)
		Weighted median	91	0.000	1.220 (1.153 to 1.290)
		Inverse-variance weighted	**91**	**0.000**	**1.186 (1.133 to 1.242)**
		Simple mode	91	0.006	1.252 (1.071 to 1.464)
		Weighted mode	91	0.001	1.248 (1.099 to 1.417)
IBD	AS	MR Egger	93	0.000	1.509 (1.235 to 1.844)
		Weighted median	93	0.000	1.351 (1.231 to 1.482)
		Inverse-variance weighted	**93**	**0.000**	**1.343 (1.248 to 1.444)**
		Simple mode	93	0.031	1.303 (1.029 to 1.651)
		Weighted mode	93	0.011	1.390 (1.083 to 1.783)
IBD	Psoriatic Arthritis	MR Egger	93	0.223	1.115 (0.937 to 1.326)
		Weighted median	93	0.031	1.094 (1.008 to 1.188)
		Inverse-variance weighted	**93**	**0.000**	**1.146 (1.072 to 1.225)**
		Simple mode	93	0.406	1.087 (0.894 to 1.321)
		Weighted mode	93	0.636	1.046 (0.870 to 1.257)
Iridocyclitis	IBD	MR Egger	7	0.204	1.118 (0.963 to 1.297)
		Weighted median	7	0.043	1.094 (1.003 to 1.194)
		Inverse-variance weighted	**7**	**0.021**	**1.103 (1.015 to 1.198)**
		Simple mode	7	0.201	1.111 (0.962 to 1.282)
		Weighted mode	7	0.114	1.097 (0.994 to 1.209)
AS	IBD	MR Egger	15	0.550	1.017 (0.963 to 1.075)
		Weighted median	15	0.004	1.063 (1.019 to 1.108)
		Inverse-variance weighted	**15**	**0.000**	**1.072 (1.038 to 1.107)**
		Simple mode	15	0.036	1.092 (1.014 to 1.176)
		Weighted mode	15	0.014	1.065 (1.019 to 1.114)

Figure 5. Bidirectional Mendelian randomization (MR) analyses between META-IBD and 4 immune-mediated diseases (ankylosing spondylitis, psoriasis, iridocyclitis, and psoriatic arthritis). Estimates and 95% confidence intervals (CIs) are shown using square plots and error bars.

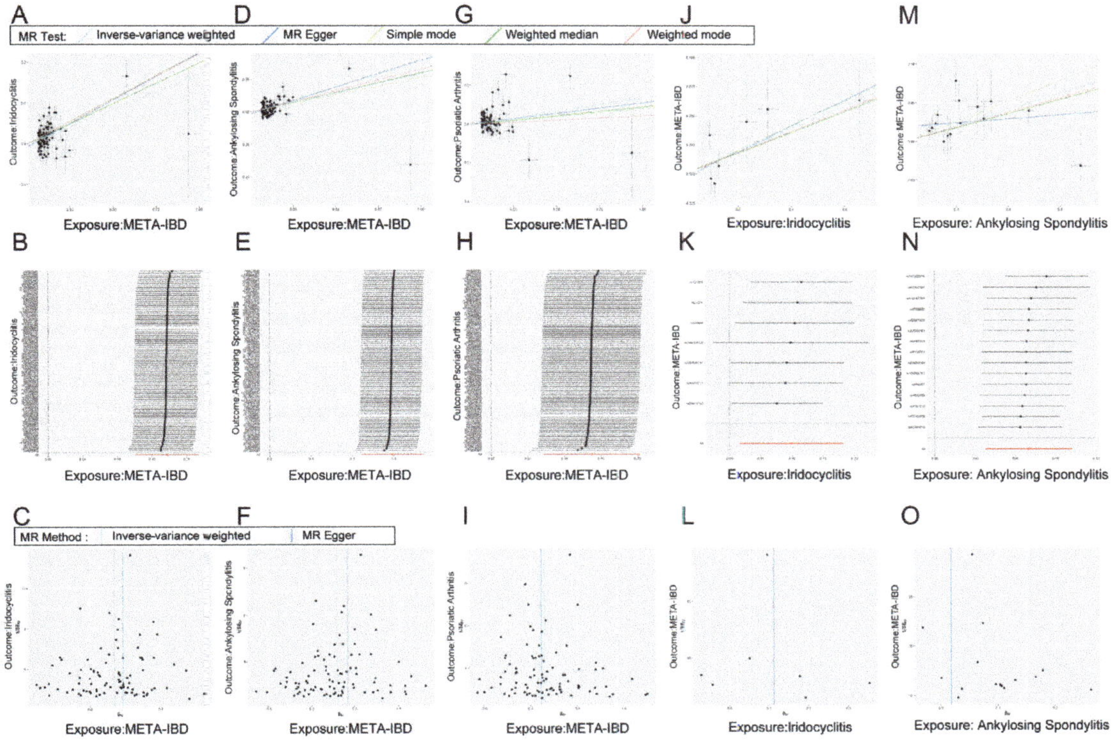

Figure 6. The scatter plot (**A**,**D**,**G**), sensitivity analysis (**B**,**E**,**H**), and funnel plot (**C**,**F**,**I**) of the effect of ankylosing spondylitis, psoriasis, and iridocyclitis on META-IBD. The scatter plot (**J**,**M**), sensitivity analysis (**K**,**N**), and funnel plot (**L**,**O**) of the effect of META-IBD on iridocyclitis and ankylosing spondylitis. In the scatter plot, five methods were employed to describe the direction of causality: IVW, Weight median, Simple Mode, Weighted Mode, and MR Egger.

3.8. Identification and Characterization of IBD Subtypes

To validate the subtypes of IBD, immunedeconv was used to quantify pleiotropic genes for each patient, and a pleiotropic gene score was created for each patient based on gene expression. Subsequently, the patients were divided into high- and low-immune-infiltration groups based on the median polytropic gene score. A histogram was generated to visualize the distinct immune cell infiltration patterns between the two groups. The proportion of most immune cell types, including activated and central memory CD4 T cells, dendritic cells, CD8-positive T cells, neutrophils, plasma cells, mast cells, and regulatory T cells (Tregs), was higher in the high-risk group. However, the proportion of M2 macrophages was higher in the low-risk group, as shown in Figure 7.

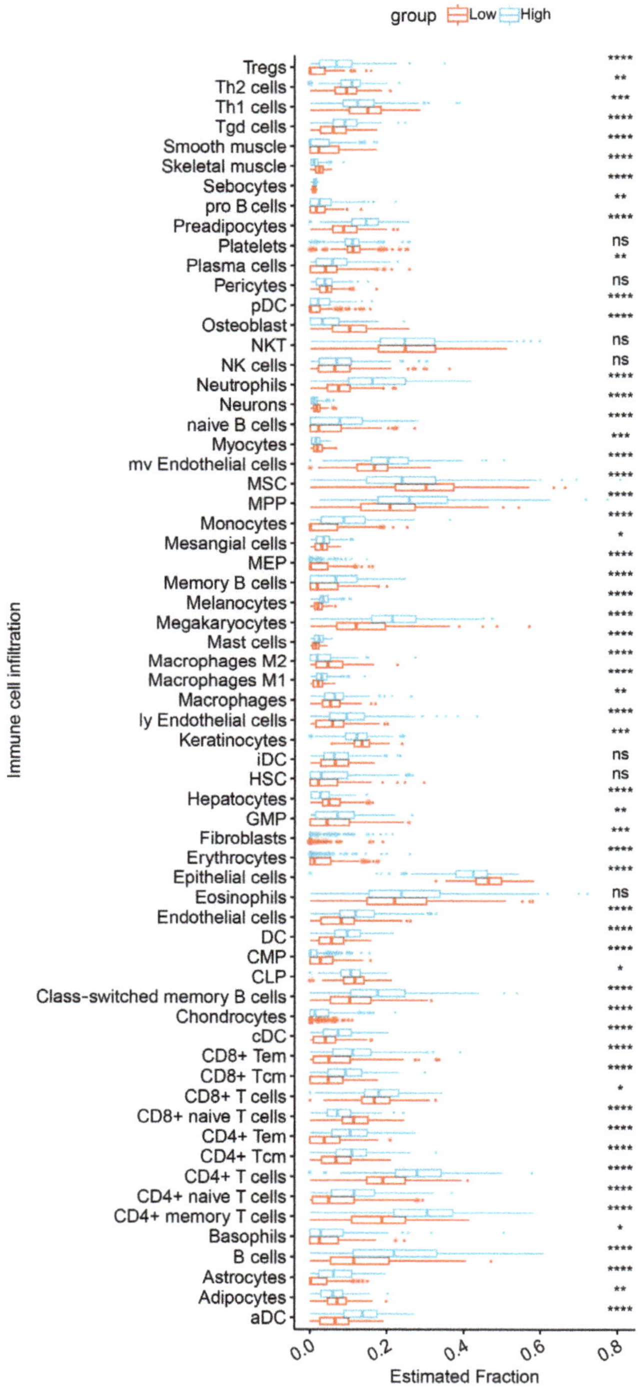

Figure 7. Immune infiltration analysis of pleiotropic genes in IBD cohort. Abundance of differences in immune cells between both groups in IBD cohort. (ns, not significant; * $p < 0.05$, ** $p < 0.01$, *** $p < 0.001$, and **** $p < 0.0001$).

4. Discussion

IBD patients often present with co-occurring immune-mediated diseases that share genetic and immunological similarities mainly driven by helper T-cell (Th) response [46,47]. A common feature of these diseases is their immune pathogenesis, characterized by hyperactivity within specific components of the immune system [48,49]. This shared, complex genetic architecture necessitates an integrated analytical approach, rather than a traditional single-disease framework, to identify genetic factors impacting both conditions. In this study, we employed an innovative, comprehensive method to investigate the genetic relationship between IBD and 16 immune-mediated diseases.

GWAS summary data from two IBD datasets were integrated into the consolidated META-IBD dataset. Of the 16 immune-mediated diseases, 4 diseases exhibited a significant genetic correlation with IBD. All of these four diseases, namely, psoriasis, AS, iridocyclitis, and PsA, are extraintestinal manifestations of IBD. These findings provide valuable insights into the treatment of extraintestinal manifestations of IBD. Among these, AS exhibits the greatest genetic overlap with IBD, with a correlation coefficient exceeding 0.5. Previous studies have indicated a positive causal relationship between IBD and its subtypes and AS. Although the mechanisms underlying their comorbidity remain incompletely understood, the "gut-joint axis" hypothesis has been proposed to explain their pathogenic connection [50]. Various environmental factors, such as dysbiosis of the gut microbiota, along with host immune factors, may lead to inflammation in genetically susceptible individuals, triggering inflammatory responses targeting both gut and joint components. These mechanisms provide important insights for understanding the comorbidity between AS and IBD [51]. The META-IBD dataset and the four immune-mediated diseases were subjected to a comprehensive multi-trait analysis aimed at enhancing the statistical scrutiny of the original IBD datasets. The results revealed 909 previously unidentified genetic loci, substantially improving the understanding of the genetic foundation of IBD. Furthermore, COJO and FUMA analyses revealed 28 independent risk loci closely associated with IBD, including 2 loci (rs1990760 and rs1990760) located in exonic regions with CADD scores exceeding 12.37. IFIH1 plays a role in the innate immune system by recognizing viruses and initiating antiviral responses [52]; however, its functional upregulation may modestly increase the risk of autoimmune diseases [53]. A meta-analysis indicated that the IFIH1 rs1990760 T allele is significantly associated with susceptibility to autoimmune diseases, including systemic lupus erythematosus, multiple sclerosis, and rheumatoid arthritis [54]. This mechanism likely involves IFIH1 enhancing IFN-α production to counteract viral infections while concurrently co-operating with IFNAR to activate the JAK-STAT pathway, thereby inducing the transcription of downstream genes and promoting the development of autoimmune diseases (AIDs) [55]. Therefore, the association of rs1990760 with IBD and other immune-mediated diseases warrants further investigation. IL-23 is secreted by activated dendritic cells, monocytes, and macrophages and is crucial for the amplification and maintenance of Th17 cell responses [56]. The IL-23/Th17 axis plays a key role in the inflammatory processes of IBD and psoriasis [57]. Studies have shown that rs11209026, a missense variant (Arg381Gln) located in the cytoplasmic tail of the IL-23 receptor (IL-23R), can alter IL-23R signaling [58]. Specifically, the IL23R polymorphism (rs11209026) has been shown to increase susceptibility to IBD in the Finnish population [59]. Additionally, the rs11209026 variant in IL23R is significantly associated with the risk of IBD, AS, and psoriasis. These findings suggest that the IL-23/Th17 pathway and its key variants play an important role in multiple immune-related diseases. Furthermore, the integrated approach used in this study not only revealed novel genetic loci but also proposed novel insights into the genetic characteristics of IBD. Genetic association analysis revealed 137 genes related to IBD. The SMR analysis further confirmed 14 genes. These include genes considered mature candidates, such as MAP3K8, IL1RL1, IL18R1, and IL18RAP, as well as less common genes like CD6. CD6 is a surface glycoprotein with a weight of 105–130 kDa, primarily expressed in mature T lymphocytes, CD56 NK cells, and some cells of the hematopoietic system [60,61].

A previous study has already identified CD6 as a negative regulatory factor in both early- and late-stage signal transduction events in T-cell responses [62]. Genetic variations in CD6 are associated with susceptibility to or severity of various immune-mediated diseases, including multiple sclerosis, Behçet's disease, and psoriasis [63–65]. Recent research also indicates that CD6 is a novel risk gene for inflammatory bowel disease (IBD). In the inflamed mucosa of active IBD patients, CD6 expression is significantly increased and positively correlated with disease severity [66,67]. CD6 knockout mice exhibit markedly decreased inflammation in experimental immune-mediated encephalomyelitis (EAE), psoriasis, and uveitis. Additionally, Th1 and Th17 cell-mediated immune responses are significantly reduced [68,69]. Additionally, humanized anti-CD6 mAb (Itolizumab) effectively treats psoriasis and rheumatoid arthritis by strongly suppressing pro-inflammatory cytokine production and Th1/17 cell proliferation [70,71]. This suggests that CD6 may be a potential therapeutic target for IBD. MAP3K8 (also known as TPL2) plays a critical role in the immune system, with its genetic polymorphisms associated with the development of IBD [72]. It promotes the migration of neutrophils to inflammation sites and enhances cytokine secretion, leading to colitis in mice [73,74]. Additionally, MAP3K8 positively regulates the MEK1/2-ERK1/2 signaling pathway, influencing the survival and proliferation of intestinal mucosal cells [75]. The inhibition of MAP3K8 has shown therapeutic potential in various inflammatory diseases, including IBD, RA, and psoriasis, highlighting its value as an important therapeutic target [76,77]. Meanwhile, RNASET2 may regulate the downstream secretion of interferon-gamma (IFN-γ) through integrin signaling pathways, positioning it as a potential therapeutic biomarker [78]. PIM3, a member of the PIM kinase family, is significant in regulating T-cell proliferation; inhibiting PIM3 can induce CD4+ T cells to halt in the G0/G1 phase, preventing their proliferation, and PIM3 inhibitors have demonstrated effectiveness in CD4+ T cell-mediated IBD models [79]. Furthermore, IL-18 and its receptors, IL18RAP and IL18R1, are crucial in immune responses, with IL-18 activating the NF-κB pathway to stimulate the production of interferon-gamma and pro-inflammatory cytokines like TNF-α and IL-1β [80]. Clinical studies show significant increases in IL-18 expression in the mucosal biopsies of IBD patients, particularly in affected lesions, suggesting a key role for IL-18 in IBD pathology [81]. Animal studies indicate that blocking IL-18 can effectively reduce intestinal inflammation [82]. Additionally, the TGF-β signaling pathway plays a vital role in promoting regulatory and inflammatory immune responses, with SMAD3, a downstream transcription factor, being essential [83]; mice lacking SMAD3 are prone to inflammation and develop IBD under environmental stimuli, underscoring the importance of this pathway in tissue repair and immune regulation [84,85]. Finally, the NKX2-3 gene has an SNP rs10883365 located 5 kb upstream of its transcriptional start site that correlates with IBD [86], although the exact mechanisms remain unclear and warrant further investigation. These findings provide significant insights into the pathogenesis of IBD and the development of novel therapeutic strategies.

Using the BLISS method, our study identified 514 proteins associated with the risk of IBD immune-mediated diseases from the deCODE, UKBPP, and ARIC databases. Encouragingly, IL1RL1 was found in multiple analyses (MAGMA, POPS, SMR, and BLISS). The ST2 receptor belongs to the interleukin (IL)-1 receptor family, encoded by the IL1RL1 gene [87]. IL-33 is the functional ligand of ST2L, capable of inducing the production of Th2 cell cytokines and enhancing Th1, Th2, and Th17 immune responses [88–90]. The IL-33/IL1RL1 pathway plays a crucial role in host defense and in the pathogenesis of immune-mediated, allergic, and chronic inflammatory diseases such as asthma, dermatitis, arthritis, and Alzheimer's disease [91].

IL1RL1 levels have been reported to be elevated in the intestines of patients with IBD, correlating with disease activity, and both IL1RL1 and IL-33 levels are higher in circulation in these patients [92]. It has been demonstrated that anti-TNF therapy reduces IL1RL1 subtype A levels while increasing soluble subtypes, providing more decoy receptors to sequester IL-33 and mitigate inflammation [93]. This suggests a potential therapeutic target within the IL-1 pathway for managing IBD and related diseases. The significance of IL1RL1 in our findings emphasizes the relevance of the IL-1 pathway, a central component of pro-inflammatory response and signaling [94]. The IL-1 pathway could be a common thread in the development of further immune-mediated diseases in patients with IBD, or at least in a subset of them, on the basis of autoinflammatory mechanisms. From a therapeutic standpoint, diseases successfully treated with IL-1 inhibitors could benefit from this insight. Furthermore, the development of anti-IL-1R1 monoclonal antibodies for rheumatoid arthritis, Still's disease, and osteoarthritis underscores the potential for targeting this pathway in IBD [95,96]. This could have significant implications for the understanding and treatment of these conditions in the context of IBD.

The immunedeconv R package was used to assess the degree of immune cell infiltration in IBD. The results indicated that the high-immune-infiltration group included not only common immune cell types observed in IBD, such as activated CD4 T cells, central memory CD4 T cells, CD8-positive T cells, plasma cells, and mast cells, but also less common cell types, such as dendritic cells, M1 macrophages, neutrophils, and Tregs, which may be involved in the onset and progression of IBD. The colonic mucosa of patients with IBD has a high infiltration and secretion of CD4 T cell-associated cytokines, which eventually impair intestinal mucosal barrier function [97,98]. Therefore, CD4 T cells play a crucial role in the pathogenesis of IBD. Neutrophils capable of producing reactive oxygen species are one of the causes of a compromised intestinal barrier in IBD [99]. B cells, dendritic cells, and macrophages can induce chronic inflammation specific to IBD through various pathways, including the regulation of immune responses, antigen processing, and the modulation of inflammation [100,101]. Additionally, mast cells, essential for maintaining homeostasis through barrier defense mechanisms, have a significantly high activity in Crohn's disease [102]. In this study, the proportion of M2 macrophages was higher in the low-immune-infiltration group. Consistently, previous studies have demonstrated that M2 macrophages can promote tissue repair and reduce inflammation, thereby alleviating the symptoms of IBD [103]. Altogether, the findings of this study highlight the importance of using polyfunctional genes in the identification of IBD subtypes and enhance the understanding of the role of various immune cells in the pathogenesis of IBD. Future drug development can be explored at the pleiotropic loci we identified to develop precise IBD drugs. However, this manuscript also has some limitations. First, the GWAS datasets used in this study were derived from individuals of European descent. Therefore, the results lack generalizability and necessitate further research involving diverse ethnic groups. Additionally, while we identified genes associated with IBD and immune-mediated disease comorbidity, the influence of epigenetic modifications on these loci remains unexplored, which could significantly impact gene expression and disease phenotypes. Furthermore, disease subgroups such as early-onset IBD may exhibit distinct genetic and biological characteristics, affecting the applicability of our results across different IBD subtypes. Future longitudinal studies and experimental investigations are essential to clarify these underlying biological mechanisms comprehensively.

5. Conclusions

In conclusion, this study highlights the strong genetic relationship between IBD and four immune-mediated diseases, revealing novel genetic risk factors. The findings improve the understanding of the genetic landscape of IBD, which may facilitate the development of innovative treatment approaches.

Supplementary Materials: The following supporting information can be downloaded at: https://www.mdpi.com/article/10.3390/biomedicines12112562/s1, Table S1: Baseline characteristics of the study population; Table S2: Genetic correlation between inflammatory bowel disease (ieu-a-31 and FinnGen database) and 16 immune-mediated diseases; Table S3: 455 independent associations identified with GCTA-COJO (conditional and joint) analysis applied to GWAS summary statistics (MTAG-IBD); Table S4: Pleiotropic genomic loci in IBD and (Ankylosing Spondylitis, Psoriasis, Iridocyclitis and Psoriatic Arthritis) identified by FUMA using PLACO results; Table S5: The annotation in fuma bassed on the result of MAGMA; Table S6: MAGMA combined with POPS screening (POPS score > 1); Table S7: SMR analysis from eQTL to MTAG-IBD (FDR < 0.05 and p_HEIDI > 0.01); Table S8: KEGG pathway and Gene ontology enrichment of pleiotropic genes; Table S9: Mammalian Phenotype ontology based on pleiotropic genes; Table S10: Bliss analysis from pQTL (ARIC, Decode and UKBPP) to MTAG-IBD (FDR < 0.05 and p_HEIDI > 0.01); Table S11: KEGG enrichment analysis of risk proteins; Table S12: Drug-Gene interaction network of the annotated genes through DGIdb; Table S13: Bidirectional Mendelian randomization estimates of the relationship between genetically instrumented inflammatory bowel disease meta and four autoimmune diseases (iridocyclitis, psoriasis, ankylosing spondylitis and psoriatic arthritis); Table S14: Heterogeneity test and Horizontal pleiotropy test.

Author Contributions: Conceptualization, X.L. and D.L.; methodology, X.L.; software, X.L.; validation, Y.Z. (Yue Zhang), H.L. and P.C.; formal analysis, X.L.; investigation, Y.Z. (Yingjie Zhao); resources, X.L.; data curation, W.Z.; writing—original draft preparation, X.L.; writing—review and editing, G.D. and P.R.; visualization, G.D.; supervision, G.D.; project administration, X.L. All authors have read and agreed to the published version of the manuscript.

Funding: This research received no external funding.

Institutional Review Board Statement: Not applicable.

Data Availability Statement: The datasets used in this study can be obtained from the corresponding author.

Conflicts of Interest: All authors declare no competing interests.

Abbreviations

GWAS	Genome-wide association study
LDSC	Linkage disequilibrium score regression
POPS	Polygenic priority score
MAGMA	Multi-marker analysis of genomic annotation
COJO	Conditional and joint analysis
BLISS	Biomarker Imputation from Summary Statistics
GSVA	Gene set variation analysis
SMR	Summary-based Mendelian randomization
MR	Mendelian randomization
IVW	Inverse-variance weighted
SNPs	Single-nucleotide polymorphisms
95% CI	95% confidence interval
AS	Ankylosing spondylitis
PsA	Psoriatic arthritis
IBD	Inflammatory bowel disease
RA	Rheumatoid arthritis
KEGG	Kyoto encyclopedia of genes and genomes
GO	Gene ontology

References

1. Ruel, J.; Ruane, D.; Mehandru, S.; Gower-Rousseau, C.; Colombel, J.F. IBD across the age spectrum: Is it the same disease? *Nat. Rev. Gastroenterol. Hepatol.* **2014**, *11*, 88–98. [CrossRef]
2. Kaplan, G.G. The global burden of IBD: From 2015 to 2025. *Nat. Rev. Gastroenterol. Hepatol.* **2015**, *12*, 720–727. [CrossRef]
3. Bernstein, C.N.; Wajda, A.; Blanchard, J.F. The clustering of other chronic inflammatory diseases in inflammatory bowel disease: A population-based study. *Gastroenterology* **2005**, *129*, 827–836. [CrossRef]
4. Wu, X.; Chen, H.; Xu, H. The genomic landscape of human immune-mediated diseases. *J. Hum. Genet.* **2015**, *60*, 675–681. [CrossRef]
5. Cotsapas, C.; Voight, B.F.; Rossin, E.; Lage, K.; Neale, B.M.; Wallace, C.; Abecasis, G.R.; Barrett, J.C.; Behrens, T.; Cho, J.; et al. Pervasive sharing of genetic effects in autoimmune disease. *PLoS Genet.* **2011**, *7*, e1002254. [CrossRef]
6. Umeno, J.; Asano, K.; Matsushita, T.; Matsumoto, T.; Kiyohara, Y.; Iida, M.; Nakamura, Y.; Kamatani, N.; Kubo, M. Meta-analysis of published studies identified eight additional common susceptibility loci for Crohn's disease and ulcerative colitis. *Inflamm. Bowel Dis.* **2011**, *17*, 2407–2415. [CrossRef]

7. Armstrong, M.J.; Hegade, V.S.; Robins, G. Advances in coeliac disease. *Curr. Opin. Gastroenterol.* **2012**, *28*, 104–112. [CrossRef]
8. Wen, Y.P.; Yu, Z.G. Identifying shared genetic loci and common risk genes of rheumatoid arthritis associated with three autoimmune diseases based on large-scale cross-trait genome-wide association studies. *Front. Immunol.* **2023**, *14*, 1160397. [CrossRef]
9. Danoy, P.; Pryce, K.; Hadler, J.; Bradbury, L.A.; Farrar, C.; Pointon, J.; Ward, M.; Weisman, M.; Reveille, J.D.; Wordsworth, B.P.; et al. Association of variants at 1q32 and STAT3 with ankylosing spondylitis suggests genetic overlap with Crohn's disease. *PLoS Genet.* **2010**, *6*, e1001195. [CrossRef] [PubMed]
10. Ji, S.G.; Juran, B.D.; Mucha, S.; Folseraas, T.; Jostins, L.; Melum, E.; Kumasaka, N.; Atkinson, E.J.; Schlicht, E.M.; Liu, J.Z.; et al. Genome-wide association study of primary sclerosing cholangitis identifies new risk loci and quantifies the genetic relationship with inflammatory bowel disease. *Nat. Genet.* **2017**, *49*, 269–273. [CrossRef] [PubMed]
11. Morrison, H.A.; Trusiano, B.; Rowe, A.J.; Allen, I.C. Negative regulatory NLRs mitigate inflammation via NF-κB pathway signaling in inflammatory bowel disease. *Biomed. J.* **2023**, *46*, 100616. [CrossRef] [PubMed]
12. Bacher, S.; Schmitz, M.L. The NF-kappaB pathway as a potential target for autoimmune disease therapy. *Curr. Pharm. Des.* **2004**, *10*, 2827–2837. [CrossRef] [PubMed]
13. Lee, C.H.; Shi, H.; Pasaniuc, B.; Eskin, E.; Han, B. PLEIO: A method to map and interpret pleiotropic loci with GWAS summary statistics. *Am. J. Hum. Genet.* **2021**, *108*, 36–48. [CrossRef] [PubMed]
14. Verbanck, M.; Chen, C.Y.; Neale, B.; Do, R. Detection of widespread horizontal pleiotropy in causal relationships inferred from Mendelian randomization between complex traits and diseases. *Nat. Genet.* **2018**, *50*, 693–698. [CrossRef]
15. Sivakumaran, S.; Agakov, F.; Theodoratou, E.; Prendergast, J.G.; Zgaga, L.; Manolio, T.; Rudan, I.; McKeigue, P.; Wilson, J.F.; Campbell, H. Abundant pleiotropy in human complex diseases and traits. *Am. J. Hum. Genet.* **2011**, *89*, 607–618. [CrossRef] [PubMed]
16. Bayardo, M.; Punzi, F.; Bondar, C.; Chopita, N.; Chirdo, F. Transglutaminase 2 expression is enhanced synergistically by interferon-γ and tumour necrosis factor-α in human small intestine. *Clin. Exp. Immunol.* **2012**, *168*, 95–104. [CrossRef]
17. Ray, D.; Chatterjee, N. A powerful method for pleiotropic analysis under composite null hypothesis identifies novel shared loci between Type 2 Diabetes and Prostate Cancer. *PLoS Genet.* **2020**, *16*, e1009218. [CrossRef] [PubMed]
18. Liu, J.Z.; van Sommeren, S.; Huang, H.; Ng, S.C.; Alberts, R.; Takahashi, A.; Ripke, S.; Lee, J.C.; Jostins, L.; Shah, T.; et al. Association analyses identify 38 susceptibility loci for inflammatory bowel disease and highlight shared genetic risk across populations. *Nat. Genet.* **2015**, *47*, 979–986. [CrossRef]
19. Kurki, M.I.; Karjalainen, J.; Palta, P.; Sipilä, T.P.; Kristiansson, K.; Donner, K.M.; Reeve, M.P.; Laivuori, H.; Aavikko, M.; Kaunisto, M.A.; et al. FinnGen provides genetic insights from a well-phenotyped isolated population. *Nature* **2023**, *613*, 508–518. [CrossRef]
20. Szekanecz, Z.; McInnes, I.B.; Schett, G.; Szamosi, S.; Benkő, S.; Szűcs, G. Autoinflammation and autoimmunity across rheumatic and musculoskeletal diseases. *Nat. Rev. Rheumatol.* **2021**, *17*, 585–595. [CrossRef]
21. Genovese, G.; Rockweiler, N.B.; Gorman, B.R.; Bigdeli, T.B.; Pato, M.T.; Pato, C.N.; Ichihara, K.; McCarroll, S.A. BCFtools/liftover: An accurate and comprehensive tool to convert genetic variants across genome assemblies. *Bioinformatics* **2024**, *40*, btae038. [CrossRef] [PubMed]
22. Võsa, U.; Claringbould, A.; Westra, H.J.; Bonder, M.J.; Deelen, P.; Zeng, B.; Kirsten, H.; Saha, A.; Kreuzhuber, R.; Yazar, S.; et al. Large-scale cis- and trans-eQTL analyses identify thousands of genetic loci and polygenic scores that regulate blood gene expression. *Nat. Genet.* **2021**, *53*, 1300–1310. [CrossRef] [PubMed]
23. Ferkingstad, E.; Sulem, P.; Atlason, B.A.; Sveinbjornsson, G.; Magnusson, M.I.; Styrmisdottir, E.L.; Gunnarsdottir, K.; Helgason, A.; Oddsson, A.; Halldorsson, B.V.; et al. Large-scale integration of the plasma proteome with genetics and disease. *Nat. Genet.* **2021**, *53*, 1712–1721. [CrossRef] [PubMed]
24. Sun, B.B.; Chiou, J.; Traylor, M.; Benner, C.; Hsu, Y.H.; Richardson, T.G.; Surendran, P.; Mahajan, A.; Robins, C.; Vasquez-Grinnell, S.G.; et al. Plasma proteomic associations with genetics and health in the UK Biobank. *Nature* **2023**, *622*, 329–338. [CrossRef]
25. Auton, A.; Brooks, L.D.; Durbin, R.M.; Garrison, E.P.; Kang, H.M.; Korbel, J.O.; Marchini, J.L.; McCarthy, S.; McVean, G.A.; Abecasis, G.R. A global reference for human genetic variation. *Nature* **2015**, *526*, 68–74. [CrossRef]
26. Willer, C.J.; Li, Y.; Abecasis, G.R. METAL: Fast and efficient meta-analysis of genomewide association scans. *Bioinformatics* **2010**, *26*, 2190–2191. [CrossRef]
27. Han, B.; Eskin, E. Random-effects model aimed at discovering associations in meta-analysis of genome-wide association studies. *Am. J. Hum. Genet.* **2011**, *88*, 586–598. [CrossRef]
28. Turley, P.; Walters, R.K.; Maghzian, O.; Okbay, A.; Lee, J.J.; Fontana, M.A.; Nguyen-Viet, T.A.; Wedow, R.; Zacher, M.; Furlotte, N.A.; et al. Multi-trait analysis of genome-wide association summary statistics using MTAG. *Nat. Genet.* **2018**, *50*, 229–237. [CrossRef]
29. Yang, J.; Ferreira, T.; Morris, A.P.; Medland, S.E.; Madden, P.A.; Heath, A.C.; Martin, N.G.; Montgomery, G.W.; Weedon, M.N.; Loos, R.J.; et al. Conditional and joint multiple-SNP analysis of GWAS summary statistics identifies additional variants influencing complex traits. *Nat. Genet.* **2012**, *44*, 369–375. [CrossRef]
30. Watanabe, K.; Taskesen, E.; van Bochoven, A.; Posthuma, D. Functional mapping and annotation of genetic associations with FUMA. *Nat. Commun.* **2017**, *8*, 1826. [CrossRef]

31. Wang, K.; Li, M.; Hakonarson, H. ANNOVAR: Functional annotation of genetic variants from high-throughput sequencing data. *Nucleic Acids Res.* **2010**, *38*, e164. [CrossRef] [PubMed]
32. Rentzsch, P.; Witten, D.; Cooper, G.M.; Shendure, J.; Kircher, M. CADD: Predicting the deleteriousness of variants throughout the human genome. *Nucleic Acids Res.* **2019**, *47*, D886–D894. [CrossRef] [PubMed]
33. Boyle, A.P.; Hong, E.L.; Hariharan, M.; Cheng, Y.; Schaub, M.A.; Kasowski, M.; Karczewski, K.J.; Park, J.; Hitz, B.C.; Weng, S.; et al. Annotation of functional variation in personal genomes using RegulomeDB. *Genome Res.* **2012**, *22*, 1790–1797. [CrossRef] [PubMed]
34. de Leeuw, C.A.; Mooij, J.M.; Heskes, T.; Posthuma, D. MAGMA: Generalized gene-set analysis of GWAS data. *PLoS Comput. Biol.* **2015**, *11*, e1004219. [CrossRef] [PubMed]
35. Weeks, E.M.; Ulirsch, J.C.; Cheng, N.Y.; Trippe, B.L.; Fine, R.S.; Miao, J.; Patwardhan, T.A.; Kanai, M.; Nasser, J.; Fulco, C.P.; et al. Leveraging polygenic enrichments of gene features to predict genes underlying complex traits and diseases. *Nat. Genet.* **2023**, *55*, 1267–1276. [CrossRef]
36. Zhu, Z.; Zhang, F.; Hu, H.; Bakshi, A.; Robinson, M.R.; Powell, J.E.; Montgomery, G.W.; Goddard, M.E.; Wray, N.R.; Visscher, P.M.; et al. Integration of summary data from GWAS and eQTL studies predicts complex trait gene targets. *Nat. Genet.* **2016**, *48*, 481–487. [CrossRef]
37. Blake, J.A.; Baldarelli, R.; Kadin, J.A.; Richardson, J.E.; Smith, C.L.; Bult, C.J. Mouse Genome Database (MGD): Knowledgebase for mouse-human comparative biology. *Nucleic Acids Res.* **2021**, *49*, D981–D987. [CrossRef]
38. Liberzon, A.; Birger, C.; Thorvaldsdóttir, H.; Ghandi, M.; Mesirov, J.P.; Tamayo, P. The Molecular Signatures Database (MSigDB) hallmark gene set collection. *Cell Syst.* **2015**, *1*, 417–425. [CrossRef]
39. Yu, G.; Wang, L.G.; Han, Y.; He, Q.Y. clusterProfiler: An R package for comparing biological themes among gene clusters. *Omics J. Integr. Biol.* **2012**, *16*, 284–287. [CrossRef]
40. Wu, C.; Zhang, Z.; Yang, X.; Zhao, B. Large-Scale Imputation Models for Multi-Ancestry Proteome-Wide Association Analysis. *bioRxiv* **2023**. [CrossRef]
41. Cannon, M.; Stevenson, J.; Stahl, K.; Basu, R.; Coffman, A.; Kiwala, S.; McMichael, J.F.; Kuzma, K.; Morrissey, D.; Cotto, K.; et al. DGIdb 5.0: Rebuilding the drug-gene interaction database for precision medicine and drug discovery platforms. *Nucleic Acids Res.* **2024**, *52*, D1227–D1235. [CrossRef] [PubMed]
42. Greenland, S. An introduction to instrumental variables for epidemiologists. *Int. J. Epidemiol.* **2000**, *29*, 722–729. [CrossRef]
43. Gusev, A.; Ko, A.; Shi, H.; Bhatia, G.; Chung, W.; Penninx, B.W.; Jansen, R.; de Geus, E.J.; Boomsma, D.I.; Wright, F.A.; et al. Integrative approaches for large-scale transcriptome-wide association studies. *Nat. Genet.* **2016**, *48*, 245–252. [CrossRef]
44. Barrett, T.; Wilhite, S.E.; Ledoux, P.; Evangelista, C.; Kim, I.F.; Tomashevsky, M.; Marshall, K.A.; Phillippy, K.H.; Sherman, P.M.; Holko, M.; et al. NCBI GEO: Archive for functional genomics data sets--update. *Nucleic Acids Res.* **2013**, *41*, D991–D995. [CrossRef]
45. Sturm, G.; Finotello, F.; Petitprez, F.; Zhang, J.D.; Baumbach, J.; Fridman, W.H.; List, M.; Aneichyk, T. Comprehensive evaluation of transcriptome-based cell-type quantification methods for immuno-oncology. *Bioinformatics* **2019**, *35*, i436–i445. [CrossRef] [PubMed]
46. Lees, C.W.; Barrett, J.C.; Parkes, M.; Satsangi, J. New IBD genetics: Common pathways with other diseases. *Gut* **2011**, *60*, 1739–1753. [CrossRef]
47. McInnes, I.B.; Schett, G. Pathogenetic insights from the treatment of rheumatoid arthritis. *Lancet* **2017**, *389*, 2328–2337. [CrossRef] [PubMed]
48. Kany, S.; Vollrath, J.T.; Relja, B. Cytokines in Inflammatory Disease. *Int. J. Mol. Sci.* **2019**, *20*, 6008. [CrossRef]
49. Schurich, A.; Raine, C.; Morris, V.; Ciurtin, C. The role of IL-12/23 in T cell-related chronic inflammation: Implications of immunodeficiency and therapeutic blockade. *Rheumatology* **2018**, *57*, 246–254. [CrossRef]
50. Brakenhoff, L.K.; van der Heijde, D.M.; Hommes, D.W.; Huizinga, T.W.; Fidder, H.H. The joint-gut axis in inflammatory bowel diseases. *J. Crohn's Colitis* **2010**, *4*, 257–268. [CrossRef]
51. Fragoulis, G.E.; Liava, C.; Daoussis, D.; Akriviadis, E.; Garyfallos, A.; Dimitroulas, T. Inflammatory bowel diseases and spondyloarthropathies: From pathogenesis to treatment. *World J. Gastroenterol.* **2019**, *25*, 2162–2176. [CrossRef] [PubMed]
52. Oliver, J.; Rueda, B.; López-Nevot, M.A.; Gómez-García, M.; Martín, J. Replication of an association between IL23R gene polymorphism with inflammatory bowel disease. *Clin. Gastroenterol. Hepatol. Off. Clin. Pract. J. Am. Gastroenterol. Assoc.* **2007**, *5*, 977–981.e2. [CrossRef] [PubMed]
53. Gorman, J.A.; Hundhausen, C.; Errett, J.S.; Stone, A.E.; Allenspach, E.J.; Ge, Y.; Arkatkar, T.; Clough, C.; Dai, X.; Khim, S.; et al. The A946T variant of the RNA sensor IFIH1 mediates an interferon program that limits viral infection but increases the risk for autoimmunity. *Nat. Immunol.* **2017**, *18*, 744–752. [CrossRef]
54. Cen, H.; Wang, W.; Leng, R.X.; Wang, T.Y.; Pan, H.F.; Fan, Y.G.; Wang, B.; Ye, D.Q. Association of IFIH1 rs1990760 polymorphism with susceptibility to autoimmune diseases: A meta-analysis. *Autoimmunity* **2013**, *46*, 455–462. [CrossRef]
55. Yoneyama, M.; Kikuchi, M.; Matsumoto, K.; Imaizumi, T.; Miyagishi, M.; Taira, K.; Foy, E.; Loo, Y.M.; Gale, M., Jr.; Akira, S.; et al. Shared and unique functions of the DExD/H-box helicases RIG-I, MDA5, and LGP2 in antiviral innate immunity. *J. Immunol.* **2005**, *175*, 2851–2858. [CrossRef] [PubMed]

56. Murphy, C.A.; Langrish, C.L.; Chen, Y.; Blumenschein, W.; McClanahan, T.; Kastelein, R.A.; Sedgwick, J.D.; Cua, D.J. Divergent pro- and antiinflammatory roles for IL-23 and IL-12 in joint autoimmune inflammation. *J. Exp. Med.* **2003**, *198*, 1951–1957. [CrossRef]
57. Yan, J.B.; Luo, M.M.; Chen, Z.Y.; He, B.H. The Function and Role of the Th17/Treg Cell Balance in Inflammatory Bowel Disease. *J. Immunol. Res.* **2020**, *2020*, 8813558. [CrossRef]
58. Di Meglio, P.; Villanova, F.; Napolitano, L.; Tosi, I.; Terranova Barberio, M.; Mak, R.K.; Nutland, S.; Smith, C.H.; Barker, J.; Todd, J.A.; et al. The IL23R A/Gln381 allele promotes IL-23 unresponsiveness in human memory T-helper 17 cells and impairs Th17 responses in psoriasis patients. *J. Investig. Dermatol.* **2013**, *133*, 2381–2389. [CrossRef]
59. Lappalainen, M.; Halme, L.; Turunen, U.; Saavalainen, P.; Einarsdottir, E.; Färkkilä, M.; Kontula, K.; Paavola-Sakki, P. Association of IL23R, TNFRSF1A, and HLA-DRB1*0103 allele variants with inflammatory bowel disease phenotypes in the Finnish population. *Inflamm. Bowel Dis.* **2008**, *14*, 1118–1124. [CrossRef]
60. Alonso-Ramirez, R.; Loisel, S.; Buors, C.; Pers, J.O.; Montero, E.; Youinou, P.; Renaudineau, Y. Rationale for Targeting CD6 as a Treatment for Autoimmune Diseases. *Arthritis* **2010**, *2010*, 130646. [CrossRef]
61. Gimferrer, I.; Calvo, M.; Mittelbrunn, M.; Farnós, M.; Sarrias, M.R.; Enrich, C.; Vives, J.; Sánchez-Madrid, F.; Lozano, F. Relevance of CD6-mediated interactions in T cell activation and proliferation. *J. Immunol.* **2004**, *173*, 2262–2270. [CrossRef] [PubMed]
62. Santos, R.F.; Oliveira, L.; Carmo, A.M. Tuning T Cell Activation: The Function of CD6 At the Immunological Synapse and in T Cell Responses. *Curr. Drug Targets* **2016**, *17*, 630–639. [CrossRef] [PubMed]
63. Krintel, S.B.; Essioux, L.; Wool, A.; Johansen, J.S.; Schreiber, E.; Zekharya, T.; Akiva, P.; Ostergaard, M.; Hetland, M.L. CD6 and syntaxin binding protein 6 variants and response to tumor necrosis factor alpha inhibitors in Danish patients with rheumatoid arthritis. *PLoS ONE* **2012**, *7*, e38539. [CrossRef] [PubMed]
64. Alonso, R.; Buors, C.; Le Dantec, C.; Hillion, S.; Pers, J.O.; Saraux, A.; Montero, E.; Marianowski, R.; Loisel, S.; Devauchelle, V.; et al. Aberrant expression of CD6 on B-cell subsets from patients with Sjögren's syndrome. *J. Autoimmun.* **2010**, *35*, 336–341. [CrossRef]
65. Ramos-Casals, M.; Font, J.; García-Carrasco, M.; Calvo, J.; Places, L.; Padilla, O.; Cervera, R.; Bowen, M.A.; Lozano, F.; Ingelmo, M. High circulating levels of soluble scavenger receptors (sCD5 and sCD6) in patients with primary Sjögren's syndrome. *Rheumatology* **2001**, *40*, 1056–1059. [CrossRef]
66. Ephraim, R.; Fraser, S.; Devereaux, J.; Stavely, R.; Feehan, J.; Eri, R.; Nurgali, K.; Apostolopoulos, V. Differential Gene Expression of Checkpoint Markers and Cancer Markers in Mouse Models of Spontaneous Chronic Colitis. *Cancers* **2023**, *15*, 4793. [CrossRef]
67. Ma, C.; Wu, W.; Lin, R.; Ge, Y.; Zhang, C.; Sun, S.; Cong, Y.; Li, X.; Liu, Z. Critical Role of CD6highCD4+ T Cells in Driving Th1/Th17 Cell Immune Responses and Mucosal Inflammation in IBD. *J. Crohn's Colitis* **2018**, *13*, 510–524. [CrossRef] [PubMed]
68. Li, Y.; Singer, N.G.; Whitbred, J.; Bowen, M.A.; Fox, D.A.; Lin, F. CD6 as a potential target for treating multiple sclerosis. *Proc. Natl. Acad. Sci. USA* **2017**, *114*, 2687–2692. [CrossRef]
69. Ishizaki, M.; Akimoto, T.; Muromoto, R.; Yokoyama, M.; Ohshiro, Y.; Sekine, Y.; Maeda, H.; Shimoda, K.; Oritani, K.; Matsuda, T. Involvement of tyrosine kinase-2 in both the IL-12/Th1 and IL-23/Th17 axes in vivo. *J. Immunol.* **2011**, *187*, 181–189. [CrossRef]
70. Krupashankar, D.S.; Dogra, S.; Kura, M.; Saraswat, A.; Budamakuntla, L.; Sumathy, T.K.; Shah, R.; Gopal, M.G.; Narayana Rao, T.; Srinivas, C.R.; et al. Efficacy and safety of itolizumab, a novel anti-CD6 monoclonal antibody, in patients with moderate to severe chronic plaque psoriasis: Results of a double-blind, randomized, placebo-controlled, phase-III study. *J. Am. Acad. Dermatol.* **2014**, *71*, 484–492. [CrossRef]
71. Rodriguez, P.C.; Torres-Moya, R.; Reyes, G.; Molinero, C.; Prada, D.; Lopez, A.M.; Hernandez, I.M.; Hernandez, M.V.; Martinez, J.P.; Hernandez, X.; et al. A clinical exploratory study with itolizumab, an anti-CD6 monoclonal antibody, in patients with rheumatoid arthritis. *Results Immunol.* **2012**, *2*, 204–211. [CrossRef] [PubMed]
72. Xu, D.; Matsumoto, M.L.; McKenzie, B.S.; Zarrin, A.A. TPL2 kinase action and control of inflammation. *Pharmacol. Res.* **2018**, *129*, 188–193. [CrossRef] [PubMed]
73. Patriotis, C.; Makris, A.; Bear, S.E.; Tsichlis, P.N. Tumor progression locus 2 (Tpl-2) encodes a protein kinase involved in the progression of rodent T-cell lymphomas and in T-cell activation. *Proc. Natl. Acad. Sci. USA* **1993**, *90*, 2251–2255. [CrossRef] [PubMed]
74. Acuff, N.V.; Li, X.; Elmore, J.; Rada, B.; Watford, W.T. Tpl2 promotes neutrophil trafficking, oxidative burst, and bacterial killing. *J. Leucoc. Biol.* **2017**, *101*, 1325–1333. [CrossRef]
75. Gantke, T.; Sriskantharajah, S.; Sadowski, M.; Ley, S.C. IκB kinase regulation of the TPL-2/ERK MAPK pathway. *Immunol. Rev.* **2012**, *246*, 168–182. [CrossRef] [PubMed]
76. Lawrenz, M.; Visekruna, A.; Kühl, A.; Schmidt, N.; Kaufmann, S.H.; Steinhoff, U. Genetic and pharmacological targeting of TPL-2 kinase ameliorates experimental colitis: A potential target for the treatment of Crohn's disease? *Mucosal Immunol.* **2012**, *5*, 129–139. [CrossRef]
77. Hu, Y.; Green, N.; Gavrin, L.K.; Janz, K.; Kaila, N.; Li, H.-Q.; Thomason, J.R.; Cuozzo, J.W.; Hall, J.P.; Hsu, S. Inhibition of Tpl2 kinase and TNFα production with quinoline-3-carbonitriles for the treatment of rheumatoid arthritis. *Bioorganic Med. Chem. Lett.* **2006**, *16*, 6067–6072. [CrossRef]
78. Gonsky, R.; Fleshner, P.; Deem, R.L.; Biener-Ramanujan, E.; Li, D.; Potdar, A.A.; Bilsborough, J.; Yang, S.; McGovern, D.P.B.; Targan, S.R. Association of Ribonuclease T2 Gene Polymorphisms with Decreased Expression and Clinical Characteristics of Severity in Crohn's Disease. *Gastroenterology* **2017**, *153*, 219–232. [CrossRef]

79. Jackson, L.J.; Pheneger, J.A.; Pheneger, T.J.; Davis, G.; Wright, A.D.; Robinson, J.E.; Allen, S.; Munson, M.C.; Carter, L.L. The role of PIM kinases in human and mouse CD4+ T cell activation and inflammatory bowel disease. *Cell. Immunol.* **2012**, *272*, 200–213. [CrossRef]
80. Corbaz, A.; ten Hove, T.; Herren, S.; Graber, P.; Schwartsburd, B.; Belzer, I.; Harrison, J.; Plitz, T.; Kosco-Vilbois, M.H.; Kim, S.H.; et al. IL-18-binding protein expression by endothelial cells and macrophages is up-regulated during active Crohn's disease. *J. Immunol.* **2002**, *168*, 3608–3616. [CrossRef]
81. Reuter, B.K.; Pizarro, T.T. Commentary: The role of the IL-18 system and other members of the IL-1R/TLR superfamily in innate mucosal immunity and the pathogenesis of inflammatory bowel disease: Friend or foe? *Eur. J. Immunol.* **2004**, *34*, 2347–2355. [CrossRef] [PubMed]
82. Sivakumar, P.; Westrich, G.; Kanaly, S.; Garka, K.; Born, T.; Derry, J.; Viney, J. Interleukin 18 is a primary mediator of the inflammation associated with dextran sulphate sodium induced colitis: Blocking interleukin 18 attenuates intestinal damage. *Gut* **2002**, *50*, 812–820. [CrossRef] [PubMed]
83. Feagins, L.A. Role of transforming growth factor-β in inflammatory bowel disease and colitis-associated colon cancer. *Inflamm. Bowel Dis.* **2010**, *16*, 1963–1968. [CrossRef] [PubMed]
84. Maggio-Price, L.; Treuting, P.; Zeng, W.; Tsang, M.; Bielefeldt-Ohmann, H.; Iritani, B.M. Helicobacter infection is required for inflammation and colon cancer in SMAD3-deficient mice. *Cancer Res.* **2006**, *66*, 828–838. [CrossRef]
85. Seamons, A.; Treuting, P.M.; Brabb, T.; Maggio-Price, L. Characterization of dextran sodium sulfate-induced inflammation and colonic tumorigenesis in Smad3$^{-/-}$ mice with dysregulated TGFβ. *PLoS ONE* **2013**, *8*, e79182. [CrossRef]
86. Yu, W.; Lin, Z.; Kelly, A.A.; Hegarty, J.P.; Poritz, L.S.; Wang, Y.; Li, T.; Schreiber, S.; Koltun, W.A. Association of a Nkx2-3 polymorphism with Crohn's disease and expression of Nkx2-3 is up-regulated in B cell lines and intestinal tissues with Crohn's disease. *J. Crohn's Colitis* **2009**, *3*, 189–195. [CrossRef]
87. Iwahana, H.; Yanagisawa, K.; Ito-Kosaka, A.; Kuroiwa, K.; Tago, K.; Komatsu, N.; Katashima, R.; Itakura, M.; Tominaga, S. Different promoter usage and multiple transcription initiation sites of the interleukin-1 receptor-related human ST2 gene in UT-7 and TM12 cells. *Eur. J. Biochem.* **1999**, *264*, 397–406. [CrossRef]
88. Schmitz, J.; Owyang, A.; Oldham, E.; Song, Y.; Murphy, E.; McClanahan, T.K.; Zurawski, G.; Moshrefi, M.; Qin, J.; Li, X.; et al. IL-33, an interleukin-1-like cytokine that signals via the IL-1 receptor-related protein ST2 and induces T helper type 2-associated cytokines. *Immunity* **2005**, *23*, 479–490. [CrossRef] [PubMed]
89. Smithgall, M.D.; Comeau, M.R.; Yoon, B.R.; Kaufman, D.; Armitage, R.; Smith, D.E. IL-33 amplifies both Th1- and Th2-type responses through its activity on human basophils, allergen-reactive Th2 cells, iNKT and NK cells. *Int. Immunol.* **2008**, *20*, 1019–1030. [CrossRef]
90. Palmer, G.; Talabot-Ayer, D.; Lamacchia, C.; Toy, D.; Seemayer, C.A.; Viatte, S.; Finckh, A.; Smith, D.E.; Gabay, C. Inhibition of interleukin-33 signaling attenuates the severity of experimental arthritis. *Arthritis Rheum.* **2009**, *60*, 738–749. [CrossRef]
91. Oboki, K.; Ohno, T.; Kajiwara, N.; Saito, H.; Nakae, S. IL-33 and IL-33 receptors in host defense and diseases. *Allergol. Int. Off. J. Jpn. Soc. Allergol.* **2010**, *59*, 143–160. [CrossRef] [PubMed]
92. Beltrán, C.J.; Núñez, L.E.; Díaz-Jiménez, D.; Farfan, N.; Candia, E.; Heine, C.; López, F.; González, M.J.; Quera, R.; Hermoso, M.A. Characterization of the novel ST2/IL-33 system in patients with inflammatory bowel disease. *Inflamm. Bowel Dis.* **2010**, *16*, 1097–1107. [CrossRef]
93. Pastorelli, L.; Garg, R.R.; Hoang, S.B.; Spina, L.; Mattioli, B.; Scarpa, M.; Fiocchi, C.; Vecchi, M.; Pizarro, T.T. Epithelial-derived IL-33 and its receptor ST2 are dysregulated in ulcerative colitis and in experimental Th1/Th2 driven enteritis. *Proc. Natl. Acad. Sci. USA* **2010**, *107*, 8017–8022. [CrossRef]
94. Dinarello, C.A. The IL-1 family of cytokines and receptors in rheumatic diseases. *Nat. Rev. Rheumatol.* **2019**, *15*, 612–632. [CrossRef] [PubMed]
95. Larid, G.; Delwail, A.; Dalle, T.; Vasseur, P.; Silvain, C.; Jégou, J.F.; Morel, F.; Lecron, J.C.; Gervais, E. Ex vivo cytokine production in psoriatic disease: Towards specific signatures in cutaneous psoriasis and peripheral psoriatic arthritis. *Front. Immunol.* **2022**, *13*, 993363. [CrossRef] [PubMed]
96. Ruscitti, P.; Cantarini, L.; Nigrovic, P.A.; McGonagle, D.; Giacomelli, R. Recent advances and evolving concepts in Still's disease. *Nat. Rev. Rheumatol.* **2024**, *20*, 116–132. [CrossRef]
97. Imam, T.; Park, S.; Kaplan, M.H.; Olson, M.R. Effector T Helper Cell Subsets in Inflammatory Bowel Diseases. *Front. Immunol.* **2018**, *9*, 1212. [CrossRef]
98. Feng, B.S.; Ma, N.; Zhang, Y.Y.; Gao, H.; Zhang, C.; Li, G.; Liu, Z.; Feng, Y.; Yu, H.Q.; Xiao, L.; et al. Survivin Impairs the Apoptotic Machinery in CD4+ T Cells of Patients with Ulcerative Colitis. *J. Innate Immun.* **2020**, *12*, 226–234. [CrossRef]
99. Drury, B.; Hardisty, G.; Gray, R.D.; Ho, G.T. Neutrophil Extracellular Traps in Inflammatory Bowel Disease: Pathogenic Mechanisms and Clinical Translation. *Cell. Mol. Gastroenterol. Hepatol.* **2021**, *12*, 321–333. [CrossRef]
100. Castro-Dopico, T.; Colombel, J.F.; Mehandru, S. Targeting B cells for inflammatory bowel disease treatment: Back to the future. *Curr. Opin. Pharmacol.* **2020**, *55*, 90–98. [CrossRef]
101. Steinbach, E.C.; Plevy, S.E. The role of macrophages and dendritic cells in the initiation of inflammation in IBD. *Inflamm. Bowel Dis.* **2014**, *20*, 166–175. [CrossRef] [PubMed]

102. Lyons, D.O.; Pullen, N.A. Beyond IgE: Alternative Mast Cell Activation Across Different Disease States. *Int. J. Mol. Sci.* **2020**, *21*, 1498. [CrossRef] [PubMed]
103. Lin, Y.; Yang, X.; Yue, W.; Xu, X.; Li, B.; Zou, L.; He, R. Chemerin aggravates DSS-induced colitis by suppressing M2 macrophage polarization. *Cell. Mol. Immunol.* **2014**, *11*, 355–366. [CrossRef] [PubMed]

biomedicines

MDPI

Review

Extraintestinal Manifestations in Inflammatory Bowel Disease: From Pathophysiology to Treatment

Ilaria Faggiani [1,2], Jacopo Fanizza [1,2], Ferdinando D'Amico [1], Mariangela Allocca [1], Alessandra Zilli [1], Tommaso Lorenzo Parigi [1,2], Alberto Barchi [1,2,*], Silvio Danese [1,2] and Federica Furfaro [1]

1 Department of Gastroenterology and Endoscopy, IRCCS San Raffaele Hospital, 20132 Milan, Italy; faggiani.ilaria@hsr.it (I.F.); fanizza.jacopo@hsr.it (J.F.); damico.ferdinando@hsr.it (F.D.); allocca.mariangela@hsr.it (M.A.); zilli.alessandra@hsr.it (A.Z.); parigi.tommaso@hsr.it (T.L.P.); sdanese@hotmail.com (S.D.); furfaro.federica@hsr.it (F.F.)

2 Gastroenterology and Endoscopy, Vita-Salute San Raffaele University, 20132 Milan, Italy

* Correspondence: barchi.alberto@hsr.it

Abstract: The inflammatory bowel diseases (IBDs) are systemic conditions that affect not only the gastrointestinal tract but also other parts of the body. The presence of extraintestinal manifestations can significantly impact the quality of life in IBD patients. Peripheral arthritis, episcleritis, and erythema nodosum are frequently associated with active intestinal inflammation and often improve with standard treatment targeting intestinal inflammation. In contrast, anterior uveitis, ankylosing spondylitis, and primary sclerosing cholangitis typically occur independently of disease flares. The incidence of these conditions in individuals with IBD can reach up to 50% of patients over the course of their lifetime. In addition, some advanced therapies utilized for the treatment of IBD potentially result in side effects that may resemble extraintestinal manifestations. This review provides a thorough analysis of the pathophysiology and treatment of extraintestinal manifestations associated with Crohn's disease and ulcerative colitis.

Keywords: extraintestinal manifestation; Crohn's disease; ulcerative colitis; inflammatory bowel diseases

1. Introduction

Inflammatory bowel diseases (IBDs) are chronic conditions including ulcerative colitis (UC) and Crohn's disease (CD). IBDs are multifaceted conditions that impact patients' lives. They require a comprehensive approach, considering not only their effects on the gastrointestinal system but also their potential extraintestinal manifestations (EIMs) [1].

EIMs can occur in up to 50% of patients with IBD, and they can be a significant cause of morbidity and, in some cases, mortality. Various organs can be affected, including the musculoskeletal, cutaneous, hepatic, ocular, and vascular systems [2]. The pathophysiology of EIMs is not yet fully understood. Possible driving forces include the extension of the immune-mediated response from the inflamed gut to other organs, changes in leukocyte trafficking, alterations to the intestinal microbiota, and underlying genetic predisposition [3].

Currently, there are numerous advanced therapies available that can effectively manage both intestinal diseases and EIMs. However, these drug side effects can sometimes be mistaken for EIMs, and the differential diagnosis is not always easy [4]. For this reason, UC and CD should be considered complex diseases that present a challenge for gastroenterologists to face within a multidisciplinary team.

In this review, we provide an overview of EIMs in IBD, from pathophysiology to treatment.

2. Materials and Methods

We conducted a comprehensive search of the Pubmed, Embase, and Scopus databases up until 30 May 2024, with the aim of identifying studies regarding extraintestinal manifestation in IBD. To achieve this, we employed specific search terms: 'extraintestinal manifestations', 'musculoskeletal manifestations', 'cutaneous manifestations', 'ocular manifestations', 'hepatic manifestations', in conjunction with 'Crohn's disease', 'ulcerative colitis', and 'inflammatory bowel disease', 'IBD', 'CD', and 'UC'. We limited our search to articles published in the English language.

Our screening process involved two independent reviewers (IF and FJ) who initially assessed titles and abstracts to identify potentially relevant studies. Subsequently, we examined the full texts of these selected articles to determine their eligibility for inclusion. Additionally, we manually scrutinized the reference lists of these articles to ensure that no relevant studies were overlooked during the electronic search. The final inclusion of abstracts and articles was based on their relevance to our research objectives.

3. Results

3.1. *Pathophysiology of EIMs*

Despite significant efforts, the pathogenesis of EIMs is not yet fully understood, given the complexity and multifactorial nature of these diseases. EIMs are characterized by either an antigen-specific immune reaction originating in the intestine and affecting a site outside the intestine, or an inflammatory process independent of intestinal involvement. These processes may be triggered or sustained by genetic or environmental factors in the host, or by the presence of IBD [3].

3.1.1. EIMs as Extension of Immune Responses from the Intestine

A potential factor contributing to EIMs is the ectopical expression of chemokine and adhesion molecules in organs and tissues outside the gut. T cells are attracted to the gut due to the expression of $\alpha4\beta7$ integrin and the CCR9 receptor, which bind to MAdCAM-1 and CCL25, respectively, expressed in the gut endothelium [5]. The altered lymphocytes homing in IBD can facilitate the upregulation of MAdCAM-1 and CCL25 expression in the liver and the migration of gut tropic T cells to sites outside of the intestine, contributing to the development of inflammation [6,7]. However, this can only partly explain EIMs, because this phenomenon does not occur in other organs, except for the liver [1].

Another theory proposes that EIMs may result from immune responses targeting antigens in the intestine but occurring outside of the intestinal tract due to cross-reactivity [8]. It has been demonstrated that enteric bacteria and host major histocompatibility complex molecules share peptide sequences [5]. The presence of a distinct microbiota in patients with primary sclerosing cholangitis (PSC) could confirm this hypothesis [9] (Figure 1).

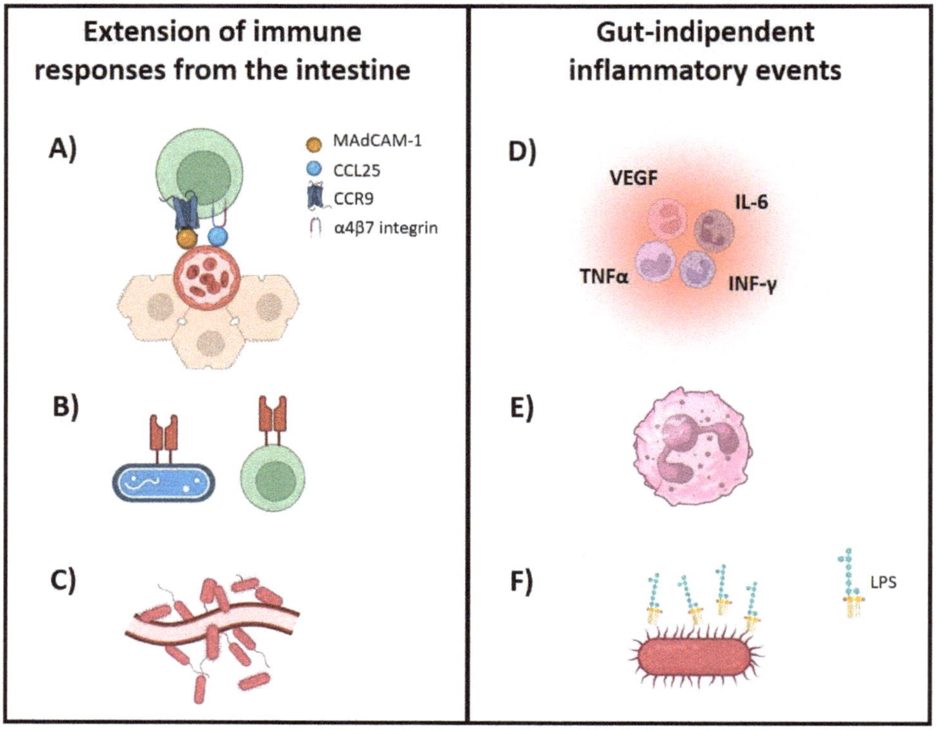

Figure 1. Potential pathophysiology of EIMs. Extension of immune responses from the intestine: (**A**) ectopic expression of adhesion molecules and chemokines, such as the abnormal expression of MAdCAM-1 and CCL25 in the vascular endothelium of the portal tract; (**B**) microbial antigen cross-reactivity, such as molecular mimicry, occurs between enteric bacteria and self-antigens presented by host's major histocompatibility complex molecules; (**C**) microbial antigen translocation [8]. EIMs as independent inflammatory events: (**D**) shift in inflammatory tone influenced by genetic, environmental, or microbial factors, or by a systemic increase in key inflammatory mediators; (**E**) systemic changes in innate immune function, for example, neutrophil priming; (**F**) gut microbiota-induced distant inflammation driven by microbial products such as lipopolysaccharide, through changes in gut permeability and microbiota-derived metabolites [8]. MAdCAM-1: mucosal vascular addressin cell adhesion molecule 1; CCL25: chemokine (C-C motif) ligand 25; CCR9: C-C motif chemokine receptor 9; VEGF: vascular endothelial growth factor; IL-6: interleukin-6; TNFα: tumor necrosis factor α; INFγ: interferon γ; LPS: lipopolysaccharide.

3.1.2. EIMs as Independent Inflammatory Events

The role of the microbiota in EIM is not yet fully defined. The potential role of molecular similarity between gut microbiota antigens and non-microbial epitopes on cells in EIM-affected organs in driving T-cell clone and immune cross-reactivity has not been definitively demonstrated [8]. Individuals with IBD and psoriatic arthritis (PsA) exhibit a relative decline in the prevalence of the *Coprococcus* and *Ruminococcus* species. These species play a crucial role in preserving the intestinal balance by generating short-chain fatty acids (SCFAs). SCFAs may have metabolic and immunomodulatory effects. Notably, in IBD patients with PsA, SCFAs are typically depleted [10]. Conversely, patients with IBD with spondyloarthritis (SpA) display elevated levels of the genus *Dialister*, a correlation that is positively linked to the activity of joint disease [11]. Finally, both IBD-associated arthropathy and rheumatoid arthritis (RA) patients have elevated levels of *Clostridiaceae*, suggesting a potential common microbial link in inflammatory arthritis [12].

Moreover, the alteration of the microbiota in patients with IBD has been observed to result in increased expression of lipopolysaccharide, thereby activating a number of proinflammatory molecules (interleukine-6, interferon γ and vascular endothelial growth factor) that could contribute to the development of EIMs [8] (Figure 1).

3.1.3. Genetic Basis of EIMs

There is a significant overlap in genetic risk loci that are shared between IBD and EIMs [13–16] (Table 1). Interestingly, the identification of associated genetic mutations and polymorphisms of key immune pathways could allow for a molecular-based classification of EIMs, which would be more precise than an organ-based classification. This would also facilitate a more comprehensive understanding of the therapeutic targets, thereby enabling the administration of more effective therapy [17].

Table 1. Genetic risk factors between inflammatory bowel disease and extraintestinal manifestations.

Genetic Risk Factors between Inflammatory Bowel Disease and Extraintestinal Manifestations	
Ankylosing spondylitis [15]	IL23R
Sacroiliitis [13]	NOD2/CARD15
Erythema nodosum [16]	PTGER4, ITGAL, SOCS5, CD207, ITGB3, rs6828740
Pyoderma gangrenosum [16]	IL8RA, PRDM1, USP15, TIMP3
Uveitis [14]	NOD2/CARD15
Primary sclerosing cholangitis [1]	SOCS1, JAK2, STAT3, TYK2, UBASSH3A, BCL2L11, FOXO1, IRF1

3.2. *Musculoskeletal EIMs*

Arthritis is the most frequent EIM of IBD, affecting axial joints, peripheral joints, or both [18]. SpA affects both sexes equally, with a higher prevalence in CD cases involving the colon than in UC, and it can occur before, simultaneously with, or after the onset of IBD [19]. Axial spondyloarthritis (axSpA) is typically characterized by symptoms such as back pain and morning stiffness of the spine. In contrast, peripheral spondyloarthritis (pSpA) is characterized by symptoms primarily affecting the upper and lower limbs [20]. Concerning prevalence, pSpA is the most common manifestation, occurring in 13% (95% CI: 12–15%) of cases, followed by sacroiliitis, at 10% (95% CI: 8–12%), and ankylosing spondylitis (AS), at 3% (95% CI: 2–4%) [18]. SpA is typically designated as 'seronegative spondyloarthropathy' due to the absence of rheumatoid factor (RF) positivity [21]. However, it is worth noting that SpA patients have a higher prevalence of positive RF test results compared to the general population (15% vs. 5%, respectively). Similarly, tests for anti-citrullinated peptide antibodies (ACPA) are typically negative, but they are positive more frequently than in the general population (8% to 12%, compared to 5%) [2,18,21].

AS commonly presents as nocturnal low back pain with morning stiffness, which is usually alleviated by physical activity, and it is often linked to uveitis. Conversely, sacroiliitis is asymptomatic in most patients [21]. The majority of patients with IBD affected by axSpA are positive for HLA-B27 (25–78%), and axial involvement can occur independently of gut pathology. It is more prevalent in CD compared to UC, with frequencies reaching up to 25% [22]. Both AS and sacroiliitis can be identified through magnetic resonance imaging (MRI) using the short-tau inversion recovery (STIR) technique [23].

pSpA can be categorized into two different types. Type 1 arthritis usually appears as acute, asymmetrical joint inflammation, affecting fewer than five joints, often involving the large knee joint [24]. It is associated with IBD activity and tends to resolve spontaneously within 10 weeks and shows a robust correlation with EIMs of IBD, such as erythema nodosum (EN) and uveitis [24]. Type 2 arthropathy is a symmetrical arthritis that affects five or more joints, often including the small metacarpophalangeal joint, and it is not associated with IBD activity and can persist for years [24].

Enthesitis, dactylitis, and tenosynovitis also occur in IBD patients as musculoskeletal EIMs [25]. Enthesitis can present as Achilles tendinitis, plantar fasciitis, or chest wall pain and is observed in 7% to 50% of adult IBD patients. Early detection can be aided by ultrasonography or MRI examination of the affected area [25].

3.3. Skin EIMs

Cutaneous manifestations are present in approximately 15–20% of patients with IBD [26]. Skin EIMs can be classified into four categories based on their pathophysiological mechanisms: skin manifestations that are reactive and have similar pathophysiological mechanisms to IBD (pyoderma gangrenosum (PG), EN, Sweet's syndrome, aphthous ulcer); cutaneous manifestation that share the same histological features as IBD (metastatic CD); skin diseases related to IBD (psoriasis, hidradenitis suppurativa, and atopic dermatitis); skin lesions induced by IBD treatment [2].

EN, a septal panniculitis, is the most reported cutaneous manifestation in IBD (15%) and usually occurs during flare-ups of IBD. It is more common in CD (4–15%) than in UC (2.8–10%) [1]. Lesions are symmetric, raised, red, and nonulcerated subcutaneous nodules of 1–5 cm in size [27]. Typically, EN is self-limiting, with skin lesions usually resolving within 2–8 weeks without sequelae [27].

PG occurs in approximately 0.5–2.6% of patients with IBD and is the second most common EIM after EN [28]. It occurs more frequently in individuals with UC, particularly in females and the elderly [29], and may run parallel to IBD activity or follow an independent course [1]. Almost 15% of PG cases pre-date the onset of IBD [30]. It typically manifests as one or more tender, inflammatory papules or pustules that rupture quickly, and the ulcers can become necrotic and painful. The lesion size ranges from 2 to 20 cm and is characterized by violaceous undermined borders and peripheral erythema [26]. The most commonly affected areas are the extensor surfaces of the legs (70–80%) and areas adjacent to postsurgical stomas (18%) [28]. Diagnosis is typically based on clinical presentation, while skin biopsy, although it is not specific to this diagnosis, can be useful in ruling out other conditions (e.g., malignancies, skin infection) [31].

Sweet's syndrome is a rare neutrophilic dermatosis that is associated with malignancies, infections, and, to a lesser extent, IBD [32]. It can manifest equally in UC and CD with erythematous papules and plaques involving the extremities, fever, and an elevation of systemic inflammatory markers [33]. The histologic feature that allows for the diagnosis is neutrophilic infiltration of the dermis without vasculitis. The management of the underlying IBD is resolutive, and systemic steroids are highly effective [2,33].

Aphthous stomatitis is characterized by multiple round or oval painful ulcers with a yellow pseudomembranous base and erythematous borders, typically found on the buccal or labial mucosa [27]. Diagnosis is clinical, although for persistent, recurrent, or refractory lesions, or in patients without a definitive IBD diagnosis, a biopsy of the ulcer borders and culture may be useful [34]. Aphthous stomatitis occurs in approximately 10% of patients with CD and UC, and in most cases, it is associated with exacerbations of IBD and the HLA-B27, so that controlling intestinal inflammation is decisive in most cases [35,36].

Metastatic CD is a rare skin EIM. Lesions usually affect the peri-genital area and they share the same characteristic of CD, such as non-caseating granuloma [26]. For mild forms, cutaneous treatments such as intralesional steroid injections and prolonged systemic metronidazole are recommended [2]. Tumor necrosis factor α (TNFα) antagonists and azathioprine (AZA) are second-line therapy [37].

3.4. Ocular EIMs

Ocular manifestations occur in 4 to 12% of IBD patients, with similar incidence in CD and UC [38].

Uveitis is the most common ocular manifestation, with a higher prevalence in CD (11.1%) than in UC (5.6%). In CD, the acute manifestation of the disease is concomitant with the intestinal disease flare, while in UC, this tight correlation does not exist [39]. Uveitis can be classified into four types: anterior, intermediate, posterior, and panuveitis based on the structures involved. Anterior uveitis affects the iris and the ciliary body and presents with conjunctival redness and photosensitivity. Intermediate and posterior uveitis are rarer and involve the vitreous and the retina, respectively, which can lead to permanent vision loss [38]. For this reason, suspected cases of uveitis require immediate referral to an ophthalmologist.

Episcleritis is an inflammation of the vascular layer between the sclera and conjunctiva that may involve the entire layer or a localized area [38], and it generally presents with hyperemia, pruritus, and burning [38]. The prevalence in CD is 3.95 [95% CI: 2.91–4.99] per 1000 patients and 4.73 [95% CI: 3.95–5.52] per 1000 patients in UC [40]. Typically, episcleritis occurs during IBD flares and can be diagnosed by the instillation of a topical vasoconstrictor [38].

Scleritis, an acute inflammation of the sclera, is a rare EIM in patients with IBD, although its incidence is increased compared to the general population (OR: 3.6; $p < 0.001$ in CD and OR: 2.2; $p < 0.001$ in UC) [41]. It can be classified as diffuse, nodular, and/or necrotizing, based on clinical manifestation, and anterior or posterior, based on location [42]. Unlike episcleritis, scleritis is not associated with intestinal disease flare-ups, and the vessels of the sclera do not whiten after the administration of vasoconstrictors, resulting in eye redness and intense pain, typically at night. Considering the risk of vision loss, an ophthalmologist should immediately be consulted, although evidence-based treatments are not available [1,43].

3.5. Hepatobiliary EIMs

PSC and autoimmune hepatitis (AIH) are immune-related liver disorders that can occur in almost 5% of IBD patients [44].

PSC is a condition characterized by the inflammation and fibrosis of the bile ducts that could culminate in end-stage liver disease [45]. The pooled prevalence in IBD is 5.01%, and it is more frequently associated with UC, 2.47%, than CD, 0.96% (OR 1.69, 95% CI 1.24–2.29) [46]. The male gender, pancolitis, non-smoking, and prior appendectomy are also risk factors for PSC [47]. Although PSC could be suspected based on elevated cholestatic liver enzymes, magnetic resonance cholangiopancreatography (MRCP) is the method of choice for the diagnosis [48]. Liver biopsy should be reserved for cases in which AIH overlap or small ducts PSC (negative MRCP) are suspected [45]. Importantly, patients with PSC and IBD should undergo yearly colonoscopy due to the 7-fold increased risk of developing colorectal cancer associated with PSC [49].

AIH occurs more frequently in patients with UC than in those with CD (OR 8 and 4, respectively) [50]. This condition should be suspected when liver enzyme levels are elevated after ruling out other causes, such as viral, alcoholic, and metabolic hepatitis. The liver biopsy is the definitive diagnostic test for AIH, presenting with features of 'interface hepatitis' on liver histology [51]. Additionally, MRCP should be performed due to the overlap syndrome with PSC (10%) [52].

3.6. Other EIMs

Patients with IBD are at an increased risk of developing venous thromboembolic events (VTE), which include deep vein thrombosis (DVT), splanchnic VTE, and pulmonary embolism [53], and the risk increases significantly during periods of disease flare-up [54]. There is no variation in the overall risk of thrombosis between genders or among patients with UC or CD [2]. Numerous studies on VTE have identified risk factors associated with IBD, including disease activity, disease phenotype, hospitalization, surgery, and corticosteroid usage, and factors unrelated to IBD, such as a history of thrombosis, obesity, pregnancy, and contraceptives [2,54]. In addition, the therapies currently employed in the treatment of IBD may be associated with an increased risk of VTE. Cases of VTE have been observed during JAK inhibitors (JAKi) trials and, although not specifically designed to assess VTE, an increased incidence of VTE events was observed in the oral surveillance trial [55]. On the other hand, two extensive meta-analyses involving patients exposed to JAKi across various immune-mediated inflammatory diseases (IMIDs) did not identify a heightened risk of VTE [56–58], and neither vedolizumab (VDZ) nor ustekinumab (UST) exhibited a heightened risk of VTE [59,60]. Anti-TNF agents may potentially reduce the risk of VTE in patients with IBD [4,58]. Nevertheless, it is recommended that all patients with IBD who are hospitalized for any reason, such as disease exacerbation or surgery, should be administered pharmacological thromboprophylaxis [2].

Anemia (defined as a hemoglobin level < 13 g/dL in men or <12 g/dL in non-pregnant women) is a prevalent EIM of IBD, with an approximate prevalence of 27% among individuals with CD and 21% among those with UC [61]. Iron deficiency and anemia of chronic disease are the predominant types observed in IBD [2]. The basic evaluation comprises red blood cell indices, such as red cell distribution width (RDW) and mean corpuscular volume (MCV), reticulocyte count, a complete blood count with differential, serum ferritin, transferrin saturation (TfS), and the concentration of C-reactive protein (CRP) [62]. A more comprehensive framing should include serum levels of vitamin B12, folic acid, haptoglobin, the proportion of hypochromic red cells, reticulocyte hemoglobin, lactate dehydrogenase, soluble transferrin receptor, creatinine, and urea [62]. For individuals with clinically active IBD, intravenous iron is the recommended initial treatment option due to its faster and more profound response, superior tolerance, and efficacy compared to oral iron supplementation [63]. Erythropoietin-stimulating agents may be contemplated for patients who exhibit an insufficient response to intravenous iron therapy [64], while intramuscular hydroxocobalamin represents the optimal intervention for the replacement of vitamin B12 in patients presenting with anemia resulting from micronutrient deficiencies [65]. Considering that anemia of chronic disease arises from reduced erythropoiesis, triggered by elevated levels of proinflammatory cytokines, the treatment of IBD may enhance bone marrow function [62,66] (Figure 2).

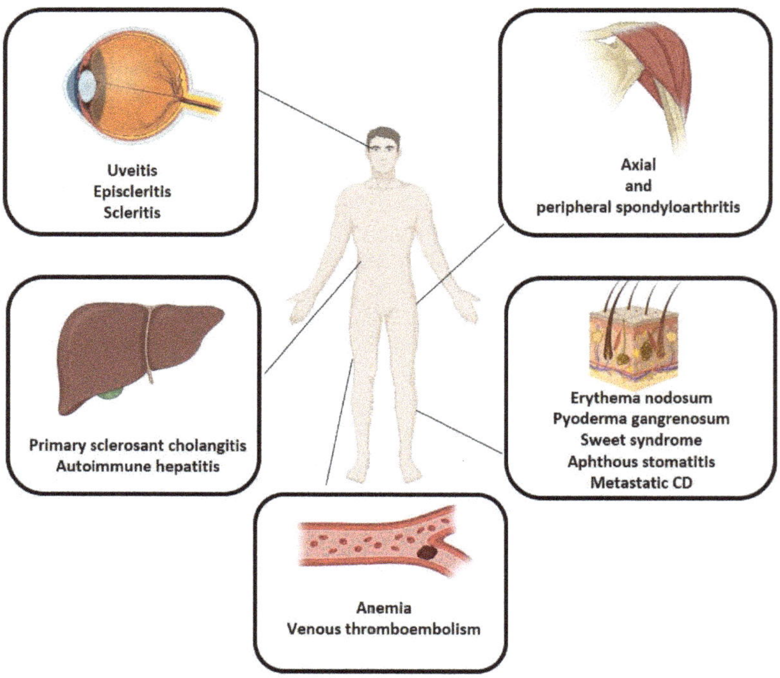

Figure 2. Main extraintestinal manifestations observed in patients with inflammatory bowel disease.

3.7. Treatments for EIMs: An Overview

Despite the high incidence of EIMs in patients with IBD, the data available on treatments are largely derived from retrospective, open-label studies and post-hoc analyses of RCTs.

Anti-TNFα are the most commonly utilized biologics in IBD and can also treat the majority of EIMs [2]. A shared effector phase is observed in immune-mediated inflammatory diseases, wherein bone marrow–derived macrophages, polymorphonuclear neutrophils, and fibroblasts are activated at the sites of inflammation, resulting in the production of TNF-α [17]. The only RCT that has been conducted thus far evaluates the use of infliximab (IFX) in PG. In the IFX group, there was a rapid and significant clinical response, with 46% of patients improving within two weeks compared to 6% in the placebo group. Overall, the response rate to IFX was 69%, with a remission rate of 21% when considering that at weeks 4 and 6, patients received open-label IFX [67]. In general, one of the most comprehensive studies on the utilization of anti-TNFα in EIMs was conducted by a Swiss cohort, which included 1249 patients, of whom 366 had at least one EIM. Of these patients, 213 (58.2%) were treated with an anti-TNFα. A clinical improvement of the EIM was observed in 71.8% of all anti-TNFα therapies. In 26.4% of cases, no response was observed, and in 1.8% of cases, a worsening of the EIM was observed. The highest response rates were observed in patients with psoriasis, aphthous stomatitis, uveitis, and peripheral arthritis, and there were no significant differences in response rates between different anti- TNFα agents [35]. With regard to the latter point, although there is a greater quantity of data available on the efficacy of IFX, adalimumab (ADA) can also be considered effective in the treatment of EIMs. In the CARE trial, 497 patients with EIMs who were treated with ADA demonstrated a 79% resolution of at least one EIM. The most efficacious outcomes were observed in the resolution of arthralgia (43%), arthritis (75%), and oral aphthous ulcers (59%) [68]. Fewer data are available for certolizumab pegol and golimumab: the approval of certolizumab pegol for RA, PA, and AS suggests that it may be efficacious in IBD-associated musculoskeletal manifestations [69–71], and it has also demonstrated efficacy in the treatment of uveitis [72]; the efficacy of golimumab in the treatment of musculoskeletal EIMs and acute uveitis is only known indirectly [73–76].

Concerning anti IL-12 and IL-23, a post hoc analysis of the UNITI trial, which included 504 patients with CD, demonstrated that there were no statistically significant differences between the UST and placebo groups at weeks 6 and 52 in terms of overall EIM resolution (36.9% vs. 39.1%, $p = 0.564$ and 76.4% vs. 80.0%, $p = 0.542$, respectively) [77]. In a recent systematic review, which included 152 IBD patients with EIMs, UST was found to be effective for arthralgia, PA, psoriasis, PG, while it exhibited poor efficacy in the axial SpA [78]. UST also demonstrated favorable outcomes in the treatment of psoriasis in a retrospective multicenter study, with a nearly 80% clinical resolution of the disease [79]. No data are currently available regarding the newly approved IL-23 inhibitors, Risankizumab, and mirikizumab.

The selective activity of VDZ on integrin α4β7, which is expressed only in the gut system, makes this drug ineffective for the treatment of pre-existing EIMs. However, there are some encouraging outcomes, indicating a lower occurrence of new EIMs under VDZ treatment [80]. Low likelihood of developing new episodes of arthralgia/arthritis in patients with CD was demonstrated in a post-hoc analysis of the GEMINI studies (VDZ vs. placebo: HR, 0.55; 95% CI 0.36–0.84). Conversely, in UC patients new/worsening arthritis/arthralgia had a similar incidence across treatment with VDZ and placebo (VDZ vs. PLA: HR, 0.99; 95% CI, 0.52–1.90) [81]. A real-life study on the use of UST and VDZ in EIMs confirmed the safe use of these drugs in patients with articular EIMs. Only a transient increased risk of developing new arthralgia was found after 6 months of VDZ treatment (VDZ 36/508 and UST 9/286; $p = 0.021$) [82].

In addition to anti-TNFα, JAKis have been demonstrated to be the most efficacious drugs for the treatment of EIMs due to their extensive spectrum of action. In a post-hoc analysis from OCTAVE trials, in both OCTAVE induction studies 1 and 2, comparable percentages of patients with active peripheral arthritis who received either tofacitinib or a placebo experienced either no change or some improvement. Specifically, 81.3% of the patients in the tofacitinib group and 85.7% of the patients in the placebo group exhibited no change or improvement, while 15.6% of the patients in the tofacitinib group and 14.3% of the patients in the placebo group demonstrated some improvement. However, by week 52 of OCTAVE Sustain, only the patients treated with tofacitinib exhibited improvements in active peripheral arthritis (16.7% and 33.3% of those receiving tofacitinib 5 mg and 10 mg twice daily, respectively) [83]. A review of the literature, which included 23 studies of tofacitinib in CD and UC, concluded that tofacitinib is an effective treatment for EIMs (dermatological, musculoskeletal, hepatological, and ophthalmological EIMs), particularly when used at higher dosages and in UC patients [84]. A recent abstract by Colombel et al. presents the findings of a pooled analysis from the U-ACHIEVE and U-ACCOMPLISH trials. The abstract demonstrates the efficacy of UPA in controlling EIMs in patients with UC: at induction (week 8), the delta in the resolution of any EIM, arthropathy, and anemia between UPA and placebo were 6.7%, 12.6%, and 5.6%, respectively. A greater difference was reached during maintenance, at week 52 (resolution of all EIM in 24.3% placebo, 41.7% UPA 15 mg, and 65.9% UPA 30 mg; $p < 0.001$, resolution of arthropathy in 22.2% placebo, 38.5% UPA 15 mg, and 66.7% UPA 30 mg; $p < 0.01$, and resolution of anemia in 36.4% placebo, 50.0% UPA 15 mg, and 70.8% UPA 30 mg; $p < 0.019$) [85] (Table 2).

Table 2. Treatments of extraintestinal manifestation in inflammatory bowel disease.

System Involved	Disease	Synchronous with IBD	Treatment That Should Be Considered	Treatment That May Be Considered	Treatment That Cannot Be Recommended
Musculoskeletal EIM 13% (12.9–13.7)	Ankylosing spondylitis	no	Anti TNF-α	JAKi	vedolizumab, ustekinumab
	Sacroiliitis	no	Anti TNF-α	JAKi	vedolizumab, ustekinumab
	Peripheral arthritis type 1	yes	Anti TNF-α, JAKi, ustekinumab	vedolizumab	-
	Peripheral arthritis type 2	no	Anti TNF-α, JAKi, ustekinumab	vedolizumab	-
Skin EIM 5% (4.7–5.2)	Erythema nodosum	yes	-	Anti TNF-α	vedolizumab
	Pyoderma gangrenosum	yes or no	systemic steroids	Anti TNF-α, JAKi, ustekinumab	vedolizumab
Ocular EIM 2.1% (1.9–2.2)	Uveitis	yes or no	topical steroids, anti TNF-α (100%)	JAKi, ustekinumab	vedolizumab
	Episcleritis	yes	topical lubricants	NSAIDs, corticosteroids	-
	Scleritis	yes or no	COX-2 inhibitors, topical NSAIDs, systemic corticosteroids	MTX, AZA, mycophenolate mofetil, calcineurin inhibitors, IFX	-
Hepatobiliary EIM 0.75% (0.6–0.8)	Primary sclerosing cholangitis	no	-	Ursodeoxycholic acid	-
	Autoimmune hepatitis	yes or no	Systemic steroids, AZA	infliximab	-

IBD: inflammatory bowel disease; EIM: extraintestinal manifestation; TNF-α: tumor necrosis factor- α; JAKi: Janus kinase inhibitor; NSAIDs: non-steroidal anti-inflammatory drugs; COX-2 inhibitors: Cyclooxygenase-2 inhibitors; MTX: methotrexate; AZA: azathioprine.

3.7.1. Treatment of Musculoskeletal EIMs

When managing axSpA in patients with IBD, there are currently no randomized controlled trials assessing the effectiveness of biologics, JAKis, or NSAIDs (non-steroidal anti-inflammatory drugs) specifically for this condition [86]. TNFα antagonists have been shown to reduce SpA associated with IBD [87–90]. Etanercept, a recombinant DNA-derived compound derived from the human immunoglobulin G1 and a TNFα antagonist, is a commonly used treatment for SpA, although it may induce paradoxical gastrointestinal inflammation and should therefore be avoided in the IBD population [91]. Considering the effectiveness of JAKis in treating AS, they may also be an option for managing axial SpA associated with IBD [92,93]. Conversely, VDZ, UST, and risankizumab are not recommended for managing axSpA in IBD [78,82,86,94]. A Sicilian cohort of 30 CD patients with SpA treated with UST demonstrated that 33.3% of patients achieved an articular response at week 8, and 43.3% at week 24. Notably, all resolution cases concerned peripheral SpA, suggesting that UST is ineffective in axial SpA [95].

Although the key trials of TNFα antagonists in IBD were not powered to assess the treatment of EIMs, the effectiveness of TNFα antagonists in treating peripheral arthritis is supported by the results of two open-label trials [68,88]. The CARE trial included 975 patients with CD who were treated with ADA. By week 20, the incidence of arthritis had decreased from 8.7% to 2.1% in comparison to the baseline [68]. Similarly, Generini et al. demonstrated a significant decrease in the incidence of arthritis (from 58% to 12.5%) in 24 patients with CD treated with IFX [88]. A systematic review of patients treated with UST for arthralgia or arthritis (nine studies included, 254) demonstrated its effectiveness in psoriatic arthropathy and arthralgia [78]. Concerning VDZ, a recently published multicenter retrospective cohort study showed an increased risk of new-onset arthralgia (adjusted OR: 2.28; 95% CI: 1.01–5.15; $p = 0.047$) [82].

3.7.2. Treatment of Cutaneous EIMs

EN should be controlled by an effective IBD therapy (anti-TNF, UST) [35,68,96,97]. Symptomatic supportive care is usually sufficient for most patients [98]. In severe or refractory cases, systemic corticosteroids (prednisone 20 mg for 7–10 days) may be used [98].

Regarding PG, mild cases can be treated with local or topical therapies, such as intralesional corticosteroid injections, although systemic steroids are often necessary during the acute phase (prednisone 0.5–2 mg/kg/day, prednisolone 0.75 mg/kg/day) [99,100]. Treatment with biologic agents, particularly IFX and ADA, has been reported as effective in improving PG [67]. Recent data also suggests the effectiveness of UST and tofacitinib [101,102].

3.7.3. Treatment of Ocular EIMs

After excluding the infectious causes of uveitis, topical steroids are the first-line of treatment for anterior uveitis, while systemic steroids are the preferred therapy for intermediate, posterior, and panuveitis [38]. Historically, medications such as AZA, cyclosporine, and cyclophosphamide have been used as second-line therapies for ocular inflammation that is unresponsive to steroid treatment [103,104]. However, the use of biologic therapy has significantly changed the way ocular EIMs are managed. ADA has shown to be effective compared to a placebo in three randomized control trials (HR: 0.50; 95% CI: 0.36–0.70; $p < 0.001$) [105–107]. Additionally, in a Swiss IBD cohort study it was found that 72% of individuals with uveitis exhibited a positive response to treatment with either IFX or ADA [35]. UST and tofacitinib have also been successfully used in treating uveitis [108,109].

Since episcleritis is a self-limiting condition, the treatment focuses on providing symptomatic relief and conservative measures. These measures include using topical lubricants such as artificial tears [110]. Additional topical NSAIDs or corticosteroids may be considered if symptoms persist or if achieving resolution of intestinal inflammation proves challenging [111].

COX-2 (cyclooxygenase-2) inhibitors and topical NSAIDs may be effective in mild forms of scleritis, while systemic corticosteroids are usually necessary, particularly in cases of posterior and necrotizing scleritis. Methotrexate (MTX), AZA, mycophenolate mofetil, calcineurin inhibitors, and IFX (5 mg/kg) are considered second-line therapy [112,113].

3.7.4. Treatment of Hepatobiliary EIMs

In PSC, corticosteroids or biologics such as VDZ, ADA, and IFX have not been shown to benefit the progression of the hepatic disease [80,114,115]. Ursodeoxycholic acid at the dose of 15–20 mg/kg/day can improve liver biochemistry, but it does not improve symptoms, the risk of cholangiocarcinoma, or mortality [116]. Liver transplantation should be considered for patients with advanced cirrhosis, recurrent cholangitis (when the palliative treatment of bile duct stenosis with endoscopic retrograde cholangiopancreatography has failed), and suspected early-stage biliary neoplasia [45]. Almost 50% of patients with PSC will require a liver transplant 15–20 years after diagnosis [117], and the overall survival rate after liver transplantation is excellent, with a 91% survival rate at 1–5 years post-transplant [118].

Systemic steroids are the first-line therapy for the AIH acute phase, while AZA is the preferred maintenance therapy. In cases of refractory disease, mycophenolate, mercaptopurine, or IFX may be considered as second-line treatment options [52,119,120].

3.7.5. Paradoxical Effects of Advanced Therapies

One crucial aspect to be taken into account in the treatment of IBD is the paradoxical effects of drugs that can be defined as the onset or worsening of a pathological condition, which typically responds to this class of drug, occurring while treating a patient for a different condition [121]. The precise mechanism by which this phenomenon occurs is not fully understood. However, it is thought that genetic predisposition, the development of antibodies against biological agents, and off-target effects may all contribute to the development of this effect [122,123]. Most of the data available on the paradoxical effects of drugs in IBD involve anti-TNF-α, with an estimated incidence of more than 10% [123]. The most common paradoxical effect observed in this class of drug is the appearance of skin manifestations, which may be psoriasis-like (1.6% to 2.7%) [124]. Skin lesions improve significantly after the discontinuation of TNF antagonists in most patients with basic hygiene practices and the use of topical treatments such as corticosteroids [123]. Other paradoxical manifestations include uveitis, vasculitis, lupus and exacerbation of IBD, CD-like [123]. Importantly, in a systematic review of 17 studies of TNFα-induced paradoxical psoriasis, switching to UST resulted in complete or partial resolution of psoriasis in 83.1% of patients (n = 89). In comparison, switching to VDZ resulted in complete resolution in 100% of patients (n = 6) [125]. Regarding other drug classes, the incidence of paradoxical effects associated with other advanced therapies is minimal: UST might cause new-onset or worsening of preexisting psoriatic lesions or other autoimmune conditions such as lupus-like syndrome [126]; JAKis have been associated with a slight increase in the risk of viral infections due to immunosuppression. For instance, the incidence of varicella-zoster virus infection has been reported to be higher with tofacitinib 10 mg (RR = 6.90; 95% CI 1.56–30.63) and upadacitinib 45 mg (RR = 7.89; 95% CI 1.04–59.59). In addition, the incidence of VTE, including DVT and pulmonary embolism, was 0.68 (95% CI 0.36–1.29), 0.44 (95% CI 0.28–0.70), and 0.59 (95% CI 0.31–1.15), respectively [127]. Additionally, there was a potential exacerbation of other autoimmune diseases and hyperlipidemia [56,128]. VDZ paradoxical effects are less common and can present with musculoskeletal symptoms in up to 30% of cases, although only half of patients had actually arthritis. Exacerbation of IBD, new-onset of psoriasis or eczema, or uveitis occur in <1% of cases [19,129]. These paradoxical reactions often improve when the medication is discontinued or switched to another agent [121].

4. Discussion

According to the most recent definition, EIMs are inflammatory conditions occurring beyond the gastrointestinal tract, where their development is either influenced by the spread of immune responses from the intestine, or it is a separate inflammatory process sustained by IBD, or they share similar genetic or environmental factors with IBD [8]. Other extraintestinal conditions may be considered complications of the disease, or the therapies given, or associated conditions with an uncertain mechanism [8].

In general, patients with IBD have a higher risk of developing other immune-mediated disease, and these are more frequent in patients with CD than UC (OR 1.48, 95% CI 1.08–1 87) [130]. In addition, EIMs occur before the diagnosis of IBD in almost 15% of cases, and in these cases, IBD has a more aggressive pattern [130] Large amount of data regarding epidemiology are obtained from the ENEIDA registry, which includes 31,077 patients with IBD. Almost 19% of these patients had at least one EIM. The registry confirms that musculoskeletal manifestations are the most frequent EIM, with a prevalence of 13% (95% CI 12.9–13.7). Cutaneous manifestations follow, with a prevalence of 5% (95% CI 4.7–5.2), while ocular manifestations and hepatobiliary manifestations have a prevalence of 2.1% (95% CI 1.9–2.2) and 0.7% (95% CI 0.6–0.8), respectively [131].

To date, the most commonly used therapies for patients presenting with EIMs are anti-TNF-α [132]. The efficacy of this class of drugs may be attributed to the fact that a common pathway of inflammation in a variety of immune-mediated diseases is the activation of TNF-α [17]. Similarly, JAKis, which exhibit a broad spectrum of action, are also efficacious pharmaceutical agents in the treatment of various types of EIMs [84]. However, they should be employed with greater caution in patients aged 65 years and older, as well as in those with a history of cardiovascular disease, in accordance with the warnings issued by the EMA and FDA [55]. In addition, the TENOR study may be able to provide insight into the efficacy of UST in the treatment of EIMs [133]. It is also essential to be aware that certain medications utilized to treat IBDs may precipitate symptoms that are analogous to those observed in EIMs [4]. Consequently, distinguishing between the etiology of symptoms is a significant challenge for both the gastroenterologist and the multidisciplinary team.

As we look to the future, it seems clear that in order to improve treatment and thus the quality of life of these patients, more and more efforts should be made to better define the etiopathogenesis of these diseases and classify them, as had already been proposed, not by organ but by the mechanism underlying the disease [17]. Furthermore, it would be beneficial to conduct prospective, randomized studies and head-to-head trials with the resolution of EIMs as an end-point, as currently, only retrospective studies and post-hoc analyses have been conducted.

Finally, a multidisciplinary approach involving collaboration with other specialists, such as rheumatologists, dermatologists, and hepatologists, is crucial to ensure high standard of care for patients with IBD, taking into account the complexity of all their comorbidities.

5. Conclusions

IBD are complex diseases that share pathogenetic mechanisms and environmental risk factors with other immune-mediated diseases. Therefore, they should not be interpreted as diseases limited to the gastrointestinal tract, but as systemic diseases requiring a multidisciplinary approach.

Author Contributions: F.F., A.B., and S.D. conceived the study. I.F. and J.F. wrote the article and created the tables and figures. S.D., F.D., M.A., F.F., A.Z., and T.L.P. critically reviewed the content of the paper. All authors have read and agreed to the published version of the manuscript.

Funding: This research received no external funding.

Institutional Review Board Statement: Not applicable.

Informed Consent Statement: Not applicable.

Data Availability Statement: No new data were generated or analyzed in support of this research.

Conflicts of Interest: F Furfaro received consulting fees from Amgen, AbbVie and lecture fees from Janssen and Pfizer, F D'Amico has served as a speaker for Abbvie, Ferring, Sandoz, Janssen, Galapagos, Takeda, Tillotts, and Omega Pharma; he also served as an advisory board member for Abbvie, Ferring, Galapagos, Janssen, and Nestlè. M Allocca has received consulting fees from Nikkiso Europe, Mundipharma, Janssen, AbbVie, Ferring, and Pfizer. S Danese has served as a speaker, consultant, and advisory board member for Schering–Plough, AbbVie, Actelion, Alphawasserman, AstraZeneca, Cellerix, Cosmo Pharmaceuticals, Ferring, Genentech, Grunenthal, Johnson and Johnson, Millenium Takeda, MSD, Nikkiso Europe GmbH, Novo Nordisk, Nycomed, Pfizer, Pharmacosmos, UCB Pharma, and Vifor. I Faggiani, J Fanizza, A Zilli, TL Parigi, and A Barchi declare no conflicts of interest.

References

1. Rogler, G.; Singh, A.; Kavanaugh, A.; Rubin, D.T. Extraintestinal Manifestations of Inflammatory Bowel Disease: Current Concepts, Treatment, and Implications for Disease Management. *Gastroenterology* **2021**, *161*, 1118–1132. [CrossRef] [PubMed]
2. Gordon, H.; Burisch, J.; Ellul, P.; Karmiris, K.; Katsanos, K.; Allocca, M.; Bamias, G.; Barreiro-de Acosta, M.; Braithwaite, T.; Greuter, T.; et al. ECCO Guidelines on Extraintestinal Manifestations in Inflammatory Bowel Disease. *J. Crohn's Colitis* **2024**, *18*, 1–37. [CrossRef] [PubMed]
3. Kim, J.M.; Cheon, J.H. Pathogenesis and clinical perspectives of extraintestinal manifestations in inflammatory bowel diseases. *Intest. Res.* **2020**, *18*, 249–264. [CrossRef] [PubMed]
4. Bhat, S.; Click, B.; Regueiro, M. Safety and Monitoring of Inflammatory Bowel Disease Advanced Therapies. *Inflamm. Bowel Dis.* **2024**, *30*, 829–843. [CrossRef] [PubMed]
5. Berlin, C.; Berg, E.L.; Briskin, M.J.; Andrew, D.P.; Kilshaw, P.J.; Holzmann, B.; Weissman, I.L.; Hamann, A.; Butcher, E.C. Alpha 4 beta 7 integrin mediates lymphocyte binding to the mucosal vascular addressin MAdCAM-1. *Cell* **1993**, *74*, 185–195. [CrossRef] [PubMed]
6. Grant, A.J.; Lalor, P.F.; Salmi, M.; Jalkanen, S.; Adams, D.H. Homing of mucosal lymphocytes to the liver in the pathogenesis of hepatic complications of inflammatory bowel disease. *Lancet* **2002**, *359*, 150–157. [CrossRef] [PubMed]
7. Chapman, R.W. Aetiology and natural history of primary sclerosing cholangitis—A decade of progress? *Gut* **1991**, *32*, 1433–1435. [CrossRef] [PubMed]
8. Hedin, C.R.H.; Vavricka, S.R.; Stagg, A.J.; Schoepfer, A.; Raine, T.; Puig, L.; Pleyer, U.; Navarini, A.; van der Meulen-de Jong, A.E.; Maul, J.; et al. The Pathogenesis of Extraintestinal Manifestations: Implications for IBD Research, Diagnosis, and Therapy. *J. Crohn's Colitis* **2019**, *13*, 541–554. [CrossRef] [PubMed]
9. Kummen, M.; Holm, K.; Anmarkrud, J.A.; Nygård, S.; Vesterhus, M.; Høivik, M.L.; Trøseid, M.; Marschall, H.-U.; Schrumpf, E.; Moum, B.; et al. The gut microbial profile in patients with primary sclerosing cholangitis is distinct from patients with ulcerative colitis without biliary disease and healthy controls. *Gut* **2017**, *66*, 611–619. [CrossRef]
10. Scher, J.U.; Ubeda, C.; Artacho, A.; Attur, M.; Isaac, S.; Reddy, S.M.; Marmon, S.; Neimann, A.; Brusca, S.; Patel, T.; et al. Decreased bacterial diversity characterizes the altered gut microbiota in patients with psoriatic arthritis, resembling dysbiosis in inflammatory bowel disease. *Arthritis Rheumatol.* **2015**, *67*, 128–139. [CrossRef]
11. Tito, R.Y.; Cypers, H.; Joossens, M.; Varkas, G.; Van Praet, L.; Glorieus, E.; Van den Bosch, F.; De Vos, M.; Raes, J.; Elewaut, D. Brief Report: Dialister as a Microbial Marker of Disease Activity in Spondyloarthritis. *Arthritis Rheumatol.* **2017**, *69*, 114–121. [CrossRef] [PubMed]
12. Muñiz Pedrogo, D.A.; Chen, J.; Hillmann, B.; Jeraldo, P.; Al-Ghalith, G.; Taneja, V.; Davis, J.M.; Knights, D.; Nelson, H.; Faubion, W.A.; et al. An Increased Abundance of Clostridiaceae Characterizes Arthritis in Inflammatory Bowel Disease and Rheumatoid Arthritis: A Cross-sectional Study. *Inflamm. Bowel Dis.* **2019**, *25*, 902–913. [CrossRef] [PubMed]
13. Peeters, H.; Vander Cruyssen, B.; Laukens, D.; Coucke, P.; Marichal, D.; Van Den Berghe, M.; Cuvelier, C.; Remaut, E.; Mielants, H.; De Keyser, F.; et al. Radiological sacroiliitis, a hallmark of spondylitis, is linked with CARD15 gene polymorphisms in patients with Crohn's disease. *Ann. Rheum. Dis.* **2004**, *63*, 1131–1134. [CrossRef] [PubMed]
14. Martin, T.M.; Smith, J.R.; Rosenbaum, J.T. Anterior uveitis: Current concepts of pathogenesis and interactions with the spondyloarthropathies. *Curr. Opin. Rheumatol.* **2002**, *14*, 337–341. [CrossRef] [PubMed]
15. Sheth, T.; Pitchumoni, C.S.; Das, K.M. Musculoskeletal manifestations in inflammatory bowel disease: A revisit in search of immunopathophysiological mechanisms. *J. Clin. Gastroenterol.* **2014**, *48*, 308–317. [CrossRef] [PubMed]
16. Weizman, A.; Huang, B.; Berel, D.; Targan, S.R.; Dubinsky, M.; Fleshner, P.; Ippoliti, A.; Kaur, M.; Panikkath, D.; Brant, S.; et al. Clinical, serologic, and genetic factors associated with pyoderma gangrenosum and erythema nodosum in inflammatory bowel disease patients. *Inflamm. Bowel Dis.* **2014**, *20*, 525–533. [CrossRef] [PubMed]
17. Schett, G.; McInnes, I.B.; Neurath, M.F. Reframing Immune-Mediated Inflammatory Diseases through Signature Cytokine Hubs. *N. Engl. J. Med.* **2021**, *385*, 628–639. [CrossRef] [PubMed]
18. Karreman, M.C.; Luime, J.J.; Hazes, J.M.W.; Weel, A.E.A.M. The Prevalence and Incidence of Axial and Peripheral Spondyloarthritis in Inflammatory Bowel Disease: A Systematic Review and Meta-analysis. *J. Crohn's Colitis* **2017**, *11*, 631–642. [CrossRef]

19. Felice, C.; Pugliese, D.; Papparella, L.G.; Pizzolante, F.; Onori, E.; Gasbarrini, A.; Rapaccini, G.L.; Guidi, L.; Armuzzi, A. Clinical management of rheumatologic conditions co-occurring with inflammatory bowel diseases. *Expert Rev. Clin. Immunol.* **2018**, *14*, 751–759. [CrossRef]
20. Dougados, M.; van der Linden, S.; Juhlin, R.; Huitfeldt, B.; Amor, B.; Calin, A.; Cats, A.; Dijkmans, B.; Olivieri, I.; Pasero, G. The European Spondylarthropathy Study Group preliminary criteria for the classification of spondylarthropathy. *Arthritis Rheum.* **1991**, *34*, 1218–1227. [CrossRef]
21. Wang, C.-R.; Tsai, H.-W. Seronegative spondyloarthropathy-associated inflammatory bowel disease. *World J. Gastroenterol.* **2023**, *29*, 450–468. [CrossRef] [PubMed]
22. Rodríguez-Reyna, T.S.; Martínez-Reyes, C.; Yamamoto-Furusho, J.K. Rheumatic manifestations of inflammatory bowel disease. *World J. Gastroenterol.* **2009**, *15*, 5517–5524. [CrossRef] [PubMed]
23. van der Heijde, D.; Ramiro, S.; Landewé, R.; Baraliakos, X.; Van den Bosch, F.; Sepriano, A.; Regel, A.; Ciurea, A.; Dagfinrud, H.; Dougados, M.; et al. 2016 update of the ASAS-EULAR management recommendations for axial spondyloarthritis. *Ann. Rheum. Dis.* **2017**, *76*, 978–991. [CrossRef] [PubMed]
24. Orchard, T.R.; Wordsworth, B.P.; Jewell, D.P. Peripheral arthropathies in inflammatory bowel disease: Their articular distribution and natural history. *Gut* **1998**, *42*, 387–391. [CrossRef]
25. Schett, G.; Lories, R.J.; D'Agostino, M.-A.; Elewaut, D.; Kirkham, B.; Soriano, E.R.; McGonagle, D. Enthesitis: From pathophysiology to treatment. *Nat. Rev. Rheumatol.* **2017**, *13*, 731–741. [CrossRef] [PubMed]
26. Greuter, T.; Navarini, A.; Vavricka, S.R. Skin Manifestations of Inflammatory Bowel Disease. *Clin. Rev. Allergy Immunol.* **2017**, *53*, 413–427. [CrossRef]
27. Antonelli, E.; Bassotti, G.; Tramontana, M.; Hansel, K.; Stingeni, L.; Ardizzone, S.; Genovese, G.; Marzano, A.V.; Maconi, G. Dermatological Manifestations in Inflammatory Bowel Diseases. *J. Clin. Med.* **2021**, *10*, 364. [CrossRef] [PubMed]
28. States, V.; O'Brien, S.; Rai, J.P.; Roberts, H.L.; Paas, M.; Feagins, K.; Pierce, E.J.; Baumgartner, R.N.; Galandiuk, S. Pyoderma Gangrenosum in Inflammatory Bowel Disease: A Systematic Review and Meta-Analysis. *Dig. Dis. Sci.* **2020**, *65*, 2675–2685. [CrossRef]
29. Xu, A.; Balgobind, A.; Strunk, A.; Garg, A.; Alloo, A. Prevalence estimates for pyoderma gangrenosum in the United States: An age- and sex-adjusted population analysis. *J. Am. Acad. Dermatol.* **2020**, *83*, 425–429. [CrossRef]
30. Hung, Y.-T.; Le, P.-H.; Kuo, C.-J.; Tang, Y.-C.; Chiou, M.-J.; Chiu, C.-T.; Kuo, C.-F.; Huang, Y.-H. The Temporal Relationships and Associations between Cutaneous Manifestations and Inflammatory Bowel Disease: A Nationwide Population-Based Cohort Study. *J. Clin. Med.* **2021**, *10*, 1311. [CrossRef]
31. Wang, E.A.; Steel, A.; Luxardi, G.; Mitra, A.; Patel, F.; Cheng, M.Y.; Wilken, R.; Kao, J.; de Ga, K.; Sultani, H.; et al. Classic Ulcerative Pyoderma Gangrenosum Is a T Cell-Mediated Disease Targeting Follicular Adnexal Structures: A Hypothesis Based on Molecular and Clinicopathologic Studies. *Front. Immunol.* **2017**, *8*, 1980. [CrossRef] [PubMed]
32. Giraudo, F.; Miraglia, E.; Garbi, M.L.; Yantorno, M.; Maradeo, M.R.; Correa, G.J.; Tufare, F. Prevalence of pyoderma gangrenosum and Sweet's syndrome in inflammatory bowel disease at a tertiary healthcare center. *Rev. Esp. Enferm. Dig.* **2021**, *113*, 691–697. [CrossRef] [PubMed]
33. Sleiman, J.; Hitawala, A.A.; Cohen, B.; Falloon, K.; Simonson, M.; Click, B.; Khanna, U.; Fernandez, A.P.; Rieder, F. Systematic Review: Sweet Syndrome Associated with Inflammatory Bowel Disease. *J. Crohn's Colitis* **2021**, *15*, 1864–1876. [CrossRef] [PubMed]
34. Zunt, S.L. Recurrent aphthous stomatitis. *Dermatol. Clin.* **2003**, *21*, 33–39. [CrossRef] [PubMed]
35. Vavricka, S.R.; Gubler, M.; Gantenbein, C.; Spoerri, M.; Froehlich, F.; Seibold, F.; Protic, M.; Michetti, P.; Straumann, A.; Fournier, N.; et al. Anti-TNF Treatment for Extraintestinal Manifestations of Inflammatory Bowel Disease in the Swiss IBD Cohort Study. *Inflamm. Bowel Dis.* **2017**, *23*, 1174–1181. [CrossRef] [PubMed]
36. Turkcapar, N.; Toruner, M.; Soykan, I.; Aydintug, O.T.; Cetinkaya, H.; Duzgun, N.; Ozden, A.; Duman, M. The prevalence of extraintestinal manifestations and HLA association in patients with inflammatory bowel disease. *Rheumatol. Int.* **2006**, *26*, 663–668. [CrossRef] [PubMed]
37. Patel, A.V.; Jones, D.M.; Hill, J.C.; MacDermott, R.P. Development of metastatic Crohn's disease of the skin while on anti-TNF biologics. *Inflamm. Bowel Dis.* **2012**, *18*, 1188–1190. [CrossRef] [PubMed]
38. Shah, J.; Shah, A.; Hassman, L.; Gutierrez, A. Ocular Manifestations of Inflammatory Bowel Disease. *Inflamm. Bowel Dis.* **2021**, *27*, 1832–1838. [CrossRef] [PubMed]
39. Biedermann, L.; Renz, L.; Fournier, N.; Rossel, J.-B.; Butter, M.; Bluemel, S.; Vavricka, S.R.; Rogler, G.; Scharl, M. Uveitis manifestations in patients of the Swiss Inflammatory Bowel Disease Cohort Study. *Ther. Adv. Gastroenterol.* **2019**, *12*, 1756284819865142. [CrossRef]
40. Yang, B.R.; Choi, N.-K.; Kim, M.-S.; Chun, J.; Joo, S.H.; Kim, H.; Lee, J. Prevalence of extraintestinal manifestations in Korean inflammatory bowel disease patients. *PLoS ONE* **2018**, *13*, e0200363. [CrossRef]
41. Braithwaite, T.; Adderley, N.J.; Subramanian, A.; Galloway, J.; Kempen, J.H.; Gokhale, K.; Cope, A.P.; Dick, A.D.; Nirantharakumar, K.; Denniston, A.K. Epidemiology of Scleritis in the United Kingdom From 1997 to 2018: Population-Based Analysis of 11 Million Patients and Association between Scleritis and Infectious and Immune-Mediated Inflammatory Disease. *Arthritis Rheumatol.* **2021**, *73*, 1267–1276. [CrossRef] [PubMed]

42. Murthy, S.I.; Sabhapandit, S.; Balamurugan, S.; Subramaniam, P.; Sainz-de-la-Maza, M.; Agarwal, M.; Parvesio, C. Scleritis: Differentiating infectious from non-infectious entities. *Indian J. Ophthalmol.* **2020**, *68*, 1818–1828. [CrossRef] [PubMed]
43. Sainz de la Maza, M.; Molina, N.; Gonzalez-Gonzalez, L.A.; Doctor, P.P.; Tauber, J.; Foster, C.S. Clinical characteristics of a large cohort of patients with scleritis and episcleritis. *Ophthalmology* **2012**, *119*, 43–50. [CrossRef] [PubMed]
44. Saich, R.; Chapman, R. Primary sclerosing cholangitis, autoimmune hepatitis and overlap syndromes in inflammatory bowel disease. *World J. Gastroenterol.* **2008**, *14*, 331–337. [CrossRef] [PubMed]
45. Chazouilleres, O.; Beuers, U.; Bergquist, A.; Karlsen, T.H.; Levy, C.; Samyn, M.; Schramm, C.; Trauner, M. EASL Clinical Practice Guidelines on sclerosing cholangitis. *J. Hepatol.* **2022**, *77*, 761–806. [CrossRef] [PubMed]
46. Barberio, B.; Massimi, D.; Cazzagon, N.; Zingone, F.; Ford, A.C.; Savarino, E.V. Prevalence of Primary Sclerosing Cholangitis in Patients with Inflammatory Bowel Disease: A Systematic Review and Meta-analysis. *Gastroenterology* **2021**, *161*, 1865–1877. [CrossRef] [PubMed]
47. Fraga, M.; Fournier, N.; Safroneeva, E.; Pittet, V.; Godat, S.; Straumann, A.; Nydegger, A.; Vavricka, S.R.; Moradpour, D.; Schoepfer, A.M.; et al. Primary sclerosing cholangitis in the Swiss Inflammatory Bowel Disease Cohort Study: Prevalence, risk factors, and long-term follow-up. *Eur. J. Gastroenterol. Hepatol.* **2017**, *29*, 91–97. [CrossRef] [PubMed]
48. Venkatesh, S.K.; Welle, C.L.; Miller, F.H.; Jhaveri, K.; Ringe, K.I.; Eaton, J.E.; Bungay, H.; Arrivé, L.; Ba-Ssalamah, A.; Grigoriadis, A.; et al. Reporting standards for primary sclerosing cholangitis using MRI and MR cholangiopancreatography: Guidelines from MR Working Group of the International Primary Sclerosing Cholangitis Study Group. *Eur. Radiol.* **2022**, *32*, 923–937. [CrossRef] [PubMed]
49. Gordon, H.; Biancone, L.; Fiorino, G.; Katsanos, K.H.; Kopylov, U.; Al Sulais, E.; Axelrad, J.E.; Balendran, K.; Burisch, J.; de Ridder, L.; et al. ECCO Guidelines on Inflammatory Bowel Disease and Malignancies. *J. Crohn's Colitis* **2023**, *17*, 827–854. [CrossRef]
50. Ghersin, I.; Khateeb, N.; Katz, L.H.; Daher, S.; Shamir, R.; Assa, A. Comorbidities in adolescents with inflammatory bowel disease: Findings from a population-based cohort study. *Pediatr. Res.* **2020**, *87*, 1256–1262. [CrossRef]
51. Lohse, A.W.; Sebode, M.; Bhathal, P.S.; Clouston, A.D.; Dienes, H.P.; Jain, D.; Gouw, A.S.H.; Guindi, M.; Kakar, S.; Kleiner, D.E.; et al. Consensus recommendations for histological criteria of autoimmune hepatitis from the International AIH Pathology Group: Results of a workshop on AIH histology hosted by the European Reference Network on Hepatological Diseases and the European Society of Pathology: Results of a workshop on AIH histology hosted by the European Reference Network on Hepatological Diseases and the European Society of Pathology. *Liver Int.* **2022**, *42*, 1058–1069. [CrossRef] [PubMed]
52. European Association for the Study of the Liver EASL Clinical Practice Guidelines: Autoimmune hepatitis. *J. Hepatol.* **2015**, *63*, 971–1004. [CrossRef] [PubMed]
53. Murthy, S.K.; Robertson McCurdy, A.B.; Carrier, M.; McCurdy, J.D. Venous thromboembolic events in inflammatory bowel diseases: A review of current evidence and guidance on risk in the post-hospitalization setting. *Thromb. Res.* **2020**, *194*, 26–32. [CrossRef] [PubMed]
54. Dhaliwal, G.; Patrone, M.V.; Bickston, S.J. Venous Thromboembolism in Patients with Inflammatory Bowel Disease. *J. Clin. Med.* **2023**, *13*, 251. [CrossRef] [PubMed]
55. Ytterberg, S.R.; Bhatt, D.L.; Mikuls, T.R.; Koch, G.G.; Fleischmann, R.; Rivas, J.L.; Germino, R.; Menon, S.; Sun, Y.; Wang, C.; et al. Cardiovascular and Cancer Risk with Tofacitinib in Rheumatoid Arthritis. *N. Engl. J. Med.* **2022**, *386*, 316–326. [CrossRef] [PubMed]
56. Yates, M.; Mootoo, A.; Adas, M.; Bechman, K.; Rampes, S.; Patel, V.; Qureshi, S.; Cope, A.P.; Norton, S.; Galloway, J.B. Venous Thromboembolism Risk with JAK Inhibitors: A Meta-Analysis. *Arthritis Rheumatol.* **2021**, *73*, 779–788. [CrossRef]
57. Olivera, P.A.; Lasa, J.S.; Bonovas, S.; Danese, S.; Peyrin-Biroulet, L. Safety of Janus Kinase Inhibitors in Patients with Inflammatory Bowel Diseases or Other Immune-mediated Diseases: A Systematic Review and Meta-Analysis. *Gastroenterology* **2020**, *158*, 1554–1573.e12. [CrossRef] [PubMed]
58. Olivera, P.A.; Zuily, S.; Kotze, P.G.; Regnault, V.; Al Awadhi, S.; Bossuyt, P.; Gearry, R.B.; Ghosh, S.; Kobayashi, T.; Lacolley, P.; et al. International consensus on the prevention of venous and arterial thrombotic events in patients with inflammatory bowel disease. *Nat. Rev. Gastroenterol. Hepatol.* **2021**, *18*, 857–873. [CrossRef] [PubMed]
59. Sandborn, W.J.; Rebuck, R.; Wang, Y.; Zou, B.; Adedokun, O.J.; Gasink, C.; Sands, B.E.; Hanauer, S.B.; Targan, S.; Ghosh, S.; et al. Five-Year Efficacy and Safety of Ustekinumab Treatment in Crohn's Disease: The IM-UNITI Trial. *Clin. Gastroenterol. Hepatol.* **2022**, *20*, 578–590.e4. [CrossRef]
60. Colombel, J.-F.; Sands, B.E.; Rutgeerts, P.; Sandborn, W.; Danese, S.; D'Haens, G.; Panaccione, R.; Loftus, E.V.; Sankoh, S.; Fox, I.; et al. The safety of vedolizumab for ulcerative colitis and Crohn's disease. *Gut* **2017**, *66*, 839–851. [CrossRef]
61. Filmann, N.; Rey, J.; Schneeweiss, S.; Ardizzone, S.; Bager, P.; Bergamaschi, G.; Koutroubakis, I.; Lindgren, S.; Morena, F.d.l.; Moum, B.; et al. Prevalence of anemia in inflammatory bowel diseases in european countries: A systematic review and individual patient data meta-analysis. *Inflamm. Bowel Dis.* **2014**, *20*, 936–945. [CrossRef] [PubMed]
62. Dignass, A.U.; Gasche, C.; Bettenworth, D.; Birgegård, G.; Danese, S.; Gisbert, J.P.; Gomollon, F.; Iqbal, T.; Katsanos, K.; Koutroubakis, I.; et al. European consensus on the diagnosis and management of iron deficiency and anaemia in inflammatory bowel diseases. *J. Crohn's Colitis* **2015**, *9*, 211–222. [CrossRef] [PubMed]
63. Gordon, M.; Sinopoulou, V.; Iheozor-Ejiofor, Z.; Iqbal, T.; Allen, P.; Hoque, S.; Engineer, J.; Akobeng, A.K. Interventions for treating iron deficiency anaemia in inflammatory bowel disease. *Cochrane Database Syst. Rev.* **2021**, *1*, CD013529. [CrossRef] [PubMed]

64. Schreiber, S.; Howaldt, S.; Schnoor, M.; Nikolaus, S.; Bauditz, J.; Gasché, C.; Lochs, H.; Raedler, A. Recombinant erythropoietin for the treatment of anemia in inflammatory bowel disease. *N. Engl. J. Med.* **1996**, *334*, 619–623. [CrossRef] [PubMed]
65. Devalia, V.; Hamilton, M.S.; Molloy, A.M. British Committee for Standards in Haematology Guidelines for the diagnosis and treatment of cobalamin and folate disorders. *Br. J. Haematol.* **2014**, *166*, 496–513. [CrossRef] [PubMed]
66. Weiss, G.; Gasche, C. Pathogenesis and treatment of anemia in inflammatory bowel disease. *Haematologica* **2010**, *95*, 175–178. [CrossRef] [PubMed]
67. Brooklyn, T.N.; Dunnill, M.G.S.; Shetty, A.; Bowden, J.J.; Williams, J.D.L.; Griffiths, C.E.M.; Forbes, A.; Greenwood, R.; Probert, C.S. Infliximab for the treatment of pyoderma gangrenosum: A randomised, double blind, placebo controlled trial. *Gut* **2006**, *55*, 505–509. [CrossRef]
68. Löfberg, R.; Louis, E.V.; Reinisch, W.; Robinson, A.M.; Kron, M.; Camez, A.; Pollack, P.F. Adalimumab produces clinical remission and reduces extraintestinal manifestations in Crohn's disease: Results from CARE. *Inflamm. Bowel Dis.* **2012**, *18*, 1–9. [CrossRef] [PubMed]
69. Smolen, J.; Landewé, R.B.; Mease, P.; Brzezicki, J.; Mason, D.; Luijtens, K.; van Vollenhoven, R.F.; Kavanaugh, A.; Schiff, M.; Burmester, G.R.; et al. Efficacy and safety of certolizumab pegol plus methotrexate in active rheumatoid arthritis: The RAPID 2 study. A randomised controlled trial. *Ann. Rheum. Dis.* **2009**, *68*, 797–804. [CrossRef]
70. Mease, P.J.; Fleischmann, R.; Deodhar, A.A.; Wollenhaupt, J.; Khraishi, M.; Kielar, D.; Woltering, F.; Stach, C.; Hoepken, B.; Arledge, T.; et al. Effect of certolizumab pegol on signs and symptoms in patients with psoriatic arthritis: 24-week results of a Phase 3 double-blind randomised placebo-controlled study (RAPID-PsA). *Ann. Rheum. Dis.* **2014**, *73*, 48–55. [CrossRef]
71. Landewé, R.; Braun, J.; Deodhar, A.; Dougados, M.; Maksymowych, W.P.; Mease, P.J.; Reveille, J.D.; Rudwaleit, M.; van der Heijde, D.; Stach, C.; et al. Efficacy of certolizumab pegol on signs and symptoms of axial spondyloarthritis including ankylosing spondylitis: 24-week results of a double-blind randomised placebo-controlled Phase 3 study. *Ann. Rheum. Dis.* **2014**, *73*, 39–47. [CrossRef] [PubMed]
72. Rudwaleit, M.; Rosenbaum, J.T.; Landewé, R.; Marzo-Ortega, H.; Sieper, J.; van der Heijde, D.; Davies, O.; Bartz, H.; Hoepken, B.; Nurminen, T.; et al. Observed Incidence of Uveitis Following Certolizumab Pegol Treatment in Patients with Axial Spondyloarthritis. *Arthritis Care Res.* **2016**, *68*, 838–844. [CrossRef] [PubMed]
73. Sieper, J.; van der Heijde, D.; Dougados, M.; Maksymowych, W.P.; Scott, B.B.; Boice, J.A.; Berd, Y.; Bergman, G.; Curtis, S.; Tzontcheva, A.; et al. A randomized, double-blind, placebo-controlled, sixteen-week study of subcutaneous golimumab in patients with active nonradiographic axial spondyloarthritis. *Arthritis Rheumatol.* **2015**, *67*, 2702–2712. [CrossRef] [PubMed]
74. Kavanaugh, A.; McInnes, I.; Mease, P.; Krueger, G.G.; Gladman, D.; Gomez-Reino, J.; Papp, K.; Zrubek, J.; Mudivarthy, S.; Mack, M.; et al. Golimumab, a new human tumor necrosis factor alpha antibody, administered every four weeks as a subcutaneous injection in psoriatic arthritis: Twenty-four-week efficacy and safety results of a randomized, placebo-controlled study. *Arthritis Rheum.* **2009**, *60*, 976–986. [CrossRef] [PubMed]
75. Tanaka, Y. A review of upadacitinib in rheumatoid arthritis. *Mod. Rheumatol.* **2020**, *30*, 779–787. [CrossRef] [PubMed]
76. van Bentum, R.E.; Heslinga, S.C.; Nurmohamed, M.T.; Gerards, A.H.; Griep, E.N.; Koehorst, C.B.J.M.; Kok, M.R.; Schilder, A.M.; Verhoef, M.; van der Horst-Bruinsma, I.E. Reduced Occurrence Rate of Acute Anterior Uveitis in Ankylosing Spondylitis Treated with Golimumab—The GO-EASY Study. *J. Rheumatol.* **2019**, *46*, 153–159. [CrossRef] [PubMed]
77. Narula, N.; Aruljothy, A.; Wong, E.C.L.; Homenauth, R.; Alshahrani, A.-A.; Marshall, J.K.; Reinisch, W. The impact of ustekinumab on extraintestinal manifestations of Crohn's disease: A post hoc analysis of the UNITI studies. *United Eur. Gastroenterol. J.* **2021**, *9*, 581–589. [CrossRef] [PubMed]
78. Guillo, L.; D'Amico, F.; Danese, S.; Peyrin-Biroulet, L. Ustekinumab for Extra-intestinal Manifestations of Inflammatory Bowel Disease: A Systematic Literature Review. *J. Crohn's Colitis* **2021**, *15*, 1236–1243. [CrossRef]
79. Pugliese, D.; Daperno, M.; Fiorino, G.; Savarino, E.; Mosso, E.; Biancone, L.; Testa, A.; Sarpi, L.; Cappello, M.; Bodini, G.; et al. Real-life effectiveness of ustekinumab in inflammatory bowel disease patients with concomitant psoriasis or psoriatic arthritis: An IG-IBD study. *Dig. Liver Dis.* **2019**, *51*, 972–977. [CrossRef]
80. Chateau, T.; Bonovas, S.; Le Berre, C.; Mathieu, N.; Danese, S.; Peyrin-Biroulet, L. Vedolizumab Treatment in Extra-Intestinal Manifestations in Inflammatory Bowel Disease: A Systematic Review. *J. Crohn's Colitis* **2019**, *13*, 1569–1577. [CrossRef]
81. Feagan, B.G.; Sandborn, W.J.; Colombel, J.-F.; Byrne, S.O.; Khalid, J.M.; Kempf, C.; Geransar, P.; Bhayat, F.; Rubin, D.T. Incidence of Arthritis/Arthralgia in Inflammatory Bowel Disease with Long-term Vedolizumab Treatment: Post Hoc Analyses of the GEMINI Trials. *J. Crohn's Colitis* **2019**, *13*, 50–57. [CrossRef] [PubMed]
82. De Galan, C.; Truyens, M.; Peeters, H.; Mesonero Gismero, F.; Elorza, A.; Torres, P.; Vandermeulen, L.; Amezaga, A.J.; Ferreiro-Iglesias, R.; Holvoet, T.; et al. The Impact of Vedolizumab and Ustekinumab on Articular Extra-Intestinal Manifestations in Inflammatory Bowel Disease Patients: A Real-Life Multicentre Cohort Study. *J. Crohn's Colitis* **2022**, *16*, 1676–1686. [CrossRef] [PubMed]
83. Rubin, D.T.; Reinisch, W.; Greuter, T.; Kotze, P.G.; Pinheiro, M.; Mundayat, R.; Maller, E.; Fellmann, M.; Lawendy, N.; Modesto, I.; et al. Extraintestinal manifestations at baseline, and the effect of tofacitinib, in patients with moderate to severe ulcerative colitis. *Ther. Adv. Gastroenterol.* **2021**, *14*, 17562848211005708. [CrossRef] [PubMed]
84. Wang, Y.; Wan, Z.; Jin, R.; Xu, T.; Ouyang, Y.; Wang, B.; Ruan, G.; Bai, X. Tofacitinib for extraintestinal manifestations of inflammatory bowel disease: A literature review. *Int. Immunopharmacol.* **2022**, *105*, 108517. [CrossRef]

85. Admin, S. European Crohn's and Colitis Organisation—ECCO—OP33 Effect of Upadacitinib (UPA) Treatment on Extraintestinal Manifestations (EIMs) in Patients with Moderate-to-Severe Ulcerative Colitis (UC): Results from the UPA Phase 3 Programme. Available online: https://www.ecco-ibd.eu/publications/congress-abstracts/item/op33-effect-of-upadacitinib-upa-treatment-on-extraintestinal-manifestations-eims-in-patients-with-moderate-to-severe-ulcerative-colitis-uc-results-from-the-upa-phase-3-programme.html (accessed on 5 September 2023).
86. Webers, C.; Ortolan, A.; Sepriano, A.; Falzon, L.; Baraliakos, X.; Landewé, R.B.M.; Ramiro, S.; van der Heijde, D.; Nikiphorou, E. Efficacy and safety of biological DMARDs: A systematic literature review informing the 2022 update of the ASAS-EULAR recommendations for the management of axial spondyloarthritis. *Ann. Rheum. Dis.* **2023**, *82*, 130–141. [CrossRef] [PubMed]
87. Barreiro-de-Acosta, M.; Lorenzo, A.; Domínguez-Muñoz, J.E. Efficacy of adalimumab for the treatment of extraintestinal manifestations of Crohn's disease. *Rev. Esp. Enferm. Dig.* **2012**, *104*, 468–472. [CrossRef] [PubMed]
88. Generini, S.; Giacomelli, R.; Fedi, R.; Fulminis, A.; Pignone, A.; Frieri, G.; Del Rosso, A.; Viscido, A.; Galletti, B.; Fazzi, M.; et al. Infliximab in spondyloarthropathy associated with Crohn's disease: An open study on the efficacy of inducing and maintaining remission of musculoskeletal and gut manifestations. *Ann. Rheum. Dis.* **2004**, *63*, 1664–1669. [CrossRef]
89. Luchetti, M.M.; Benfaremo, D.; Ciccia, F.; Bolognini, L.; Ciferri, M.; Farinelli, A.; Rossini, M.; Mosca, P.; Triolo, G.; Gabrielli, A. Adalimumab efficacy in enteropathic spondyloarthritis: A 12-mo observational multidisciplinary study. *World J. Gastroenterol.* **2017**, *23*, 7139–7149. [CrossRef]
90. Rispo, A.; Scarpa, R.; Di Girolamo, E.; Cozzolino, A.; Lembo, G.; Atteno, M.; De Falco, T.; Lo Presti, M.; Castiglione, F. Infliximab in the treatment of extra-intestinal manifestations of Crohn's disease. *Scand. J. Rheumatol.* **2005**, *34*, 387–391. [CrossRef]
91. Iriarte, A.; Zaera, C.; Bachiller-Corral, J.; López-Sanromán, A. Inflammatory bowel disease as a paradoxical effect of anti-TNF alpha therapy. *Gastroenterol. Hepatol.* **2017**, *40*, 117–121. [CrossRef]
92. Deodhar, A.; Sliwinska-Stanczyk, P.; Xu, H.; Baraliakos, X.; Gensler, L.S.; Fleishaker, D.; Wang, L.; Wu, J.; Menon, S.; Wang, C.; et al. Tofacitinib for the treatment of ankylosing spondylitis: A phase III, randomised, double-blind, placebo-controlled study. *Ann. Rheum. Dis.* **2021**, *80*, 1004–1013. [CrossRef]
93. van der Heijde, D.; Baraliakos, X.; Sieper, J.; Deodhar, A.; Inman, R.D.; Kameda, H.; Zeng, X.; Sui, Y.; Bu, X.; Pangan, A.L.; et al. Efficacy and safety of upadacitinib for active ankylosing spondylitis refractory to biological therapy: A double-blind, randomised, placebo-controlled phase 3 trial. *Ann. Rheum. Dis.* **2022**, *81*, 1515–1523. [CrossRef] [PubMed]
94. Dubash, S.; Marianayagam, T.; Tinazzi, I.; Al-Araimi, T.; Pagnoux, C.; Weizman, A.V.; Richette, P.; Tran Minh, M.-L.; Allez, M.; Singh, A.; et al. Emergence of severe spondyloarthropathy-related entheseal pathology following successful vedolizumab therapy for inflammatory bowel disease. *Rheumatology* **2019**, *58*, 963–968. [CrossRef] [PubMed]
95. Macaluso, F.S.; Fries, W.; Viola, A.; Costantino, G.; Muscianisi, M.; Cappello, M.; Guida, L.; Giuffrida, E.; Magnano, A.; Pluchino, D.; et al. Effectiveness of Ustekinumab on Crohn's Disease Associated Spondyloarthropathy: Real-World Data from the Sicilian Network for Inflammatory Bowel Diseases (SN-IBD). *Expert Opin. Biol. Ther.* **2020**, *20*, 1381–1384. [CrossRef] [PubMed]
96. Clayton, T.H.; Walker, B.P.; Stables, G.I. Treatment of chronic erythema nodosum with infliximab. *Clin. Exp. Dermatol.* **2006**, *31*, 823–824. [CrossRef] [PubMed]
97. Biemans, V.B.C.; van der Meulen-de Jong, A.E.; van der Woude, C.J.; Löwenberg, M.; Dijkstra, G.; Oldenburg, B.; de Boer, N.K.H.; van der Marel, S.; Bodelier, A.G.L.; Jansen, J.M.; et al. Ustekinumab for Crohn's Disease: Results of the ICC Registry, a Nationwide Prospective Observational Cohort Study. *J. Crohn's Colitis* **2020**, *14*, 33–45. [CrossRef] [PubMed]
98. Pagani, K.; Lukac, D.; Bhukhan, A.; McGee, J.S. Cutaneous Manifestations of Inflammatory Bowel Disease: A Basic Overview. *Am. J. Clin. Dermatol.* **2022**, *23*, 481–497. [CrossRef] [PubMed]
99. Maverakis, E.; Marzano, A.V.; Le, S.T.; Callen, J.P.; Brüggen, M.-C.; Guenova, E.; Dissemond, J.; Shinkai, K.; Langan, S.M. Pyoderma gangrenosum. *Nat. Rev. Dis. Primer* **2020**, *6*, 81. [CrossRef]
100. Funayama, Y.; Kumagai, E.; Takahashi, K.-I.; Fukushima, K.; Sasaki, I. Early diagnosis and early corticosteroid administration improves healing of peristomal pyoderma gangrenosum in inflammatory bowel disease. *Dis. Colon Rectum* **2009**, *52*, 311–314. [CrossRef]
101. Phillips, F.M.; Verstockt, B.; Sebastian, S.; Ribaldone, D.; Vavricka, S.; Katsanos, K.; Slattery, E.; de Suray, N.; Flores, C.; Fries, W.; et al. Inflammatory Cutaneous Lesions in Inflammatory Bowel Disease Treated with Vedolizumab or Ustekinumab: An ECCO CONFER Multicentre Case Series. *J. Crohn's Colitis* **2020**, *14*, 1488–1493. [CrossRef]
102. Vavricka, S.R.; Galván, J.A.; Dawson, H.; Soltermann, A.; Biedermann, L.; Scharl, M.; Schoepfer, A.M.; Rogler, G.; Prinz Vavricka, M.B.; Terracciano, L.; et al. Expression Patterns of TNFα, MAdCAM1, and STAT3 in Intestinal and Skin Manifestations of Inflammatory Bowel Disease. *J. Crohn's Colitis* **2018**, *12*, 347–354. [CrossRef]
103. Thomas, A.S.; Lin, P. Ocular manifestations of inflammatory bowel disease. *Curr. Opin. Ophthalmol.* **2016**, *27*, 552–560. [CrossRef]
104. Singh, R.B.; Sinha, S.; Saini, C.; Elbasiony, E.; Thakur, S.; Agarwal, A. Recent advances in the management of non-infectious posterior uveitis. *Int. Ophthalmol.* **2020**, *40*, 3187–3207. [CrossRef] [PubMed]
105. Jaffe, G.J.; Dick, A.D.; Brézin, A.P.; Nguyen, Q.D.; Thorne, J.E.; Kestelyn, P.; Barisani-Asenbauer, T.; Franco, P.; Heiligenhaus, A.; Scales, D.; et al. Adalimumab in Patients with Active Noninfectious Uveitis. *N. Engl. J. Med.* **2016**, *375*, 932–943. [CrossRef]
106. Nguyen, Q.D.; Merrill, P.T.; Jaffe, G.J.; Dick, A.D.; Kurup, S.K.; Sheppard, J.; Schlaen, A.; Pavesio, C.; Cimino, L.; Van Calster, J.; et al. Adalimumab for prevention of uveitic flare in patients with inactive non-infectious uveitis controlled by corticosteroids (VISUAL II): A multicentre, double-masked, randomised, placebo-controlled phase 3 trial. *Lancet* **2016**, *388*, 1183–1192. [CrossRef] [PubMed]

107. Suhler, E.B.; Adán, A.; Brézin, A.P.; Fortin, E.; Goto, H.; Jaffe, G.J.; Kaburaki, T.; Kramer, M.; Lim, L.L.; Muccioli, C.; et al. Safety and Efficacy of Adalimumab in Patients with Noninfectious Uveitis in an Ongoing Open-Label Study: VISUAL III. *Ophthalmology* **2018**, *125*, 1075–1087. [CrossRef]
108. Mugheddu, C.; Atzori, L.; Del Piano, M.; Lappi, A.; Pau, M.; Murgia, S.; Zucca, I.; Rongioletti, F. Successful ustekinumab treatment of noninfectious uveitis and concomitant severe psoriatic arthritis and plaque psoriasis. *Dermatol. Ther.* **2017**, *30*, e12527. [CrossRef]
109. Paley, M.A.; Karacal, H.; Rao, P.K.; Margolis, T.P.; Miner, J.J. Tofacitinib for refractory uveitis and scleritis. *Am. J. Ophthalmol. Case Rep.* **2019**, *13*, 53–55. [CrossRef]
110. Williams, C.P.R.; Browning, A.C.; Sleep, T.J.; Webber, S.K.; McGill, J.I. A randomised, double-blind trial of topical ketorolac vs artificial tears for the treatment of episcleritis. *Eye* **2005**, *19*, 739–742. [CrossRef]
111. Mintz, R.; Feller, E.R.; Bahr, R.L.; Shah, S.A. Ocular manifestations of inflammatory bowel disease. *Inflamm. Bowel Dis.* **2004**, *10*, 135–139. [CrossRef]
112. Juillerat, P.; Manz, M.; Sauter, B.; Zeitz, J.; Vavricka, S.R. Swiss IBDnet, an official working group of the Swiss Society of Gastroenterology Therapies in Inflammatory Bowel Disease Patients with Extraintestinal Manifestations. *Digestion* **2020**, *101* (Suppl. S1), 83–97. [CrossRef] [PubMed]
113. Abdel-Aty, A.; Gupta, A.; Del Priore, L.; Kombo, N. Management of noninfectious scleritis. *Ther. Adv. Ophthalmol.* **2022**, *14*, 25158414211070879. [CrossRef] [PubMed]
114. Caron, B.; Peyrin-Biroulet, L.; Pariente, B.; Bouhnik, Y.; Seksik, P.; Bouguen, G.; Caillo, L.; Laharie, D.; Carbonnel, F.; Altwegg, R.; et al. Vedolizumab Therapy is Ineffective for Primary Sclerosing Cholangitis in Patients with Inflammatory Bowel Disease: A GETAID Multicentre Cohort Study. *J. Crohn's Colitis* **2019**, *13*, 1239–1247. [CrossRef] [PubMed]
115. Tse, C.S.; Loftus, E.V.; Raffals, L.E.; Gossard, A.A.; Lightner, A.L. Effects of vedolizumab, adalimumab and infliximab on biliary inflammation in individuals with primary sclerosing cholangitis and inflammatory bowel disease. *Aliment. Pharmacol. Ther.* **2018**, *48*, 190–195. [CrossRef] [PubMed]
116. Shi, J.; Li, Z.; Zeng, X.; Lin, Y.; Xie, W.-F. Ursodeoxycholic acid in primary sclerosing cholangitis: Meta-analysis of randomized controlled trials. *Hepatol. Res.* **2009**, *39*, 865–873. [CrossRef] [PubMed]
117. Boonstra, K.; Weersma, R.K.; van Erpecum, K.J.; Rauws, E.A.; Spanier, B.W.M.; Poen, A.C.; van Nieuwkerk, K.M.; Drenth, J.P.; Witteman, B.J.; Tuynman, H.A.; et al. Population-based epidemiology, malignancy risk, and outcome of primary sclerosing cholangitis. *Hepatology* **2013**, *58*, 2045–2055. [CrossRef] [PubMed]
118. Adam, R.; Karam, V.; Cailliez, V.; O Grady, J.G.; Mirza, D.; Cherqui, D.; Klempnauer, J.; Salizzoni, M.; Pratschke, J.; Jamieson, N.; et al. 2018 Annual Report of the European Liver Transplant Registry (ELTR)—50-year evolution of liver transplantation. *Transpl. Int.* **2018**, *31*, 1293–1317. [CrossRef]
119. Lohse, A.W.; Sebode, M.; Jørgensen, M.H.; Ytting, H.; Karlsen, T.H.; Kelly, D.; Manns, M.P.; Vesterhus, M.; European Reference Network on Hepatological Diseases (ERN RARE-LIVER); International Autoimmune Hepatitis Group (IAIHG). Second-line and third-line therapy for autoimmune hepatitis: A position statement from the European Reference Network on Hepatological Diseases and the International Autoimmune Hepatitis Group. *J. Hepatol.* **2020**, *73*, 1496–1506. [CrossRef]
120. Weiler-Normann, C.; Schramm, C.; Quaas, A.; Wiegard, C.; Glaubke, C.; Pannicke, N.; Möller, S.; Lohse, A.W. Infliximab as a rescue treatment in difficult-to-treat autoimmune hepatitis. *J. Hepatol.* **2013**, *58*, 529–534. [CrossRef]
121. Mihai, I.R.; Burlui, A.M.; Rezus, I.I.; Mihai, C.; Macovei, L.A.; Cardoneanu, A.; Gavrilescu, O.; Dranga, M.; Rezus, E. Inflammatory Bowel Disease as a Paradoxical Reaction to Anti-TNF-α Treatment—A Review. *Life* **2023**, *13*, 1779. [CrossRef]
122. Jostins, L.; Ripke, S.; Weersma, R.K.; Duerr, R.H.; McGovern, D.P.; Hui, K.Y.; Lee, J.C.; Philip Schumm, L.; Sharma, Y.; Anderson, C.A.; et al. Host–microbe interactions have shaped the genetic architecture of inflammatory bowel disease. *Nature* **2012**, *491*, 119–124. [CrossRef] [PubMed]
123. Fiorino, G.; Danese, S.; Pariente, B.; Allez, M. Paradoxical immune-mediated inflammation in inflammatory bowel disease patients receiving anti-TNF-α agents. *Autoimmun. Rev.* **2014**, *13*, 15–19. [CrossRef] [PubMed]
124. Afzali, A.; Wheat, C.L.; Hu, J.K.; Olerud, J.E.; Lee, S.D. The association of psoriasiform rash with anti-tumor necrosis factor (anti-TNF) therapy in inflammatory bowel disease: A single academic center case series. *J. Crohn's Colitis* **2014**, *8*, 480–488. [CrossRef] [PubMed]
125. Revankar, R.; Patel, H.; Rojas, M.; Walsh, S.; McGee, J.S. Systematic review of TNFα-induced paradoxical psoriasis: Treatment outcomes of switching to alternative biologic therapies in inflammatory bowel disease patients. *J. Dermatol. Treat.* **2023**, *34*, 2133533. [CrossRef] [PubMed]
126. Puig, L. Paradoxical Reactions: Anti-Tumor Necrosis Factor Alpha Agents, Ustekinumab, Secukinumab, Ixekizumab, and Others. In *Adverse Reactions to Biologics*; Karger Publishers: Basel, Switzerland, 2017. [CrossRef]
127. Din, S.; Selinger, C.P.; Black, C.J.; Ford, A.C. Systematic review with network meta-analysis: Risk of Herpes zoster with biological therapies and small molecules in inflammatory bowel disease. *Aliment. Pharmacol. Ther.* **2023**, *57*, 666–675. [CrossRef] [PubMed]
128. Panés, J.; Sandborn, W.J.; Schreiber, S.; Sands, B.E.; Vermeire, S.; D'Haens, G.; Panaccione, R.; Higgins, P.D.R.; Colombel, J.-F.; Feagan, B.G.; et al. Tofacitinib for induction and maintenance therapy of Crohn's disease: Results of two phase IIb randomised placebo-controlled trials. *Gut* **2017**, *66*, 1049–1059. [CrossRef] [PubMed]
129. Dupré, A.; Collins, M.; Nocturne, G.; Carbonnel, F.; Mariette, X.; Seror, R. Articular manifestations in patients with inflammatory bowel disease treated with vedolizumab. *Rheumatology* **2020**, *59*, 3275–3283. [CrossRef] [PubMed]

130. García, M.J.; Pascual, M.; Del Pozo, C.; Díaz-González, A.; Castro, B.; Rasines, L.; Crespo, J.; Rivero, M. Impact of immune-mediated diseases in inflammatory bowel disease and implications in therapeutic approach. *Sci. Rep.* **2020**, *10*, 10731. [CrossRef] [PubMed]
131. Algaba, A.; Guerra, I.; Ricart, E.; Iglesias, E.; Mañosa, M.; Gisbert, J.P.; Guardiola, J.; Mínguez, M.; Castro, B.; de Francisco, R.; et al. Extraintestinal Manifestations in Patients with Inflammatory Bowel Disease: Study Based on the ENEIDA Registry. *Dig. Dis. Sci.* **2021**, *66*, 2014–2023. [CrossRef]
132. Guillo, L.; D'Amico, F.; Serrero, M.; Angioi, K.; Loeuille, D.; Costanzo, A.; Danese, S.; Peyrin-Biroulet, L. Assessment of extraintestinal manifestations in inflammatory bowel diseases: A systematic review and a proposed guide for clinical trials. *United Eur. Gastroenterol. J.* **2020**, *8*, 1013–1030. [CrossRef]
133. Janssen Cilag, S.A.S. Effectiveness of Ustekinumab in Patients Suffering from Inflammatory Bowel Disease (Crohn's Disease or Ulcerative Colitis) with Extra-Intestinal Manifestations or Immune-Mediated Inflammatory Diseases in a Real-World Setting. clinicaltrials.gov, Clinical Trial Registration NCT03606499, October 2023. Available online: https://clinicaltrials.gov/study/NCT03606499 (accessed on 1 January 2024).

biomedicines

MDPI

Review

Ocular Manifestations of IBD: Pathophysiology, Epidemiology, and Iatrogenic Associations of Emerging Treatment Strategies

Holly Richardson [1,†], Giho Yoon [1,†], George Moussa [2], Aditi Kumar [3] and Philip Harvey [3,*]

[1] Department of Undergraduate Medical Education, The Royal Wolverhampton NHS Trust, Wolverhampton WV10 0QP, UK
[2] Manchester Royal Eye Hospital, Manchester M13 9WL, UK; george.moussa@mft.nhs.uk
[3] Department of Gastroenterology, The Royal Wolverhampton NHS Trust, Wolverhampton WV10 0QP, UK; aditi.kumar@nhs.net
* Correspondence: philipharvey@nhs.net
† These authors contributed equally to this work.

Abstract: Inflammatory bowel disease (IBD) is a complex, multisystemic disease and is associated with ocular pathology in 4–12% of patients. In general, ocular disease affects Crohn's patients more frequently than those with ulcerative colitis. Episcleritis and uveitis are the most common presentations, with episcleritis often correlating with IBD flares, whereas uveitis presents independently of IBD activity and, in some cases, may even alert clinicians to a new diagnosis of IBD. Corneal EIMs encompass a range of pathologies, such as the common and benign keratoconjunctivitis sicca (dry eye disease), which nevertheless causes significant patient discomfort, and the rarer condition of peripheral ulcerative keratitis, which warrants urgent review due to the risk of corneal perforation. Alongside EIMs, clinicians should also be aware of the iatrogenic consequences to the eye following treatment of IBD. Corticosteroids may cause cataracts, glaucoma, and—indirectly via hyperglycaemia—diabetic retinopathy. Methotrexate is irritating to ocular tissues and may cause conjunctivitis and blepharitis. Biologic medications, such as anti-TNFα agents, overlap in their use as treatment of both IBD and uveitis, and yet in some patients may also increase the risk of acute uveitis flares, as well as opportunistic, sight-threatening infections. With integrated care between gastroenterology and ophthalmology, patient outcomes can be improved by facilitating earlier detection and management of ocular disease. This narrative review summarises the ocular extraintestinal manifestations of IBD, including pathophysiology, epidemiology, and current treatment strategies.

Keywords: inflammatory bowel disease; Crohn's disease; ulcerative colitis; extraintestinal manifestations; episcleritis; scleritis; uveitis; keratoconjunctivitis sicca; peripheral ulcerative keratitis

1. Introduction

Inflammatory bowel disease (IBD) is a complex disease affecting the gastrointestinal tract with multisystemic effects. It is immune mediated, chronic, and follows a remitting-relapsing pattern [1]. These characteristics are shared by the two discrete conditions that IBD encompasses, ulcerative colitis (UC) and Crohn's disease (CD).

Although IBD predominantly affects the gastrointestinal tract, its effects on other organ systems, known as extraintestinal manifestations (EIMs), carry significant morbidity. These include, but are not limited to, the musculoskeletal, dermatological, hepatobiliary, and ophthalmic systems [1,2]. The literature varies regarding the prevalence of EIMs [3–6]; however, it is likely that up to half of patients will be affected by an EIM in the 30 years following IBD diagnosis [7]. Ocular manifestations are the third most common EIM, following musculoskeletal and mucocutaneous pathologies [8].

Ocular manifestations are more common in patients with CD than UC, those with a longer disease duration, and smokers [9]. They typically affect 4–12% of patients [2]; however, in some studies, the prevalence is as high as 29% [10]. Although episcleritis and anterior uveitis are the most common [6], manifestations such as scleritis are also important to recognise due to the risk of damage to ocular structures [1,6] (Figure 1 shows the anatomic structures of the eye and their relationships). The temporal association of IBD and ocular EIMs is frequently unpredictable. Ocular disease may precede intestinal symptoms in some cases, and, therefore, may facilitate early diagnosis of IBD [1]. Iatrogenic eye disease is another important consideration, as corticosteroids, immunomodulators, and biologic therapies may cause unintended ocular sequelae.

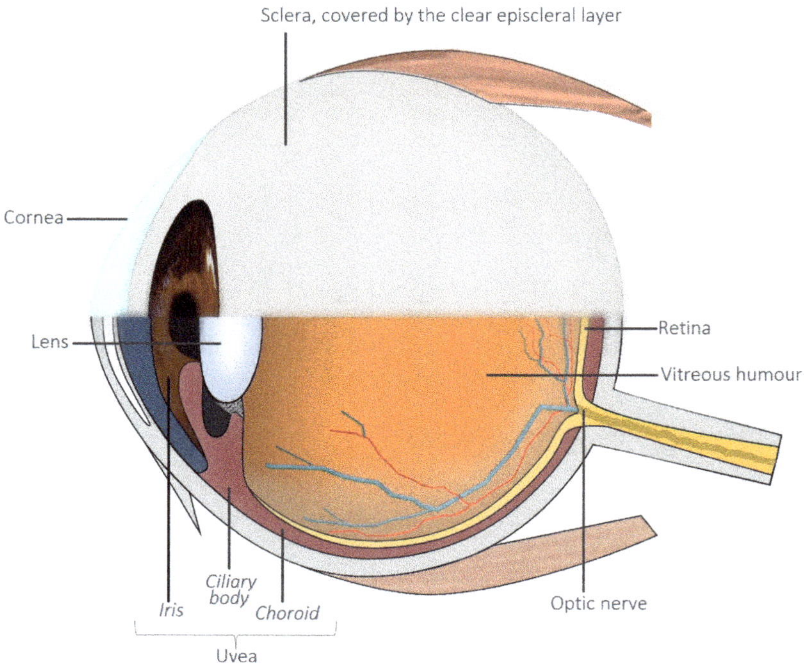

Figure 1. An illustration of important ocular anatomical structures. The uveal tract comprises the iris, ciliary body, and choroid. Original image.

This narrative review will provide an overview of the common ocular manifestations of IBD, including the pathophysiology, epidemiology, presentation, and current management options. It will additionally consider the emerging evidence on associations between new IBD treatment strategies and ocular disease.

2. Episcleritis

2.1. Overview

Episcleritis is an inflammatory condition of the episcleral vascular layer between the sclera and conjunctiva. It can be simple or nodular, but with up to 75% being simple, this is the most common subtype [11]. The pathophysiology of the condition is characterised as a non-granulomatous inflammation of the episcleral layer [12].

2.2. Epidemiology

Episcleritis is the most common ocular manifestation of IBD, typically seen in 2–5% of patients [13]. It often manifests during acute phases of IBD and, therefore, serves as a useful indicator of disease activity [12,14]. Globally, episcleritis is seen in equal frequency in CD and UC; however, in European populations, it is more than twice as prevalent in CD compared with UC (pooled OR 2.40, 95% CI 1.11–5.19, $p = 0.026$) [15]. Proposed explanations for this include greater inflammation in CD, reduced fibre intake, increased meat intake, and urbanisation [15,16].

Interestingly, within the demographics of race, age, and gender, there are no significant differences between episcleritis and the more severe scleritis [17]. Due to the similar patient risk factors and demographics that present with each condition, the distinction between the two must be made clinically.

2.3. Presentation

Simple episcleritis presents with symptoms of grittiness and occasionally photophobia, with sectoral or diffuse redness of the eye on examination. This condition is milder in symptomatology compared with other causes of red eye, such as scleritis, and typically does not affect visual acuity. Furthermore, up to half of patients with simple episcleritis have no ocular discomfort and at worst report moderate discomfort [11].

Nodular episcleritis is similar but is slower in onset and longer in duration. Patients report a characteristic painful red nodule, usually within the interpalpebral fissure [11].

Episcleritis can be mistaken for other conditions causing an acute red eye, such as conjunctivitis and scleritis. It is imperative to be able to differentiate between these conditions, as accurate recognition directly affects treatment and prevention of complications [12,17]. Episcleritis can be distinguished from scleritis by the application of 10% phenylephrine drops, which will blanche the dilated episcleral vessels, resulting in the sclera returning to a healthy white colour. This contrasts with scleritis in which the eye will remain hyperaemic and red [11].

2.4. Management

Both simple and nodular episcleritis are usually self-limiting, with patients advised to use cool compresses and topical lubrication for symptomatic relief as the conservative first-line therapy [1,11]. Reassuringly, patients will often see resolution of episcleritis with appropriate treatment of underlying IBD [14,18,19]. Topical or oral non-steroidal anti-inflammatory drugs (NSAIDs) and topical corticosteroids can be used in refractory cases, although NSAIDs may predispose to IBD exacerbations and adverse gastrointestinal effects and are not currently recommended by the European Crohn's and Colitis Organisation (ECCO) [14,20,21]. In a case study, infliximab was shown to be effective in treating refractory episcleritis in a patient with CD [14].

3. Scleritis

3.1. Overview

Scleritis is an inflammatory disease of the sclera, which is the opaque white layer of the eye, and the underlying scleral vasculature [12,14]. The condition has historically been classified into anterior scleritis and posterior scleritis, with the former being further subdivided into diffuse, nodular, necrotising with inflammation, and necrotising without inflammation [22].

While the role of the immune system in the development of scleritis is well recognised, there is limited understanding as to its precise pathophysiology and relationship with other systemic autoimmune diseases [23]. Similarities in predisposing genes and autoimmunity due to overlap in the composition of organ tissue are proposed hypotheses that require further exploration [23].

3.2. Epidemiology

Scleritis is rarer than episcleritis, occurring in less than 1% of IBD patients [3,13], with older patients, female patients, and those of Black or South Asian ethnicity at higher risk [24–26]. Scleritis is associated with multiple immune-mediated inflammatory diseases, with scleritis patients in the UK over three times more likely to have a diagnosis of CD than a control group (OR 3.60 95% CI 2.28–5.67) and more than twice as likely to have UC than controls (OR 2.20 95% CI 1.49–3.27) [25].

3.3. Presentation

Scleritis presents with redness of the sclera which progresses to severe eye pain, commonly described as deep or throbbing in character, with blurred vision and ocular tenderness [11,12,22]. Compared to episcleritis, the symptoms are typically more severe, may wake patients from sleep, and improve throughout the day [11]. Examination reveals redness of the sclera, which remains unchanged with application of topical phenylephrine and displays a characteristic 'blue hue' with recurrent disease [1,20] (see Figure 2). A further diagnostic test is the manipulation of the inflamed vasculature with cotton tip applicators, which will be movable in episcleritis, but it is not possible to manipulate in scleritis due to the anchoring of the scleral vasculature to the globe [1]. The hyperaemia may be restricted to a specific area of the sclera or diffusely distributed across the eye. Scleral nodules may also be observed, usually in the interpalpebral region [11].

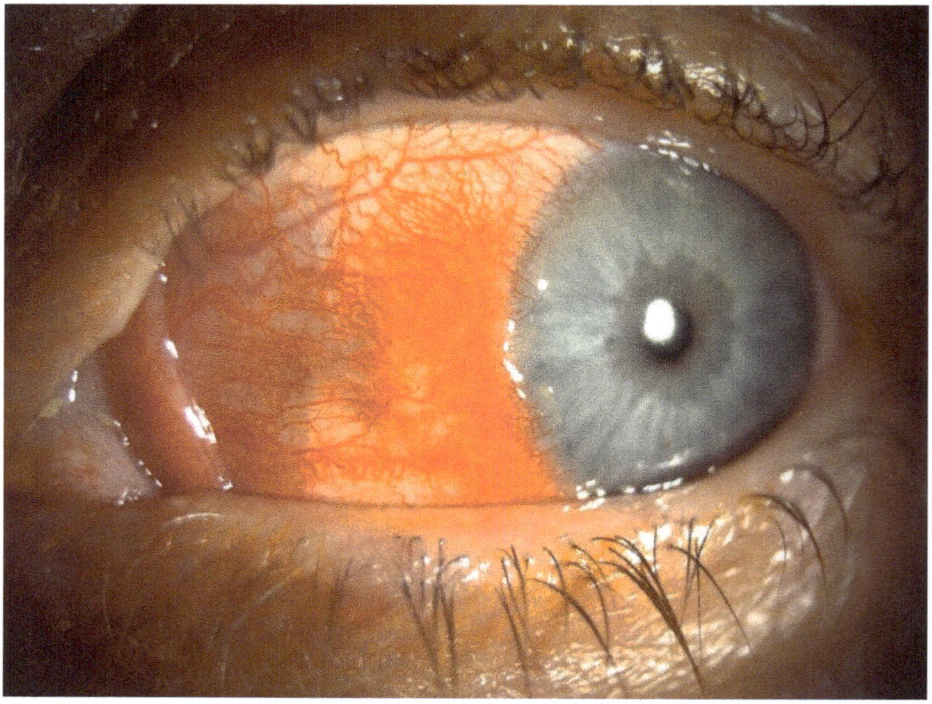

Figure 2. Episcleritis (pictured) and scleritis both present with dilation and increased visibility of the vascular congestion of the superficial episcleral plexus and deep vascular plexus. Application of phenylephrine drops would cause constriction of the superficial vessels involved in episcleritis but not the deeper vascular plexus as with scleritis. *Image kindly provided by the Manchester Royal Eye Infirmary.*

Clinicians should be vigilant of the challenges in recognising posterior scleritis, which can be investigated using ultrasound imaging to detect fluid in the subtenon space [11]. The non-distinct presentation, with inflammation occurring behind the examinable aspects of the sclera, can lead to difficulty in diagnosing this subcategory of scleritis [27,28]. Some cases may present with more significant signs such as ptosis, retinal detachment, diplopia due to restriction of extraocular muscles, or raised intraocular pressure [27]. Although posterior scleritis is a less common form of scleritis, the high risk of visual impairment suggests a low threshold is needed to investigate patients with atypical presentation, such as those with disproportional levels of pain or double or reduced vision [17,29]. Younger patients, female patients, and those with a history of anterior scleritis are more predisposed to posterior scleritis [30,31].

3.4. Management

Scleritis, when associated with systemic disease, is more likely to necessitate extensive and aggressive management [32], while also being more likely to lead to visual impairment [17]. This is particularly pertinent, as up to 50% of patients with scleritis have an associated systemic disorder [17]. An IBD patient with suspected scleritis (for example, waking from sleep due to eye pain) thus warrants urgent referral to an ophthalmologist [14,21]. Scleritis should be treated aggressively with oral NSAIDs (first line) and oral corticosteroids (second line) [13,14,21,32]. Immunosuppressants and biologics are considered in refractory cases [21,32]. In a retrospective study, nearly 90% of patients required systemic therapy (NSAIDs, prednisolone, or systemic immunosuppressants), with around 25% of patients requiring immunosuppressants [17]. This study was undertaken in a tertiary centre and, therefore, included more complex cases; yet, it highlights the frequent inevitability of systemic scleritis treatment.

Topical therapies such as topical NSAIDs and topical corticosteroids, are also occasionally used [1,21]; however, evidence is weak on the effectiveness of topical NSAIDs [33]. In contrast, topical corticosteroids have demonstrated effectiveness in symptom improvement as an adjunct to systemic therapies but should be used with caution due to the risk of developing cataracts and ocular hypertension [1,33].

In aggressive cases, for example, necrotising scleritis, in chronic disease, or in cases refractory to NSAIDs and corticosteroids, immunotherapy may be used to improve visual prognosis [11,32]. However, the evidence base for selecting immunotherapy regimes is not robust [32]. Methotrexate is considered an appropriate starting point, or azathioprine or mycophenolate mofetil may be alternatively used if there are significant side effects or refractory cases [18,32]. These suggestions are echoed by the ECCO consensus [18].

The use of biologics can also be beneficial in the treatment of scleritis. Infliximab is effective and may improve visual acuity or inflammation in over 90% of cases, with 64% of patients able to reduce or discontinue corticosteroid treatment and 36% able to discontinue infliximab entirely [32]. Ultimately, when associated with a systemic disease, such as IBD, it is important to ensure adequate treatment of the underlying condition to ensure the chance of recurrence is minimised [33].

Scleritis is not always present during periods of active intestinal flares and can occasionally precede systemic disease [20,34]. Due to its association with other systemic inflammatory diseases, such as rheumatoid arthritis and vasculitis, it is important to ensure a thorough examination and appropriate speciality referrals wherever necessary [20,24]. The complications of recurrent scleritis are significant, as it may eventually cause ocular perforation [1]; therefore, early recognition, treatment, and control of underlying autoimmune systemic conditions, including IBD, is imperative in the long-term management of this condition [20].

4. Uveitis

4.1. Overview

Uveitis is a group of inflammatory diseases affecting the middle layer of vascular structures of the eye. It is the most common ocular EIM and frequently precedes IBD diagnosis [35]. Importantly, uveitis is independent of the activity of the intestinal disease [7,12].

Uveitis may be categorised according to aetiology. Around 30–40% of cases are non-infective and associated with autoimmune inflammatory diseases, such as IBD, psoriatic arthritis, or Behçet disease. Infection, including bacterial, viral, and fungal, and trauma is a separate but significant cause [36,37]. Uveitis may be further subdivided according to the structures that are affected. Anterior uveitis is the most commonly associated with IBD and involves inflammation of the iris (iritis) and sometimes also with involvement of the ciliary body (iridocyclitis). Rarer forms of the disease include intermediate uveitis, which affects the vitreous humour, and posterior uveitis (chorioretinitis), which is inflammation of the retina and/or the underlying choroid—the network of blood vessels supplying the retina [12]. A combination of diseases may be referred to as panuveitis [1].

The pathophysiology of uveitis is complex and multi-factorial. Studies suggest that multiple genetic factors are involved and likely triggered by a pro-inflammatory gut microbiome, including *Prevotella* and *Streptococcus* species [12]. These gut flora are thought to trigger the activation of autoreactive T cells, which have a causal link with uveitis [38]. Cytokines, including interleukins IL-6, IL-10, and IL-17, play a role in the pathophysiology of both uveitis and IBD, suggesting that these may circulate to the eye and cause uveal inflammation [39]. Additionally, a reduction in *Clostridioides* and *Bacteroides* in patients with IBD can lead to a decrease in de-hydroxylated bile acids, which are suggested to have an anti-inflammatory effect in preventing uveitis [40]. A disrupted microbiome can similarly lead to decreased production in the gut of short-chain fatty acids (SCFAs), which are associated with lower rates of uveitis [12].

Despite anti-inflammatory properties, anti-TNFα agents, including those used for the treatment of IBD, such as infliximab and adalimumab, have also paradoxically been demonstrated to trigger uveitis, which will be further discussed below [8,13].

4.2. Epidemiology

Uveitis is a common ocular EIM, with an incidence of 0.5–3.5% in IBD patients [12]. The typical presentation of uveitis in IBD patients is of anterior uveitis, whereas intermediate and posterior uveitis are less associated with IBD [12]. There is a significant overlap between uveitis, arthritis, and ankylosing spondylitis, which are associated with the HLA-B27 allele [41], with 50–80% of acute anterior uveitis patients possessing the HLA-B27 gene [42,43]. Uveitis in IBD patients is also associated with HLA-B58 and HLA-DR103 [8,44].

Uveitis is significantly more common in patients with CD, with a prevalence of 3.27% (95% CI 2.15–4.39%), compared to a prevalence of 1.60% (95% CI 0.93–2.27%) in UC [35]. Uveitis can appear in all age groups, but cases tend to increase with age [37]. Uveitis is the most common EIM in children with IBD and particularly affects male patients, those with colonic involvement, and those with CD [45]. However, children with IBD are unlikely to develop ocular complications from untreated uveitis, which differs from the more aggressive nature of uveitis in children which is associated with juvenile idiopathic arthritis [45].

4.3. Presentation

Patients with anterior uveitis classically present with photophobia, red eye, blurred vision, headache, and ocular pain [39] (Figure 3). Ciliary injection or "perilimbal flush" around the limbus (prominent blood vessels visible around the cornea) is a key feature [1]. Inflammation of the iris may cause adhesions to the lens, known as posterior synechiae, which distort the circular shape of the pupil, leading to irregularity. Patients with IBD tend to present with bilateral uveitic disease (albeit not necessarily simultaneously) and insidious onset of symptoms [8,13].

4.4. Management

Patients with suspected uveitis should be referred urgently to the ophthalmology department for management. The inflammation and pain associated with anterior uveitis may be treated with topical corticosteroids and topical cycloplegics, which have the analgesic effect of paralysing the iris and ciliary body as well as reducing the formation of posterior synechiae [8]. It is important to rule out infectious uveitis before commencing steroid treatment [46]. In persistent disease, systemic steroids or immunosuppression are indicated [8].

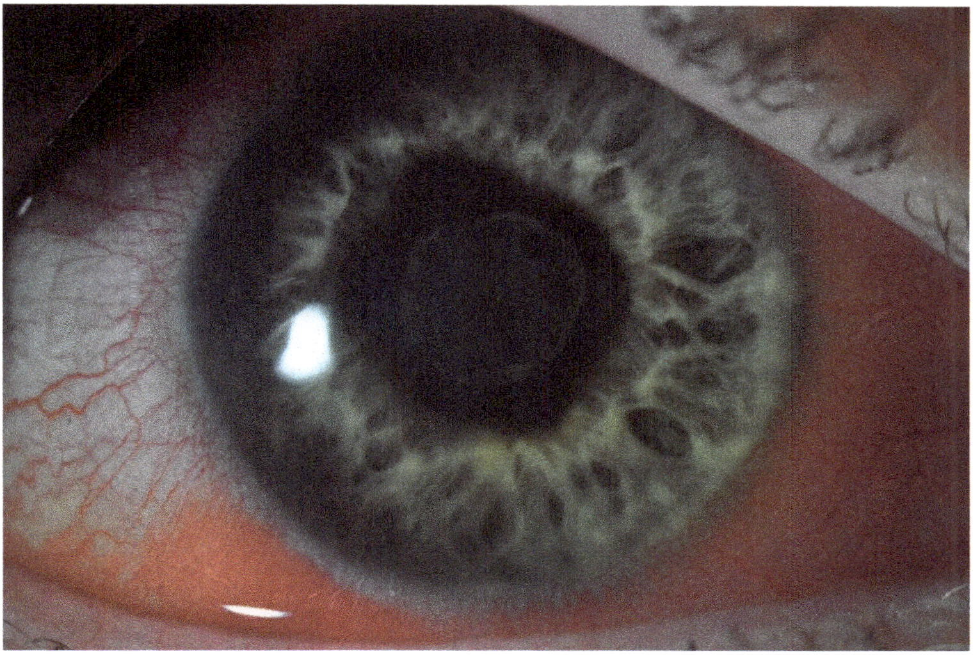

Figure 3. This image demonstrates the irregularly shaped pupil due to posterior synechiae, fibrin formation on the anterior lens surface, and perilimbal flush (redness of the sclera immediately adjacent to the cornea), which is a characteristic of anterior uveitis. The patient will also complain of ocular pain and photophobia. *Image kindly provided by the Manchester Royal Eye Infirmary.*

5. Corneal Disease

5.1. Overview

Patients with IBD exhibit significant corneal thinning and reduced corneal volume compared to healthy controls [47], lacrimal gland dysfunction [48], and increased risk of corneal inflammation [49]. This combination of factors can lead to dry eye disease, marginal keratitis, and peripheral ulcerative keratitis (PUK) [11]. Recognition of the risk of corneal disease is, therefore, an important part of IBD work up [50].

The pathophysiology leading to corneal EIMs is not fully understood but in general is believed to result from the complex interaction between immune dysregulation, genetic factors, and environmental factors present in IBD [47]. The breakdown of immune tolerance and release of pro-inflammatory cytokines, such as TNF-α and interleukins, can disrupt the normal immune balance of the cornea [51]. Other contributing factors to corneal disease include nutritional deficiencies due to malabsorption. For example, vitamin A deficiency in short bowel syndrome can cause keratoconjunctivitis sicca and keratitis [52,53].

5.2. Epidemiology

Corneal disease, or keratopathy, is slightly more prevalent in patients with CD compared to UC, with precise rates varying by pathology [54]. For example, dry eye disease has an incidence rate of 8.18 per 1000 person years in IBD compared to 5.42 per 1000 person years in a healthy population ($p < 0.01$), with more serious corneal damage affecting 2.34 IBD patients per 1000 person years and 2.02 healthy patients per 1000 person years ($p < 0.01$) [48]. Patients are at higher risk of corneal complications during periods of heightened disease activity, as well as in patients with longer disease duration and higher severity. Corneal disease rarely precedes the IBD diagnosis [12]. Patients with extensive colonic disease and those with other EIMs (for example, rheumatological or dermatological) are also at increased risk [8].

5.3. Keratoconjunctivitis Sicca

The most common corneal manifestation of IBD is keratoconjunctivitis sicca (KCS), also known as dry eye disease (DED), which leads to dryness of both the cornea and conjunctiva. KCS in IBD patients has an adjusted hazard ratio of 1.43 (95% CI 1.35–1.51) compared to the healthy population and is particularly prevalent in older patients, females, and those with long-standing IBD [48,54]. The use of 5-aminosalicylates is also correlated with increased rates of KCS [13].

The symptoms of irritation, dryness, and foreign body sensation are caused by inflammation of the lacrimal glands and reduced tear production. Mild cases can be managed with artificial tears, punctal plugs (inserted into the lacrimal duct to reduce tear drainage), or topical immunosuppressive agents, including cyclosporine [55]. Vitamin A replacement, taken either orally or intramuscularly, may be effective in cases of deficiency [56]. Severe cases are an indication that further systemic control of IBD is required. Although often considered a mild disease, KCS can have a debilitating impact on quality of life, physical function, and productivity loss, and should, therefore, prompt consideration of onward referral [48].

5.4. Peripheral Ulcerative Keratitis

Peripheral ulcerative keratitis (PUK) is a rare but serious inflammatory condition in which ulceration of the peripheral cornea leads to thinning. Its aetiology can be idiopathic or in association with systemic inflammatory conditions [57]. The corneal periphery is particularly susceptible to ulceration due to its physiology, relating to the presence of collagen bundles and the vasculature [58]. PUK frequently presents with unilateral disease but can affect both eyes [12].

PUK can be suspected in patients presenting with painful vision loss who may also complain of excessive tearing and photophobia. A peripheral corneal ulcer may be seen on slit lamp examination with the use of fluorescein to visualise epithelial defects, as well as inflammatory cells in the anterior chamber. Severe cases associated with IBD have led to corneal perforation [59]. Concurrent scleritis, episcleritis, conjunctivitis, or iritis may also be seen [57].

PUK warrants an urgent referral to the ophthalmology department due to the need to treat it early to reduce the risk of corneal perforation. Management during the acute phase involves systemic immunosuppression using corticosteroids, followed by tapering of steroids to prevent disease recurrence. Topical antibiotics prevent bacterial superinfection, and topical lubrication is also used to minimise stromal loss and maintain ocular surface health [60]. If there are concerns about corneal perforation or worsening ulceration despite maximum medical therapy, early surgical intervention is necessary [57]. Surgical interventions may include a lamellar patch graft, conjunctival resection, or amniotic membrane transplant [60].

6. Posterior Segment

While rare, it is also pertinent to note the association of IBD with pathology in the posterior segment of the eye due to its significant risk of irreversible loss of vision [61]. It is well recognised that IBD is linked with an increased risk of thromboembolic vascular events with the deep leg and pulmonary veins the most affected [62,63]. However, albeit rare, this can also occur in both venous and arterial retinal vessels [64–67]. Alongside this, a further pathology related to the retinal vasculature is retinal vasculitis, which is sporadically presented in literature emphasising its uncommon nature [68].

7. Iatrogenic Ocular Disease in IBD

Common anti-inflammatory medications used in IBD can have effects on the eye that the gastroenterologist should be aware of. This section provides an overview of iatrogenic ocular conditions associated with IBD therapies, including steroids, immunomodulators, and biologic agents.

The long-term use of systemic corticosteroids is a well-documented risk factor for the development of cataracts in IBD patients, affecting approximately one-third of patients on long-term corticosteroid treatment [69,70]. Cataracts involve the clouding of the eye's natural lens, leading to impaired vision. Patients on prolonged corticosteroid therapy may experience gradual vision loss and require regular ophthalmic monitoring to detect early cataract formation. Management typically involves surgical intervention, such as phacoemulsification with intraocular lens implantation, when cataracts significantly impair vision [71].

Long-term corticosteroid use can also lead to glaucoma, a condition characterised by irreversible optic neuropathy due to increased intraocular pressure (IOP). A trial of 50 IBD patients treated with prednisolone or budesonide for >4 weeks found 24% of patients developed ocular hypertension, which is the primary risk factor for glaucoma, compared to 2.7–3.8% of the general population who have ocular hypertension [72]. CD patients are more at risk than those with UC [72]. If left untreated, glaucoma leads to permanent loss of vision; therefore, early detection through IOP monitoring in patients on long-term steroids is important. Treatment of glaucoma aims to reduce disease progression and involves a variety of IOP-lowering medications or surgical interventions, such as trabeculectomy, to relieve the pressure [72].

Indirectly, steroid use, which leads to the dysregulation of glycaemic control, can have ophthalmic effects in diabetic patients through the development of diabetic retinopathy [20]. Retinopathy can lead to symptoms such as blurred vision, floaters, or sudden vision loss in the case of vitreous haemorrhage. Retinal detachment can also occur, leading to permanent loss of vision unless surgical intervention is undertaken. Management is focused on optimising glycaemic control, with further anti-VEGF therapies recommended for advanced disease to prevent neovascularisation of the retina [73].

IBD treatment may include methotrexate, azathioprine, and 6-mercaptopurine. Of these, methotrexate is most frequently associated with ocular side effects. Methotrexate is a dihydrofolate reductase inhibitor and reduces the synthesis of purine. Methotrexate can be passed into the composition of tears and is irritating to the cornea and conjunctiva, causing burning, irritation, and general pruritis [8]. Patients on methotrexate may also be at risk of conjunctivitis and blepharitis (inflammation of the eyelid margin) [74]. Azathioprine and 6-mercaptopurine are purine analogues that interrupt DNA and RNA synthesis. They have few documented ocular adverse effects. Azathioprine is in fact commonly used to treat ocular inflammatory conditions, such as scleritis and uveitis [75]. However, there have been isolated cases of ocular toxoplasmosis reactivation and cytomegalovirus retinitis in patients with immunosuppression due to azathioprine treatment [74,76].

Ozanimod is a sphingosine l-phosphate (S1P) receptor modulator used in UC. In a phase 1 placebo-controlled study [77] and a phase 2 uncontrolled trial 'STEPSTONE' [78], evaluating the use of ozanimod in healthy volunteers and CD patients, respectively, there were no significant ophthalmological disturbances. However, there were concerns of macular oedema in further trials, with 2 out of 170 patients in a phase 2 placebo-controlled trial and 3 out of 1026 patients in a phase 3 placebo-controlled trial developing this pathology [79,80]. Reassuringly, macular oedema resolved after treatment discontinuation, and the overall incidence is low [80,81]. Macular oedema manifests as blurred vision and occasionally with the visual distortion of objects to appear smaller than they really are [11]. Given there is an association, albeit rare, between ozanimod and macular oedema, an ophthalmology referral for investigation and treatment alongside consideration of discontinuation of ozanimod would be recommended in potential cases [81]. For this reason, consideration of an ophthalmological review for patients with diabetes, uveitis, or a known history of macular oedema before commencing treatment with ozanimod may be appropriate [81,82].

Vedolizumab, an $\alpha4\beta7$ integrin-targeting monoclonal antibody, and ustekinimab, a human IL-12 and IL-23 antagonist, are biologic agents used in IBD. The phase 3 open-label long-term safety study 'GEMINI' assessed the risk of vedolizumab in IBD and noted 4.2 (95% CI 1.8–6.6) episodes of uveitis per 1000 person years in UC patients and 3.4 (95% CI 1.5–5.2) in CD [83]. No ocular adverse effects were recorded in the 'UNITI' placebo-controlled trial exploring the role of ustekinimab during induction and maintenance therapy for CD [84].

Additionally, in a systematic review, the proportion of patients with IBD taking vedolizumab and ustekinimab who developed new ocular manifestations (episcleritis, scleritis, or uveitis) was similar for each drug. The vedolizumab group had an incidence of 1% (95% CI, 0–2%, I^2 = 36%, 95% CI 0–71%), and the incidence for ustekinimab was also 1% (95% CI, 0–5%, I^2 = 61%, 95% CI 0–87%), with no significant difference between the groups (p = 0.834) [6,85]. In addition, ustekinimab was also associated with an improvement of pre-existing ocular EIMs in 59% of cases (95% CI 32–81%, I^2 = 0%, 95% CI 0–85%), and there was no worsening of ocular disease. There is similar improvement seen in patients taking vedolizumab; however, this is limited by a significantly smaller sample size [85].

It is pertinent to note that despite the positives mentioned, the choice of medication may influence the likelihood of a patient developing EIMs in the first place. This is highlighted in a study comparing the use of vedolizumab against anti-TNFα medication, where it was noted that patients with CD treated with vedolizumab were more likely to develop episcleritis or scleritis (incidence rate ratio 2.51, 95% CI, 1.02–6.14) and uveitis (incidence rate ratio, 2.89; 95% CI, 1.35–6.18) when compared with those taking anti-TNFα medication [86]. Though this was similarly seen in UC, the results were not statistically significant [86]. It is notable that vedolizumab is a gut-selective agent without systemic immunomodulatory effects, and, therefore, the significant association between the drug and ocular inflammation is not fully understood. It is suggested that the higher likelihood of uveitis, scleritis and episcleritis in patients treated with vedolizumab is due to either unmasked IBD flares in patients with loss of response to therapy or by the mechanism of action of vedolizumab, in which the binding of leukocyte $\alpha4\beta7$ integrin to mucosal addressing cellular adhesion molecule-1 (MAdCAM-1) reduces leukocyte migration to the GI tract. This may redirect $\alpha4\beta7$-expressing lymphocytes systemically, thus causing extraintestinal effects [86].

Anti-TNFα medications, commonly used for IBD, are also often used in the treatment of various ophthalmic conditions. Golimumab [87–89], adalimumab [90,91], and infliximab [32] have all been utilised in the treatment of scleritis and uveitis. However, ocular complications are among the variety of paradoxical autoimmune reactions that can be induced by anti-TNFα drugs (paradoxical because they mimic the autoimmune conditions they are designed to suppress). Paradoxical autoimmune reactions come in many forms, commonly psoriasiform skin lesions and arthralgia [92], but may less commonly include ocular inflammatory diseases, such as uveitis [93]. Literature reviews of anti-TNFα drugs also reference cases of ocular malignancy, herpes zoster keratosis, scleritis, necrotising fasciitis, retinal vein occlusions, optic neuritis, and de novo or relapse of existing chronic uveitis [93,94]. The majority of these cases were in relation to adalimumab, infliximab, or both. However, one study found optic neuritis occurring in a small proportion of patients treated with golimumab or certolizumab [95]. Further investigation is warranted to determine whether this is a true association, as golimumab and certolizumab were licensed more recently than adalimumab and infliximab, so there are less data available regarding the safety profile [93,96]. Alongside this, many of the cases reported are those in which anti-TNFα medications were used to treat a range of systemic inflammatory conditions, such as rheumatoid arthritis and psoriasis, so it remains difficult to identify the risk for ocular adverse side effects in those with IBD as the main treatment indication.

Upadacitinib is a selective JAK-1 inhibitor used in both UC and CD. Filgotinib, also a selective JAK-1 inhibitor, and tofacitinib, a pan-JAK inhibitor, are utilised in the treatment of UC. There were no reported ocular adverse effects in the randomised controlled trials evaluating the respective medications for induction and maintenance of UC and CD (for upadacitinib) and UC (for filgotinib and tofacitinib) [97–100].

Interestingly, there have been case studies, albeit rare, of patients developing cytomegalovirus (CMV) retinitis following upadacitinib and tofacitinib treatment [101]. CMV retinitis is an opportunistic infection that is sight threatening and warrants urgent referral to ophthalmology. Furthermore, there was one case of retinal vein occlusion out of 102 patients who reported treatment-emergent adverse effects in 'FINCH 2', a phase 3 RCT evaluating the effects of filgotinib in patients with rheumatoid arthritis (RA) [102]. Clinicians may be concerned about the increased risk of venous thromboembolism (VTE) seen in IBD patients [103] and the potential role of JAK inhibitors in increasing said risk from an ocular perspective; however, the evidence to support the association of JAK inhibitors and the increased risk of VTE in this population remains ambiguous [62]. This is reinforced by the lack of ocular VTE events reported in the RCTs specific to IBD patients [97–100].

It must be highlighted that in all the cases mentioned above, the patients were being treated for RA, and further evaluation into the specific cumulative risks of CMV retinitis and RVO for those who are being treated for IBD would be useful to understand whether there is any difference in the risks to this specific population.

In many of the biologic medications currently used in IBD, there is an increased risk of opportunistic infections [97,98,100], such as CMV, which can present with ocular manifestations [104]. Therefore, any patient presenting with symptoms of reduced visual acuity and visual field loss during treatment should be appropriately assessed and referred for urgent investigation wherever necessary.

8. The Role of Ophthalmology

In the Emergency Eye Care Commissioning Guidelines published by the Royal College of Ophthalmologists in 2020, there is acknowledgment of the association scleritis and uveitis have with systemic inflammatory conditions [105]. The recommendation as part of management includes early assessment for potential systemic disorders and collaboration with respective specialists. However, there are no specific guidelines on referral pathways or investigations, which may further prompt clinicians to explore this possibility. The lack of a similar recommendation for episcleritis is likely due to the self-limiting nature of the condition; although, the aforementioned recommendation may be relevant in refractory cases.

This recommendation is supported by a large UK-based cohort analysis, showing that patients diagnosed with ocular conditions, including anterior uveitis, episcleritis, and scleritis, are at a twofold increased risk of subsequent diagnosis of IBD, especially CD [106]. The delay between the diagnosis of the ocular condition to the diagnosis of IBD was, on average, greater than two years [106]. This demonstrates a significant delay in possible diagnosis and treatment of IBD. The non-specific correlation of symptoms highlights the importance of a thorough history and systems review in both the ophthalmology setting and in general practice. Further simple investigations, such as faecal calprotectin, and onward gastroenterology referral should be considered to reduce the risk of delayed diagnosis and treatment, especially in those presenting with gastrointestinal symptoms, including rectal bleeding, anaemia, and loose stool, which were common in patients presenting for the first time with ocular EIMs but without a formal IBD diagnosis [106].

9. Conclusions

In summary, understanding and addressing ocular EIMs is important to help aid early diagnosis and improve comprehensive IBD management (see Table 1). Advanced therapies used to treat IBD carry an increased risk of developing ocular complications, ranging from the common conditions, such as cataracts and glaucoma, to the less common but severe manifestations, such as optic neuritis.

Table 1. A summary of ocular extraintestinal manifestations of inflammatory bowel disease, including relevant epidemiological and clinical information for the gastroenterologist.

EIM	Incidence in IBD	Risk Factors	Presentation	Management
Episcleritis	2–5% CD > UC in European populations CD = UC globally	Active IBD flares Other autoimmune diseases	Mild–moderate ocular discomfort Episcleral hyperaemia, itching	Conservative management + treatment of underlying disease Cool compress, topical lubrication Topical NSAID, topical corticosteroids Oral NSAIDs
Scleritis	<1% CD > UC	Other autoimmune diseases Long-term corticosteroids Increased age Female Black/South Asian	Moderate–severe ocular pain Scleral hyperaemia Blurred vision Ocular tenderness	Oral NSAIDs Oral corticosteroids Systemic immunosuppressants, e.g., methotrexate +/− topical corticosteroid
Uveitis	0.5–3.5% CD > UC	Ankylosing spondylitis HLA-B27, HLA-B58, HLA-DR103 Increased age Male Colonic involvement Anti-TNFα agents Not associated with active IBD flares	Photophobia Red eye Blurred vision Headache Eye pain Conjunctival injection	Topical steroids Topical cycloplegics Systemic steroids and immunosuppression if severe
KCS	Up to 44%	Increased age Females Long-standing IBD Use of 5-ASA	Irritation Dryness Foreign body sensation	Artificial tears Punctal plugs Topical immunosuppressants Vit A replacement
PUK	Rare	Increased age Systemic autoimmune disease	Ocular pain Vision loss Ulceration seen on slit lamp examination with fluorescein	Corticosteroids Topical antibiotics Lubrication

There are aspects of this topic that require further research. It is suggested that future research may focus on addressing the precise pathophysiological mechanisms of ocular EIMs, in particular scleritis and corneal disease. Broader research into the risks of new IBD medications, such as ozanimod, vedolizumab, and JAK inhibitors, is also a priority. This may focus on establishing the underlying mechanism of ocular side effects and differentiating risks that are specific to IBD patients from those that have been found for the same drugs used in other autoimmune conditions. For example, is there a significant association between the anti-TNFα agents golimumab and certolizumab and the development of optic neuritis? And, do JAK inhibitors increase the risk of retinal vein occlusion or CMV retinitis?

The development of protocols for both ophthalmological monitoring of high-risk IBD patients and GI investigations for patients with recurrent ocular activity suspicious of underlying systemic disease would also be welcome. Ongoing surveillance and vigilant assessment will be essential as newer therapies become more widely used, especially in patients with pre-existing risk factors for ocular disease. A thorough history and systems review will facilitate the early detection of patients who will benefit from an ophthalmology referral, thus improving holistic management and enhancing patient outcomes. Indeed, as the prevalence of IBD continues to rise, collaboration between the gastroenterology and ophthalmology teams is imperative to allow earlier recognition and treatment of these conditions.

Author Contributions: P.H. conceptualised the manuscript outline. H.R. and G.Y. were equally involved in writing the main draft of the manuscript. G.M., A.K. and P.H. were involved in critical revisions of the manuscript. All authors have read and agreed to the published version of the manuscript.

Funding: This research received no external funding.

Acknowledgments: The authors would like to acknowledge the support of the Manchester Royal Eye Hospital Imaging Department for providing images in Figures 2 and 3.

Conflicts of Interest: A.K. has received speaker fees for Abbvie and Ferring and has been on the advisory board for Abbvie and Dr. Falk (unrelated to this work). P.H. has received speaker fees for Abbvie and Alphasigma, received conference support from Tillots and Abbvie, and been on advisory boards for Dr. Falk (unrelated to this work). All other authors declare no conflict of interest.

References

1. Mady, R.; Grover, W.; Butrus, S. Ocular complications of inflammatory bowel disease. *Sci. World J.* **2015**, *2015*, 438402. [CrossRef] [PubMed]
2. Greuter, T.; Vavricka, S.R. Extraintestinal manifestations in inflammatory bowel disease–epidemiology, genetics, and pathogenesis. *Expert. Rev. Gastroenterol. Hepatol.* **2019**, *13*, 307–317. [CrossRef]
3. Harbord, M.; Annese, V.; Vavricka, S.R.; Allez, M.; de Acosta, M.B.; Boberg, K.M.; Burisch, J.; De Vos, M.; De Vries, A.M.; Dick, A.D.; et al. The first european evidence-based consensus on extra-intestinal manifestations in inflammatory bowel disease. *J. Crohns Colitis.* **2016**, *10*, 239–254. [CrossRef] [PubMed]
4. Mendoza, J.L.; Lana, R.; Taxonera, C.; Alba, C.; Izquierdo, S.; Díaz-Rubio, M. Extraintestinal manifestations in inflammatory bowel disease: Differences between Crohn's disease and ulcerative colitis. *Med. Clin.* **2005**, *125*, 297–300.
5. Vavricka, S.R.; Brun, L.; Ballabeni, P.; Pittet, V.; Prinz Vavricka, B.M.; Zeitz, J.; Rogler, G.; Schoepfer, A.M. Frequency and risk factors for extraintestinal manifestations in the swiss inflammatory bowel disease cohort. *Am. J. Gastroenterol.* **2011**, *106*, 110–119. [CrossRef] [PubMed]
6. Hedin, C.R.H.; Vavricka, S.R.; Stagg, A.J.; Schoepfer, A.; Raine, T.; Puig, L.; Pleyer, U.; Navarini, A.; Van Der Meulen-de Jong, A.E.; Maul, J.; et al. The Pathogenesis of Extraintestinal Manifestations: Implications for IBD Research, Diagnosis, and Therapy. *J. Crohns Colitis.* **2019**, *13*, 541–554. [CrossRef] [PubMed]
7. Vavricka, S.R.; Rogler, G.; Gantenbein, C.; Spoerri, M.; Vavricka, M.P.; Navarini, A.A.; French, L.E.; Safroneeva, E.; Fournier, N.; Straumann, A.; et al. Chronological order of appearance of extraintestinal manifestations relative to the time of IBD diagnosis in the Swiss Inflammatory Bowel Disease Cohort. *Inflamm. Bowel Dis.* **2015**, *21*, 1794–1800. [CrossRef]
8. Pytrus, W.; Akutko, K.; Pytrus, T.; Turno-Kręcicka, A. A Review of Ophthalmic Complications in Inflammatory Bowel Diseases. *J. Clin. Med.* **2022**, *11*, 7457. [CrossRef]
9. Roberts, H.; Rai, S.N.; Pan, J.; Rao, J.M.; Keskey, R.C.; Kanaan, Z.; Short, E.P.; Mottern, E.; Galandiuk, S. Extraintestinal manifestations of inflammatory bowel disease and the influence of smoking. *Digestion* **2014**, *90*, 122–129. [CrossRef]
10. Yilmaz, S.; Aydemir, E.; Maden, A.; Unsal, B. The prevalence of ocular involvement in patients with inflammatory bowel disease. *Int. J. Color. Dis.* **2007**, *22*, 1027–1030. [CrossRef]
11. Bowling, B. *Kanski's Clinical Ophthalmology a Systemic Approach*; Elsevier: Amsterdam, The Netherlands, 2016; Volume 897.
12. Migliorisi, G.; Vella, G.; Dal Buono, A.; Gabbiadini, R.; Busacca, A.; Loy, L.; Bezzio, C.; Vinciguerra, P.; Armuzzi, A. Ophthalmological Manifestations in Inflammatory Bowel Diseases: Keep an Eye on It. *Cells* **2024**, *13*, 142. [CrossRef]
13. Troncoso, L.L.; Biancardi, A.L.; De Moraes, H.V.; Zaltman, C. Ophthalmic manifestations in patients with inflammatory bowel disease: A review. *World J. Gastroenterol.* **2017**, *23*, 5836–5848. [CrossRef] [PubMed]
14. Mintz, R.; Feller, E.R.; Bahr, R.L.; Shah, S.A. Ocular manifestations of inflammatory bowel disease. *Inflamm. Bowel Dis.* **2004**, *10*, 135–139. [CrossRef] [PubMed]
15. Li, J.X.; Chiang, C.C.; Chen, S.N.; Lin, J.M.; Tsai, Y.Y. The Prevalence of Ocular Extra-Intestinal Manifestations in Adults Inflammatory Bowel Disease: A Systematic Review and Meta-Analysis. *Int. J. Environ. Res. Public Health* **2022**, *19*, 15683. [CrossRef] [PubMed]
16. Beaugerie, L.; Langholz, E.; Nyboe-Andersen, N.; Pigneur, B.; Sokol, H. Differences in epidemiological features between ulcerative colitis and Crohn's disease: The early life-programmed versus late dysbiosis hypothesis. *Med. Hypotheses* **2018**, *115*, 19–21. [CrossRef] [PubMed]
17. Jabs, D.A.; Mudun, A.; Dunn, J.P.; Marsh, M.J. Episcleritis and scleritis: Clinical features and treatment results. *Am. J. Ophthalmol.* **2000**, *130*, 469–476. [CrossRef]
18. Gordon, H.; Burisch, J.; Ellul, P.; Karmiris, K.; Katsanos, K.; Allocca, M.; Bamias, G.; De Acosta, M.B.; Braithwaite, T.; Greuter, T.; et al. ECCO Guidelines on Extraintestinal Manifestations in Inflammatory Bowel Disease. *J. Crohns Colitis* **2024**, *18*, 1–37. [CrossRef] [PubMed]
19. Evans, P.E.; Pardi, D.S. Extraintestinal manifestations of inflammatory bowel disease: Focus on the musculoskeletal, dermatologic, and ocular manifestations. *MedGenMed* **2007**, *9*, 55. [PubMed]

20. Shah, J.; Shah, A.; Hassman, L.; Gutierrez, A. Ocular Manifestations of Inflammatory Bowel Disease. *Inflamm. Bowel Dis.* **2021**, *27*, 1832–1838. [CrossRef]
21. Maaser, C.; Sturm, A.; Vavricka, S.R.; Kucharzik, T.; Fiorino, G.; Annese, V.; Calabrese, E.; Baumgart, D.C.; Bettenworth, D.; Nunes, P.B.; et al. ECCO-ESGAR Guideline for Diagnostic Assessment in IBD Part 1: Initial diagnosis, monitoring of known IBD, detection of complications. *J. Crohns Colitis* **2019**, *13*, 144–164K. [CrossRef]
22. Watson, P.; Hayreh, S. Scleritis and episcleritis. *Br. J. Ophthalmol.* **1976**, *60*, 163–191. [CrossRef] [PubMed]
23. Vergouwen, D.P.C.; Rothova, A.; Berge, J.C.T.; Verdijk, R.M.; van Laar, J.A.M.; Vingerling, J.R.; Schreurs, M.W.J. Current insights in the pathogenesis of scleritis. *Exp. Eye Res.* **2020**, *197*, 108078. [CrossRef]
24. de-la-Torre, A.; Cabrera-Pérez, M.; Durán, C.; García, S.; Cuevas, M.; Carreño, N.; Rangel, C.M.; Pachón-Suárez, D.I.; Martínez-Ceballos, M.A.; Mejía, M.E.; et al. Clinical patterns and risk factors in scleritis: A multicentric study in Colombia. *Graefe's Arch. Clin. Exp. Ophthalmol.* **2022**, *260*, 3957–3967. [CrossRef] [PubMed]
25. Braithwaite, T.; Adderley, N.J.; Subramanian, A.; Galloway, J.; Kempen, J.H.; Gokhale, K.; Cope, A.P.; Dick, A.D.; Nirantharakumar, K.; Denniston, A.K. Epidemiology of Scleritis in the United Kingdom From 1997 to 2018: Population-Based Analysis of 11 Million Patients and Association Between Scleritis and Infectious and Immune-Mediated Inflammatory Disease. *Arthritis Rheumatol.* **2021**, *73*, 1267–1276. [CrossRef]
26. Homayounfar, G.; Nardone, N.; Borkar, D.S.; Tham, V.M.; Porco, T.C.; Enanoria, W.T.A.; Parker, J.V.; Vinoya, A.C.; Uchida, A.; Acharya, N.R. Incidence of scleritis and episcleritis: Results from the pacific ocular inflammation study. *Am. J. Ophthalmol.* **2013**, *156*, 752–758.e3. [CrossRef]
27. Galor, A.; Thorne, J.E. Scleritis and Peripheral Ulcerative Keratitis. *Rheum. Dis. Clin. N. Am.* **2007**, *33*, 835–854. [CrossRef]
28. Dutta Majumder, P.; Agrawal, R.; McCluskey, P.; Biswas, J. Current Approach for the Diagnosis and Management of Noninfective Scleritis. *Asia-Pac. J. Ophthalmol.* **2021**, *10*, 212–223. [CrossRef] [PubMed]
29. Gonzalez-Gonzalez, L.A.; Molina-Prat, N.; Doctor, P.; Tauber, J.; Sainz De La Maza, M.; Foster, C.S. Clinical features and presentation of posterior scleritis: A report of 31 cases. *Ocul. Immunol. Inflamm.* **2014**, *22*, 203–207. [CrossRef]
30. Benson, W.E.; Shields, J.A.; Tasman, W.; Crandall, A.S. Posterior Scleritis A Cause of Diagnostic Confusion. *Arch. Ophthalmol.* **1979**, *97*, 1482–1486. [CrossRef] [PubMed]
31. McCluskey, P.J.; Watson, P.G.; Lightman, S.; Haybittle, J.; Restori, M.; Branley, M. Posterior scleritis: Clinical features, systemic associations, and outcome in a large series of patients. *Ophthalmology* **1999**, *106*, 2380–2386. [CrossRef] [PubMed]
32. Abdel-Aty, A.; Gupta, A.; Del Priore, L.; Kombo, N. Management of noninfectious scleritis. *Ther. Adv. Ophthalmol.* **2022**, *14*, 25158414211070879. [CrossRef]
33. Rogler, G.; Singh, A.; Kavanaugh, A.; Rubin, D.T. Extraintestinal Manifestations of Inflammatory Bowel Disease: Current Concepts, Treatment, and Implications for Disease Management. *Gastroenterology* **2021**, *161*, 1118–1132. [CrossRef]
34. Sainz De La Maza, M.; Molina, N.; Gonzalez-Gonzalez, L.A.; Doctor, P.P.; Tauber, J.; Foster, C.S. Clinical characteristics of a large cohort of patients with scleritis and episcleritis. *Ophthalmology* **2012**, *119*, 43–50. [CrossRef] [PubMed]
35. Lin, H.; Zhang, J.; Liang, C.; Wu, D.; Tan, Y.; Luo, L.; Liu, Z. Differences in the prevalence of uveitis between Crohn's disease and ulcerative colitis: A systematic review and meta-analysis. *Acta Ophthalmol.* **2024**, *102*, e485–e492. [CrossRef]
36. Jadon, D.R.; Corp, N.; van der Windt, D.A.; Coates, L.C.; Soriano, E.R.; Kavanaugh, A.; Raine, T.; Rieder, F.; Siebert, S.; Zummer, M.; et al. Management of Concomitant Inflammatory Bowel Disease or Uveitis in Patients with Psoriatic Arthritis: An Updated Review Informing the 2021 GRAPPA Treatment Recommendations. *J. Rheumatol.* **2023**, *50*, 438–450. [CrossRef]
37. Joltikov, K.A.; Lobo-Chan, A.M. Epidemiology and Risk Factors in Non-infectious Uveitis: A Systematic Review. *Front. Med.* **2021**, *8*, 695904. [CrossRef]
38. Horai, R.; Zárate-Bladés, C.R.; Dillenburg-Pilla, P.; Chen, J.; Kielczewski, J.L.; Silver, P.B.; Jittayasothorn, Y.; Chan, C.C.; Yamane, H.; Honda, K.; et al. Microbiota-Dependent Activation of an Autoreactive T Cell Receptor Provokes Autoimmunity in an Immunologically Privileged Site. *Immunity* **2015**, *43*, 343–353. [CrossRef] [PubMed]
39. Meng, Y.; Tan, Z.; Liu, C.; Dong, W.; Chen, C. Association between Inflammatory Bowel Disease and Iridocyclitis: A Mendelian Randomization Study. *J. Clin. Med.* **2023**, *12*, 1282. [CrossRef] [PubMed]
40. Hu, J.; Wang, C.; Huang, X.; Yi, S.; Pan, S.; Zhang, Y.; Yuan, G.; Cao, Q.; Ye, X.; Hong, L. Gut microbiota-mediated secondary bile acids regulate dendritic cells to attenuate autoimmune uveitis through TGR5 signaling. *Cell Rep.* **2021**, *36*, 109726. [CrossRef]
41. Ghanchi, F.D.; Rembacken, B.J. Inflammatory bowel disease and the eye. *Surv. Ophthalmol.* **2003**, *48*, 663–676. [CrossRef]
42. Huang, X.F.; Brown, M.A. Progress in the genetics of uveitis. *Genes Immun.* **2022**, *23*, 57–65. [CrossRef]
43. Wakefield, D.; Clarke, D.; McCluskey, P. Recent Developments in HLA B27 Anterior Uveitis. *Front. Immunol.* **2021**, *11*, 608134. [CrossRef] [PubMed]
44. Orchard, T.R.; Chua, C.N.; Ahmad, T.; Cheng, H.; Welsh, K.I.; Jewell, D.P. Uveitis and erythema nodosum in inflammatory bowel disease: Clinical features and the role of HLA genes. *Gastroenterology* **2002**, *123*, 714–718. [CrossRef]
45. Ottaviano, G.; Salvatore, S.; Salvatoni, A.; Martelossi, S.; Ventura, A.; Naviglio, S. Ocular Manifestations of Paediatric Inflammatory Bowel Disease: A Systematic Review and Meta-analysis. *J. Crohns Colitis* **2018**, *12*, 870–879. [CrossRef] [PubMed]
46. Wu, X.; Tao, M.; Zhu, L.; Zhang, T.; Zhang, M. Pathogenesis and current therapies for non-infectious uveitis. *Clin. Exp. Med.* **2023**, *23*, 1089–1106. [CrossRef] [PubMed]
47. Czompa, L.; Barta, Z.; Ziad, H.; Nemeth, G.; Rentka, A.; Aszalos, Z.; Zold, E.; Gesztelyi, R.; Zsuga, J.; Szodoray, P.; et al. Corneal Manifestations of Inflammatory Bowel Disease. *Semin. Ophthalmol.* **2019**, *34*, 543–550. [CrossRef] [PubMed]

48. Ko, Y.T.; Wu, Y.M.; Wu, H.L.; Lai, S.C.; Dai, Y.X.; Chen, T.J.; Cherng, Y.G.; Tai, Y.H.; Kao, C.Y. Inflammatory bowel disease and the associated risk of dry eye and ocular surface injury: A nationwide matched cohort study. *BMC Ophthalmol.* **2023**, *23*, 415. [CrossRef] [PubMed]
49. Janardhana, P.; Al-Kadhi, S. A review of ophthalmic manifestations of inflammatory bowel disease and associated treatments. *Curr. Opin. Ophthalmol.* **2021**, *32*, 549–554. [CrossRef] [PubMed]
50. Agrawal, M.; Jess, T. Implications of the changing epidemiology of inflammatory bowel disease in a changing world. *United Eur. Gastroenterol. J.* **2022**, *10*, 1113–1120. [CrossRef]
51. Perez, V.L.; Stern, M.E.; Pflugfelder, S.C. Inflammatory basis for dry eye disease flares. *Exp. Eye Res.* **2020**, *201*, 108294. [CrossRef]
52. Khan, Z.; Cox, V.; Creagmile, J.; Oboh-Weilke, A. Nyctalopia and Xerophthalmia in a Patient With Crohn's Induced Vitamin A Deficiency. *Cureus* **2023**, *15*, e42961. [CrossRef] [PubMed]
53. Gilbert, C. The eye signs of vitamin A deficiency. *Community Eye Health J.* **2013**, *26*, 66–67.
54. Barta, Z.; Czompa, L.; Rentka, A.; Zold, E.; Remenyik, J.; Biro, A.; Gesztelyi, R.; Zsuga, J.; Szodoray, P.; Kemeny-Beke, A. Evaluation of Objective Signs and Subjective Symptoms of Dry Eye Disease in Patients with Inflammatory Bowel Disease. *BioMed Res. Int.* **2019**, *2019*, 8310583. [CrossRef]
55. Golden, M.I.; Meyer, J.J.; Zeppieri, M.; Patel, B.C. Dry Eye Syndrome. In *StatPearls*; StatPearls Publishing: Treasure Island, FL, USA, 2024.
56. Fogagnolo, P.; De Cilla, S.; Alkabes, M.; Sabella, P.; Rossetti, L. A review of topical and systemic vitamin supplementation in ocular surface diseases. *Nutrients* **2021**, *13*, 1998. [CrossRef]
57. Hassanpour, K.; ElSheikh, R.H.; Arabi, A.; Frank, C.R.; Elhusseiny, A.M.; Eleiwa, T.K.; Arami, S.; Djalilian, A.R.; Kheirkhah, A. Peripheral Ulcerative Keratitis: A Review. *J. Ophthalmic Vis. Res.* **2022**, *17*, 252–275. [CrossRef]
58. Gomes, B.F.; Santhiago, M.R. Biology of peripheral ulcerative keratitis. *Exp. Eye Res.* **2021**, *204*, 108458. [CrossRef] [PubMed]
59. Tan, M.H.; Chen, S.D.M.; Rubinstein, A.; Bron, A.J. Corneal perforation due to severe peripheral ulcerative keratitis in Crohn disease. *Cornea* **2006**, *25*, 628–630. [CrossRef] [PubMed]
60. Gupta, Y.; Kishore, A.; Kumari, P.; Balakrishnan, N.; Lomi, N.; Gupta, N.; Vanathi, M.; Tandon, R. Peripheral ulcerative keratitis. *Surv. Ophthalmol.* **2021**, *66*, 977–998. [CrossRef] [PubMed]
61. Nakayama, L.F.; Bergamo, V.C.; Conti, M.L.; Bueno, L.; Moraes, N.S.; Ambrogini, O., Jr. Frequency of ophthalmological posterior segment findings in patients with inflammatory bowel disease. *Arq. De Gastroenterol.* **2018**, *55*, 188–191. [CrossRef] [PubMed]
62. Sharma, N.; Tewatia, P.; Harvey, P.R.; Kumar, A. Controversies in Venous Thromboembolism Risk Assessment in Inflammatory Bowel Disease: A Narrative Review. *Diagnostics* **2024**, *14*, 2112. [CrossRef]
63. Kohoutova, D.; Moravkova, P.; Kruzliak, P.; Bures, J. Thromboembolic complications in inflammatory bowel disease. *J. Thromb. Thrombolysis.* **2015**, *39*, 489–498. [CrossRef]
64. Wu, L.A.; Chu, Y.C.; Wang, J.K.; Hsu, Y.R. Bilateral Retinal Artery Occlusions and Uveitis as the First Manifestation of Crohn's Disease. *Ocul. Immunol. Inflamm.* **2024**, *32*, 767–770. [CrossRef]
65. Rouleau, J.; Longmuir, R.; Lee, A.G. Optic disc edema with adjacent cilioretinal artery occlusion in a male with ulcerative colitis. *Semin. Ophthalmol.* **2007**, *22*, 25–28. [CrossRef]
66. Seo, Y.; Kim, M.; Kim, J.H.; Park, J.J.; Lee, S.C. Central retinal vein occlusion associated with ulcerative colitis. *Optom. Vis. Sci.* **2016**, *93*, 1567–1570. [CrossRef] [PubMed]
67. Figueiredo, L.; Rothwell, R.; Brandão, A.; Fonseca, S. Central retinal vein occlusion in a patient with retinal vasculitis and Crohn's disease. *Case Rep. Ophthalmol. Med.* **2014**, *2014*, 967878. [CrossRef]
68. Sy, A.; Khalidi, N.; Dehghan, N.; Barra, L.; Carette, S.; Cuthbertson, D.; Hoffman, G.S.; Koening, C.L.; Langford, C.A.; McAlear, C.; et al. Vasculitis in patients with inflammatory bowel diseases: A study of 32 patients and systematic review of the literature. Seminars in arthritis and rheumatism. *WB Saunders* **2016**, *45*, 475–482.
69. Urban, R.C.; Cotlier, E. Corticosteroid-induced cataracts. *Surv. Ophthalmol.* **1986**, *31*, 102–110. [CrossRef]
70. Blackwell, J.; Selinger, C.; Raine, T.; Parkes, G.; Smith, M.A.; Pollok, R. Steroid use and misuse: A key performance indicator in the management of IBD. *Frontline Gastroenterol.* **2021**, *12*, 207–213. [CrossRef] [PubMed]
71. Lee, H.J.; Song, H.J.; Jeong, J.H.; Kim, H.U.; Boo, S.J.; Na, S.Y. Ophthalmologic manifestations in patients with inflammatory bowel disease. *Intest. Res.* **2017**, *15*, 380–387. [CrossRef]
72. Gil, A.; Alizadeh, M.; Yarmovsky, D.; Swamy, R.; Wong, U. Use of Systemic Steroids for Inflammatory Bowel Disease Can Increase Intraocular Pressure. *Gastro Hep Adv.* **2024**, *3*, 536–538. [CrossRef]
73. Mansour, S.E.; Browning, D.J.; Wong, K.; Flynn, H.W.; Bhavsar, A.R. The evolving treatment of diabetic retinopathy. *Clin. Ophthalmol.* **2020**, *14* 653–678. [CrossRef]
74. Castillejo Becerra, C.M.; Ding, Y.; Kenol, B.; Hendershot, A.; Meara, A.S. Ocular side effects of antirheumatic medications: A qualitative review. *BMJ Open Ophthalmol.* **2020**, *5*, e000331. [CrossRef]
75. Pasadhika, S.; Kempen, J.H.; Newcomb, C.W.; Liesegang, T.L.; Pujari, S.S.; Rosenbaum, J.T.; Thorne, J.E.; Foster, C.S.; Jabs, D.A.; Levy-Clarke, G.; et al. Azathioprine for Ocular Inflammatory Diseases. *Am. J. Ophthalmol.* **2009**, *148*, 500–509. [CrossRef]
76. Puga, M.; Carpio, D.; Sampil, M.; Zamora, M.J.; Fernandez-Salgado, E. Ocular Toxoplasmosis Reactivation in a Patient with Inflammatory Bowel Disease under Treatment with Azathioprine. *J. Clin. Gastroenterol.* **2016**, *50*, 610. [CrossRef] [PubMed]

77. Tran, J.Q.; Hartung, J.P.; Peach, R.J.; Boehm, M.F.; Rosen, H.; Smith, H.; Brooks, J.L.; Timony, G.A.; Olson, A.D.; Gujrathi, S.; et al. Results From the First-in-Human Study With Ozanimod, a Novel, Selective Sphingosine-1-Phosphate Receptor Modulator. *J. Clin. Pharmacol.* **2017**, *57*, 988–996. [CrossRef] [PubMed]
78. Feagan, B.G.; Sandborn, W.J.; Danese, S.; Wolf, D.C.; Liu, W.J.; Hua, S.Y.; Minton, N.; Olson, A.; D'Haens, G. Ozanimod induction therapy for patients with moderate to severe Crohn's disease: A single-arm, phase 2, prospective observer-blinded endpoint study. *Lancet Gastroenterol. Hepatol.* **2020**, *5*, 819–828. [CrossRef] [PubMed]
79. Sandborn, W.J.; Feagan, B.G.; D'Haens, G.; Wolf, D.C.; Jovanovic, I.; Hanauer, S.B.; Ghosh, S.; Petersen, A.; Hua, S.Y.; Lee, J.H.; et al. Ozanimod as Induction and Maintenance Therapy for Ulcerative Colitis. *N. Engl. J. Med.* **2021**, *385*, 1280–1291. [CrossRef] [PubMed]
80. Sandborn, W.J.; Feagan, B.G.; Hanauer, S.; Vermeire, S.; Ghosh, S.; Liu, W.J.; Petersen, A.; Charles, L.; Huang, V.; Usiskin, K.; et al. Long-Term Efficacy and Safety of Ozanimod in Moderately to Severely Active Ulcerative Colitis: Results from the Open-Label Extension of the Randomized, Phase 2 TOUCHSTONE Study. *J. Crohns Colitis* **2021**, *15*, 1120–1129. [CrossRef] [PubMed]
81. Becher, N.; Swaminath, A.; Sultan, K. A Literature Review of Ozanimod Therapy in Inflammatory Bowel Disease: From Concept to Practical Application. *Ther. Clin. Risk Manag.* **2022**, *18*, 913–927. [CrossRef]
82. Lassiter, G.; Melancon, C.; Rooney, T.; Murat, A.M.; Kaye, J.S.; Kaye, A.M.; Kaye, R.J.; Cornett, E.M.; Kaye, A.D.; Shah, R.J.; et al. Ozanimod to treat relapsing forms of multiple sclerosis: A comprehensive review of disease, drug efficacy and side effects. *Neurol. Int.* **2020**, *12*, 89–108. [CrossRef] [PubMed]
83. Loftus, E.V.; Feagan, B.G.; Panaccione, R.; Colombel, J.F.; Sandborn, W.J.; Sands, B.E.; Danese, S.; D'Haens, G.; Rubin, D.T.; Shafran, I.; et al. Long-term safety of vedolizumab for inflammatory bowel disease. *Aliment. Pharmacol. Ther.* **2020**, *52*, 1353–1365. [CrossRef]
84. Feagan, B.G.; Sandborn, W.J.; Gasink, C.; Jacobstein, D.; Lang, Y.; Friedman, J.R.; Blank, M.A.; Johanns, J.; Gao, L.L.; Miao, Y.; et al. Ustekinumab as Induction and Maintenance Therapy for Crohn's Disease. *N. Engl. J. Med.* **2016**, *375*, 1946–1960. [CrossRef]
85. Tímár, Á.E.; Párniczky, A.; Budai, K.A.; Hernádfoi, M.V.; Kasznár, E.; Varga, P.; Hegyi, P.; Váncsa, S.; Tóth, R.; Veres, D.S.; et al. Beyond the Gut: A Systematic Review and Meta-Analysis of Advanced Therapies for Inflammatory Bowel Disease-Associated Extraintestinal Manifestations. *J. Crohns Colitis* **2024**, *18*, 851–863. [CrossRef]
86. Dubinsky, M.C.; Cross, R.K.; Sandborn, W.J.; Long, M.; Song, X.; Shi, N.; Ding, Y.; Eichner, S.; Pappalardo, B.; Ganguli, A.; et al. Extraintestinal Manifestations in Vedolizumab and Anti-TNF-Treated Patients with Inflammatory Bowel Disease. *Inflamm. Bowel Dis.* **2018**, *24*, 1876–1882. [CrossRef] [PubMed]
87. Tosi, G.M.; Sota, J.; Vitale, A.; Rigante, D.; Emmi, G.; Lopalco, G.; Guerriero, S.; Orlando, I.; Iannone, F.; Frediani, B.; et al. Efficacy and safety of certolizumab pegol and golimumab in the treatment of non-infectious uveitis. *Clin. Exp. Rheumatol.* **2019**, *37*, 680–683. [PubMed]
88. Jin, Y.; Lu, S.; Lin, Y.; Mou, X. The efficacy and safety of TNF inhibitor (golimumab) as salvage treatment in patients with refractory noninfectious uveitis. *Inflammopharmacology* **2022**, *30*, 1363–1368. [CrossRef]
89. Dutta Majumder, P.; Jayshree David, R.; Kaushik, V. A case of idiopathic necrotizing scleritis with secondary glaucoma treated successfully with golimumab and Ahmed valve implantation. *Indian. J. Ophthalmol.* **2019**, *67*, 1360–1362. [CrossRef] [PubMed]
90. Jaffe, G.J.; Dick, A.D.; Brézin, A.P.; Nguyen, Q.D.; Thorne, J.E.; Kestelyn, P.; Barisani-Asenbauer, T.; Franco, P.; Heiligenhaus, A.; Scales, D.; et al. Adalimumab in Patients with Active Noninfectious Uveitis. *N. Engl. J. Med.* **2016**, *375*, 932–943. [CrossRef] [PubMed]
91. Lawuyi, L.E.; Gurbaxani, A. Refractory necrotizing scleritis successfully treated with adalimumab. *J. Ophthalmic Inflamm. Infect.* **2016**, *6*, 37. [CrossRef] [PubMed]
92. Kremenevski, I.; Sander, O.; Sticherling, M.; Raithel, M.; LastName, F.M. Paradoxical Reactions to Biologicals in Chronic Inflammatory Systemic Diseases. *Dtsch. Arztebl. Int.* **2022**, *119*, 88–95. [CrossRef]
93. Nicolela Susanna, F.; Pavesio, C. A review of ocular adverse events of biological anti-TNF drugs. *J. Ophthalmic Inflamm. Infect.* **2020**, *10*, 11. [CrossRef]
94. Kowalski, T.; Mack, H.G. Ocular complications of tumour necrosis factor alpha inhibitors. *Clin. Exp. Optom.* **2020**, *103*, 148–154. [CrossRef] [PubMed]
95. Winthrop, K.L.; Chen, L.; Fraunfelder, F.W.; Ku, J.H.; Varley, C.D.; Suhler, E.; Hills, W.L.; Gattey, D.; Baddley, J.W.; Liu, L.; et al. Initiation of anti-TNF therapy and the risk of optic neuritis: From the safety assessment of biologic ThERapy (SABER) study. *Am. J. Ophthalmol.* **2013**, *155*, 183–189.e1. [CrossRef]
96. Lis, K.; Kuzawińska, O.; Bałkowiec-Iskra, E. Tumor necrosis factor inhibitors—State of knowledge. *Arch. Med. Sci.* **2014**, *10*, 1175–1185. [CrossRef] [PubMed]
97. Danese, S.; Vermeire, S.; Zhou, W.; Pangan, A.L.; Siffledeen, J.; Greenbloom, S.; Hébuterne, X.; D'Haens, G.; Nakase, H.; Panés, J.; et al. Upadacitinib as induction and maintenance therapy for moderately to severely active ulcerative colitis: Results from three phase 3, multicentre, double-blind, randomised trials. *Lancet* **2022**, *399*, 2113–2128. [CrossRef] [PubMed]
98. Loftus, E.V.; Panés, J.; Lacerda, A.P.; Peyrin-Biroulet, L.; D'Haens, G.; Panaccione, R.; Reinisch, W.; Louis, E.; Chen, M.; Nakase, H.; et al. Upadacitinib Induction and Maintenance Therapy for Crohn's Disease. *N. Engl. J. Med.* **2023**, *388*, 1966–1980. [CrossRef] [PubMed]
99. Feagan, B.G.; Danese, S.; Loftus, E.V.; Vermeire, S.; Schreiber, S.; Ritter, T.; Fogel, R.; Mehta, R.; Nijhawan, S.; Kempiński, R.; et al. Filgotinib as induction and maintenance therapy for ulcerative colitis (SELECTION): A phase 2b/3 double-blind, randomised, placebo-controlled trial. *Lancet* **2021**, *397*, 2372–2384. [CrossRef]

100. Sandborn, W.J.; Su, C.; Sands, B.E.; D'Haens, G.R.; Vermeire, S.; Schreiber, S.; Danese, S.; Feagan, B.G.; Reinisch, W.; Niezychowski, W.; et al. Tofacitinib as Induction and Maintenance Therapy for Ulcerative Colitis. *N. Engl. J. Med.* **2017**, *376*, 1723–1736. [CrossRef]
101. Hirai, H.; Akai, Y.; Ogata, N.; Ueda, T. Cytomegalovirus Retinitis in a Patient Taking Upadacitinib: A Case Report. *Cureus* **2023**, *15*, e48337. [CrossRef]
102. Genovese, M.C.; Kalunian, K.; Gottenberg, J.E.; Mozaffarian, N.; Bartok, B.; Matzkies, F.; Gao, J.; Guo, Y.; Tasset, C.; Sundy, J.S.; et al. Effect of Filgotinib vs Placebo on Clinical Response in Patients with Moderate to Severe Rheumatoid Arthritis Refractory to Disease-Modifying Antirheumatic Drug Therapy: The FINCH 2 Randomized Clinical Trial. *JAMA—J. Am. Med. Assoc.* **2019**, *322*, 315–325. [CrossRef]
103. Arvanitakis, K.D.; Arvanitaki, A.D.; Karkos, C.D.; Zintzaras, E.; Germanidis, G.S. The risk of venous thromboembolic events in patients with inflammatory bowel disease: A systematic review and meta-analysis. *Ann. Gastroenterol.* **2021**, *34*, 680. [CrossRef] [PubMed]
104. Bloom, J.N.; Palestine, A.G. The diagnosis of cytomegalovirus retinitis. *Ann. Intern. Med.* **1988**, *109*, 963–969. [CrossRef]
105. The Royal College of Ophthalmologists. Commissioning Guidance: Emergency Eye Care. 2020. Available online: https://www.rcophth.ac.uk/resources-listing/emergency-eye-care-commissioning-guidance/ (accessed on 11 December 2024).
106. King, D.; Chandan, J.S.; Thomas, T.; Denniston, A.K.; Braithwaite, T.; Niranthrankumar, K.; Reulen, R.; Adderley, N.; Trudgill, N.J. Risk of a subsequent diagnosis of inflammatory bowel disease in subjects with ophthalmic disorders associated with inflammatory bowel disease: A retrospective cohort analysis of UK primary care data. *BMJ Open* **2022**, *12*, e052833. [CrossRef] [PubMed]

biomedicines

MDPI

Article

Disease Acceptance and Control from the Subjective Health Experience Model as Health Perception Predictors in Immune-Mediated Inflammatory Diseases

Tessa S. Folkertsma [1,2,3,*], Sjaak Bloem [4], Robert M. Vodegel [1], Reinhard Bos [2] and Greetje J. Tack [3]

1 Department of Dermatology, Medisch Centrum Leeuwarden, MCL—Medical Center Leeuwarden, Henri Dunantweg 2, 8934 AD Leeuwarden, The Netherlands; r.vodegel@mcl.nl

2 Department of Rheumatology, Medisch Centrum Leeuwarden, MCL—Medical Center Leeuwarden, Henri Dunantweg 2, 8934 AD Leeuwarden, The Netherlands; r.bos@mcl.nl

3 Department of Gastroenterology, Medisch Centrum Leeuwarden, MCL—Medical Center Leeuwarden, Henri Dunantweg 2, 8934 AD Leeuwarden, The Netherlands; greetje.tack@mcl.nl

4 Center for Marketing & Supply Chain Management, Nyenrode Business University, 3621 BG Breukelen, The Netherlands; s.bloem@nyenrode.nl

* Correspondence: tessa.folkertsma@mcl.nl; Tel.: +31-582868594

Abstract: Background/Objectives: The multifactorial nature of immune-mediated inflammatory diseases (IMIDs) requires integrating pathophysiological understanding with subjective patient experiences. Patient-reported outcome measures (PROMs) are a useful tool for incorporating this in routine clinical practice. However, current PROMs do not fully encompass the complete subjective health experiences (SHE) of patients and are thus insufficient for guiding truly personalised care. The SHE model provides insights into SHE through the determinants of disease acceptance and perceived control. While validated across various demographics, its predictive power in IMIDs cohorts remains unexplored. This study aims to assess whether acceptance and perceived control in the SHE model predict health experiences in patients with IMID and how these immunological conditions compare. **Methods:** Questionnaires regarding health perception, acceptance, control, and subjective health experiences were distributed to 450 Dutch citizens. Descriptive statistics, reliability checks, and partial least squares structural equation modelling were used to examine relationships between variables. **Results:** Health perception strongly predicts SHE through acceptance and control. Across all conditions, the pathway moves from health perception to control, then to acceptance, and finally to SHE. However, the roles of acceptance and control differ by condition. In burdensome diseases like inflammatory bowel disease and rheumatoid arthritis, acceptance plays a greater role, while control has a stronger influence in conditions like psoriasis. **Conclusions:** This study supports the predictive validity of the SHE model for IMIDs, showing that disease acceptance and control affect health experiences differently across conditions. These insights improve the understanding of psychological factors in health experiences and call for tailored interventions for patients with IMID.

Keywords: immune-mediated inflammatory diseases (IMIDs); immunology; subjective health experience; health perception; personalised supportive healthcare; patient-reported outcomes; structural equation modelling; psoriasis (PsO); rheumatoid arthritis (RA); inflammatory bowel disease (IBD)

1. Introduction

The impact of immune-mediated inflammatory diseases (IMIDs) extends beyond their physical manifestations, profoundly affecting quality of life (QoL) [1,2]. While the physical complications of these diseases are well documented, ranging from cardiovascular issues in rheumatoid arthritis (RA) [3] and psoriasis (PsO) [4] to fistulas [5] and malnutrition [6,7] in inflammatory bowel disease (IBD), the psychological impact is equally significant. Individuals with IMID often struggle with depression, anxiety, stigmatisation, and social withdrawal, underscoring the need for comprehensive care strategies [8–10]. The multifactorial nature of these conditions requires the integration of pathophysiological understanding with subjective patient experiences. A patient's overall subjective perception of how illness and treatment impact their physical, psychological, and social well-being is referred to as health-related QoL (HRQoL) [11]. Despite advances in treatment, managing IMIDs remains challenging due to variations in disease mechanisms and individual responses to therapy. Emerging research highlights that while IMIDs share common inflammatory pathways, differences in cytokine function and immune regulation contribute to variability in treatment effectiveness [12]. Many individuals remain unresponsive or intolerant to current therapies, underscoring the need for novel approaches that target multiple inflammatory pathways simultaneously.

The use of patient-reported outcome measures (PROMs) could be a useful tool for incorporating HRQoL in daily healthcare [13]. However, their application into routine clinical practice is limited in its suitability as a tool for tailoring patient-specific care. Transforming PROMs results into effective, personalised interventions remains challenging. Broekharst et al. highlight this in their study of a cohort of IBD patients [14], emphasising the need to integrate a general HRQoL measure alongside traditional disease activity assessments. According to Broekharst et al., while current PROMs (like the EuroQol Five-dimensions Five-level; EQ-5D-5L) reflect health perception, they do not fully encompass the complete HRQoL. This distinction is critical, as health perception primarily addresses how patients perceive specific aspects of their illness, such as pain, limitations, or emotional distress, but it falls short of capturing the broader, subjective experience of health itself. As a result, current PROMs are insufficient to guide truly personalised care.

Bloem and Stalpers developed a model that does provide insights into the complete Subjective Health Experience (SHE) of patients [15]. They characterise SHE as an individual's physical and mental functioning, aligned with their desired lifestyle, yet constrained by the realities of their existence. SHE goes beyond health perception, capturing not only how patients perceive their illness but also how they subjectively experience their overall health. Therefore, SHE provides a more accurate representation of HRQoL. For example, two individuals with the same disease burden may experience vastly different levels of subjective health, with one perceiving their condition as far worse than the other. Stalpers found that in chronically ill patients, including patients with asthma, rheumatoid arthritis, various types of cancer, and psoriasis, the most important psychological determinants of subjective health were disease acceptance and perceived control [16]. Increased acceptance, indicative of a patient's ability to integrate their health condition into everyday life, combined with a sense of control, reflecting their capacity to improve their health, positively influences SHE. In the SHE model, the evaluation of disease acceptance and perceived control involves three specific questions each, making the model simple and highly applicable in routine clinical practice.

The SHE model has previously demonstrated its versatility and has been validated across various patient demographics and disease domains [17,18]. In addition, the SHE model has recently been adapted to address the specific needs of patients with IMID [19]. Despite the previously demonstrated value of the SHE model in healthcare, the predictive power of the model has yet to be examined in immunological patient cohorts. Therefore, this study aims to determine whether the disease acceptance and control parameters of the SHE model can predict experiences of health and illness in patients with IMID

(IBD, PsO, and RA) and whether or not these conditions show similarities. The findings from this study could further legitimise and support the integration of the SHE model for the easy evaluation of health experiences in routine clinical practice for patients with IMID.

2. Materials and Methods

This study is part of an extensive research project aiming to offer and monitor more personalised supportive care related to IMIDs and treatments based on PROMs. The study protocol was reviewed by the accredited Independent Ethics Committee and approved by the Board of Directors of the Medical Centre Leeuwarden (RTPO, nWMO 20200091, January 2021). This study utilised a cross-sectional research design featuring online questionnaires. An overview of the research process is presented in Figure 1. The questionnaires were distributed to a panel of Dutch citizens by the market research firm IPSOS between February and December 2023. To tailor distribution, IPSOS used responses from a general pre-screening questionnaire to identify potential participants with predefined diagnoses. Questionnaires were then sent until a predetermined quota was reached. Panel members received comprehensive information about the study and were asked to provide formal consent prior to participation. Only respondents who consented to the use of their data for research purposes and who reported an official diagnosis (by a physician) of IBD (Crohn's disease or ulcerative colitis), PsO, or RA were included in the study. Although spondyloarthropathy was initially included as a diagnosis in the study, the number of respondents was too small for meaningful analysis, and therefore, it was excluded from the final sample. The final sample consisted of 450 Dutch participants. IPSOS supplied the full dataset, including only those who completed the survey in its entirety.

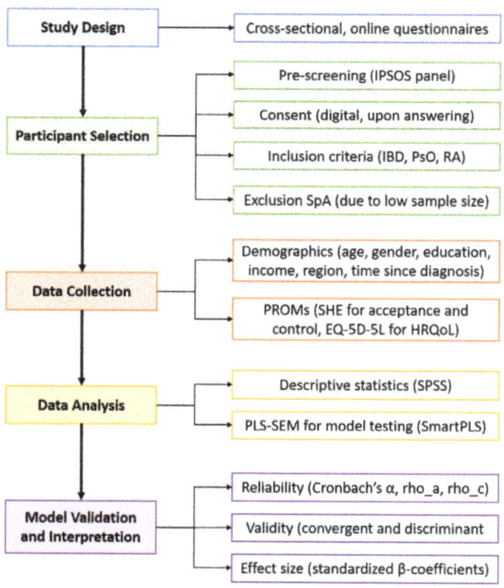

Figure 1. Analytical process chart.

Questionnaires included various items on sample characteristics as well as PROMs. Demographics, including age, gender, residential region, area population density, education level, annual income, and time since diagnosis, were used to describe the study population. These items were measured on nominal scales containing binary response categories, as well as ordinal scales containing ascending response categories. The EQ-5D-5L questionnaire was used to measure health perception [20]. The dimensions (i.e., mobility, self-care, usual activities, pain and discomfort, and anxiety and depression) were measured with a five-point scale. The SHE questionnaire was used to determine acceptance, control, and SHE [16]. Acceptance and control were measured using three items equipped with a seven-point Likert scale ranging from 1 = fully disagree to 7 = fully agree. SHE was measured as the average perception of health for the previous month by marking a ladder with 11 levels, in which level 0 indicates the worst day of the previous month and level 10 indicates the best day of the previous month.

The characteristics of the study population were analysed using descriptive statistics, with percentages reported for categorical variables and means for continuous variables. Cut-off values were based on statistical data from the general Dutch population [21–23]. Partial least squares structural equation modelling (PLS-SEM) was employed to determine the relationships between the instruments (subsamples: 5000). Criteria for the reliability and validity of the instruments, as well as model interpretation, followed the guidelines outlined by Hair et al. [24]. The construct reliability of the instruments was assessed using Cronbach's alpha (α), rho_A, and rho_C coefficients and was deemed reliable if their values exceeded 0.70. Construct validity was assessed by establishing convergent and discriminant validity. Convergent validity was examined using the average variance extracted (AVE) coefficient and considered sufficient if it surpassed 0.50. Discriminant validity was analysed using the heterotrait–monotrait (HTMT) ratio, which was sufficient if below 0.90, and the Fornell–Larcker (FL) criterion, which was satisfied if the AVE of a construct was greater than its correlation with any other construct. Effect sizes were determined using standardised beta coefficients (β), which were classified as small if below 0.30, average if between 0.30 and 0.50, and large if above 0.50. Significance levels were assessed using *p*-values, which were considered significant if below 0.05. Explained variance was analysed using R-squared (R^2) coefficients, which were considered small if below 0.30, average if between 0.30 and 0.50, and large if above 0.50. IBM SPSS Statistics Version 28 was used for describing the final sample, and SmartPLS Version 4.1 was deployed for analysing the instruments and models.

3. Results

3.1. Participant Characteristics

For this study, 450 panel members were included, comprising 100 individuals with IBD (50 with Crohn's disease and 50 with ulcerative colitis), 200 with PsO, and 150 with RA. Although SpA was initially included as a diagnosis, the number of respondents was too small to allow for a meaningful analysis. As a result, SpA was excluded from the final analysis. The cohort resembled the general Dutch population in terms of the residential region and population density (Table 1). However, the population was relatively older, slightly more female-dominated, and had a lower education level and lower income [25]. These cohort characteristics are, however, representative of the characteristics of individuals with IMID [26,27]. The differences in sample sizes between diagnoses were due to limitations in the availability of participants within the IPSOS panel. Despite this, the patient demographics were relatively comparable across diagnoses.

3.2. Instrument Characteristics

To verify the accuracy and credibility of the models, the reliability and validity of the instruments were determined. The instruments of health perception (α = 0.78–0.82; rho_A = 0.79–0.84; rho_C = 0.85–0.87), acceptance (α = 0.89–0.90; rho_A = 0.90–0.92; rho_C = 0.93–0.94), and control (α = 0.90–0.93; rho_A = 0.90–0.93; rho_C = 0.93–0.96) demonstrated reliability, with coefficients exceeding 0.70. The instruments of health perception, acceptance, and control had sufficient construct validity, as all their items loaded on a single component. The instruments of health perception (AVE = 0.53–0.59), acceptance (AVE = 0.81–0.83), and control (AVE = 0.82–0.88) demonstrated sufficient convergent validity, with coefficients exceeding 0.50. The instruments of health perception (HTMT = 0.50–0.74), acceptance (HTMT = 0.57–0.83), control (HTMT = 0.50–0.83), and SHE (HTMT = 0.50–0.79) demonstrated sufficient discriminant validity, as coefficients remained below 0.90, and the FL criterion was satisfied.

Table 1. Sample characteristics of the total study population and per diagnosis.

	Total Study Population	***n* = 450**		
Age	61.0 years (22–87 years)			
Gender	58.9% Female	41.1% Male		
Residential region	35.3% North and East NL	40.7% West NL	24.0% South NL	
Area population density	12.0% $\leq$ 200 inhab/km^2	40.7% 200–999 inhab/km^2	47.3% $\geq$ 1000 inhab/km^2	
Education level *	28.4% Low	38.9% Middle	32.4% High	
Annual income	49.5% < EUR 36,500	17.0% EUR 36,500–EUR 43,500	33.5% > EUR 43,500	
Time since diagnosis	36.7% 0–10 years	21.4% 11–20 years	18.1% 21–30 years	23.8% > 30 years
	IBD	*n* = 100		
Age	57.1 years (30–81 years)			
Gender	53.0% Female	47.0% Male		
Residential region	39.0% North and East NL	30% West NL	31.0% South NL	
Area population density	9.0% $\leq$ 200 inhab/km^2	42.0% 200–999 inhab/km^2	49.0% $\geq$ 1000 inhab/km^2	
Education level *	23.0% Low	40.0% Middle	37.0% High	
Annual income	37.4% < EUR 36,500	20.4% EUR 36,500–EUR 43,500	42.2% > EUR 43,500	
Time since diagnosis	25.0% 0–10 years	29.0% 11–20 years	23.0% 21–30 years	23.0% > 30 years
	PsO	*n* = 200		
Age	61.1 years (22–83 years)			
Gender	53.0% Female	47.0% Male		
Residential region	35.0% North and East NL	43.5% West NL	21.5% South NL	
Area population density	17.5% $\leq$ 200 inhab/km^2	39.5% 200–999 inhab/km^2	43.0% $\geq$ 1000 inhab/km^2	
Education level *	25.5% Low	37.5% Middle	37.0% High	
Annual income	46.2% < EUR 36,500	18.5% EUR 36,500–EUR 43,500	35.3% > EUR 43,500	
Time since diagnosis	32.4% 0–10 years	21.4% 11–20 years	12.1% 21–30 years	34.1% > 30 years
	RA	*n* = 150		
Age	63.5 years (32–87 years)			
Gender	70.7% Female	29.3% Male		
Residential region	33.3% North & East NL	44.0% West NL	22.7% South NL	
Area population density	6.7% $\leq$ 200 inhab/km^2	41.3% 200–999 inhab/km^2	52% $\geq$ 1000 inhab/km^2	
Education level *	36.2% Low	40.3% Middle	23.5% High	
Annual income	61.9% < EUR 36,500	12.7% EUR 36,500–EUR 43,500	25.4% > EUR 43,500	
Time since diagnosis	50.7% 0–10 years	15.9% 11–20 years	22.5% 21–30 years	10.9% > 30 years

* Low education level: primary education level, VMBO, the first three years of HAVO/VWO, and entrance training, including the former assistant training (MBO1). Middle education level: upper levels of HAVO/VWO, basic vocational training (MBO2), vocational training (MBO3), or middle management and specialist training (MBO4). High education level: education at higher vocational or university level.

3.3. Model Characteristics

The model for predicting SHE with health perception via acceptance and control was first examined for the total study population, followed by the IBD, PsO, and RA subsets.

3.3.1. Total Study Population Model

The total IMID sample model (Figure 2; Model 1) showed statistically significant relationships between all variables. Health perception was a strong predictor ($\beta = 0.59$, $p < 0.01$) of control, which was a strong predictor ($\beta = 0.52$, $p < 0.01$) of acceptance, which was a strong predictor ($\beta = 0.52$, $p < 0.01$) of SHE. The effect of health perception on acceptance ($\beta = 0.28$, $p < 0.01$) and control on SHE ($\beta = 0.19$, $p < 0.01$) was considered small. The model explained 35%, 51%, and 44% of variance in control, acceptance, and SHE, respectively, which is considered moderate to large.

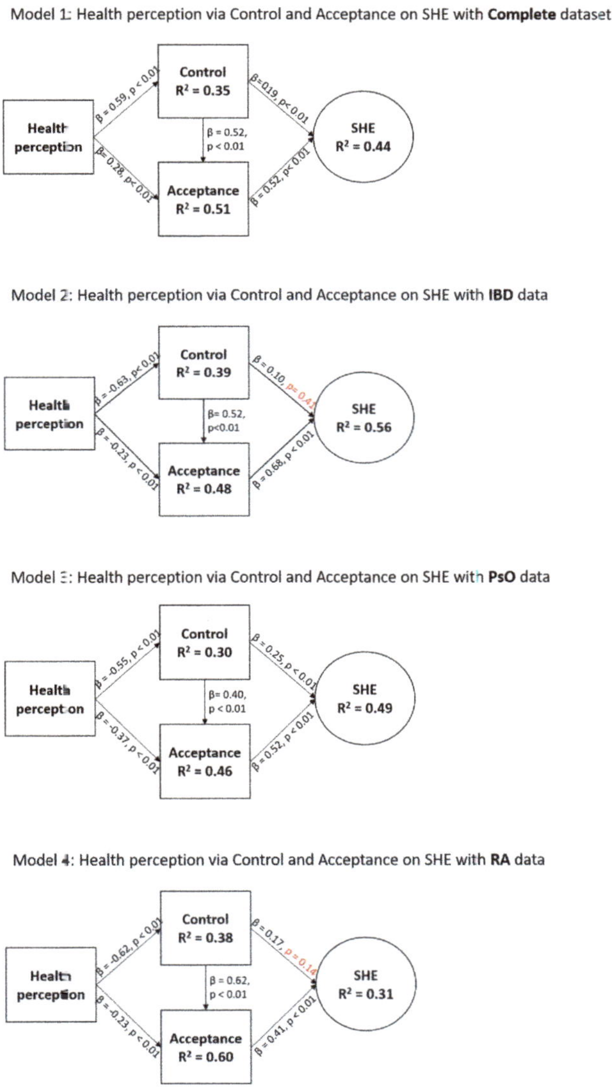

Figure 2. Characteristics of the SHE model for the total study population and for disease-specific data. Health perception was measured via the EQ-5D-5L questionnaire, and acceptance, control, and SHE were measured via the SHE questionnaire. Non-significant p-values ($p > 0.05$) are indicated in red.

3.3.2. IBD Model

The IBD sample model (Figure 2; Model 2) demonstrated statistically significant relationships between all variables except for the relationship between control and SHE. Again, health perception was a strong predictor of control ($\beta = 0.63$, $p < 0.01$), which was a strong predictor of acceptance ($\beta = 0.52$, $p < 0.01$), which was a strong predictor of SHE ($\beta = 0.68$, $p < 0.01$). The effect of health perception on acceptance ($\beta = 0.23$, $p < 0.01$) and control on SHE ($\beta = 0.10$, $p = 0.41$) was considered small. The model explained 39%, 48%, and 56% of variance in control, acceptance, and SHE, respectively, which is considered moderate to large.

3.3.3. PsO Model

The PsO sample model (Figure 2; model 3) demonstrated statistically significant relationships between all variables. As with previous findings, health perception was a strong predictor of control ($\beta = 0.55$, $p < 0.01$), and acceptance was a strong predictor of SHE ($\beta = 0.52$, $p < 0.01$). However, in this sample, the effect of health perception on acceptance ($\beta = 0.37$, $p < 0.01$) and control on acceptance ($\beta = 0.40$, $p < 0.01$) were considered moderate. The effect of control on SHE ($\beta = 0.25$, $p < 0.01$) was considered small. The model explained 30%, 46%, and 49% of variance in control, acceptance, and SHE, respectively, which is considered moderate.

3.3.4. RA Model

The RA sample model (Figure 2; model 4) showed statistically significant relationships between all variables, except for the relationship between control and SHE. As with the PsO sample, health perception was a strong predictor of control ($\beta = 0.62$, $p < 0.01$), which in turn strongly predicted acceptance ($\beta = 0.62$, $p < 0.01$). The effect of acceptance on SHE was moderate ($\beta = 0.41$, $p < 0.01$). The effects of health perception on acceptance ($\beta = 0.23$, $p < 0.01$) and control on SHE ($\beta = 0.17$, $p = 0.41$) were considered small. The model explained 38%, 60%, and 31% of variance in control, acceptance, and SHE, respectively, which is considered moderate to large.

4. Discussion

The aim of this study was to determine whether the disease acceptance and control parameters of the SHE model can predict experiences of health and illness in patients with IMIDs (restricted here to IBD, PsO, and RA) and whether or not these conditions show similarities. This study demonstrates that disease acceptance and perceived control are key psychological mechanisms mediating the relationship between health perception and subjective health experience (SHE) in patients with IMID, with notable variations in the roles of these factors across different conditions.

The total study population model indicates that the impact of health perception, measured via the EQ-5D-5L questionnaire, on SHE through disease acceptance and control is strong within this population, confirming the significant relationships between all variables. This means that the relationship between health perception (specifically the effect of illness and intervention) and SHE is mediated by the psychological variables of disease acceptance and perceived control over disease. This result aligns with the findings of Stalpers [15], confirming their earlier conclusions regarding the importance of these factors in mediating SHE.

Acceptance and control emerge as crucial mechanisms for optimising SHE, a pattern that is consistent with studies by Bloem et al. and Broekharst et al. [16,17], further underscoring the reliability of these constructs in health outcomes. Notably, we also observe a significant indirect effect, where perceived control influences SHE via acceptance, highlighting the importance of perceived control in indirectly shaping health experiences through its impact on acceptance. This indirect effect will be explored in more detail in subsequent sections.

When analysing the PsO model, a similar trend to the total study population model emerges. Both acceptance and control play pivotal roles in predicting SHE. However, in PsO the influence of acceptance and control is slightly more balanced. This suggests that while the route from perception to SHE remains significant, the roles of control and acceptance are more proportionate, making their combined influence more synergistic.

In contrast to PsO, the models for IBD and RA reveal a distinct pathway in which acceptance predominantly mediates SHE, with no significant direct relationship between control and SHE. This confirms earlier work by van Erp [28], which established a relationship between control and acceptance in IBD and is further supported by Teugels et al. [29]. Our findings extend this understanding by showing that the same pattern applies to RA, indicating that in both IBD and RA, acceptance plays a central mediating role. However, while Teugels focused only on correlations, our study goes beyond, testing a more comprehensive model that also accounts for indirect effects. In this context, control is indeed related to SHE but indirectly through its influence on acceptance. This provides a more nuanced understanding of the relationship between control and SHE in IBD, contrasting with Teugels' conclusions.

One possible explanation for the more prominent role of disease acceptance in IBD and RA compared to PsO is that the disease burden is generally higher in gastroenterological (including IBD) and rheumatological conditions (including RA) [17]. These variations in acceptance and control levels could explain the proportional effect sizes (β) observed in the models. As Broekharst et al. noted, the greater disease burden may require IBD and RA patients to expend more energy or time to achieve higher levels of acceptance, which in turn influences SHE [17]. Further research is needed to confirm this assumption.

Additionally, PsO patients may have access to more treatment options or perceive greater support, which could directly improve their SHE without requiring as much psychological adaptation via acceptance. Further research is currently underway to explore this hypothesis in greater detail.

Looking at the models and the causal pathway with the strongest effects, a common pattern is observed across all models: health perception influences perceived control, which in turn affects acceptance, ultimately leading to SHE. This suggests that interventions aimed at improving patients' perceived control could directly contribute to better acceptance and, ultimately, better SHE. Supporting this, our recent qualitative study examined the type of information and support that patients with IBD, RA, and PsO need for their treatment [19]. The study found that support, tailored for improving both acceptance and control, can play a crucial role in optimising SHE, reinforcing the importance of these psychological variables in patient care.

Generally, improving acceptance tends to take more time than improving control. Furthermore, support for enhancing control is typically more practical and instrumental, such as providing information about the diagnosis and defining the treatment plan. In contrast, improving acceptance requires more patient-centred guidance. Given this, focusing on control in the initial stages of treatment may be more time-efficient and immediately beneficial. Further research is currently exploring the relationship between the time since diagnosis and levels of acceptance and control, potentially identifying whether the pathways in the SHE model differ across varying stages of diagnosis.

A key strength of this study lies in the high reliability and validity of the measurement instruments used, which enhances the accuracy and credibility of the findings. Furthermore, the use of partial least squares structural equation modelling for this study instead of multiple correlations has a number of advantages. Structural equation modelling accounts for the measurement error of latent variables and avoids inadmissible solutions and factor indeterminacy [30,31].

Another strength is the ability to show meaningful relationships within the SHE model, even with smaller sample sizes, as demonstrated in this study. Although the effect of control on SHE for IBD and RA was not significant, the significance of models with larger sample sizes suggests that this issue could be addressed by increasing the sample size.

However, there are some limitations to consider. The final sample may be biased due to a relatively older age group, a slight overrepresentation of females, and lower education levels among respondents, which could potentially distort or misrepresent the findings. Additionally, this study's focus on a Dutch population may limit the interpretability and generalisation of the results to other contexts.

The findings of this study have important implications for clinical practice. They suggest that the SHE model is applicable within different types of IMIDs, making it a useful general tool for managing the treatment of multiple immune-mediated disorders. The simplicity of the model makes it well-suited for clinical settings. Furthermore, the results indicate that improving health perception can be achieved by specifically targeting the levels of acceptance and control perceived by patients, offering a strategic approach to enhancing patient outcomes. In the initial stages of treatment, the focus should be on improving control rather than acceptance for disorders with a high disease burden.

At least four main directions for future research may be pursued. The first direction focuses on further segmenting this model based on other important demographic variables, such as annual income and character traits. Stalpers found in an exploratory study that these factors could influence the model, but it remains to be explored whether this holds true within the IMID population [15].

The second direction involves validating the model using disease-specific PROMs to assess health perception. Since these PROMs are more tailored to the individual patient, they may provide a more accurate representation of their health perception, potentially improving the model's predictive accuracy.

The third direction highlights the need for validation of this model in various countries to better understand the impact of geographical location and cultural differences on its applicability.

The fourth direction centres on integrating this model into clinical practice. By using the model to personalise healthcare, the goal would be to improve health perception through targeted strategies that focus on disease acceptance and control.

5. Conclusions

In conclusion, while health perception consistently predicts SHE across all disorders, the roles of acceptance and control vary between IMIDs, with acceptance playing a larger role in more burdensome diseases like IBD and RA and control having a more direct influence in conditions like PsO. These insights not only confirm existing findings but also contribute to a deeper understanding of how psychological factors mediate health experiences in patients with IMID.

Author Contributions: S.B., G.J.T., R.B. and R.M.V. conceived and planned the study. S.B., G.J.T., R.B. and R.M.V. developed the protocol. The questionnaires were distributed by the IPSOS research agency. T.S.F. contributed to the analysis. T.S.F. and S.B. worked on the interpretation of the results. T.S.F. wrote the manuscript. All authors provided critical feedback and helped shape the research, analysis, and manuscript. All authors have read and agreed to the published version of the manuscript.

Funding: TF received a grant from the MSB-VCL (a partnership of different medical specialists) to stimulate multidisciplinary innovation in the daily clinical care of the MCL.

Institutional Review Board Statement: This study was performed in accordance with the Declaration of Helsinki and the Dutch ethical laws, rules, and regulations. The study protocol was reviewed by the accredited Independent Ethics Committee and approved by the Board of Directors of the Medical Centre Leeuwarden (RTPO, nWMO 20200091, January 2021, https://wetten.overheid.nl/BWBR0009408/2022-07-01, accessed on 16 October 2024).

Informed Consent Statement: The IPSOS panel members were comprehensively informed about the study and were asked for their consent before participation. Panel members were only included in this study if they consented to the use of their responses for research purposes.

Data Availability Statement: The raw data used during this study are not publicly available but are available from the corresponding author upon reasonable request.

Acknowledgments: The authors would like to acknowledge the support of the participants who engaged in this project.

Conflicts of Interest: The authors declare no conflicts of interest. The funders had no role in the design of the study; in the collection, analysis, or interpretation of data; in the writing of the manuscript; or in the decision to publish the results.

References

1. Han, S.W.; McColl, E.; Barton, J.R.; James, P.; Steen, I.N.; Welfare, M.R. Predictors of Quality of Life in Ulcerative Colitis.: The Importance of Symptoms and Illness Representations. *Inflamm. Bowel Dis.* **2005**, *11*, 24–34. [CrossRef] [PubMed]
2. Rahman, P.; Inman, R.D.; El-Gabalawy, H.; Krause, D.O. Pathophysiology and pathogenesis of immune-mediated inflammatory diseases: Commonalities and differences. *J. Rheumatol. Suppl.* **2010**, *85*, 11–26. [CrossRef] [PubMed]
3. Bullock, J.; Rizvi, S.A.A.; Saleh, A.M.; Ahmed, S.S.; Do, D.P.; Ansari, R.A.; Ahmed, J. Rheumatoid Arthritis: A Brief Overview of the Treatment. *Med. Princ. Pract. Int. J. Kuwait Univ. Health Sci. Cent.* **2018**, *27*, 501–507. [CrossRef] [PubMed]
4. Garshick, M.S.; Ward, N.L.; Krueger, J.G.; Berger, J.S. Cardiovascular Risk in Patients with Psoriasis: JACC Review Topic of the Week. *J. Am. Coll. Cardiol.* **2021**, *77*, 1670–1680. [CrossRef]
5. Makowiec, F.; Jehle, E.C.; Starlinger, M. Clinical course of perianal fistulas in Crohn's disease. *Gut* **1995**, *37*, 696–701. [CrossRef]
6. Donnellan, C.F.; Yann, L.H.; Lal, S. Nutritional management of Crohn's disease. *Ther. Adv. Gastroenterol.* **2013**, *6*, 231–242. [CrossRef]
7. Goh, J.; O'Morain, C.A. Review article: Nutrition and adult inflammatory bowel disease. *Aliment. Pharmacol. Ther.* **2003**, *17*, 307–320. [CrossRef]
8. Leon Mateos, L. Psychosocial aspects of rheumatic and musculoskeletal diseases. *Reumatol. Clínica (Engl. Ed.)* **2020**, *16*, 1–2. [CrossRef]
9. Bacconnier, L.; Rincheval, N.; Flipo, R.M.; Goupille, P.; Daures, J.P.; Boulenger, J.P.; Combe, B. Psychological distress over time in early rheumatoid arthritis: Results from a longitudinal study in an early arthritis cohort. *Rheumatology* **2015**, *54*, 520–527. [CrossRef] [PubMed]
10. Tarar, Z.I.; Zafar, M.U.; Farooq, U.; Ghous, G.; Aslam, A.; Inayat, F.; Ghouri, Y.A. Burden of depression and anxiety among patients with inflammatory bowel disease: Results of a nationwide analysis. *Int. J. Color. Dis.* **2022**, *37*, 313–321. [CrossRef]
11. EUnetHTA. Endpoints used for relative effectiveness assessment of pharmaceuticals. In *Health-Related Quality of Life and Utility Measures*; EUnetHTA: Diemen, The Netherlands, 2013.
12. Monteleone, G.; Moscardelli, A.; Colella, A.; Marafini, I.; Salvatori, S. Immune-mediated inflammatory diseases: Common and different pathogenic and clinical features. *Autoimmun. Rev.* **2023**, *22*, 103410. [CrossRef]
13. Krogsgaard, M.R.; Brodersen, J.; Christensen, K.B.; Siersma, V.; Kreiner, S.; Jensen, J.; Hansen, C.F.; Comins, J.D. What is a PROM and why do we need it? *Scand. J. Med. Sci. Sports* **2021**, *31*, 967–971. [CrossRef] [PubMed]
14. Broekharst, D.S.; Thomas, P.W.; Russel, M.G.; West, R.L.; Jansen, J.M.; Bloem, S.; Römkens, T.E. Health State Questionnaires Deployed in Ulcerative Colitis Patients: The Medical, Psychological, and Economic Perspective-ScienceDirect. *Gastro Hep Adv.* **2023**, *2*, 770–777. [CrossRef]
15. Bloem, S.; Stalpers, J. Subjective Experienced Health as a Driver of Health Care Behavior. *Nyenrode Res. Pap. Ser.* **2012**, *12*, 1–22. [CrossRef]
16. Stalpers, J. *Psychological Determinants of Subjective Health*; Nyenrode Business Universiteit: Breukelen, The Netherlands, 2009.
17. Bloem, S.; Stalpers, J.; Groenland, E.A.G.; van Montfort, K.; van Raaij, W.F.; de Rooij, K. Segmentation of health-care consumers: Psychological determinants of subjective health and other person-related variables. *BMC Health Serv. Res.* **2020**, *20*, 726. [CrossRef]

18. Broekharst, D.S.; Bloem, S.; Groenland, E.A.G.; Folkertsma, T.S.; Carlsone, J.I.; Folkvorde, F.; Everittg, C.; Lupiáñez-Villanuevae, F.; Liefveld, A.R. Explaining health behaviour: A new model centred around health experience and its determinants. *Soc. Sci. Med.* 2024; submitted.
19. Folkertsma, T.S.; Bos, R.; Vodegel, R.M.; Bloem, S.; Liefveld, A.R.; Tack, G.J. Personalizing supportive healthcare for immunological disorders-A qualitative exploration of patient needs and behaviours based on the Subjective Health Experience model. *Int. J. Integr. Care* **2024**. submitted.
20. Group, E. EuroQol-a new facility for the measurement of health-related quality of life. *Health Policy* **1990**, *16*, 199–208. [CrossRef]
21. Zorg, V.E. Bevolkingsdichtheid 2024. Available online: https://www.vzinfo.nl/bevolking/regionaal (accessed on 22 October 2024).
22. CBS. What Is Working People's Income? Available online: https://longreads.cbs.nl/the-netherlands-in-numbers-2023/what-is-working-peoples-income/ (accessed on 22 October 2024).
23. Ministerie van Onderwijs, C.e.W. Opleidingsniveau van de Bevolking. Available online: https://www.ocwincijfers.nl/sectoren/hoger-onderwijs/kwaliteit/onderwijs-en-arbeidsmarkt/kwantitatieve-aansluiting-op-de-arbeidsmarkt/opleidingsniveau-van-de-bevolking#:~:text=Gegevens%20in%20een%20tabel&text=19,8-,Gemiddeld%20was%20in%202020%20bijna%2028%25%20van%20de%2015-%20tot,dan%20gemiddeld%20in%20de%20EU (accessed on 22 October 2024).
24. Hair, J.F.; Risher, J.J.; Sarstedt, M.; Ringle, C.M. When to use and how to report the results of PLS-SEM. *Eur. Bus. Rev.* **2019**, *31*, 2–24. [CrossRef]
25. CBS. Regionale Kerncijfers Nederland. Available online: https://opendata.cbs.nl/#/CBS/nl/dataset/70072ned/table?ts=1726750501721 (accessed on 25 September 2024).
26. Calixto, O.-J.; Anaya, J.-M. Socioeconomic status. The relationship with health and autoimmune diseases. *Autoimmun. Rev.* **2014**, *13*, 641–654. [CrossRef]
27. Fairweather, D.; Frisancho-Kiss, S.; Rose, N.R. Sex Differences in Autoimmune Disease from a Pathological Perspective. *Am. J. Pathol.* **2008**, *173*, 600–609. [CrossRef] [PubMed]
28. van Erp, L.W.; van Gerven, J.; Bloem, S.; Groenen, M.J.M.; Wahab, P.J. Acceptance and Perceived Control are Independently Associated With Quality of Life in Inflammatory Bowel Disease: Introduction of a New Segmentation Model. *J. Crohn's Colitis* **2021**, *15*, 1837–1845. [CrossRef] [PubMed]
29. Teugels, A.; van den Eijnden, I.; Keersmaekers, B.; Verstockt, B.; Sabino, J.; Vermeire, S.; Guadagnoli, L.; Van Diest, I.; Ferrante, M. Disease Acceptance, but not Perceived Control, is Uniquely Associated with Inflammatory Bowel Disease-related Disability. *J. Crohn's Colitis* **2024**, *18*, 1025–1033. [CrossRef] [PubMed]
30. Falk, R.F.; Miller, N.B. *A Primer for Soft Modeling*; University of Akron Press: Akron, OH, USA, 1992; p. 103.
31. Chin, W.W. The Partial Least Squares Approach to Structural Equation Modeling. In *Modern Methods for Business Research*, 1st ed.; Marcoulides, G.A., Ed.; Lawrence Erlbaum Associates: Mahwah, NJ, USA, 1998.

biomedicines

Review

Managing Crohn's Disease Postoperative Recurrence Beyond Prophylaxis: A Comprehensive Review with Meta-Analysis

Andrei Ovidiu Olteanu [1,2,†], Artsiom Klimko [3,†], Eugen Nicolae Tieranu [4,*], Andreea Daniela Bota [1,2,*], Carmen Monica Preda [1,5], Ioana Tieranu [6], Christopher Pavel [1,7], Mihai Radu Pahomeanu [1,8], Cristian Valentin Toma [9], Adrian Saftoiu [1,2], Elena Mirela Ionescu [1,2] and Cristian George Tieranu [1,2]

1 Department of Gastroenterology, "Carol Davila" University of Medicine and Pharmacy, 020021 Bucharest, Romania; ovidiu-andrei.olteanu@drd.umfcd.ro (A.O.O.); carmen.preda@umfcd.ro (C.M.P.); christopher.pavel@gmail.com (C.P.); adrian.saftoiu@umfcd.ro (A.S.); mirela.ionescu@umfcd.ro (E.M.I.); cristian.tieranu@umfcd.ro (C.G.T.)
2 Department of Gastroenterology, ELIAS Emergency University Hospital, 011461 Bucharest, Romania
3 Laboratory of Molecular Neuro-Oncology, Department of Neurology, University Hospital Zurich, 8091 Zurich, Switzerland; klimkoartiom@gmail.com
4 Department of Cardiology, University of Medicine and Pharmacy, 200349 Craiova, Romania
5 Department of Gastroenterology, Fundeni Clinical Institute, 022328 Bucharest, Romania
6 Department of Pediatrics, "Marie Sklodowska Curie" Children Emergency Hospital, 077120 Bucharest, Romania; dr.cindeaioana@yahoo.ro
7 Department of Gastroenterology, Clinical Emergency University Hospital, 014461 Bucharest, Romania
8 Department of Internal Medicine and Gastroenterology, Bucharest Emergency University Hospital, 050098 Bucharest, Romania
9 Department of Innovation and e-Health, "Carol Davila" University of Medicine and Pharmacy, 020021 Bucharest, Romania; cristian.toma@umfcd.ro
* Correspondence: tieranueugen@gmail.com (E.N.T.); andreeadbota@gmail.com (A.D.B.)
† These authors contributed equally to this paper and thus share first authorship.

Abstract: Background and Aims: Postoperative recurrence in Crohn's disease remains a significant clinical challenge, with high recurrence rates despite advancements in medical therapy. This study aims to evaluate the efficacy of various treatments for managing postoperative recurrence following ileocolonic resection in Crohn's disease. Methods: A comprehensive search of PubMed, Cochrane, and Scopus databases was performed to identify studies reporting on the therapeutic management of postoperative recurrence in Crohn's disease. Studies encompassing patients with an endoscopic Rutgeerts score of at least I2 were included. Results: Ustekinumab showed promise, achieving significant endoscopic and clinical success in difficult-to-treat patients. Anti-TNF agents demonstrated superior endoscopic and clinical remission rates compared to mesalamine and azathioprine. Retreatment with anti-TNF therapy remained effective even after preoperative failure. Thalidomide showed efficacy in refractory Crohn's disease, but carries significant toxicity risks, necessitating careful patient selection and monitoring. Combination therapies and non-pharmacologic strategies like enteral nutrition offer additional options, though patient compliance remains challenging. Conclusions: Personalized treatment plans based on individual risk factors and biomarkers are crucial. Infliximab is recommended as the first-line treatment, with ustekinumab and vedolizumab as alternatives in case of anti-TNF failure or intolerance. Early intervention, patient education, and ongoing evaluation are essential for optimizing long-term outcomes in managing postoperative recurrence in Crohn's disease.

Keywords: postoperative recurrence; Crohn's disease; biologic therapy; infliximab; ustekinumab; azathioprine; anti-TNF agents; endoscopic remission

1. Introduction

Crohn's disease (CD) is a chronic, relapsing autoimmune inflammatory bowel disease that can affect any part of the gastrointestinal tract. It is phenotypically classified into inflammatory, stricturing, or penetrating types [1]. Despite significant advancements in medical therapy, approximately 75% of patients with penetrating or stricturing CD affecting the terminal ileum and/or right colon will require intestinal resection at some point [2]. Even after resection, recurrence is common [3]. The Third European Evidence-based Consensus on the Diagnosis and Management of Crohn's Disease of the European Crohn's and Colitis Organization (ECCO) defines recurrence as the reappearance of lesions after surgical resection, while relapse is a flare of symptoms in a patient previously in clinical remission [4].

Several risk factors for postoperative recurrence (POR) of CD are well established. These include younger age at diagnosis, active smoking, ileal disease, a perforating phenotype, and repeated surgeries due to CD [3]. Additional clinical risk factors are active perianal disease, continuous ileocolonic disease, and the NOD2/CARD15 genetic variant. Histological markers such as positive resection margins, granulomas in the resected tissue, and myenteric and submucosal plexitis also predict POR [5]. Bacterial dysbiosis and low levels of *Faecalibacterium prausnitzii* in both resected and postoperative ileal mucosa are associated with an increased risk of endoscopic recurrence, although antibiotic use in the perioperative period can affect the utility of microbiota in predicting recurrence [6].

The American Gastroenterological Association (AGA) defines high-risk patients for POR as those with ≥1 of the following: age at diagnosis < 30 years, current smoking, ≥2 previous surgeries for penetrating disease, with or without perianal disease. Low-risk patients are those diagnosed at >50 years of age, non-smokers, and with a first surgery for a short segment (10–20 cm) of fibrostenotic disease after a longer disease duration (>10 years) [7]. The ECCO guidelines are similar, defining high-risk patients for POR as those with ≥1 of the following: smoking, prior intestinal surgery, absence of prophylactic treatment, penetrating disease at index surgery, perianal location, granulomas in resection specimen, and myenteric plexitis [8].

After ileocecal resection, postoperative endoscopic recurrence without treatment occurs in approximately 65% to 90% of patients within one year and 80% to 100% within three years [9]. Histological recurrence can be detected in all patients within the first week post-surgery, with more than 70% developing endoscopic recurrence in the first postoperative year and up to 35% experiencing clinical relapse after three years. As postoperative endoscopic recurrence typically precedes clinical relapse, ileocolonoscopy is the gold standard for assessing POR of CD and is recommended 6–12 months post-surgery [3]. The Rutgeerts score (RS) evaluates the severity of endoscopic recurrence in postoperative CD patients and is a predictor of future clinical relapse [7,10]. The RS assesses the progression risk of CD based on the postsurgical endoscopic appearance, grading the severity of endoscopic lesions in the neo-terminal ileum and ileocolonic anastomosis. A score of ≥i1 signifies endoscopic recurrence, and escalation of medical therapy is recommended for scores ≥i2. A score of ≥i2 is a reliable predictor of subsequent clinical recurrence [7]. Thus early postoperative reduction of endoscopic inflammation with medications in this scenario can delay symptomatic recurrence [10]. Recently, lesions confined to the anastomosis have been separated from those in the neo-terminal ileum in a modified RS, with subscores i2a (anastomosis lesions) and i2b (>5 aphthous lesions in the neo-terminal ileum) [6]. The implementation of this modified score has yielded contradictory results, and until further prospective trials are available, the same treatment strategy should be applied to all i2 group patients [11].

ECCO and AGA guidelines are also concordant in recommending medical prophylaxis with thiopurines or anti-TNF drugs for patients with at least one risk factor for recurrence. Other options include high-dose mesalamine for patients with isolated ileal resection and imidazole antibiotics, which are less well tolerated. Addressing risk factors is crucial, with smoking cessation being particularly important [8,12]. In severe recurrence or complications, surgery may be necessary. The technique of anastomosis is also critical; Kono et al. introduced Kono-S anastomosis, which is based on the theory that inflammation in CD begins in the mesentery, and thus the anastomosis should be created away from it [13].

A randomized control trial comparing Kono-S anastomosis with conventional side-to-side anastomosis showed significant reductions in postoperative surgical and endoscopic recurrence rates and lower clinical recurrence rates, with no safety issues [14].

The management of POR in CD involves endoscopic monitoring, medical prophylaxis, and occasionally surgical intervention. The goals of treatment in CD are to achieve and maintain remission, improve long-term prognosis by limiting complications, and enhance the patient's quality of life [10]. Traditionally, the focus was on inducing and maintaining symptomatic remission, but this approach did not prevent bowel damage or alter disease progression. Studies indicate that up to 50% of patients in clinical remission still exhibit objective inflammation [15]. Treatment goals have evolved with the STRIDE consensus to include 'deep remission'—achieving both symptomatic and endoscopic remission [16].

Although numerous studies have examined the effects of prophylactic therapy on maintaining post-surgery remission, data on treating the established endoscopic POR to prevent clinical relapse are less consistent. This study aims to evaluate the efficacy and safety of different management strategies for POR of CD through a comprehensive review of the current literature.

2. Literature Review—Search Strategy

This review was conducted following the guidelines of the Preferred Reporting Items for Systematic Reviews and Meta-Analyses group (PRISMA) (Figure 1) in order to capture as many papers of interest as possible. A comprehensive search of PubMed, Cochrane, and Scopus databases was performed in March 2024. The search strategy included: (post-operative OR postoperative OR "post operative" OR "ileocolic resection" OR "ileo-colic resection" OR "ileocolonic resection" OR "ileo-colonic resection") AND recurrence AND Crohn's AND (biologic OR biologics OR "anti-tumor necrosis factor" OR "anti-tumour necrosis factor" OR anti-TNF OR infliximab OR adalimumab OR vedolizumab OR ustekinumab OR azathioprine OR 5-aminosalicylates).

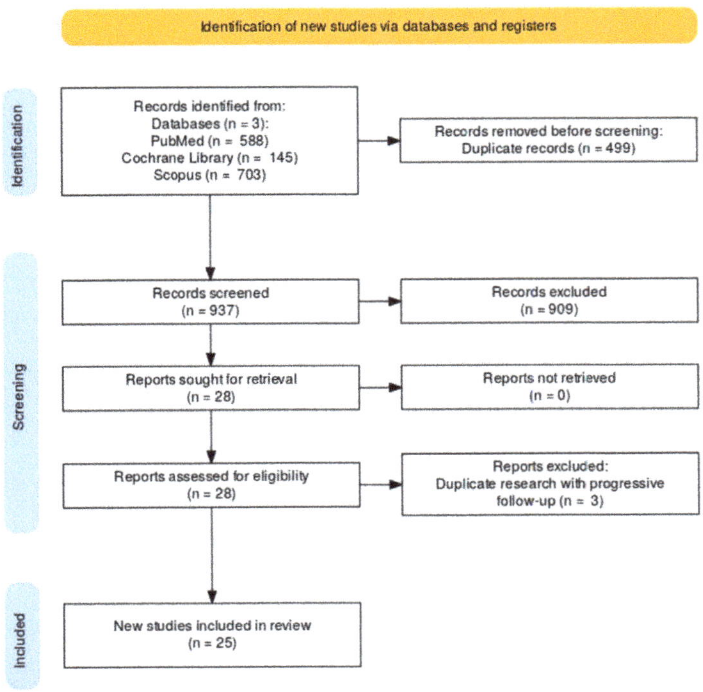

Figure 1. Flow chart showing the PRISMA methodology.

We included studies that met the following eligibility criteria: (1) reporting data on the therapeutic management of established POR after ileocolonic resection in CD, (2) defining POR as RS ≥i2, and (3) study types including case reports, retrospective/prospective studies, and randomized controlled trials (RCTs). Excluded studies were those referring strictly to prophylaxis of POR and reviews.

Two authors independently reviewed all titles and abstracts to identify relevant studies, selecting articles that met the inclusion and exclusion criteria. They used Rayyan software, available online at https://new.rayyan.ai. Duplicates were semi-automatically removed by the software, after double-checking with the reviewers. For discrepant decisions between the two individual researchers, a third researcher reviewed the full-text papers and decided upon inclusion.

3. Meta-Analysis Methodology and Risk of Bias Assessment

We decided to perform a network meta-analysis (NMA) to compare the efficacy of different treatments for postoperative recurrence (POR) of Crohn's disease. The analysis was performed using R software within the RStudio integrated development environment (Version 2024.9.0.375), specifically the "netmeta" package version 2.9.0. [17]. The included studies met the following criteria: (a) reporting on therapeutic management of postoperative recurrence in Crohn's disease following ileocolonic resection and (b)reporting the endoscopic Rutgeerts score of at least i2.

The primary outcome selected was endoscopic improvement, defined as a reduction of at least one point in the Rutgeerts score. For the studied outcome, the odds ratios (ORs) with 95% confidence intervals (CIs) were calculated using a random-effects model to account for heterogeneity across studies.

The "netmeta" package in RStudio was used to create a network plot, illustrating the direct and indirect comparisons between treatments. The relative treatment effects were estimated using a frequentist approach, which calculates odds ratios for each treatment comparison. The network plot (Figure 2) and the forest plot (Figure 3) were generated using the same software package to visually present the relationships between treatments and the comparative odds ratios.

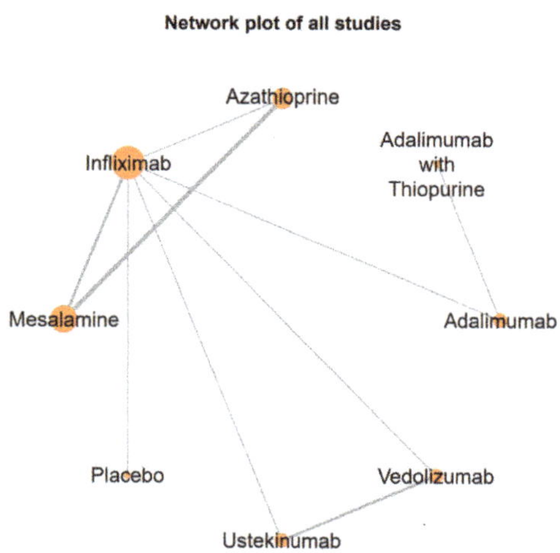

Figure 2. The network plot of included treatments illustrates the comparative relationships between treatments analyzed in the network meta-analysis. Each node represents a treatment, with the size of the nodes corresponding to the number of studies that examined each treatment. The edges (lines) connecting the nodes represent direct comparisons made between treatments, with the thickness of the edges indicating the number of studies that made each comparison. IFX is centrally located, which highlights its extensive evaluation against various other treatments.

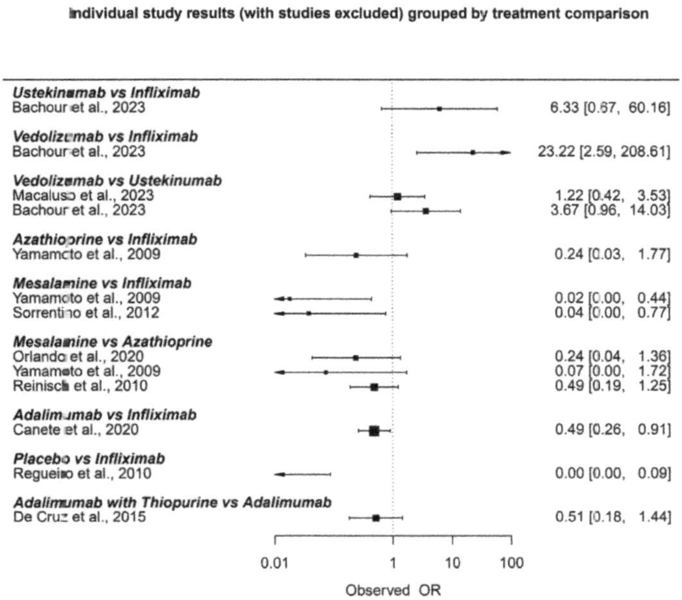

Figure 3. Individual study results grouped by treatment comparison [10,18–25].

To verify the validity of our findings, we performed a risk of bias assessment. The quality of the included randomized controlled trials (RCTs) was assessed using the Cochrane Risk of Bias tool, while cohort and case-control studies were evaluated using the Newcastle-Ottawa Scale. Case reports were assigned, by default, a high risk of bias due to various reasons such as lack of control group, selection bias, confounding factors, and lack of blinding. Studies with a high risk of bias or insufficient reporting of endoscopic outcomes were excluded from the meta-analysis [26,27].

4. Results

A total of 1436 studies were initially identified (588 Pubmed, 145 Cochrane, and 703 Scopus). After the elimination of duplicates, 937 studies were assessed for eligibility, and 25 were included in the final review. The primary reason for such a high exclusion rate (909 articles, 97.01%) was the specific focus of these papers limited to prophylactic measures rather than the treatment of established POR.

The detailed study inclusion process can be summarized in the following flow diagram based on the PRISMA methodology (Figure 1).

The results are presented in Table 1, which includes the following columns: "Author and Study Year", "Outcome", "Type of Trial", "Drug vs. Placebo/Drug Efficacy Comparison", "Number of Patients", "Endoscopic Response", "Clinical Response", "Primary Endpoint", "Secondary Endpoint", "Duration of Follow-up", "Adverse Events", and "Comments". The primary endpoint was defined as the main outcome measure of each study, while the secondary endpoint included any additional outcomes used to evaluate the results. The "Comments" column in the review table provided additional context and insights that were not captured by the other columns, such as specific observations made by the authors, notable limitations, or unique findings relevant to the interpretation of the study results.

Table 1. Summary of the studies reporting on the management of Crohn's disease postoperative recurrence.

Author and Study Year	Outcome	Type of Trial	Drug vs. Placebo/Drug Efficacy Comparison	Number of Patients	Endoscopic Response	Clinical Response	Primary Endpoint	Secondary Endpoint	Duration of Follow-up	Adverse Events	Comments
Macaluso et al., 2023 [18]	Endoscopic and clinical response	Real-world observational study	UST	44	50% achieved a reduction of at least one point in RS	72.7% clinical success	Reduction of at least one point in RS	Clinical success (absence of clinical failure)	17.8 ± 8.4 months	No adverse events reported	UST initiated for endoscopically documented POR, with significant rates of endoscopic and clinical success
Huinink et al., 2023 [28]	Retreatment with anti-TNF therapy for postoperative Crohn's disease recurrence is valid. Combination therapy is more effective than monotherapy.	Retrospective cohort study	Anti-TNF therapy vs. combination therapy	364	Not specified	Not specified	Treatment failure rate (need for reintroduction of corticosteroids, immunosuppressants, or biologicals or need for re-resection)	Treatment failure rate at 1 and 2 years, analysis of preoperative anti-TNF failure, combination therapy vs. monotherapy, retreatment with the same or different anti-TNF agent	1 and 2 years	Not specified	Retreatment with anti-TNF therapy post-ICR is effective, especially with combination therapy. The study highlights the importance of combination therapy to reduce treatment failure rates
Bachour et al., 2023 [19]	Change in Biologic Class Promotes Endoscopic Remission Following Endoscopic Postoperative Crohn's Disease Recurrence	Retrospective Cohort Study	New Biologic Class vs. Therapy Optimization/Continuation	81	Initiation of a new biologic class was associated with a higher rate of endoscopic improvement	60 patients (74.1%) experienced composite recurrence (persistent ePOR or surgical recurrence)	Composite endoscopic or surgical recurrence	Reduction of modified RS	Median follow-up from ePOR to subsequent endoscopy: 426.5 days	Not specified specifically for each intervention	The study emphasizes the benefit of changing the biologic class after the detection of ePOR despite prophylactic biologic therapy
Ueda et al., 2023 [29]	Endoscopic and clinical response	Retrospective cohort study	Biologic era treatments	267	Postoperative anastomotic lesions were detected in 61.0% at index ileo-colonoscopy and 74.9% at follow-up ileo-colonoscopy	Patients with intermediate or severe lesions required significantly more interventions (endoscopic dilation or surgery)	Frequency and severity of postoperative anastomotic lesions	Interventions required (endoscopic dilation or surgery)	~1 year, follow-up duration not specified	Not reported	Frequent and increasing severity of anastomotic lesions observed, prospective studies needed to evaluate treatment enhancement
De Cruz et al., 2022 [30]	Endoscopic and clinical response	Randomized controlled trial	Thiopurine/ADA vs. Placebo	85	A combination of ulcer depth and circumference at 6 months was associated with endoscopic recurrence at 18 months	38% remission at 12 months for patients who stepped up treatment at 6 months, 39% recurrence at 6 months	A combination of ulcer depth and circumference at 6 months was associated with endoscopic recurrence at 18 months	N/A	18 months	N/A	The combination of ulcer depth and circumference at anastomosis at 6 months was predictive of endoscopic recurrence at 18 months

Table 1. *Cont.*

Author and Study Year	Outcome	Type of Trial	Drug vs. Placebo/Drug Efficacy Comparison	Number of Patients	Endoscopic Response	Clinical Response	Primary Endpoint	Secondary Endpoint	Duration of Follow-up	Adverse Events	Comments
Marquez Cami et al., 2022 [31]	Endoscopic and clinical response	Case report	Ruxolitinib	1	More than 50% reduction of ulcerated mucosa in both ileocolonic anastomosis and neoileum	Clinical remission for six months, no further budesonide cycles needed	Reduction of ulcerated mucosa, clinical remission	Fecal calprotectin levels, blood test normalization	6 months	No adverse events reported	Patient showed significant clinical and endoscopic improvement related to ruxolitinib treatment, with satisfactory evolution of polycythemia vera
Macaluso et al., 2022 [32]	Endoscopic and clinical response	Cohort study	VDZ	58	Endoscopic success in 47.6% (reduction of at least one point of RS)	Clinical failure in 19.0% at one year, 32.8% at the end of follow-up, 12.1% required new resection	Endoscopic success (reduction of at least one point RS)	Clinical failure, need for new resection	Mean 24.8 ± 13.1 months	Not reported	VDZ shows potential effectiveness in treating POR of CD
Orlando et al., 2020 [20]	Endoscopic and clinical response	Randomized double-blind double-dummy trial	AZA vs. High-dose 5-aminosalicylic acid (5-ASA)	46	AZA: 6 (27.3%) with RS decrease ≥ 2 points, 8 (36.4%) with decrease ≥ 1 point; 5-ASA: 2 (8.3%) with RS decrease ≥ 2 points, 2 (8.3%) with decrease ≥ 1 point	AZA: 3 (13.6%) clinical recurrence; 5-ASA: 5 (20.8%) clinical recurrence	Therapeutic failure (clinical recurrence or drug discontinuation due to adverse events) at 12 months	10-year post-trial analysis of clinical and endoscopic outcomes	12 months	AZA: 3 adverse events leading to drug discontinuation (fever, hyper-amylasemia, mild pancreatitis)	No significant difference in treatment failure between 5-ASA and AZA, AZA has a less favorable safety profile but may be more effective in preventing clinical recurrence
Canete et al., 2020 [21]	Endoscopic and clinical response	Multicenter retrospective observational study	IFX vs. ADA	179	Endoscopic improvement in 61%, endoscopic remission in 42%	59% clinical remission in patients with clinical POR at the start of therapy	Effectiveness of anti-TNF agents in improving mucosal lesions	Endoscopic improvement, clinical remission	Median 31 months (IQR 13–54)	Not specified	IFX showed higher rates of endoscopic response and remission compared to ADA; concomitant thiopurine use increased efficacy
Riviere et al., 2021 [33]	Clinical and surgical recurrence	Retrospective cohort study	Immunosuppressants and biologics	365	RS ≥ i2 associated with increased risk of clinical and surgical recurrence	48% clinical POR, 26% modified surgical POR within a median follow-up of 88 months	Clinical POR rates, surgical POR rates	Impact of endoscopy-guided therapy modification	Median 88 months	Not reported	RS ≥ i2 patients more likely to receive new therapy; modest decrease in clinical POR for RS i3 and i4 with immunosuppres-sants or biologics; no benefit for RS i2

Table 1. *Cont.*

Author and Study Year	Outcome	Type of Trial	Drug vs. Placebo/Drug Efficacy Comparison	Number of Patients	Endoscopic Response	Clinical Response	Primary Endpoint	Secondary Endpoint	Duration of Follow-up	Adverse Events	Comments
Hu et al., 2016 [34]	Endoscopic and clinical response	Case report	Thalidomide	1	Mucosal healing achieved at 9 months; RS declined from i2 to i1	Clinical remission at 15 months	Mucosal healing (MH) of anastomotic ulcers	Endoscopic and clinical improvement	15 months	No adverse effects reported	Thalidomide is effective in inducing mucosal healing in postoperative CD endoscopic recurrence
De Cruz et al., 2015 [22]	Endoscopic and clinical response	Randomized controlled trial	Thiopurine/ADA vs. Metronidazole alone	174	60 (49%) in the active care group had endoscopic recurrence at 18 months vs. 35 (67%) in standard care	33 (27%) in the active care group had clinical recurrence (CDAI > 200) vs. 21 (40%) in standard care	Endoscopic recurrence at 18 months	Clinical recurrence, C-reactive protein levels, need for further surgery	18 months	No significant differences between active care and standard care groups	Early colonoscopy and treatment step-up for recurrence is better than conventional drug therapy alone
Zabana et al., 2014 [35]	Endoscopic and clinical response	Case-control study	Thiopurines with mesalamine vs. Thiopurines alone	37	Endoscopic improvement in 49%, no difference between groups	32% clinical recurrence in cases, 11% in controls (p = 0.2)	Development of clinical recurrence	Change in RS, mucosal lesions	Median 59 months (IQR 22–100)	No specific adverse effects reported for mesalamine	Mesalamine addition showed no benefit over thiopurine alone for endoscopic improvement or clinical recurrence rates
Reinisch et al., 2013 [36]	Clinical recurrence	Follow-up survey of randomized double-blind double-dummy trial	AZA vs. Mesalamine	46	N/A	36% clinical recurrence with AZA, 25% with mesalamine within 24 months post-treatment	Clinical recurrence within 24 months post-treatment	Long-term prevention of clinical recurrence	Approximately 4 years	N/A	No significant difference in time to clinical recurrence between AZA and mesalamine
Yamamoto et al., 2013 [37]	Endoscopic and clinical response	Prospective cohort study	Enteral nutrition (EN) vs. Control	40	56% (EN) vs. 82% (control) endoscopic recurrence	30% (EN) vs. 60% (control) clinical recurrence	Recurrence requiring biologic therapy or reoperation	Clinical recurrence rate, reoperation rate	5 years	Diarrhea and abdominal distension in the EN group	EN significantly reduced the incidence of recurrence requiring biologic therapy, though compliance issues noted
Papamichael et al., 2012 [3]	Endoscopic and clinical response	Prospective, single-center, open-label, two-year pilot study	ADA	23	60% (9/15) achieved complete (RS-i0) or near-complete (RS-i1) mucosal healing at 24 months	56% (5/9) of patients with clinical relapse at study enrolment achieved and maintained clinical and serological remission	Prevention of early (at 6 months) and late (at 24 months) PO-ER (Group I) and rate of complete mucosal healing (Group II)	Endoscopic and clinical improvement (Group II)	24 months	No serious adverse events reported	ADA is effective in preventing and treating PO-ER and PO-CR in high-risk CD patients

Table 1. *Cont.*

Author and Study Year	Outcome	Type of Trial	Drug vs. Placebo/Drug Efficacy Comparison	Number of Patients	Endoscopic Response	Clinical Response	Primary Endpoint	Secondary Endpoint	Duration of Follow-up	Adverse Events	Comments
Sorrentino et al., 2012 [23]	Endoscopic and clinical response	Prospective open-label multicenter pilot study	IFX vs. Mesalamine	24	IFX: 54% endoscopic remission, 69% improvement in endoscopic score; Mesalamine: 0% endoscopic remission, no improvement in endoscopic score	IFX: 0% clinical recurrence; Mesalamine: 18% clinical recurrence at 8 and 9 months	Proportion of patients with endoscopic remission (score < 2) after 54 weeks	Improvements in endoscopic scores, clinical recurrence at 54 weeks	54 weeks	Flu-like symptoms in 3 patients in the IFX group, new positivity for anti-DNA and lupus anticoagulant antibodies in 2 patients	IFX is superior to mesalamine in treating postoperative endoscopic recurrence of CD, though prophylactic use of IFX may be more effective
Reinisch et al., 2010 [24]	Clinical and endoscopic recurrence	Randomized double-blind double-dummy multicenter trial	AZA vs. Mesalamine	78	63.3% of AZA patients showed ≥1 point reduction RS vs. 34.4% of mesalamine patients	22.0% therapeutic failure in the AZA group vs. 10.8% in the mesalamine group; clinical recurrence: 0% (AZA) vs. 10.8% (mesalamine)	Therapeutic failure during 1 year (CDAI ≥ 200 and increase of ≥60 points from baseline or drug discontinuation due to lack of efficacy/adverse reaction)	Endoscopic improvement at month 12, CDAI score change, IBDQ score change, CRP level change, mucosal healing	12 months	Adverse drug reactions led to discontinuation in 22.0% of AZA patients (e.g., pancreatitis, leucopenia)	AZA showed superior endoscopic improvement but higher adverse event-related discontinuations compared to mesalamine
Regueiro et al., 2010 [25]	Endoscopic and clinical response	Long-term follow-up of randomized controlled trial	IFX vs. Placebo	24	71% remission in the placebo group switched to INF at 2 years; recurrence in all INF patients who stopped at 1 year	Not specified	Long-term endoscopic remission and recurrence rates after surgery	Effectiveness of INF beyond the first postoperative year, response to INF after recurrence	Up to 4.5 years	Infusion reactions leading to switch to (ADA) in some patients	INF maintains remission with ongoing infusions; recurrence if stopped; effective in treating endoscopic recurrence in anti-TNF naive patients post-surgery
Yamamoto et al., 2009 [10]	Endoscopic and clinical response	Prospective pilot study	IFX vs. Mesalamine vs. AZA	26	75% endoscopic improvement with IFX, 38% with AZA, 0% with mesalamine	0% clinical recurrence with IFX, 38% with AZA, 70% with mesalamine	Clinical recurrence (CDAI > 150) at 6 months	Endoscopic improvement, changes in mucosal cytokine levels	6 months	No serious adverse events reported	IFX significantly reduced clinical and endoscopic recurrence and mucosal cytokine levels compared to AZA and mesalamine
Biancone et al., 2006 [38]	Endoscopic and clinical response	Pilot open-label study	Local injection of IFX	8	Endoscopic score improved in 3/8 patients, reduced number and extent of lesions in 7/8 patients	No clinical relapse observed during the follow-up period	Feasibility and safety of local iIFXnfliximab injection for CD recurrence	Clinical remission, histologic score, and assessment of local side effects	Median 20 months (range 14–21 months)	No local or systemic side effects reported	IFX injections were feasible and safe, with reduced lesion extent in most patients; further placebo-controlled studies needed to assess efficacy

Table 1. *Cont.*

Author and Study Year	Outcome	Type of Trial	Drug vs. Placebo/Drug Efficacy Comparison	Number of Patients	Endoscopic Response	Clinical Response	Primary Endpoint	Secondary Endpoint	Duration of Follow-up	Adverse Events	Comments
Alves et al., 2004 [39]	Clinical recurrence	Retrospective cohort study	Immunosuppressive (IS) drugs (AZA, 6-mercaptopurine, or methotrexate) vs. Control (salicylates or no treatment)	26	N/A	Clinical recurrence rate at 3 years: IS group 25%, Control group 60%	Clinical recurrence rate at 3 years	Recurrence rate at follow-up, third intestinal resection rate	Mean follow-up of 80 ± 46 months	No specific IS complications reported	IS drugs lowered clinical recurrence and third resection rates after the second resection for ileocolonic anastomotic recurrence in CD patients
Dejaco et al., 2004 [40]	Endoscopic and clinical response	Open-label pilot study	(rhG-CSF)	5	Complete mucosal healing in 2 patients (40%); Partial response in 4 patients (80%)	All patients remained in clinical remission for 12 months	Complete mucosal healing (RSi0)	Intestinal permeability, cytokine levels, quality of life (IBDQ)	12 months	Transient headache, mild bone and muscle pain observed in 2 patients	rhG-CSF was well tolerated and demonstrated potential efficacy in treating severe endoscopic POR in CD patients
De Cruz et al., 2013 [41]	Endoscopic and clinical response	Multicenter randomized controlled trial	Immediate postoperative ADA vs. Step-up ADA at 6 months	60	43% endoscopic recurrence with immediate Adalimumab, 59% with step-up Adalimumab	32% complete mucosal normality with immediate ADA, 22% with step-up ADA	Endoscopic recurrence at 18 months	Severe disease recurrence rates, mucosal healing	18 months	Not specifically reported	No significant difference in recurrence; step-up anti-TNF therapy based on endoscopic findings viable for high-risk patients
Reinisch et al., 2008 [42]	Clinical and endoscopic response	Randomized double-blind double-dummy multicenter trial	AZA vs. Mesalamine	78	46.3% endoscopic improvement with AZA vs. 29.7% with mesalamine (ITT); 63.3% vs. 34.4% (completer analysis)	Not specified	Therapeutic failure (CDAI ≥ 200 or drug discontinuation due to lack of efficacy or intolerable adverse reaction)	Endoscopic improvement (≥ 1 point drop in RS)	52 weeks	Not specified	No significant difference in therapeutic failure rates; higher endoscopic improvement with AZA

Abbreviations: CD—Crohn's disease, RS—Rutgeerts score, POR—postoperative recurrence, rhG-CSF—granulocyte colony-stimulating factor, AZA—azathioprine, IFX—infliximab, ADA—adalimumab, UST—Ustekinumab, VDZ—vedolizumab.

This search strategy ultimately identified 25 eligible studies, encompassing randomized controlled trials (RCTs), cohort studies, and case reports, focusing on the therapeutic management of established POR of CD after ileocolonic resection. The total number of patients across these studies was 2140, with a diverse range of follow-up durations and endpoints. The average follow-up duration varied significantly, with some studies providing short-term (6 months) and others long-term (up to 10 years) outcomes. The common endpoints evaluated included endoscopic improvement, clinical remission, and the incidence of adverse events.

The studies included multiple designs: 6 randomized controlled trials (RCTs), 5 retrospective cohort studies, 2 prospective cohort studies, 2 case reports, 1 case-control study, and 9 other various study types including observational studies, pilot studies, and follow-up surveys. These studies collectively involved patients with moderate to severe CD, primarily focusing on those with RS $\geq$ i2, consistent with the diagnosis of endoscopic POR. Patient demographics were diverse, with many studies including patients who had undergone previous resections and those with a history of failure of prior biological therapies.

The primary outcomes measured were endoscopic and clinical responses. Endoscopic improvement was typically defined as a reduction in the RS with at least 1 point, while clinical remission was measured by the absence of clinical symptoms and the need for additional intervention. For example, Macaluso et al. (2023) reported that 50% of patients achieved a reduction of at least one point in the RS, and 72.7% attained clinical success with UST [18]. Similarly, Bachour et al. (2023) noted that 60% of patients treated with UST achieved endoscopic improvement, and 55% achieved clinical remission at 12 months [19].

The efficacy of different treatments varied across the studies. Azathioprine (AZA) and high-dose 5-aminosalicylic acid (5-ASA) were compared in several studies, with AZA generally showing higher rates of endoscopic and clinical improvement but also a higher incidence of adverse events [20,24]. Anti-TNF agents, such as infliximab (IFX) and adalimumab (ADA), demonstrated superior efficacy compared to mesalamine and AZA in multiple studies, with higher rates of endoscopic remission and clinical success [10,23].

Biologic therapies, including ustekinumab (UST), vedolizumab (VDZ), and anti-TNF agents, showed significant promise in managing POR. UST was particularly effective, with studies showing significant rates of endoscopic and clinical success [18,19]. VDZ also showed potential effectiveness, with 47.6% of patients achieving endoscopic success and a clinical failure rate of 19.0% at one year [32].

Combination therapies, particularly those involving anti-TNF agents and immunomodulators, were found to be more effective than monotherapy. Huinink et al. (2023) reported that combination therapy significantly reduced the treatment failure rate at 2 years compared to anti-TNF monotherapy (30% vs. 49%, $p = 0.02$) [28]. This highlights the importance of combination therapy in maintaining remission and reducing the need for additional interventions.

Non-pharmacologic strategies, such as enteral nutrition (EN), also played a role in managing POR. Yamamoto et al. (2012) demonstrated that EN significantly reduced the incidence of recurrence requiring biologic therapy or reoperation compared to the control, though compliance issues were noted [37]. Novel treatments like thalidomide and ruxolitinib were explored for their potential in refractory cases. Thalidomide was effective in inducing mucosal healing in a case report by Hu et al. (2016), and ruxolitinib showed significant clinical and endoscopic improvement in a single patient [31,34].

Adverse events varied across the studies, with some treatments associated with higher rates of adverse reactions. For example, AZA was linked to myelosuppression, hepatotoxicity, and increased risk of lymphoma, while thalidomide posed risks of teratogenicity and peripheral neuropathy [24,43]. However, some biologics like UST reported no serious adverse events, underscoring their favorable safety profile [18].

We conducted a network meta-analysis enrolling nine studies with a total of 561 patients to determine which clinical treatment is most likely to produce an endoscopic response, defined as an improvement of at least one point in the RS. The studies included in our initial study were highly heterogeneous, with varied definitions of clinical response, relapse, and therapeutic failure. Therefore, we focused on more objective outcomes like the endoscopic response, as the definitions were more consistent across studies, which limited the number of studies included.

For this shortlist analysis, we excluded case reports, incomplete abstracts from congress presentations, and studies with variable step-up treatment protocols, where patients were initially treated with one drug and subsequently added another upon relapse. Additionally, studies that segregated patients into low- or high-risk cohorts with conditional treatment plans were excluded.

The network plot (Figure 2) demonstrates the interconnectedness of the various treatments evaluated. IFX was compared with multiple therapies, including AZA, mesalamine, ADA, UST, and VDZ. The plot underscores the comprehensive nature of the analysis and highlights the robust network of evidence supporting these findings.

Figure 3 provides an overview of the observed odds ratios (OR) and the comparative effectiveness of the treatments in inducing endoscopic response.

A frequentist network meta-analysis was performed, with IFX chosen as the reference treatment. IFX was selected as the reference drug because it is widely used and well studied, minimizing the effects of outliers and providing a robust baseline for comparison.

The network meta-analysis revealed that compared to IFX, several treatments showed varying degrees of effectiveness in producing endoscopic response (Figure 4). Adalimumab (OR: 0.49; 95% CI: 0.26–0.91), ADA combined with thiopurine (OR: 0.25; 95% CI: 0.08–0.83), and AZA (OR: 0.16; 95% CI: 0.03–0.80) were all associated with significantly lower odds of achieving endoscopic response compared to IFX. Conversely, UST (OR: 9.30; 95% CI: 1.06–81.50) and VDZ (OR: 17.35; 95% CI: 2.03–148.66) demonstrated higher odds of achieving endoscopic response, suggesting their potential efficacy in this setting.

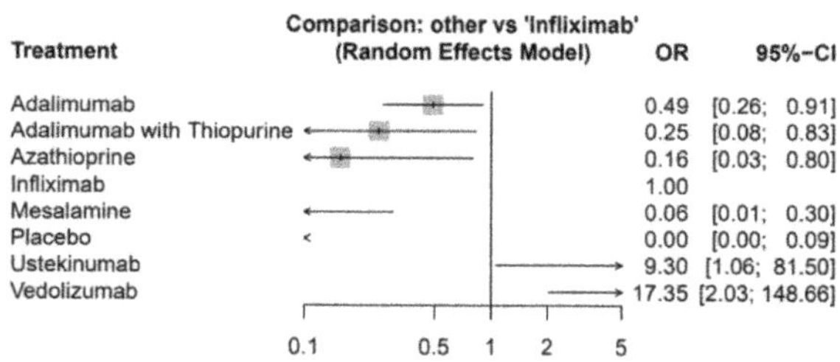

Figure 4. Random effects model—comparison of treatments to infliximab.

However, this last observation should be interpreted with restraint due to the low number of patients in these studies. An overview of these results is presented in Table 2.

In the current review, the risk of bias assessment for the randomized controlled trials (RCTs) was performed using the Cochrane Risk of Bias 2 (RoB 2) tool, while observational studies were assessed using the Newcastle-Ottawa Scale (NOS). Overall, the majority of RCTs demonstrated a low to moderate risk of bias. The existing randomization processes reduced performance and selection bias in most trials. Possible drawbacks regarding missing outcome data were present in several studies, particularly in Regueiro et al. (2009) [25] and Cruz et al. (2014) [41], where long follow-up periods generated the potential for attrition bias. The outcomes, measured using standardized criteria like the Rutgeerts score, were similarly applied across studies, thus reducing measurement bias.

For observational studies assessed using NOS, the majority showed a low to moderate risk of bias. Well-defined cohorts and control for confounders were the main attributes mitigating the risk of bias. However, studies like Yamamoto et al. (2009) [10] and Sorrentino et al. (2012) [44] faced a moderate risk of bias due to the absence of control groups and limited adjustment for confounders.

Table 2. Overview of the effectiveness of different drugs compared to IFX.

Treatment	Odds Ratio	95% Confidence Interval	Comparative Effectiveness to IFX	Comments
Infliximab (IFX)	Reference		Baseline	Widely used and well studied; serves as the reference treatment in this analysis
Adalimumab (ADA)	0.49	0.26–0.91	Less effective than IFX	ADA combined with thiopurine shows better outcomes compared to ADA alone
ADA + Thiopurine	0.25	0.08–0.83	Less effective than IFX	Combination therapy is more effective than monotherapy
Azathioprine (AZA)	0.16	0.03–0.80	Less effective than IFX	AZA shows lower effectiveness but may have a higher adverse event profile
Ustekinumab	9.3	1.06–81.50	More effective than IFX	Significant endoscopic and clinical success; favorable safety profile
Vedolizumab	17.35	2.03–148.66	More effective than IFX	High odds of achieving endoscopic response; promising alternative to anti-TNF therapies
Mesalamine	0.1	0.02–0.45	Less effective than IFX	Significantly less effective in inducing endoscopic response compared to IFX; safer profile but limited efficacy

Lastly, the two included case reports, Marques Cami et al. (2022) [31] and Hu et al. (2016) [34], while thorough in their documentation of patient information and outcomes, carry an inherently high risk of bias due to their descriptive nature, lack of control groups, and absence of blinding.

The overall low to moderate risk of bias in both randomized controlled trials and observational studies included in this review suggests that the findings provide a reliable foundation for clinical decision-making. Even though there were limitations identified, particularly in studies with moderate bias, the use of standardized outcome measures, such as the Rutgeerts score, reinforces the reliability of the results.

5. Discussion

POR in CD remains a significant clinical challenge, as surgery is not curative, and recurrence rates remain high despite advancements in medical therapy. Despite numerous studies exploring the efficacy of various treatments in preventing and managing POR, there is a lack of consensus on how to manage relapsing patients. The severity of endoscopic lesions within the first year following ileocolic resection is a well-documented predictor of clinical recurrence. Patients with endoscopic recurrence (ER) higher than i1 in the neoterminal ileum face an increased risk of early symptoms and complications. A significant proportion of ER is detectable as early as six months post-resection, with many cases being very severe [31].

5.1. 5-Aminosalicylates Versus Azathioprine

Once severe ER is documented, it is crucial to treat patients to avoid clinical and surgical recurrence. Studies have shown the efficacy of 5-ASA or AZA versus placebo in preventing clinical recurrence after surgically induced remission. However, only one previous randomized controlled trial compared the efficacy of 5-ASA versus AZA for clinical recurrence prevention in CD patients with severe postsurgical ER [20].

A multicenter randomized double-blind double-dummy trial by Orlando et al. (2020) evaluated the efficacy of high-dose 5-ASA and AZA in 46 patients with early severe postsurgical endoscopic recurrence (ER) (RS ≥ i2). In this high-risk population, 17.4% of patients experienced therapeutic failure, defined as clinical recurrence or drug discontinuation due to adverse events, within 12 months from randomization, with no significant difference between the 5-ASA and AZA groups (20.8% vs. 13.6%, respectively, $p = 0.702$). Therapeutic failure with 5-ASA was primarily due to clinical recurrence, while with AZA, it was related to adverse events. Additionally, AZA led to an RS decrease of ≥2 points in 27.3% and ≥1 point in 36.4% of patients, whereas 5-ASA achieved similar decreases in only 8.3% of patients. Clinical recurrence was encountered only in 5-ASA treated patients (20.8%), while AZA had a less favorable safety profile, with three adverse events leading to drug discontinuation, indicating a trade-off between efficacy and safety. Clinical relapse rates were 17% at 12 months and 53% up to 10 years post-trial, with no significant adverse events recorded [20]. A similar randomized double-blind double-dummy multicenter trial involving 78 patients found that AZA patients showed a ≥1 point reduction in the RS in 63.3% of cases, compared to 34.4% for mesalamine. Additionally, 5-ASA was less effective than AZA in preventing clinical recurrence ($p = 0.031$). Therapeutic failure was higher in the AZA group (22.0%) compared to the mesalamine group (10.8%), with adverse drug reactions leading to discontinuation in all these AZA patients [24]. AZA appears to have superior efficacy in reducing ER compared to mesalamine, although its use is limited by a higher incidence of adverse events.

The combination of mesalamine and thiopurine did not significantly enhance therapeutic outcomes compared to thiopurine alone. Endoscopic improvement was seen in 49% of patients, with no differences between the groups. Clinical recurrence occurred in 32% of cases and 11% of controls, with no specific adverse effects reported, indicating that adding mesalamine to thiopurine therapy does not significantly improve outcomes in POR management [20].

5.2. *AntiTNF Agents Versus Azathioprine and 5-Aminosalicylates*

The adverse event profile that limits the use of thiopurines, such as AZA, includes myelosuppression, hepatotoxicity, and increased risk of lymphoma, which often preclude adherence [34]. Within this context, an IFX-based regimen may be more effective than AZA/5-ASA protocols in reducing clinical and endoscopic disease activity. Yamamoto et al. found that six months after treatment, none of the IFX-treated patients developed postoperative clinical recurrence (PO-CR) compared with 38% of AZA-treated and 70% of 5-ASA-treated patients. Endoscopic inflammation improved in 75% of IFX-treated vs. 38% of AZA-treated and none of the 5-ASA-treated patients. Complete mucosal healing was achieved in 38% of IFX patients, 13% of AZA patients, and none of the 5-ASA patients. This reinforces the superiority of IFX in managing early endoscopic lesions and preventing clinical recurrence [10]. Treatment with mesalamine alone, although safer than AZA, is less effective—in a comparison study, 7 out of 13 patients treated with IFX achieved remission, while none did while being treated with mesalamine [23].

Moreover, retreatment with anti-TNF therapy, such as IFX or adalimumab (ADA), even after preoperative anti-TNF therapy failure, can be an effective strategy for managing postoperative CD. Adverse events were reported in 15% of patients receiving combination therapy and 18% receiving monotherapy, indicating a comparable safety profile. This finding is particularly important for patients who have previously failed anti-TNF therapy, suggesting that retreatment remains a viable option [28].

Over the past decade, the use of biological drugs, especially anti-TNFs, has increased for the prevention and treatment of postsurgical recurrence. This has led to the ECCO guidelines introducing the recommendation for prophylactic treatment with thiopurines or anti-TNFs after ileocolonic resection in patients with at least one risk factor for postsurgical recurrence. However, limited data are available on managing severe postsurgical ER. The POCER study found step-up treatment, meaning escalating therapy from 'no treatment' to a thiopurine or adalimumab, for early severe ER to be the best option for preventing clinical recurrence [22]. Compared to metronidazole alone, the active treatment approach improved endoscopic remission (33% vs. 51%) and recurrence (67% vs. 49%) profiles at 18 months. Within this trial, a higher proportion of patients in the 5-ASA group underwent treatment escalation compared to the AZA group, affirming the limited efficacy of mesalamine. Patients with severe postsurgical ER benefitted from prompt postsurgical treatment, as early AZA use did affect long-term clinical outcomes in high-risk patients [22].

Anti-TNF therapy may have some efficacy in preventing as well as in treating POR in CD. In a prospective, single-center, open-label pilot study, Papamichael et al. (2012) assessed ADA's short- and long-term efficacy in the postoperative setting for patients at high risk for early POR and in patients with established POR. The study involved 23 patients treated with ADA following curative intestinal resection for complications of CD, divided into two subgroups of 8 and 15 patients respectively, receiving a standard induction regimen and maintenance therapy either straightaway following surgery or after endoscopic documentation of POR (RS $\geq$ 2). After one year of treatment, no clinical recurrences were observed, although 10% had PO-ER, and 45% had at least moderate histologic recurrence. Regarding the POR subgroup, at 24 months of ADA treatment, 60% of patients achieved complete or near-complete mucosal healing, and 56% maintained clinical remission [3].

Similarly, IFX in combination with low-dose oral methotrexate (10 mg/week) may have preventive potential for PO-ER and clinical recurrence of CD. None of the CD patients treated with scheduled IFX maintenance therapy in the immediate postoperative period experienced PO-ER for 24 months. However, 83% developed PO-ER within four months after discontinuing IFX. Re-treatment with lower doses of IFX successfully restored and maintained endoscopic remission for one year [45].

In the only randomized placebo-controlled trial to date, one-year treatment with the classical IFX regimen after surgery was far more effective than placebo in preventing endoscopic and histologic recurrence of CD (9.1% and 27.3% vs. 84.6% and 84.6%, respectively). The rate of PO-CR was likewise lower in the IFX arm compared to the placebo-treated patients (20.0% vs. 46.2%). This study also suggested that improved outcomes could be maintained in subjects who continued IFX therapy. Local injections of low-dose IFX into the sites of endoscopic recurrence prevented short- and medium-term clinical relapses of CD without compromising safety, improving both Rutgeerts endoscopic and histologic scores [25,38].

IFX was also more effective than AZA and mesalamine in managing early postoperative recurrence, as quantified by endoscopic improvement (75% with IFX, 38% with AZA, and 0% with mesalamine) and clinical recurrence (0% with IFX, 38% with AZA, and 70% with mesalamine) [10].

The comparative efficacy of IFX is higher than ADA in the postoperative period, which can be further augmented by thiopurines, resulting in higher trough levels of IFX and decreased underexposure rates. Canete et al. found that roughly 25 months after surgery, IFX patients had higher rates of endoscopic remission (57% vs. 29%) and marginally improved rates of clinical response (61% vs. 57%) compared to ADA patients [21].

Several studies further examined whether combinatorial anti-TNF therapy may augment outcomes. Postsurgical anti-TNF therapy reduced treatment failure rates by 19% at 2 years when combined with immunomodulators compared to anti-TNF monotherapy (30% vs. 49%, $p = 0.02$). The cumulative rates of treatment failure were 28% at 1 year and 47% at 2 years, with combination therapy proving superior in maintaining remission [28]. In an RCT, De Cruz et al. compared thiopurine/ADA versus placebo in 85 patients, finding that step-up treatment results in a 38% remission rate at 12 months., suggesting that the combination of thiopurine and ADA can provide significant benefits in early intervention, potentially reducing long-term recurrence rates [30].

5.3. New Biologic Agents

Ustekinumab (UST) shows promise as a therapeutic option for treating POR. In a multicenter real-world study, 50% of patients achieved endoscopic success, and 72.7% attained clinical success among difficult-to-treat patients, even those with high rates of previous resections and failures to prior biological therapies. Approximately 50% of patients achieved at least a one-point reduction in the RS, and 27.3% reported an absence of POR (RS $\leq$ i1) at the first post-treatment colonoscopy. UST may slow or halt the progression of POR, particularly for severe (i3 or i4) and intermediate severity (i2) lesions [18]. Similar results were reported by Bachour et al., where UST therapy for POR-CD resulted in a 60% endoscopic response and a 55% clinical remission rate at 12 months [19]. Both studies did not report any adverse events and present UST as a viable treatment option for patients with moderate to severe postsurgical disease activity [18,19].

When comparing UST to vedolizumab (VDZ), both drugs showed similar rates of endoscopic success (50.0% for UST vs. 47.6% for VDZ) and clinical failure (27.3% for UST vs. 32.8% for VDZ). However, UST demonstrated a slightly lower rate of surgical recurrence (9.1%) over a mean follow-up of approximately 18 months. UST may offer a slight advantage in terms of long-term outcomes, although further research is needed to confirm these findings and determine factors that could guide treatment selection [18]. VDZ monotherapy was assessed by Macaluso et al. in a 58-patient cohort study, where endoscopic success was 47.6% and clinical failure was 19.0% at one year, which increased to 32.8% at roughly two years [32].

5.4. Other Non-Biologic Agents

Several other treatment strategies have been explored for their efficacy in managing POR, including thalidomide and ruxolitinib. The ECCO/ESPGHAN consensus guidelines recommend thalidomide as an alternative for patients who do not tolerate or lose response to anti-TNF agents [46]. Simon et al. reported 54% of their 77 patients with active refractory CD to achieve clinical remission within the first year of thalidomide treatment [47]. Although thalidomide's use in surgical CD is less documented, Hershfield et al. reported significant improvement in terminal ileal ulcers in a CD patient who failed other treatments [48]. There are also several case reports that document excellent responses to thalidomide in patients with refractory disease, with clinical remission being maintained for up to 15 months without adverse effects [34]. Thalidomide, similarly to thiopurines, is limited by its toxicity profile—the former drug may cause peripheral neuropathy, thromboembolism, sedation, and dermatitis. It is also a notorious teratogen [34].

Evidence examining ruxolitinib, a JAK inhibitor, is limited—a case report documented a 50% reduction in mucosal ulceration, along with a six-month clinical remission in a refractory POR patient [31].

Long-term enteral nutrition (EN) with an elemental diet showed promise in reducing recurrence incidence and the need for biologic therapy, although patient compliance remains a challenge. Motivated patients who have maintained EN therapy for over five years demonstrated its potential feasibility for long-term management in select populations. Yamamoto et al. (2012) demonstrated that EN significantly reduced the incidence of recurrence requiring biologic therapy or reoperation compared to controls in a cohort of 40 patients. Endoscopic recurrence was lower in the EN group (56%) compared to the control group (82%), and clinical recurrence was also reduced (30% vs. 60%). However, compliance issues were noted, impacting the long-term efficacy of EN [37].

Within this complex treatment landscape, identifying predictive factors and understanding long-term outcomes are critical for improving management strategies for POR. Treatment timing recommendations are somewhat discordant. The POCER study suggested that initiating optimum drug therapy based on endoscopic detection is preferable to waiting for clinical symptoms to appear [22]. Conversely, Riviere et al. found that using immunosuppressants and tumor necrosis factor antagonists to treat asymptomatic endoscopic postoperative recurrence of CD did not significantly reduce long-term clinical recurrence risk in patients with Rutgeerts scores of i2 but had a small effect in those with scores of i3 or i4. An RS $\geq$ i2 increases the risk of clinical and endoscopic CD recurrence. Riviere et al. reported clinical and surgical POR rates of 48% and 26%, respectively, within a median follow-up of 88 months [33].

The findings of our review suggest that IFX is the preferred treatment for managing early endoscopic lesions post-resection in CD patients, particularly those at high risk for severe endoscopic recurrence. Proactive monitoring and timely step-up therapeutic adjustments are integral to therapeutic success. AZA can be considered for patients at lower risk for adverse events and those preferring an immunomodulatory approach, while mesalamine should be limited to those with mild disease or contraindications to other treatments. EN therapy is a viable option for motivated patients who can maintain the regimen, with education and support enhancing compliance. For clinical practice, IFX is recommended as the first-line treatment for high-risk patients, with new biologic agents such as UST and VDZ as a second-line option in case of anti-TNF contraindications, failure, or intolerance. Moderate-risk patients may start with AZA, considering their risk profile and potential for adverse events, and mesalamine or long-term EN as alternatives for those with low risk and good compliance. Patients preferring non-pharmacologic approaches can consider long-term EN with an elemental diet, supported by educational and compliance strategies.

Our study has limitations that may interfere with the general applicability of our findings. Firstly, there is significant heterogeneity in defining clinical outcomes across studies. To address this, we focused our network meta-analysis on studies with endoscopic outcomes based on Rutgeerts scores (RS). Secondly, the low number of patients in studies evaluating the efficacy of vedolizumab (VDZ) and ustekinumab (UST) may falsely infer their superiority over infliximab (IFX). Lastly, variable follow-up intervals can influence drug efficacy interpretations, as initial suboptimal endoscopic responses may improve with longer follow-up.

6. Conclusions

Managing POR in CD remains challenging despite advancements in medical therapy. This review highlights the efficacy of biologic therapies, particularly IFX, in reducing recurrence rates. Personalized treatment plans based on individual risk factors and biomarkers are crucial. For high-risk patients, IFX is recommended as the first-line treatment, with UST and VDZ as second-line options. Early intervention and proactive monitoring are essential for optimizing long-term outcomes in the postoperative setting of CD.

Author Contributions: A.O.O., A.K. and A.D.B. contributed to data collection, screening of relevant literature, and drafting of the manuscript; C.M.P., I.T. and C.P. contributed to data interpretation and statistical analysis; M.R.P., E.N.T. and C.V.T. contributed to the study design and drafting of the manuscript; A.S., E.M.I. and C.G.T. supervised the writing process, critically reviewed the draft, and contributed to writing the final version of the manuscript. All authors have read and agreed to the published version of the manuscript.

Funding: This research received no external funding.

Informed Consent Statement: Patient consent was waived due to the type of this paper—a review of previously published studies.

Data Availability Statement: The data supporting this article are available within the manuscript.

Acknowledgments: The publication of this manuscript was supported by the "Carol Davila" University of Medicine and Pharmacy through the institutional program "Publish not Perish".

Conflicts of Interest: The authors declare no conflicts of interest.

References

1. Gasche, C.; Grundtner, P. Genotypes and phenotypes in Crohn's disease: Do they help in clinical management? *Gut* **2005**, *54*, 162–167. [CrossRef] [PubMed]
2. Cosnes, J.; Bourrier, A.; Nion-Larmurier, I.; Sokol, H.; Beaugerie, L.; Seksik, P. Factors affecting outcomes in Crohn's disease over 15 years. *Gut* **2012**, *61*, 1140–1145. [CrossRef] [PubMed]
3. Papamichael, K.; Archavlis, E.; Lariou, C.; Mantzaris, G. Adalimumab for the prevention and/or treatment of post-operative recurrence of Crohn's disease: A prospective, two-year, single center, pilot study. *J. Crohns Colitis* **2012**, *6*, 924–931. [CrossRef] [PubMed]
4. Gomollón, F.; Dignass, A.; Annese, V.; Tilg, H.; van Assche, G.; Lindsay, J.O.; Peyrin-Biroulet, L.; Cullen, G.J.; Daperno, M.; Kucharzik, T.; et al. 3rd European Evidence-based Consensus on the Diagnosis and Management of Crohn's Disease 2016, Part 1, Diagnosis and Medical Management. *J. Crohns Colitis* **2017**, *11*, 3–25. [CrossRef] [PubMed]
5. Rao, G.V.; Pal, P.; Sekaran, A.; Rebala, P.; Tandan, M.; Nageshwar Reddy, D. Proposal of novel staging system CNM (Crohn's primary site, nodes, mesentery) to predict postoperative recurrence of Crohn's disease. *Intest. Res.* **2023**, *21*, 196–204. [CrossRef] [PubMed]
6. Dasharathy, S.S.; Limketkai, B.N.; Sauk, J.S. What's New in the Postoperative Management of Crohn's Disease? *Dig. Dis. Sci.* **2022**, *67*, 3508–3517. [CrossRef]
7. Ble, A.; Renzulli, C.; Cenci, F.; Grimaldi, M.; Barone, M.; Sedano, R.; Chang, J.; Nguyen, T.M.; Hogan, M.; Zou, G.; et al. The Relationship Between Endoscopic and Clinical Recurrence in Postoperative Crohn's Disease: A Systematic Review and Meta-analysis. *J. Crohns Colitis* **2022**, *16*, 490–499. [CrossRef]
8. Gionchetti, P.; Dignass, A.; Danese, S.; Magro Dias, F.J.; Rogler, G.; Lakatos, P.L.; Adamina, M.; Ardizzone, S.; Buskens, C.J.; Sebastian, S.; et al. 3rd European Evidence-based Consensus on the Diagnosis and Management of Crohn's Disease 2016, Part 2, Surgical Management and Special Situations. *J. Crohns Colitis* **2017**, *11*, 135–149. [CrossRef]
9. Maaser, C.; Sturm, A.; Vavricka, S.R.; Kucharzik, T.; Fiorino, G.; Annese, V.; Calabrese, E.; Baumgart, D.C.; Bettenworth, D.; Borralho Nunes, P.; et al. ECCO-ESGAR Guideline for Diagnostic Assessment in IBD Part 1, Initial diagnosis, monitoring of known IBD, detection of complications. *J. Crohns Colitis* **2019**, *13*, 144–164. [CrossRef]
10. Yamamoto, T.; Umegae, S.; Matsumoto, K. Impact of infliximab therapy after early endoscopic recurrence following ileocolonic resection of Crohn's disease: A prospective pilot study. *Inflamm. Bowel Dis.* **2009**, *15*, 1460–1466. [CrossRef]
11. Rivière, P.; Pekow, J.; Hammoudi, N.; Wils, P.; De Cruz, P.; Pu Wang, C.; Manosa, M.; Ollech, J.; Allez, M.; Nachury, M.; et al. Comparison of the Risk of Crohn's Disease Postoperative Recurrence Between Modified Rutgeerts Score i2a and i2b Categories: An Individual Patient Data Meta-analysis. *J. Crohns Colitis* **2023**, *17*, 269–276. [CrossRef] [PubMed]
12. Nguyen, G.C.; Loftus, E.V.; Hirano, I.; Falck-Ytter, Y.; Singh, S.; Sultan, S.; AGA Institute Clinical Guidelines Committee. American Gastroenterological Association Institute Guideline on the Management of Crohn's Disease After Surgical Resection. *Gastroenterology* **2017**, *152*, 271–275. [CrossRef] [PubMed]
13. Kelm, M.; Reibetanz, J.; Kim, M.; Schoettker, K.; Brand, M.; Meining, A.; Germer, C.T.; Flemming, S. Kono-S Anastomosis in Crohn's Disease: A Retrospective Study on Postoperative Morbidity and Disease Recurrence in Comparison to the Conventional Side-To-Side Anastomosis. *J. Clin. Med.* **2022**, *11*, 6915. [CrossRef] [PubMed]
14. Luglio, G.; Rispo, A.; Tropeano, F.P.; Giglio, M.C.; Cricrì, M.; Imperatore, N.; De Sire, R.; Guarino, A.D.; Bucci, L.; Castiglione, F. P522 Kono-S anastomosis reduces endoscopic and surgical post-operative recurrence in Crohn's disease. The SuPREMe-CD Trial Update. *J. Crohns Colitis* **2023**, *17*, i650. [CrossRef]
15. Garcia, N.M.; Cohen, N.A.; Rubin, D.T. Treat-to-target and sequencing therapies in Crohn's disease. *United Eur. Gastroenterol. J.* **2022**, *10*, 1121–1128. [CrossRef]
16. Chateau, T.; Peyrin-Biroulet, L. Evolving therapeutic goals in Crohn's disease management. *United Eur. Gastroenterol. J.* **2020**, *8*, 133–139. [CrossRef]
17. RStudio Team. RStudio: Integrated Development for R. 2020. Available online: http://www.rstudio.com/ (accessed on 24 August 2024).
18. Macaluso, F.S.; Grova, M.; Mocciaro, F.; Di Mitri, R.; Privitera, A.C.; Distefano, M.E.; Vitello, A.; Camilleri, S.; Ferracane, C.; Pluchino, D.; et al. Ustekinumab is a promising option for the treatment of postoperative recurrence of Crohn's disease. *J. Gastroenterol. Hepatol.* **2023**, *38*, 1503–1509. [CrossRef]
19. Bachour, S.P.; Shah, R.S.; Joseph, A.; Syed, H.; Ali, A.H.; Rieder, F.; Barner, E.L.; Axelrad, J.; Holubar, S.D.; Regueiro, M.; et al. Change in Biologic Class Promotes Endoscopic Remission Following Endoscopic Postoperative Crohn's Disease Recurrence. *J. Clin. Gastroenterol.* **2024**, *58*, 810–817. [CrossRef]
20. Orlando, A.; Mocciaro, F.; Ventimiglia, M.; Renna, S.; Rispo, A.; Scribano, M.L.; Testa, A.; Aratari, A.; Bossa, F.; Angelucci, E.; et al. Azathioprine for prevention of clinical recurrence in Crohn's disease patients with severe endoscopic recurrence: An IG-IBD randomized double-blind trial. *Eur. Rev. Med. Pharmacol. Sci.* **2020**, *24*, 11356–11364.
21. Cañete, F.; Mañosa, M.; Pérez-Martínez, I.; Barreiro-de-Acosta, M.; Gonzalez-Sueyro, R.C.; Nos, P.; Iglesias-Flores, E.; Gutierrez, A.; Bujanda, L.; Gordillo, J.; et al. Antitumor Necrosis Factor Agents to Treat Endoscopic Postoperative Recurrence of Crohn's Disease: A Nationwide Study With Propensity-Matched Score Analysis. *Clin. Transl. Gastroenterol.* **2020**, *11*, e00218. [CrossRef]

22. De Cruz, P.; Kamm, M.A.; Hamilton, A.L.; Ritchie, K.J.; Krejany, E.O.; Gorelik, A.; Liew, D.; Prideaux, L.; Lawrance, I.C.; Andres, J.M.; et al. Crohn's disease management after intestinal resection: A randomised trial. *Lancet* **2015**, *385*, 1406–1417. [CrossRef] [PubMed]
23. Sorrentino, D.; Terrosu, G.; Paviotti, A.; Geraci, M.; Avellini, C.; Zoli, G.; Fires, W.; Danese, S.; Occhipinti, P.; Croatto, T.; et al. Early Diagnosis and Treatment of Postoperative Endoscopic Recurrence of Crohn's Disease: Partial Benefit by Infliximab—A Pilot Study. *Dig. Dis. Sci.* **2012**, *57*, 1341–1348. [CrossRef] [PubMed]
24. Reinisch, W.; Angelberger, S.; Petritsch, W.; Shonova, O.; Lukas, M.; Bar-Meir, S.; Teml, A.; Schaeffeler, E.; Schwab, M.; Dilger, K.; et al. Azathioprine versus mesalazine for prevention of postoperative clinical recurrence in patients with Crohn's disease with endoscopic recurrence: Efficacy and safety results of a randomised, double-blind, double-dummy, multicentre trial. *Gut* **2010**, *59*, 752–759. [CrossRef] [PubMed]
25. Regueiro, M.; Schraut, W.H.; Baidoo, L.; Kip, K.E.; Sepulveda, A.R.; Pesci, M.; Harrison, J.; Plevy, S.E. T1207 Two Year Postoperative Follow-Up of Patients Enrolled in the Randomized Controlled Trial (RCT) of Infliximab (IFX) for Prevention of Recurrent Crohn's Disease (CD). *Gastroenterology* **2009**, *136*, A-522. [CrossRef]
26. Sterne Jonathan, A.C.; Savović, J.; Page Matthew, J.; Elbers, R.G.; Blencowe, N.S.; Boutron, I.; Cates, C.J.; Cheng, H.-Y.; Corbett, M.S.; Eldridge, S.M.; et al. RoB 2, A revised tool for assessing risk of bias in randomised trials. *BMJ* **2019**, *366*, l4898. [CrossRef] [PubMed]
27. Wells, G.A.; Shea, B.; O'Connell, D.; Peterson, J.; Welch, V.; Losos, M.; Tugwell, P. The Newcastle-Ottawa Scale (NOS) for Assessing the Quality of Nonrandomised Studies in Meta-Analyses. Available online: http://www.ohri.ca/programs/clinical_epidemiology/oxford.asp (accessed on 12 October 2024).
28. Ten Bokkel Huinink, S.; Beelen, E.M.J.; Ten Bokkel Huinink, T.; Hoentjen, F.; Bodelier, A.G.L.; Dijkstra, G.; Romberg-Camps, M.; de Boer, N.K.; Stassen, L.P.S.; van der Meulen, A.E.; et al. Retreatment with anti-tumor necrosis factor therapy in combination with an immunomodulator for recurrence of Crohn's disease after ileocecal resection results in prolonged continuation as compared to anti-tumor necrosis factor monotherapy. *Eur. J. Gastroenterol. Hepatol.* **2023**, *35*, 45–51. [CrossRef]
29. Ueda, T.; Koyama, F.; Sugita, A.; Ikeuchi, H.; Futami, K.; Fukushima, K.; Nezu, R.; Iijima, H.; Mizushima, T.; Itabashi, M.; et al. Endoscopic Lesions of Postoperative Anastomotic Area in Patients With Crohn's Disease in the Biologic Era: A Japanese Multi-Centre Nationwide Cohort Study. *J. Crohns Colitis* **2023**, *17*, 1968–1979. [CrossRef]
30. De Cruz, P.; Hamilton, A.L.; Burrell, K.J.; Gorelik, A.; Liew, D.; Kamm, M.A. Endoscopic Prediction of Crohn's Disease Postoperative Recurrence. *Inflamm. Bowel Dis.* **2022**, *28*, 680–688. [CrossRef]
31. Marquès-Camí, M.; García-Guiñón, A.; Garreta, J.; Volta, T.; Torres, G.; Sese, E. A 61-year-old patient with Crohn's disease and severe postoperative recurrence responding to JAK inhibitor ruxolitinib for polycythemia vera treatment. *Gastroenterol. Hepatol.* **2022**, *45*, 16–17. [CrossRef]
32. Macaluso, F.S.; Cappello, M.; Crispino, F.; Grova, M.; Privitera, A.C.; Piccillo, G.; Magnano, A.; Ferracane, C.; Belluardo, N.; Giangreco, E.; et al. Vedolizumab may be an effective option for the treatment of postoperative recurrence of Crohn's disease. *Dig. Liver Dis.* **2022**, *54*, 629–634. [CrossRef]
33. Rivière, P.; Vermeire, S.; Irles-Depe, M.; van Assche, G.; Rutgeerts, P.; Denost, Q.; Wolthuis, A.; D'Hoore, A.; Laharie, D.; Ferrante, M. Rates of Postoperative Recurrence of Crohn's Disease and Effects of Immunosuppressive and Biologic Therapies. *Clin. Gastroenterol. Hepatol.* **2021**, *19*, 713–720.e1. [CrossRef] [PubMed]
34. Hu, H.; Wang, X.; Liu, S. Thalidomide induces mucosal healing in postoperative Crohn disease endoscopic recurrence: Case report and literature review. *Medicine* **2016**, *95*, e4799. [CrossRef] [PubMed]
35. Zabana, Y.; Mañosa, M.; Cabré, E.; Bernal, I.; Marin, L.; Lorenzo-Zuniga, V.; Moreno, V.; Boix, J.; Domenech, E. Addition of mesalazine for subclinical post-surgical endoscopic recurrence of C rohn's disease despite preventive thiopurine therapy: A case–control study. *J Gastroenterol. Hepatol.* **2014**, *29*, 1413–1417. [CrossRef] [PubMed]
36. Reinisch, W.; Angelberger, S.; Petritsch, W.; Shonova, O.; Lukas, M.; Bar-Meir, S.; Teml, A.; Schaeffeler, E.; Schwab, M.; Dilger, K.; et al. P608 Azathioprine versus mesalazine for prevention of postoperative clinical recurrence in Crohn's disease patients with endoscopic recurrence: Follow-up data of a randomised, double-blind, double-dummy, 1-year, multicentre trial. *J. Crohns Colitis* **2013**, *7*, S254. [CrossRef]
37. Yamamoto, T.; Shiraki, M.; Nakahigashi, M.; Umegae, S.; Matsumoto, K. Enteral nutrition to suppress postoperative Crohn's disease recurrence: A five-year prospective cohort study. *Int. J. Color. Dis.* **2013**, *28*, 335–340. [CrossRef]
38. Biancone, L.; Cretella, M.; Tosti, C.; Palmieri, G.; Petruzziello, C.; Geremia, A.; Calabrese, E.; Pallone, F. Local injection of infliximab in the postoperative recurrence of Crohn's disease. *Gastrointest. Endosc.* **2006**, *63*, 486–492. [CrossRef]
39. Alves, A.; Panis, Y.; Joly, F.; Pocrad, M.; Lavergne-Slove, A.; Bouhnik, Y.; Valleur, P. Could Immunosuppressive Drugs Reduce Recurrence Rate After Second Resection for Crohn Disease? *Inflamm. Bowel Dis.* **2004**, *10*, 491–495. [CrossRef]
40. Dejaco, C.; Lichtenberger, C.; Miehsler, W.; Oberhuber, G.; Herbst, F.; Vogelsang, H.; Gangl, A.; Reinisch, W. An Open-Label Pilot Study of Granulocyte Colony-Stimulating Factor for the Treatment of Severe Endoscopic Postoperative Recurrence in Crohn's Disease. *Digestion* **2003**, *68*, 63–70. [CrossRef]
41. Cruz, P.D.; Kamm, M.A.; Ritchie, K.J.; Hamilton, A.L.; Krejany, S.; Gorelik, A.; Liew, D.; Prideaux, L.; Lawrance, I.C.; Andrews, J.M.; et al. Strategic timing of anti-TNF therapy in postoperative Crohn's disease: Comparison of routine use immediately postoperatively with selective use after demonstrated recurrence at 6 month endoscopy. Results from POCER. *J. Gastroenterol. Hepatol.* **2013**, *28*, 92.

42. Reinisch, W.; Angelberger, S.; Petritsch, W.; Herrlinger, R.K.; Shonova, O.; Lukas, M.; Bar-Meir, S.; Schwab, M.; Greinwald, R.; Mueller, R.; et al. 504 A Double-Blind, Double-Dummy, Randomized, Controlled, Multicenter Trial On the Efficacy and Safety of Azathioprine vs. mesalamine for Prevention of Clinical Relapses in Crohn's Disease Patients with Postoperative Moderate or Severe Endoscopic Recurrence. *Gastroenterology* **2008**, *134*, A-70.
43. Lazzerini, M. Association between orofacial granulomatosis and Crohn's disease in children: Systematic review. *World J. Gastroenterol.* **2014**, *20*, 7497. [CrossRef] [PubMed]
44. Rutgeerts, P.; Geboes, K.; Vantrappen, G.; Beyls, J.; Kerremans, R.; Hiele, M. Predictability of the postoperative course of Crohn's disease. *Gastroenterology* **1990**, *99*, 956–963. [CrossRef] [PubMed]
45. Sorrentino, D. Infliximab With Low-Dose Methotrexate for Prevention of Postsurgical Recurrence of Ileocolonic Crohn Disease. *Arch. Intern. Med.* **2007**, *167*, 1804. [CrossRef] [PubMed]
46. Ruemmele, F.M.; Veres, G.; Kolho, K.L.; Griffiths, A.; Levine, A.; Escher, J.C.; Amil Dias, J.; Barabino, A.; Braegger, C.P.; Bronsky, J.; et al. Consensus guidelines of ECCO/ESPGHAN on the medical management of pediatric Crohn's disease. *J. Crohns Colitis* **2014**, *8*, 1179–1207. [CrossRef]
47. Simon, M.; Pariente, B.; Lambert, J.; Cosnes, J.; Bouhnik, Y.; Marteau, P.; Allez, M.; Colombel, J.F.; Gornet, J.M. Long-term Outcomes of Thalidomide Therapy for Adults With Refractory Crohn's Disease. *Clin. Gastroenterol. Hepatol.* **2016**, *14*, 966–972.e2. [CrossRef]
48. Hershfield, N. Disappearance of Crohn's Ulcers in the Terminal Ileum after Thalidomide Therapy. *Can. J. Gastroenterol.* **2004**, *18*, 101–104. [CrossRef]

biomedicines

MDPI

Article

The Diagnostic Significance of SLC26A2 and Its Potential Role in Ulcerative Colitis

Lijuan Qian [1,†], Shuo Hu [2,†], Haizhou Zhao [2], Ye Han [2], Chenguang Dai [1], Xinquan Zan [2,*], Qiaoming Zhi [2,*] and Chunfang Xu [1,*]

1 Department of Gastroenterology, The First Affiliated Hospital of Soochow University, Suzhou 215006, China; zzxmd@126.com (L.Q.); daicg_soochow@163.com (C.D.)

2 Department of General Surgery, The First Affiliated Hospital of Soochow University, Suzhou 215006, China; hushuo1996@163.com (S.H.); zhz19950125@163.com (H.Z.); hanyeor@163.com (Y.H.)

* Correspondence: zanxinquan@163.com (X.Z.); strexboy@163.com (Q.Z.); xcf601@163.com (C.X.)

† These authors contributed equally to this work.

Abstract: Background/Objectives: The solute carrier family 26, member 2 (SLC26A2) gene, which belongs to the family of SLC26 transporters, can be detected in multiple tissues. However, the studies of SLC26A2 in colon-related diseases are still limited and incompletely understood, especially in ulcerative colitis (UC). **Methods:** In this study, we attempted to search and identify putative UC candidate genes within a large number of known genes by multiple bioinformatics analyses. The potential cellular characteristics and biological functions of SLC26A2 in the pathogenesis of UC were also elucidated. **Results:** Notably, SLC26A2 was representative and down-regulated in the intestinal mucosa of patients with active UC, compared to healthy controls. Decreased levels of SLC26A2 were proved to have a more value in diagnosis of UC patients, and closely correlated with some UC characteristics, including the Mayo score and Paediatric Ulcerative Colitis Activity Index (PUCAI). Mechanistically, subsequent results from published datasets and our validated clinical data all strongly implied that SLC26A2 was negatively correlated with the IL-17 signaling pathway, and positively associated with the tight junction, which led to abnormal immune cell infiltration and inflammatory injuries. After establishing the UC mice models in vivo by orally administration of DSS in portable water, SLC26A2 was significantly down-regulated at the mRNA or protein level, when compared to that in the control groups. Furthermore, the correlation analyses confirmed that SLC26A2 was positively associated with CLDN3, and negatively correlated with IL-17A expression in colon tissues. In addition, according to the SLC26A2 expression, UC patients were divided into different subgroups. The potential target drugs for UC treatment, such as progesterone, tetradioxin, and dexamethasone, were initially predicted and exerted anti-inflammatory effects via the common molecule-SLC26A2. **Conclusions:** SLC26A2 might be served as a protective candidate in the UC pathogenesis as well as a potential drug target for UC treatment.

Keywords: SLC26A2; diagnosis; ulcerative colitis; IL-17 signaling pathway; tight junction

1. Introduction

Ulcerative colitis (UC) is a chronic, relapsing, and remitting inflammatory disorder of the colon. It starts from the rectum and can extend proximally to involve the whole colon. Based on the anatomic extent of involvement, patients can be divided into proctitis (E1, disease limited to the rectum), left-sided colitis (E2, distal to splenic flexure) and extensive colitis (E3, disease extends proximal to splenic flexure [1,2]. In recent decades, the incidence and prevalence rates of UC have steadily increased in several regions of the world, especially in developing countries, which have placed a heavy health and economic burden on society [3]. Traditionally, the methods of UC detection include patient-reported symptoms, basic clinical and laboratory tests, as well as endoscopic, histologic and imaging assessments [4,5]. However, those traditionally used methods, such as the most commonly used laboratory markers, including C-reactive protein (CRP), the erythrocyte sedimentation rate (ESR), fecal lactoferrin (FL) and fecal calprotectin (FC), are often nonspecific, inaccurate, or unsatisfactory in the diagnosis and monitoring of this disease [6]. Therefore, searching better biomarkers for predicting the UC prognostication and development are still urgently needed [7].

The solute carrier family 26, member 2 (SLC26A2) gene, which belongs to the family of SLC26 transporters and encodes for a sulfate/chloride antiporter of the cell membrane, is pivotal to the uptake of inorganic sulfate [8]. Previous studies had confirmed that a strong signal for SLC26A2 mRNA and protein immunostaining could be detected in developing fetal hyaline cartilage [9]. Patients with different phenotypes of inherited chondrodysplasias experienced skeletal defects mainly due to SLC26A2 mutations or pathogenic variants, resulting in defective sulfate absorption and uptake in enterocytes and chondrocytes [10]. Furthermore, SLC26A2 expression might also be detected in multiple tissues, such as the eccrine sweat glands, bronchial glands, placental villi, exocrine pancreas, and adrenal cortex [9,11]. As early as 2001, SLC26A2 mRNA expression could be detected in the normal colon, mainly in the absorptive epithelial and goblet cells [12]. Pitule et al. firstly found that SLC26A2 expression was significantly down-regulated in colorectal cancer (CRC) tissues, and patients with a higher expression of SLC26A2 in tumor tissues had a longer overall survival (OS) and disease-free interval (DFI) [13]. However, the studies of SLC26A2 in colon-related diseases are still limited and incompletely understood, especially in inflammatory bowel disease (IBD). In 2009, Comelli et al. identified some novel ileal and colonic genes in Crohn's disease (CD) and/or UC patients, and SLC26A2 was found to be up-regulated only in Crohn's colon, but not in Crohn's ileum or an UC-inflamed ileum and colon, compared to the healthy epithelium [14]. The opposite results of the study by Bjerrum et al. reported that the expression of SLC26A2 was decreased in patients with IBD as having UC or CD [15]. In 2025, a recent study from Zhang et al. firstly focused on nicotinamide adenine dinucleotide (NAD+)-related genes to reveal their potential pivotal roles in UC. SLC26A2 was strongly associated with respiratory electron transport. However, their PCR data for SLC26A2 did not show any significant statistical differences, which could be attributed to an insufficient sample size and differences in patient medication (the authors only selected five UC and five control patients for PCR validation) [16].

Since the first publication two decades ago describing the use of microarray in IBD, this method appears as a good possibility for finding more information on differentially expressed genes and isoforms in UC [17–19]. Subsequently, other novel technologies or advances, such as high-throughput next-generation sequencing (NGS) or single-cell RNA sequencing (scRNA-seq) have been applied and transformed biological research, allowing them to collect more accurate and proficient information during the UC initiation and development, and elucidate biological mechanisms even at the cellular level [20–23]. In this study, we attempted to identify the UC-associated molecules by WGCNA analyses, and evaluate the potential clinical significance of these involved genes in UC colon samples. SLC26A2 was significantly down-regulated in UC colon tissues, and selected for our further experiment. Then, enrichment analyses in GSE87466 and GSE109142 demonstrated the potential relationships between SLC26A2 levels and inflammation signals. Subsequently, using the GSE231993 dataset, multiple bioinformatics analyses at the level of a single-cell RNA-seq further revealed the potential cellular characteristics and biological functions of

SLC26A2 in the pathogenesis of UC. According to the SLC26A2 expression, UC patients were divided into different subgroups, and potential target drugs for UC treatment were also initially predicted. In addition, using the UC mice models by oral administration of DSS in portable water, the potential relationships between SLC26A2 and some related molecules of tight junctions (and IL-17 signals) were discussed in vivo.

2. Materials and Methods

2.1. Data Acquisition and Sample Collection

We obtained the data from the Gene Expression Omnibus (GEO) database (https://www.ncbi.nlm.nih.gov/geo/ (accessed on 22 November 2024) and followed the principles outlined below: (1) Microarray, RNA-seq, and single-cell sequencing data were comprehensively included to ensure reliable results. (2) The dataset for bulk RNA-seq analysis of UC must contain more than 100 samples. (3) The samples of UC must be accompanied by detailed clinical characteristics. For discovery, we selected GSE87466, GSE109142, and GSE56298. For validation, we used GSE92415. The detailed information of the included datasets was is presented in Table 1. The raw data were downloaded, and if not available, the series matrix files were downloaded. The RNA-seq data were normalized to transcripts per kilobase per million mapped reads (TPM) format. In detail, gene exon length information was obtained using the "GenomicFeatures" package (version 1.58.0) in R. Reads per kilobase (RPK) values were calculated using the formula: counts/(exon_lengths/1000). Subsequently, RPK values were scaled by the sample-specific scaling factor and multiplied by one million to derive TPM values.

Table 1. Data information in this study.

GEO ID	Source	Platform	Participants	Tissues	Attribute
GSE87466	Array	GPL13158	87 active UC and 21 controls	Mucosal	Discovery
GSE109142	RNA-seq	GPL16791	206 active UC and 20 controls	Mucosal	Discovery
GSE231993	Single cell RNA-seq	GPL18573	4 active UC and 4 controls containing 37,967 cells	Mucosal	Discovery
GSE92415	Array	GPL13158	87 active UC with clinical characteristics	Mucosal	Validation

In addition, 57 colonic mucosa samples from patients diagnosed with UC through digestive endoscopy and pathology were collected. These patients were registered in the Department of Gastroenterology (or General Surgery) at the First Affiliated Hospital of Soochow University from April 2019 to December 2022. Simultaneously, 20 colonic mucosa samples were collected from healthy individuals. Samples were immediately stored in liquid nitrogen upon removal during endoscopy or surgery. The clinical characteristics were collected concurrently. This research work was granted approval by the ethics committee of the First Affiliated Hospital of Soochow University (2022-431) on 20 March 2022.

2.2. Weighted Gene Co-Expression Network Analysis (WGCNA)

We performed a WGCNA to identify gene clusters with similar expression patterns, and to identify the most relevant gene clusters associating with UC. Cluster trees of the samples were constructed to exclude any abnormal samples. Subsequently, we selected the top 15,000 genes with a high standard deviation for analysis. The soft threshold power β was determined using the "pickSoftThreshold" function in the R package "WGCNA" (version 1.72.1), which served as the primary tool for this analysis [24]. Genes in the module that showed the highest correlation with UC traits were selected for further analysis.

2.3. Identification of Differentially Expressed Genes (DEGs)

We used the R package "limma" (version 3.56.2) to identify genes that were differentially expressed in a statistically significant manner. Genes with an adjusted p value < 0.05 and a $|\text{logFC}| > 2$ were selected.

2.4. Quantitative Real-Time Polymerase Chain Reaction (qRT-PCR)

RNA extraction from fresh frozen tissues was performed using a TRIzol reagent (Invitrogen, Waltham, MA, USA), and complementary DNA (cDNA) was synthesized using a Prime Script RT Master Mix (Takara, Osaka, Japan). Primers were designed using the "Primer-BLAST" website (https://www.ncbi.nlm.nih.gov/tools/primer-blast/index.cgi (accessed on 20 November 2024)). The reaction and quantification were performed using a FastStart Universal SYBR Green Master (Roche, Mannheim, Germany), and data processing was carried out on a LightCycler 96 System. The expressing levels were quantified using ΔCt, which meant the average Ct value of target genes minus the Ct value of GAPDH. The primers applied for PCR analysis were listed as follows: ABCB1 (Human): forward, 5′-TTGCTGCTTACATTCAGGTTTCA-3′, reverse, 5′-AGCCTATCTCCTGTCGCATTA-3′; AQP8 (Human): forward, 5′-GCGAGTGTCCTGGTACGAAC-3′, reverse, 5′-CAGGCACCC GATGAAGATGAA-3′; SLC26A2 (Human): forward, 5′-GGCTCCCAAAATACGACCTAAA-3′, reverse, 5′-GGCACCAATAATATGCCCACAA-3′; CFTR (Human): forward, 5′-AAAAGG CCAGCGTTGTCTCC-3′, reverse, 5′-AAACATCGCCGAAGGGCATTA-3′; CLDN3 (Human): forward: 5′- AACACCATTATCCGGGACTTCT-3′, reverse, 5′-GCGGAGTAGACGAC CTTGG-3′; CLDN7 (Human): forward: 5′-AGCTGCAAAATGTACGACTCG-3′, reverse, 5′-GGAGACCACCATTAGGGCTC-3′; MYL6 (Human): forward, 5′-GAAGACCAGACCGCA GAGTTC-3′; reverse, 5′-TCCAGCACCTTCACATTCATC-3′; SLC9A3R1 (Human): forward, 5′-GGCTGGCAACGAAAATGAGC-3′; reverse, 5′-TGTCGCTGTGCAGGTTGAAG-3′; GAPDH (Human): forward, 5′-GGAGCGAGATCCCTCCAAAAT-3′, reverse, 5′-GGCTGTTGTCATACTTCTCATGG-3′; SLC26A2 (Mice): forward, 5′-AAGAGCAGCATGA CCTCTCAC-3′, reverse, 5′-CTGCCTCAAGTCAGTGCCT-3′; CLDN3 (Mice): forward, 5′-ACCAACTGCGTACAAGACGAG-3′, reverse, 5′-CGGGCACCAACGGGTTATAG-3′; IL-17A (Mice): forward, 5′-TTTAACTCCCTTGGCGCAAAA-3′, reverse, 5′-CTTTCCCTCCGC ATTGACAC-3′; and GAPDH (Mice): forward, 5′-AGGTCGGTGTGAACGGATTTG-3′, reverse, 5′-TGTAGACCATGTAGTTGAGGTCA-3′.

2.5. Correlation Analysis

We performed correlation analysis between genes and clinical characteristics using the Spearman method, considering p-values less than 0.01 as statistically significant. After that, we calculated the scores for the IL-17 signaling pathway and immune cell subtypes using the ssGSEA method, and determined their correlation values using the Spearman method. In addition, a similar correalation method was also employed to reveal the relationships between gene or protein expressions in vivo.

2.6. Single-Gene Gene Set Enrichment Analysis (Single-Gene GSEA)

The UC samples were evenly divided into the high and low expression groups based on the expressing levels of the target gene. Gene Set Enrichment Analysis (GSEA) was performed based on the gene set "c2.cp.kegg.v7.2.symbols.gmt" using the R package "clusterProfiler" (version 4.8.2) [25]. Pathways that ranked among the top 50% based on adjusted p-values less than 0.05 were considered statistically significant.

2.7. Single Sample Gene Set Enrichment Analysis (ssGSEA)

The enrichment scores for the IL-17 signaling pathway were determined using the gene set "IL-17 Family Signaling Pathways" from the "GeneCards" database (https://www.genecards.org/ (accessed on 20 November 2024)). Furthermore, the enrichment scores for 28 immune cell subtypes were evaluated using an annotated gene set downloaded from the "MSigDB" database (https://www.gsea-msigdb.org/gsea/msigdb/index.jsp (accessed on 20 November 2024)). The above enrichment analysis was performed using the R packages "GSEABase" (version 1.62.0) and "GSVA" (version 1.48.3).

2.8. Data Processing of Single-Cell Sequencing and Cell Communication Analysis

We used the R package "Seurat" (version 4.3.0.1) to process the data from single-cell sequencing. Firstly, we excluded cells with a gene expression count of less than 200 or more than 7000, and retained cells with a mitochondrial gene expression ratio greater than 20%. Subsequently, we selected the top 2000 highly variable genes using the "FindVariableFeatures" function, and normalized them using the "vst" method. After that, we eliminated the batch effect using the R package "harmony" (version 0.1.1) [26]. Finally, we performed cell clustering using the "FindClusters" function, and assigned labels to the clusters using the R package "singleR" (version 2.2.0) [27]. In addition, we utilized the R package "cellchat" (version 1.1.3) [28], which relied on the "CellChatDB" database, to study intercellular communications between epithelial cells and other cells in the UC colonic mucosa.

2.9. High-Dimension Weighted Gene Co-Expression Network Analysis (hdWGCNA)

Due to the sparse matrix nature of the single-cell sequencing data, we employed hdWGCNA to explore the co-expression of genes with SLC26A2 and the specific functions of the gene cluster involving SLC26A2 in epithelial cells. We utilized the R package "hdWGCNA" (version 0.2.19) to accomplish the task [29]. Genes expressed in epithelial cells (at least 5%) were included based on the "SetupForWGCNA" function by setting up the fraction threshold as 0.05. Subsequently, metacells were constructed using the "MetacellsByGroups" function based on the KNN algorithm. The metacells should contain more than 50 cells and fewer than 15 cells shared with others. The optimal soft power value was determined using the "TestSoftPowers" function, which was employed to construct the co-expression network.

2.10. Construction of PPI Network

We queried the "STRING" database (https://cn.string-db.org/ (accessed on 20 November 2024)) to explore the interaction network of target proteins, which encompasses a comprehensive collection of known and predicted proteins, as well as their potential relationships [30–33]. We uploaded proteins associated with SLC26A2, the IL-17 signaling pathway, tight junctions, and other effectors activated in epithelial cells of UC. The results were exported to Cytoscape software (version 3.9.1), and the nodes were ranked based on their "Degree" scores, which were calculated using "Hytohubba" [34]. The darker color indicated a higher "Degree" value, which signified a more prominent position in the network.

2.11. Pathway Enrichment and Drug Prediction Analysis

We conducted KEGG pathway enrichment and drug prediction analysis using the online tool "Enrichr" (https://maayanlab.cloud/Enrichr/ (accessed on 20 November 2024)), a comprehensive platform that encompassed over 400,000 terms [35–37]. We uploaded the DEGs ($|logFC| > 1$, adjusted p value < 0.05) obtained from comparing samples with high expression levels of SLC26A2 to those with low expression levels. Subsequently, drugs targeting these DEGs were enriched using the "DSigDB" library within the "Enrichr" platform.

2.12. Establishment of UC Model In Vivo

UC was induced by oral administration of 3% DSS in portable water. A total of 20 6-week-old male mice (BALB/c, 18–20 g in weight) were divided into the Control (n = 10) and UC group (n = 10). Mice in the Control or UC groups drank water or 3.0% DSS (35,000–50,000, MW, MP Biomedicals, Santa Ana, CA, USA) for 7 days, respectively. On the seventh day, all mice were sacrificed, and colons were collected from the ileocecal junction to the anus, and opened longitudinally. Half of the colon was fixed in 4% paraformaldehyde for hematoxylin and eosin (H&E) and immunofluorescence (IF) staining; the other half was frozen in liquid nitrogen for qRT-PCR. All experimental procedures were granted approval by the Experimental Animal Care and Use Committee (the First Affiliated Hospital of Soochow University) (2024-658) on 20 December 2024.

2.13. Hematoxylin and Eosin (H&E) and Immunofluorescence (IF) Staining

Colon tissues were fixed in 10% neutral buffered formalin. Paraffin-embedded tissues were prepared, cut into sections (4-μm thickness) and stained with H&E. Then, H&E-stained sections were observed by two blinded pathologists, and the histological scores were determined according to the crypt damage, infiltration of neutrophils, and foci of ulceration in the detected colons [38]. For IF staining, colon slides were dewaxed, and the primary SLC26A2 (1:200, PA5-76918, Invitrogen, USA), CLDN3 (1:300, YT0949, Immunoway, San Jose, CA, USA), or IL-17A (1:500, ab302922, Abcam, Waltham, MA, USA) antibody was added for 2 h at 37 °C. Then, the slides were incubated with the secondary antibody (BS10007, 1:100, Bioworld, Tulare County, CA, USA). Finally, the slides were counter-stained with DAPI and imaged. The fluorescence intensity was calculated by Image J software (version 1.54k).

2.14. Statistical Analyses

All statistical analyses were conducted using R software (version 4.2.2) and GraphPad Prism 9 (version 9.5.1). The Spearman correlation method was employed for correlation analysis. The data from different groups were compared by a Student's t test. The p-values were adjusted using the default Benjamini–Hochberg correction method, with a significance level of 0.05 for all analyses unless otherwise specified. The flowchart was drawn by Figdraw (https://www.figdraw.com/static/index.html#/ (accessed on 20 November 2024)) (Figure 1).

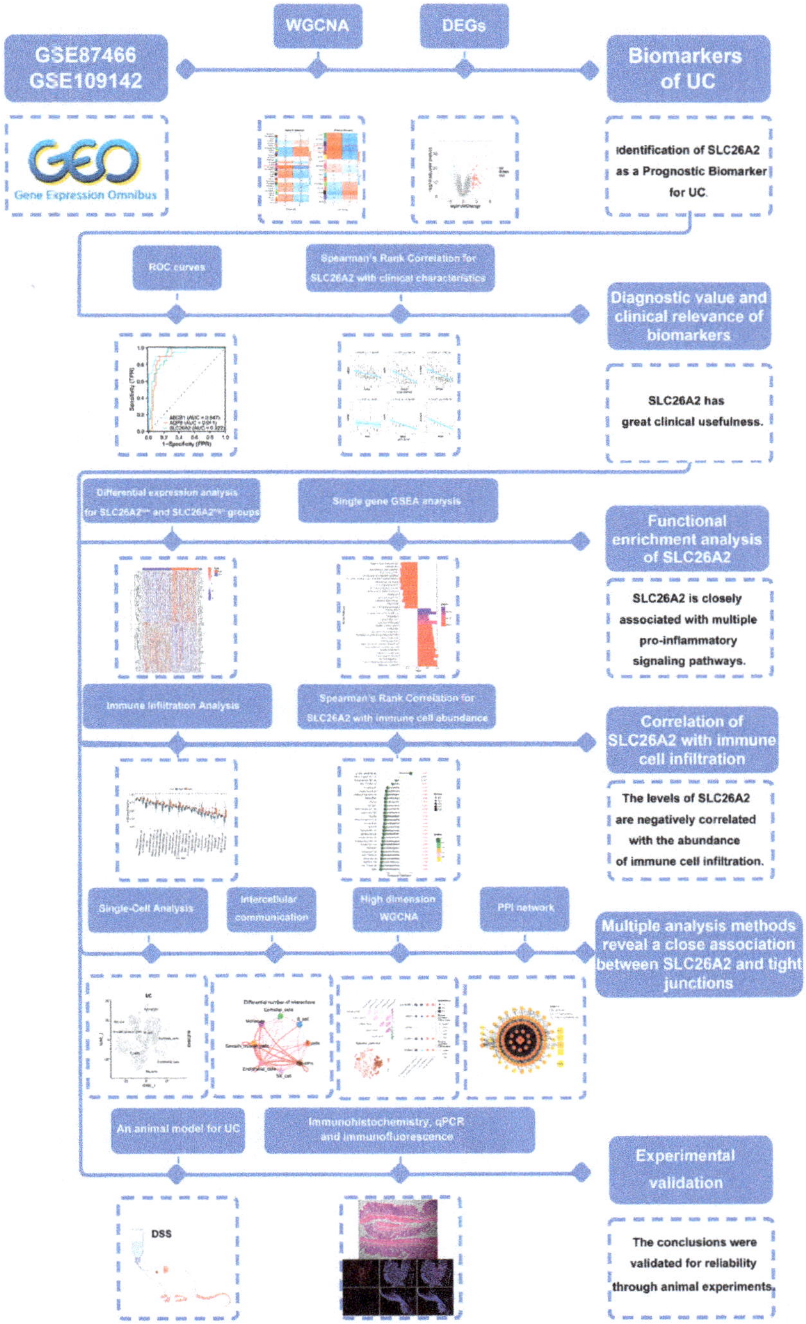

Figure 1. The flowchart of the analysis process.

3. Results

3.1. The Screening of Potential UC-Related Molecules by WGCNA Analyses

WGCNA analyses were conducted on the datasets GSE87466 and GSE109142 after excluding abnormal samples, and the resulting cluster trees were depicted in Figure S1A.

Soft thresholds of 14 and 18 were selected to achieve a scale-free degree distribution for genes in GSE87466 and GSE109142, resulting in the identification of 30 and 16 modules, respectively (Figures 2A and S1B). Subsequently, correlation analysis was performed, revealing that the magenta module in GSE87466 and purple module in GSE109142 exhibited the strongest correlations with UC (Figure 2B). Genes within the magenta module (n = 429, cor = 0.78, $p = 8.1 \times 10^{-92}$) and purple module (n = 348, cor = 0.83, $p = 9.6 \times 10^{-90}$) demonstrated strong correlations with UC, and were chosen for our subsequent studies (Figure 2C). In addition, differential expression analyses were conducted. A total of 134 (85 up-regulated and 49 down-regulated) in GSE87466 and 320 DEGs (242 up-regulated genes and 78 down-regulated) in GSE109142 were screened as possible UC related genes (Figure 2D). Finally, using the Venn analysis, three genes (ABCB1, AQP8, and SLC26A2) were identified through intersection analysis of genes from DEGs and WGCNA modules, and considered as potential UC-associated molecules (Figure 2E).

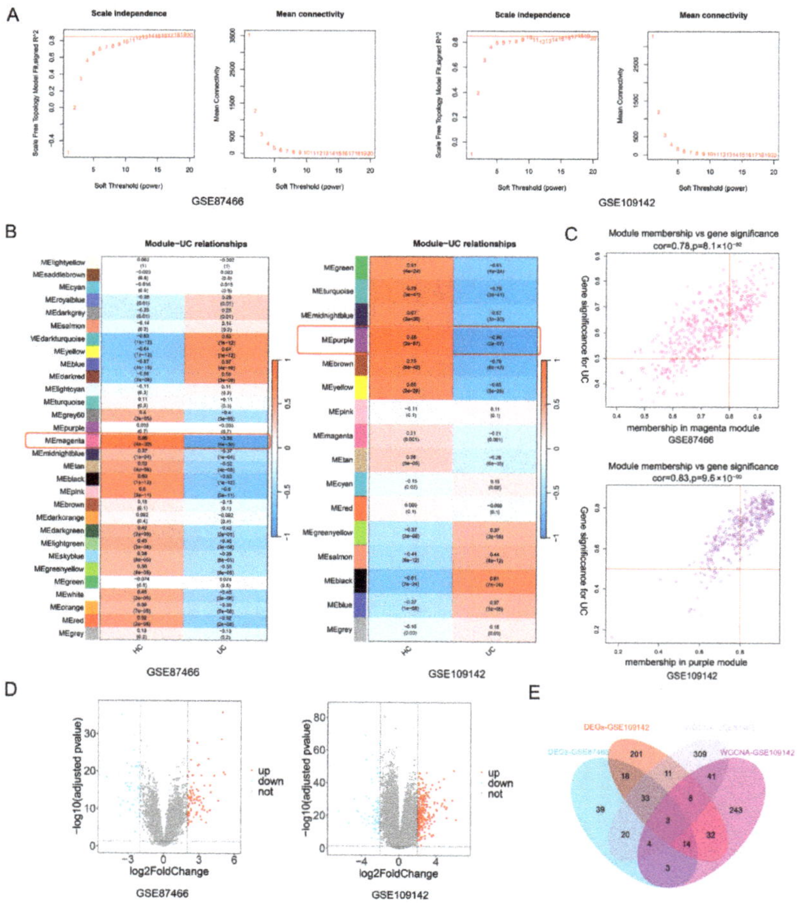

Figure 2. Screening of potential UC-related molecules. (**A**) Selection of the soft threshold for WGCNA (GSE87466 and GSE109142). (**B**) The heatmaps indicated the correlations between modules and UC. Red boxes indicate that magenta module in GSE87466 and purple module in GSE109142 exhibited the strongest correlations with UC. (**C**) The scatterplots showed the relationships between gene significance and module membership in the magenta module of GSE87466 and purple module of GSE109142. (**D**) The volcano plots displayed all the DEGs. (**E**) The Venn diagram illustrates the overlapping genes.

3.2. Clinical Significance of Potential UC-Related Molecules

The expressing levels of these three genes were validated between healthy controls and UC samples. In GSE87466 and GSE109142, the mRNA expressions of ABCB1, AQP8, and SLC26A2 were all significantly down-regulated in UC samples, when compared to healthy controls (Figure 3A,B). Fortunately, the same results were also observed in our collected UC samples, and these three genes were all down-regulated with all *p*-values < 0.0001 (*t*-test) (Figure 3C). Then, the receiver operating characteristic (ROC) curves were used to evaluate the potential usages and values of tissue-derived ABCB1, AQP8, and SLC26A2 as novel biomarkers for UC diagnosis. As shown in Figure 3D, the areas under the curve (AUC) for three datasets (GSE87466, GSE109142, and our validated clinical samples) all exceeded 0.9. These data strongly confirmed the remarkable diagnostic performances of these down-regulated genes in UC diagnosis.

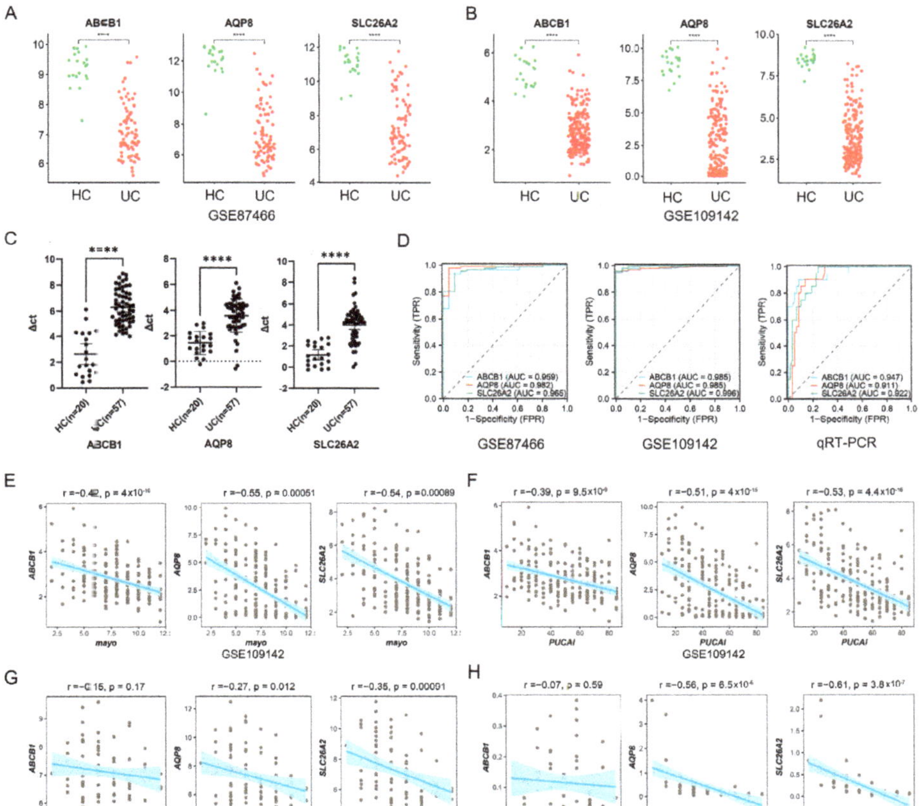

Figure 3. Validate the clinical significance of potential UC related molecules. (**A**,**B**) The boxplots illustrated the expressing levels of 3 UC-related molecules between healthy controls and UC samples in the GSE87466 (**A**) and GSE109142 (**B**) datasets, respectively. (**C**) The ABCB1, AQP8, and SLC26A2 mRNA expressions in our collected UC samples were also determined by the RT-PCR. (**D**) ROC curves were used to evaluate the potential usages and values of tissue-derived ABCB1, AQP8, and SLC26A2 as invasive biomarkers for UC diagnosis. (**E**–**H**) The Spearman correlation analyses revealed the possible relationships between 3 UC-related genes (ABCB1, AQP8, and SLC26A2) and some significant clinical characteristics, including the Mayo and PUCAI scores in UC samples from GSE109142, GSE92415, and our collected UC samples, respectively. (**** $p < 0.0001$).

We further examined the relationships between these three UC-related genes (ABCB1, AQP8, and SLC26A2) and some significant clinical characteristics. For instance, Spearman correlation analyses revealed that down-regulated ABCB1, AQP8, and SLC26A2 were all negatively correlated with the Mayo scores as well as the PUCAI scores in UC samples from GSE109142 (Figure 3E,F). However, ABCB1 and AQP8 exhibited poor performance in GSE92415 ($p > 0.01$), and ABCB1 was not associated with the Mayo score according to our self-test statistics (Figure 3G,H). Consequently, we selected SLC26A2 for our further investigations due to its outstanding diagnostic performance and clinical significance.

3.3. Enrichment Analysis of SLC26A2 and Its Potential Role in the UC Pathogenesis

Single-gene GSEA analysis was conducted on SLC26A2. Samples were reorganized based on their expressing levels and divided into two groups (SLC26A2 high and low expression) according to the median value. The heatmaps in Figure 4A depicted the top 30 up- and 30 down-regulated genes from GSE87466 and GSE109142, respectively. The DEGs were then utilized for KEGG enrichment analyses. Surprisingly, the IL-17 signaling pathway played a prominent role in both GSE87466 and GSE109142, which was also supported by the subsequent GSEA analysis (Figure 4B,C). Additionally, the GSEA results revealed that SLC26A2 positively or negatively associated with different signaling pathways. Among them, some inflammation- or immune-related signals, such as the IL-17 signaling pathway, NF-kappa B signaling pathway, Toll-like receptor signaling pathway, TNF signaling pathway, and JAK-STAT signaling pathway, were negatively associated with the levels of SLC26A2. However, the tight junction and some metabolism-related signals were positively correlated with SLC26A2 (Figure 4D). These intriguing findings motivated us to further investigate the possible role of SLC26A2 in UC. Next, we took the IL-17 signaling pathway as an example. The scores of the IL-17 signaling pathway in each sample were calculated using the ssGSEA method. Interestingly, the ssGSEA data showed that the scores of the IL-17 signaling pathway were significantly lower in the high SLC26A2 expression group, when compared to the low expression group (Figure 5A). Furthermore, we also observed a strong negative–correlation between the SLC26A2 expressing levels and scores of the IL-17 signaling pathway (Figure 5B). Since SLC26A2 was proved to negatively regulate the inflammation- or immune-related signaling pathways, we speculated that this novel gene might influence the immune cell infiltration during the UC pathogenesis. Thus, a subsequent immune cell infiltration analysis was conducted, and the results revealed that low SLC26A2 levels might lead to more recruitment of immune cells, including different types of innate- and adaptive-immune related cells (Figure 5C). In addition, the scores of involved immune cells were also found to negatively correlate with the SLC26A2 levels (Figure 5D). Based on the above enrichment analyses from GSE87466 and GSE109142, we proposed SLC26A2 as a novel negatively regulated gene in the UC development. Decreased SLC26A2 expression might activate some inflammation- or immune-related signals, and loosen the tight junction between intestinal epithelial cells, finally leading to more immune cell infiltration and inflammatory injuries.

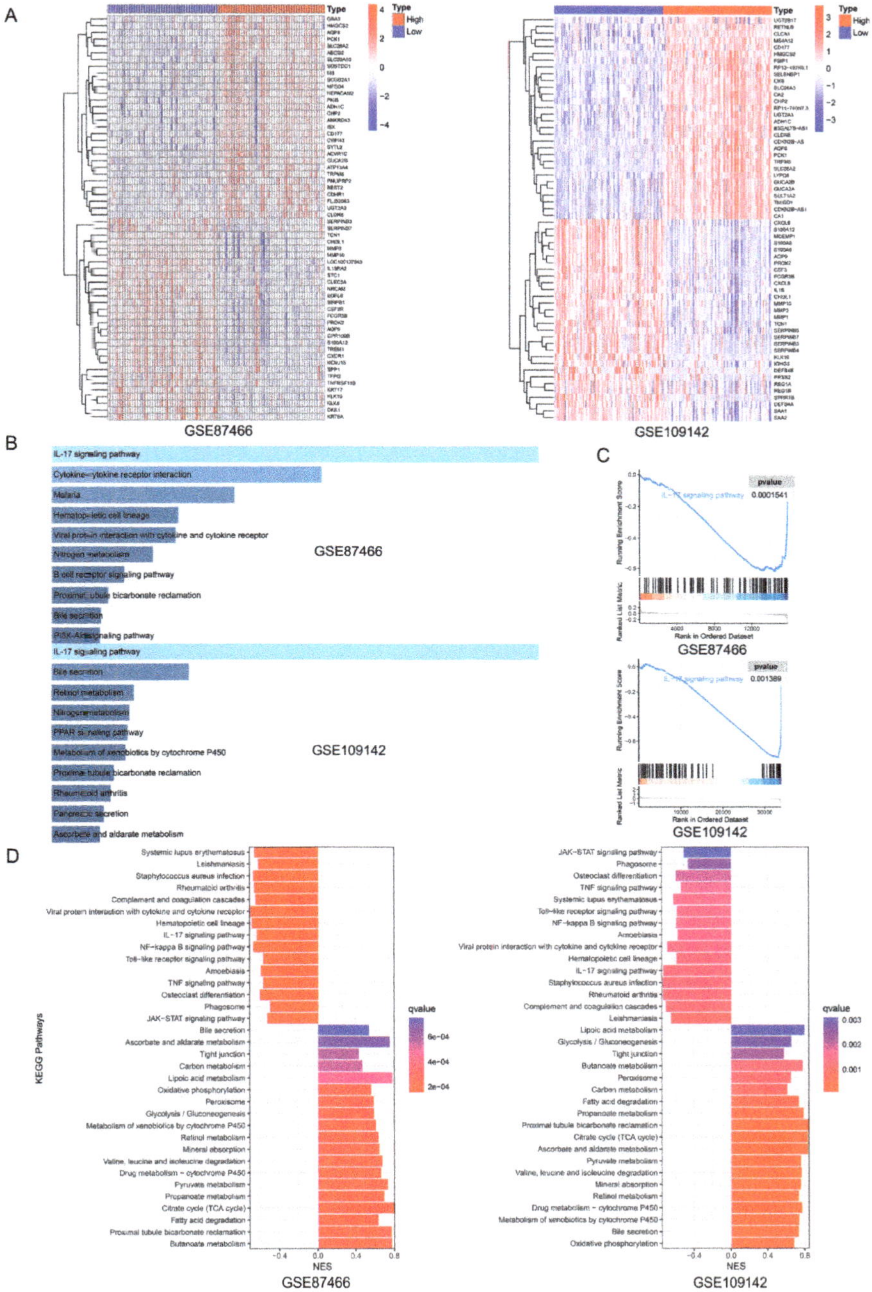

Figure 4. Single gene GSEA analysis was conducted on SLC26A2. (**A**) The heatmaps displayed the top 30 up-regulated and 30 down-regulated genes in the high-SLC26A2 expressed groups, compared to the low-expressed groups. (**B**) The KEGG pathway enrichment analyzed the DEGs in the GSE87466 and GSE109142 datasets. (**C**) The GSEA implied that SLC26A2 was negatively associated with the IL-17 signaling pathway. (**D**) The barplots illustrated the top 50% of enriched pathways in the GSE87466 and GSE109142 datasets.

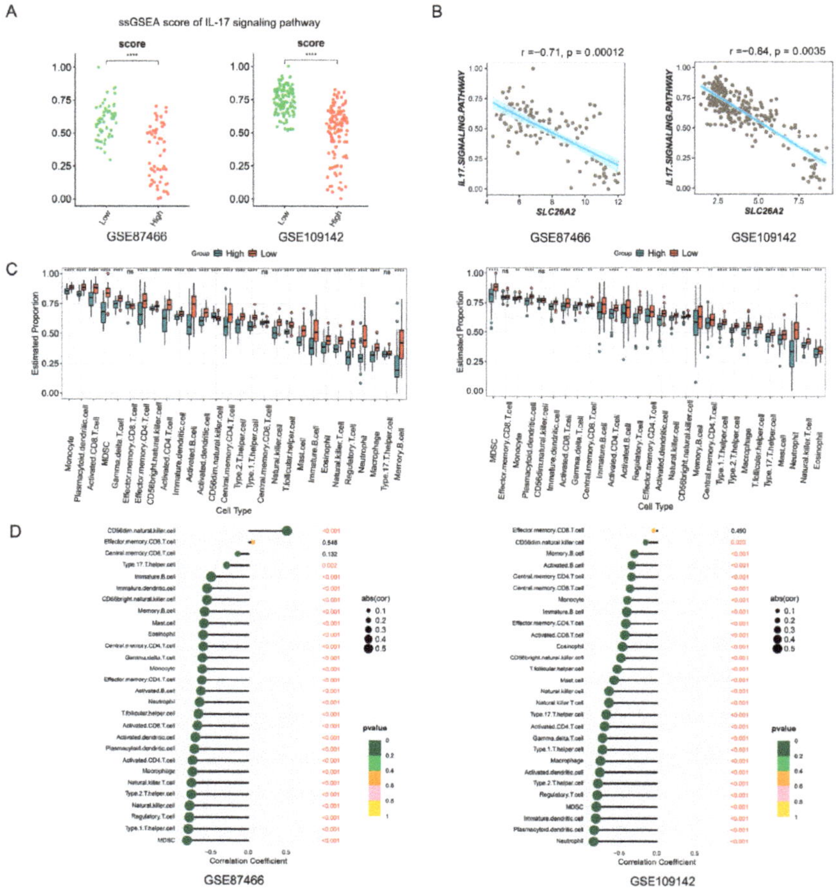

Figure 5. According to the expressing levels of SLC26A2, ssGSEA of the IL-17 signaling pathway and immune cell clusters were performed in the GSE87466 and GSE109142 datasets, respectively. (**A**) The scores of the IL-17 signaling pathway were significantly lower in the high SLC26A2 expression group, compared to the low expression group. (**B**) A strong negative correlation between the SLC26A2 expressing levels and scores of the IL-17 signaling pathway was observed by the Spearman correlation analyses. (**C**) The boxplots illustrated the differences in immune infiltration between the high and low expression groups of SLC26A2. (**D**) The correlations between immune cell infiltration and SLC26A2 were also estimated. (* $p < 0.05$, ** $p < 0.01$, *** $p < 0.001$, **** $p < 0.0001$ and ns: no significance).

3.4. Localization Analysis of SLC26A2 in Single-Cell Sequencing Data During the UC Pathogenesis

Single-cell RNA sequencing (scRNAseq) is a powerful approach for allowing researchers to profile the transcriptomes of thousands of cells simultaneously and study the genetic makeup of individual cells. In GSE231993, the gene count, mRNA count, and mitochondrion ratio in each cell were presented in Figure S1C. The number of principal components (PCs) was initially set to 30 based on the elbow plot (Figure S1D). Following the computation of "FindNeighbors" and "FindClusters", cells from eight samples were segregated into 16 clusters based on their principal components, rather than samples, as shown in Figure 6A,B. Subsequently, clusters were signed as T cells, B cell, Epithelial cells, Monocyte, Smooth muscle cells, Endothelial cells, NK cells, and Neurons using the "SingleR" package by comparing cell characteristics with its five internal databases (Figure 6C).

As shown in Figure 6D,E, we observed that SLC26A2 was predominantly expressed in healthy intestinal epithelial cells, while its expression was relatively lower in epithelial cells of UC (Figure 6D,E). Thus, we focused on the epithelial cells and conducted further analysis of cell–cell interactions, which revealed numerous differential expression patterns of signaling pathways between healthy individuals and individuals with UC (Figure 6F). In UC epithelial cells, the MIF, APP, and MK signaling pathways were activated, compared to healthy colonic epithelial cells, whereas GALECTIN was inactivated in UC (Figure 6G). Further in-depth analysis showed the relatively activated signaling pathways in UC epithelial cells communicating with others, compared to other cell types, with particular relevance to epithelial cells, monocytes, smooth muscle cells, endothelial cells, and NK cells (Figure 6H). All the above data aroused our interest in understanding the role of SLC26A2 in intestinal epithelial cells during the UC pathogenesis.

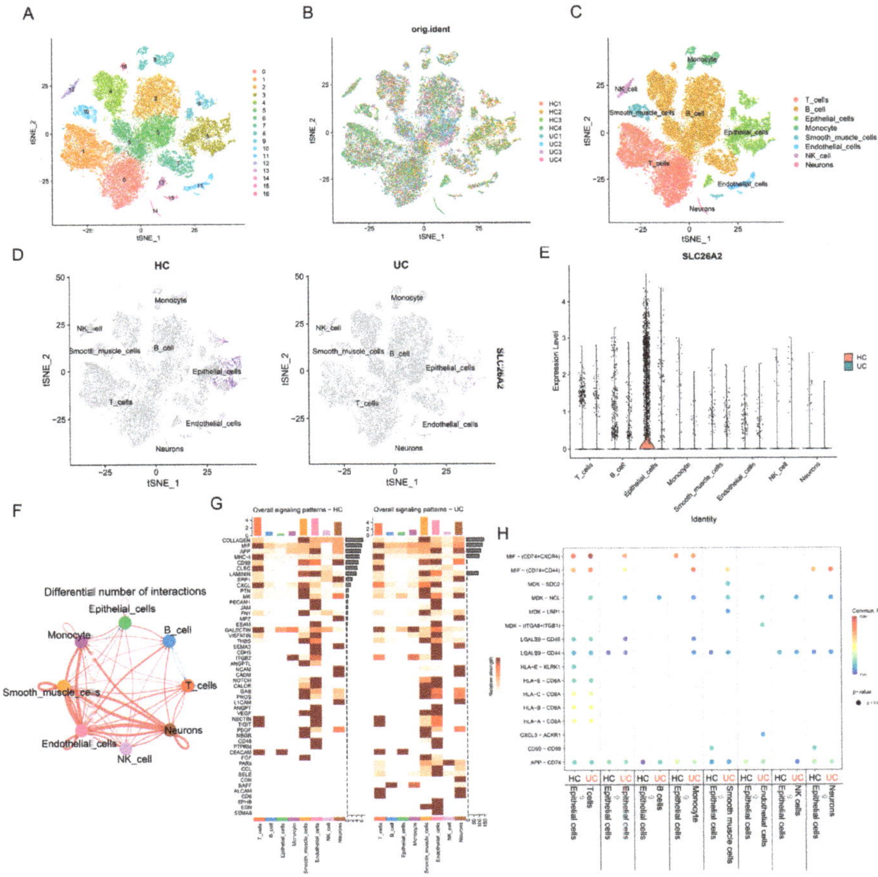

Figure 6. Localization analysis of SLC26A2 in single-cell sequencing data. (**A–D**) tSNE plots visualized the cell clusters, original identities, cell annotation, and localization of SLC26A2 in healthy controls and individuals with UC, respectively. (**E**) The distribution of SLC26A2 in cells with annotation was visualized as a violin plot. (**F**) Integrated map of the different numbers of interactions detected between each cell and other cells was presented. (**G**) Intensity demonstration of cell populations in different pathways in healthy controls and individuals with ulcerative colitis. (**H**) Differential signaling pathways in epithelial cells between healthy controls and individuals with UC revealed the diverse biological functions of epithelial cells.

3.5. High-Dimensional Weighted Gene Co-Expression Network Analysis (hdWGCNA) Revealed the Potential Biological Functions of SLC26A2 at the Level of Single-Cell RNA-Seq

Accordingly, we conducted hdWGCNA to identify the gene clusters, which were associated with SLC26A2, and gained deeper insights into its biological functions in UC. Metacells were generated from a large population of epithelial cells, and genes expressed in more than 5% of cells were selected for WGCNA. The genes displayed a scale-free degree distribution when the soft power was set to 5 (Figure 7A). As a result, these genes were clustered into five distinct modules, along with a grey module in which genes had no co-expressed partners (Figure 7B). As shown in Figure 7C, the brown module, in which SLC26A2 was located, presented significant correlations with "nFeature_RNA" (number of detected genes in cells), "nCount_RNA" (number of detected mRNAs in cells) and "tissue type" (healthy controls or ulcerative colitis). Furthermore, we conducted KEGG pathway enrichment analysis on the genes in the brown module. Notably, the tight junction pathway was once again found to be enriched, as previously observed in the analysis of bulk RNA sequencing data using single gene GSEA (Figures 4D and 7D). The correlation analysis indicated indicates that the brown module exhibited weak correlations with other modules, and the gene scores calculated by UCells in the brown module were highest in epithelial cells, implying a distinct biological function this module possessed (Figure 7E,F). Taking all factors into consideration, our attention was primarily directed towards the IL-17 signaling pathway and the tight junction pathways. Subsequent correlation analysis of bulk RNA sequencing data among genes involved in the tight junction, IL-17 signaling pathway, and immune cells validated our hypothesis. SLC9A3R1, MYL6, CLDN7, and CLDN3, which were involved in the tight junction pathway in the brown module, displayed negative correlations with the IL-17 signaling pathway and the majority of immune cells, while exhibiting a positive correlation with SLC26A2 (Figure 7G,H).

3.6. PPI Network Construction and Drug Prediction

In order to elucidate the underlying mechanisms of SLC26A2 in tight junction regulation, we constructed the protein-protein interaction (PPI) network involving SLC26A2, tight junction proteins, IL-17 signaling pathway-related proteins, and activated proteins in epithelial cells from individuals with UC. The network revealed the possibility that SLC26A2 might primarily interact with CFTR, thereby influencing the related proteins, which were involved in the IL-17 signaling pathway and downstream tight junction proteins. Furthermore, the activated proteins in the epithelial cells of individuals with UC also played a pivotal role in the interaction network (Figure 8A). In addition, we determined the expressions of downstream tight junction genes in our collected colonic samples by qRT-PCR. The data demonstrated that the expressions of CFTR, CLDN3, CLDN7, and SLC9A3R1 were all down-regulated in UC tissues, in comparison with healthy controls, except for MYL6 (Figure 8B). Subsequent correlation analysis confirmed that the SLC26A2 levels in 57 UC samples were positively correlated with the expressions of CFTR, CLDN3, SLC9A3R1, and MYL6 (Figure 8C). These data partly re-confirmed SLC26A2 as a tight junction-associated gene during the UC development.

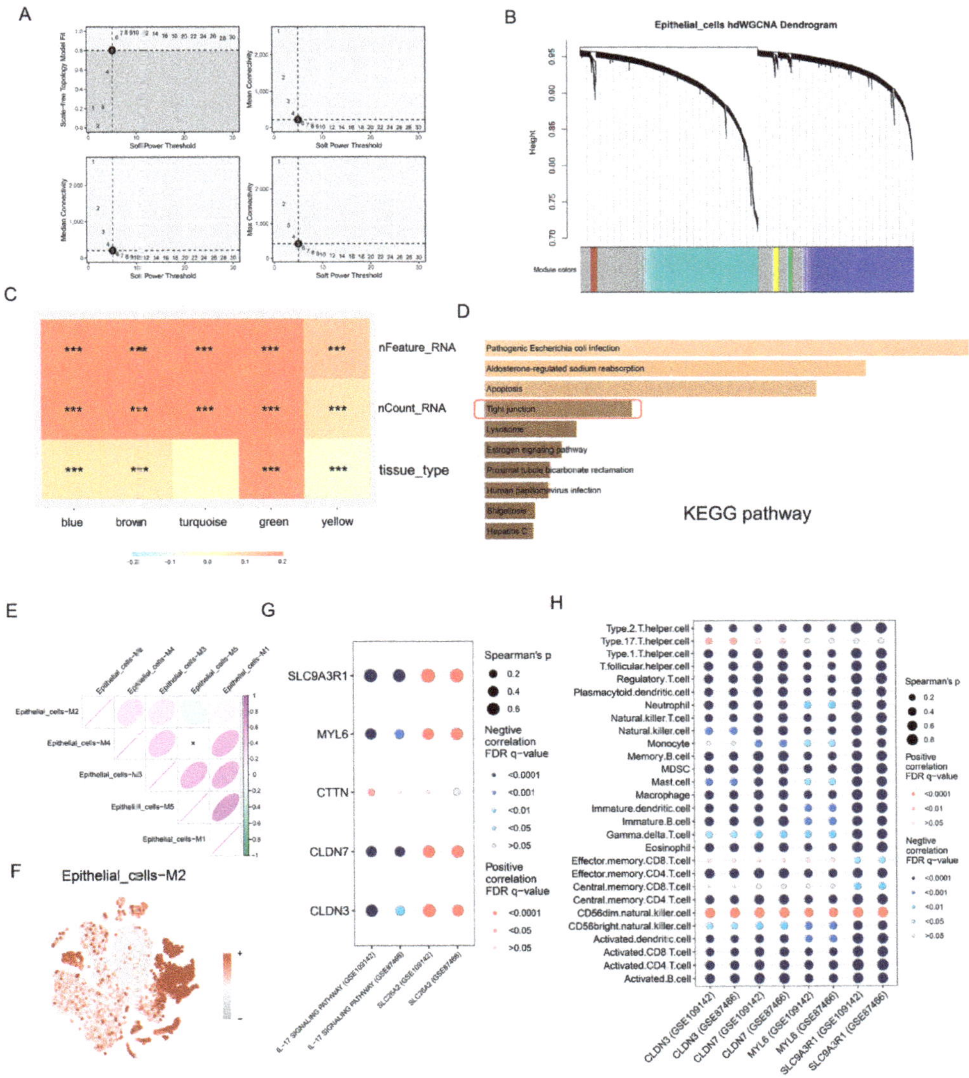

Figure 7. hdWGCNA revealed the potential biological functions of SLC26A2 at the level of single-cell RNA-seq. (**A**) The scale-free topology model displayed the scale-free fit index and the mean connectivity for various soft-thresholding powers. (**B**) The dendrogram illustrated illustrates the different modules in which genes are clustered. (**C**) The correlations between traits and modules were are shown in the correlation heatmap. (**D**) The KEGG pathways enriched by the genes in the brown module were listed, and the tight junction pathway (marked by a red box) was enriched. (**E**) The potential correlations among modules were calculated using the Pearson method. (**F**) Gene scores of the brown module were calculated using the UCell algorithm and presented in each cell. (**G**) The correlations between the genes involved in the tight junction in the brown module and SLC26A2 (as well as the IL-17 signaling pathway), were analyzed using the Spearman method. (**H**) Similar Spearman analyses were conducted between the genes involved in the tight junction in the brown module and immune cell subtypes. (*** $p < 0.001$).

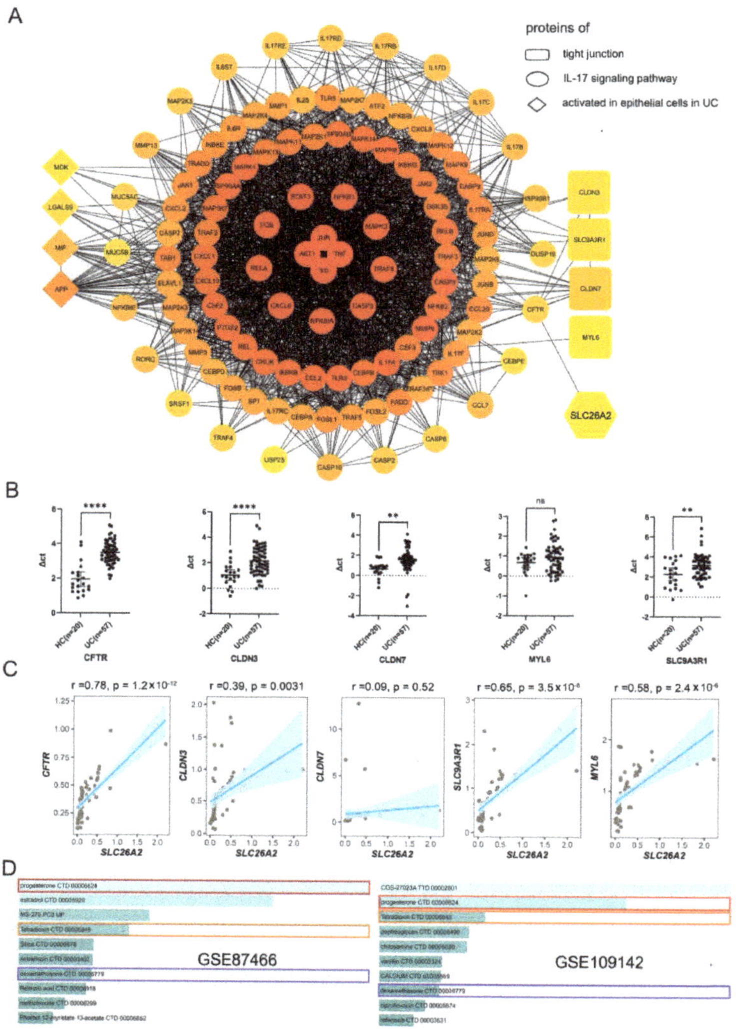

Figure 8. The relationship between SLC26A2 and tight junction genes. (**A**) The PPI network demonstrated the relationships among involved proteins, including SLC26A2, tight junction proteins, the IL-17 signaling pathway, and activated molecules in epithelial cells in UC. (**B**) The mRNA expressing levels of CFTR, CLDN3, CLDN7, MYL6, SLC26A3R1, and SLC26A2 were determined by the qRT-PCR. (**C**) The potential correlations between SLC26A2 and CFTR (CLDN3, CLDN7, MYL6, SLC26A3R1 and SLC26A2, respectively) were analyzed. (**D**) According to the expressing levels of SLC26A2 in GSE87466 and GSE109142 datasets, putative drugs were predicted, and the top 10 drugs were described. Progesterone CTD 00006624, tetradioxin CTD 00006848, and dexamethasone CTD 00005779 were highly co-enriched and indicated by the red, orange and blue boxes respectively. (** $p < 0.01$, **** $p < 0.0001$, and ns: no significance).

Moreover, we identified drugs that targeted the DEGs between the high and low expressing groups of SLC26A2 in GSE87466 and GSE109142 datasets. The results listed the top 10 potential targeted drugs through SLC26A2. Among them, progesterone CTD 00006624, tetradioxin CTD 00006848, and dexamethasone CTD 00005779 were highly co-enriched (Figure 8D). This meant that these involved drugs might exerted anti-UC effects through the common molecule-SLC26A2.

3.7. SLC26A2 Closely Associated with Tight Junctions and IL-17 Signals In Vivo

To further reveal the potential relationships between SLC26A2 and tight junctions (or IL-17 signals) in vivo. Firstly, we established the UC mice models by the oral administration of DSS in portable water, and colon length and histological score were calculated (Figure 9A–D). Then, we determined the mRNA expressions of SLC26A2, CLDN3, and IL-17A in all mice colons. The data showed that SLC26A2 was significantly down-regulated in the UC colon tissues, compared to that in the control groups (Figure 9E). The correlation analysis initially implied that the colon SLC26A2 expression was negatively correlated with the inflammatory injury score, which indicated SLC26A2 as a protective factor in the occurrence of UC (Figure 9F). Subsequent PCR results also showed that the CLDN3 mRNA expression was significantly down-regulated, while IL-17A was up-regulated during the UC development (Figure 9G,H). Interestingly, subsequent correlation analyses also confirmed that SLC26A2 was positively associated with CLDN3, and negatively correlated with IL-17A expression in colon tissues (Figure 9I,J). To further observe the potential relationships between SLC26A2 and CLDN3 (or IL-17A) at protein levels, we performed the IF staining and their corresponding fluorescence intensities of SLC26A2, CLDN3, and IL-17A were calculated (Figure 10A–F). Fortunately, the data was consistent with our results of the PCR analyses, which partly implied that decreased SLC26A2 expression might disrupt the tight junctions between colonic epithelial cells, and positively associated the activation of the IL-17 signaling pathway in vivo (Figure 10G,H).

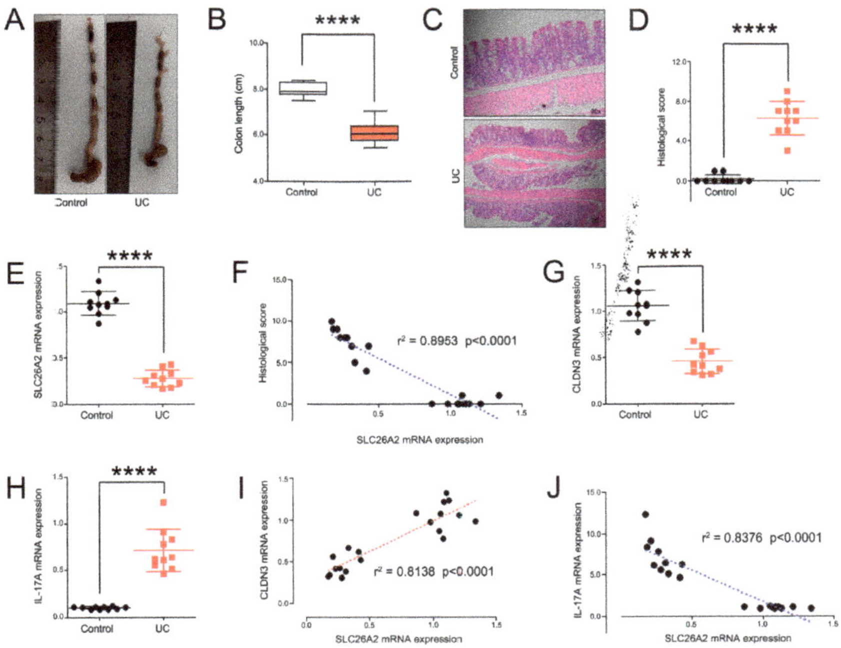

Figure 9. The relationships between SLC26A2 and CLDN3 (or IL-17A) at mRNA levels in vivo. (**A**) Photos of mice colon in each group. (**B**) The colon length of mice on 7th day in the control and UC groups. (**C**,**D**) The colons were stained by H&E, and the corresponding histological scores were compared. (**E**,**F**) The SLC26A2 mRNA expressions in each group were detected by qRT-PCR, and correlation analysis showed the potential relationships between SLC26A2 and histological scores. (**G–J**) The CLDN3 and IL-17A mRNA expressions in each group were also determined by qRT-PCR, and the relationships between SLC26A2 and CLDN3 (or IL-17A) were evaluated. (**** $p < 0.0001$).

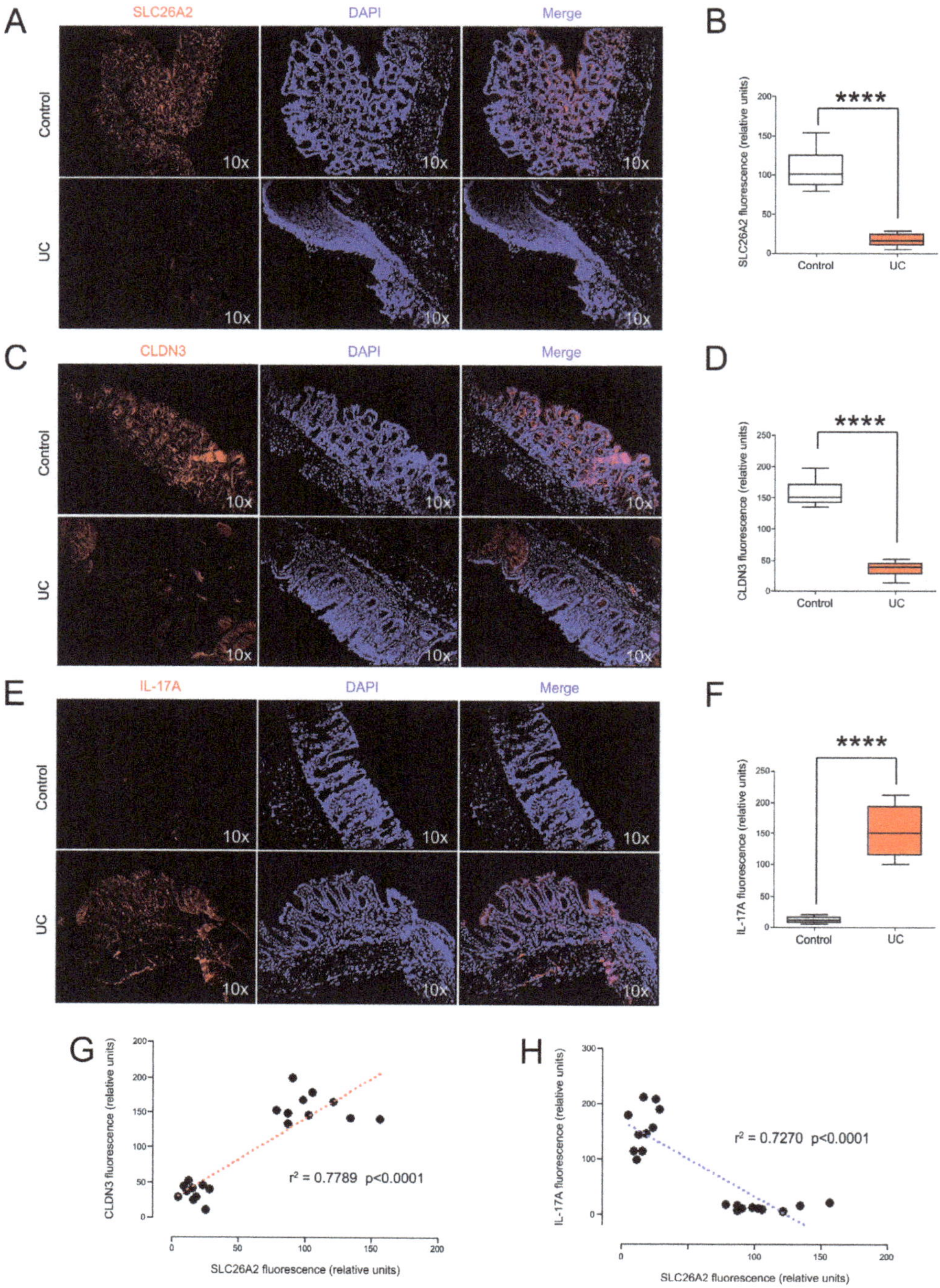

Figure 10. The relationships between SLC26A2 and CLDN3 (or IL-17A) at protein levels in vivo. (**A–F**) The protein expressions of SLC26A2, CLDN3 and IL-17A in mice colon were determined by immunofluorescence, and the fluorescence quantification was compared. (**G**,**H**) Spearman–Pearson correlation between SLC26A2 and CLDN3 (or IL-17A) fluorescence intensity in mice was analyzed. (**** $p < 0.0001$).

4. Discussion

Despite the progresses in the management of UC over the past few centuries, much less has been achieved in the diagnosis, detection, and monitoring of this disease. Fortunately, we have entered a new era for transcriptome analysis, due to the advances and applications of newly developed technologies, such as microarrays, NGS, next-generation sequencing (TGS), scRNA-seq, and spatial transcriptomics (ST). Many investigators have now noticed the significance of available big data and used multiple analysis methods to disclose the new causes or mechanisms of diverse diseases [39–42]. Recently, we combined long-read sequencing technology with short-read RNA-seq methods to investigate the transcriptome complexity in CRC. Newly identified splicing isoform TIMP1 Δ4–5 was proved to play a crucial role in mediating the CRC progression, and might be a potential therapy target in CRC [43]. Similarly, we also made attempts at IBD detection. For instance, we successfully used the method of the K-means clustering algorithm to identify human PRKAR2A-derived circRNAs as novel candidates for predicting colitis-associated cancer (CAC). However, the data between UC and healthy controls are not satisfactory, and RTEL1-derived circRNAs had no clinical significance in human UC patients [19]. In this study, to identify putative UC candidate genes within a large number of known genes, differential expression analysis on microarray and RNA-seq datasets were performed from the GSE87466 and GSE109142, including 107 UC and 227 healthy control samples. WGCNA analyses were conducted, and the corresponding modules were selected. The Venn analysis initially considered ABCB1, AQP8, and SLC26A2 as potential UC-associated molecules. This was very interesting and significant. For instance, the ABCB1 expression was strongly diminished in the intestinal mucosa of patients with active UC [44,45]. Similarly, the putative gene AQP8 was also found to be down-regulated in UC tissues, and possibly correlates with the immune cell infiltration of neutrophils, monocytes, and macrophages [46,47]. These published results were consistent with our validated data from the GSE87466, GSE109142, and our collected colon samples.

Notably, in this study, SLC26A2 presented a more statistical significance and clinical value in diagnosis and correlation analysis of some clinical features, including the Mayo score and PUCAI in multiple validated colon samples. However, the potential mechanisms of SLC26A2 in the occurrence and development of UC has not been fully elucidated. Both single-gene GSEA analysis from GSE87466 and GSE109142, and the subsequent KEGG enrichment analyses all implied that the SLC26A2 expression negatively associated with some inflammatory signaling pathways, including the IL-17 signaling pathway, NF-kappa B signaling pathway, Toll-like receptor signaling pathway, TNF signaling pathway, and JAK-STAT signaling pathway. Taking the IL-17 signaling pathway, for example, IL-17 functions as a pivotal pro-inflammatory cytokine predominantly secreted by Th17 cells, and the levels of IL-17 are significantly increased in the intestinal mucosa and serum of active UC patients [48–50]. The potential inflammatory effects of IL-17 were partly derived from its synergistic functions with other cytokines and its ability to recruit excessive inflammatory cells, such as neutrophils and the production of chemokines, which in turn intensified the tissue injuries of colon mucosa [51,52]. Fortunately, our ssGSEA data showed that scores of the IL-17 signaling pathway were significantly lower in the high SLC26A2 expression group, and a strong negative correlation between the SLC26A2 expressing levels and scores of the IL-17 signaling pathway was also observed. These results strongly implied that SLC26A2 could be proposed as a protective candidate in the UC pathogenesis, and reduced levels of SLC26A2 might activate the pro-inflammatory cytokines and signaling pathways, finally leading to more immune cell infiltration and inflammatory injuries.

Of course, we need more evidence to support our hypothesis that decreased SLC26A2 expression is a major underlying cause in the initiation and progression of UC. Analyzing the obtained scRNA-seq information from the GSE231993 dataset, SLC26A2 was found to be predominantly expressed in healthy intestinal epithelial cells, compared to other types of cells, such as T cells, B cell, epithelial cells, monocyte, smooth muscle cells, endothelial cells, NK cells, and neurons. Meanwhile, its expressing levels in epithelial cells of UC were significantly decreased, in comparison with healthy intestinal epithelial cells. This meant means that SLC26A2 might play a suppressing role in UC mainly through the intestinal epithelial cells. In addition, the existed existing cell—cell interactions, and potential communicated signals between epithelial cells and other cell types, were explicitly displayed. To further reveal the putative mechanism of SLC26A2 at the level of single-cell RNA-seq, hdWGCNA was conducted. Our data showed that the brown module, in which SLC26A2 was also involved, was most representative with the features of UC. Importantly, results of KEGG from the brown module implied that the tight junction pathway was closely involved. Previous studies have indicated that tight junctions, adherens junctions, and desmosomes are essential components for the contacts between adjacent intestinal epithelial cells [53]. Tight junctions act as the "kissing points" between neighboring cells, which can form a continuous protective seal to maintain the correct regulation of the intestinal barrier. In the pathogenesis of UC, the intestinal tight junction disruption, including its composition and integrity, can be clearly observed in the inflamed colonic mucosa [54–56]. To confirm our hypothesis, we selected the representative genes involved in the tight junction pathway of the brown module, including SLC9A3R1, MYL6, CTTN and CLDN3. The subsequent correlation analyses strongly demonstrated that these tight junction pathway-related genes negatively correlated with the IL-17 signaling pathway and majority of immune cells, while they positively associated with the SLC26A2 expressions. Then, the PPI network and our validated results of PCR analysis all showed that SLC26A2 actually interacted with CFTR, thereby influencing the tight junction-related proteins and IL-17 signaling pathway. Furthermore, we successfully established the mice models by oral administration of DSS in portable water, and found that SLC26A2 was significantly down-regulated in colons, when compared to the control groups. More importantly, correlation analyses showed that SLC26A2 was positively associated with CLDN3, and negatively correlated with IL-17A expression in colon tissues. These data provided us with new evidence of SLC26A2 as a protective factor during the UC pathogenesis in vivo.

We had proved SLC26A2 as a putative biomarker and target in the pathogenesis of UC. According to the SLC26A2 expression, UC patients were divided into different subgroups, and potential target drugs were also initially predicted. Progesterone, tetradioxin, and dexamethasone demonstrated the potential for use in the treatment of UC. The data implied that these three predicted drugs might exert an anti-inflammatory effect through the potential target SLC26A2 gene. In fact, this study has certain limitations. Firstly, the potential and usage of SLC26A2 target drugs for UC treatment is only a speculation. The exact mechanisms remain elusive, which still need more experimental evidence to support in the future. Secondly, the causal relationships between SLC26A2 and tight junctions (or the IL-17 signaling pathway) remain unclear. We still need a series of experiments, such as constructing an SLC26A2 transgenic mice model in vivo and SLC26A2 over-expressing colon epithelial cells in vitro, to reveal its possible upstream or downstream relationships with tight junctions as well as IL-17 signals. Thirdly, our data in this study only included a total of 57 UC patients. An insufficient sample size might affect the statistical analyses of the corresponding clinical data. Finally, our study only included some existing published databases for data mining and analysis. If more data platforms can be added in the future for supplementation, they may provide us with a more in-depth understanding of SLC26A2 in UC.

5. Conclusions

In conclusion, our data identified some putative UC candidate genes within a large number of known genes by multiple bioinformatics analyses, including ABCB1, AQP8, and SLC26A2. Notably, SLC26A2 was representative and down-regulated in the intestinal mucosa of patients with active UC, compared to healthy controls. Decreased levels of SLC26A2 were proven to have a more value in the diagnosis of UC patients, and closely correlated with some UC characteristics, including the Mayo score and PUCAI. Mechanistically, the results strongly showed that SLC26A2 was negatively correlated with the IL-17 signaling pathway, and positively associated with the tight junction, which led to abnormal immune cell infiltration and inflammatory injuries during the pathogenesis of UC. Though larger well-designed studies with more clinical and experimental data are required, to the best of our knowledge, this study is the first report to evaluate the potential role of SLC26A2 in UC. SLC26A2 can be served as a novel protective candidate in the UC pathogenesis as well as a putative drug target for UC treatment.

Supplementary Materials: The following supporting information can be downloaded at: https://www.mdpi.com/article/10.3390/biomedicines13020461/s1, Figure S1: Sample clusters and quality control. (A) The cluster tree showed the clusters of samples after removing the outliers. (B) The dendrogram displayed the different modules in which genes were clustered. (C) The violin plot presented the gene count, mRNA count, and the ratio of mitochondrion in each cell in single-cell RNA sequencing (scRNA-seq) data. (D) The elbow plot indicated the relationship between the count of principal components and standard deviation.

Author Contributions: L.Q., S.H. and Y.H. designed the study and wrote the manuscript. H.Z. provided the technical and writing support. C.D., X.Z., Q.Z. and C.X. designed the study and revised the manuscript. All authors have read and agreed to the published version of the manuscript.

Funding: This research was funded by the Natural Science Foundation of the Jiangsu Higher Education Institutions of China (24KJA320005), Suzhou Gusu Medical Youth Talent (GSWS2019032), Suzhou Medical and Health Technology Innovation Application Basic Research Project (SKJY2021060), Science and Technology Program of Suzhou (SKY2022139), and Horizontal Cooperation Project of Soochow University (H230753 and H241466).

Institutional Review Board Statement: This study was approved by the ethics committee of The First Affiliated Hospital of Soochow University (2022-431) on 20 March 2022. All experimental procedures were granted approval by the Experimental Animal Care and Use Committee (the First Affiliated Hospital of Soochow University) (2024-658) on 20 December 2024.

Informed Consent Statement: Written informed consent was obtained from all participants before recruitment.

Data Availability Statement: The datasets (Nos. GSE87466, GSE109142, GSE56298 and GSE92415) generated and/or analyzed during the current study are available in the Gene Expression Omnibus (GEO) database (https://www.ncbi.nlm.nih.gov/geo/ (accessed on 22 November 2024)).

Conflicts of Interest: The authors declare no conflicts of interest.

References

1. Suarez Ferrer, C.; Mendoza, M.I.V.; Roman, L.A.S.; Lama, Y.G.; Moya, M.C.; Casas, M.G.; Garcia, L.A. Risk of thromboembolic phenomena in patients with inflammatory bowel disease. *Gastroenterol. Hepatol.* **2012**, *35*, 634–639. [PubMed]
2. Narang, V.; Kaur, R.; Garg, B.; Mahajan, R.; Midha, V.; Sood, N.; Sood, A. Association of endoscopic and histological remission with clinical course in patients of ulcerative colitis. *Intest. Res.* **2018**, *16*, 55–61. [CrossRef]
3. Buie, M.J.; Quan, J.; Windsor, J.W.; Coward, S.; Hansen, T.M.; King, J.A.; Kotze, P.G.; Gearry, R.B.; Ng, S.C.; Mak, J.W.Y.; et al. Global Hospitalization Trends for Crohn's Disease and Ulcerative Colitis in the 21st Century: A Systematic Review with Temporal Analyses. *Clin. Gastroenterol. Hepatol.* **2023**, *21*, 2211–2221. [CrossRef]

4. M'Koma, A.E. Inflammatory Bowel Disease: Clinical Diagnosis and Surgical Treatment-Overview. *Medicina* **2022**, *58*, 567. [CrossRef] [PubMed]
5. Feuerstein, J.D.; Cheifetz, A.S. Ulcerative colitis: Epidemiology, diagnosis, and management. *Mayo Clin. Proc.* **2014**, *89*, 1553–1563. [CrossRef] [PubMed]
6. Matowicka-Karna, J. Markers of inflammation, activation of blood platelets and coagulation disorders in inflammatory bowel diseases. *Postepy. Hig. Med. Dosw. (Online)* **2016**, *70*, 305–312. [CrossRef] [PubMed]
7. Liu, D.; Saikam, V.; Skrada, K.A.; Merlin, D.; Iyer, S.S. Inflammatory bowel disease biomarkers. *Med. Res. Rev.* **2022**, *42*, 1856–1887. [CrossRef]
8. Li, J.; Xia, F.; Reithmeier, R.A. N-glycosylation and topology of the human SLC26 family of anion transport membrane proteins. *Am. J. Physiol. Cell. Physiol.* **2014**, *306*, C943–C960. [CrossRef]
9. Haila, S.; Hästbacka, J.; Böhling, T.; Karjalainen-Lindsberg, M.L.; Kere, J.; Saarialho-Kere, U. SLC26A2 (diastrophic dysplasia sulfate transporter) is expressed in developing and mature cartilage but also in other tissues and cell types. *J. Histochem. Cytochem.* **2001**, *49*, 973–982. [CrossRef] [PubMed]
10. Biji, I.K.; Yadav, S.; Kulshrestha, S.; Saxena, R.; Kohli, S.; Verma, I.C.; Kumar, B.; Puri, R.D. Computational biology insights into genotype-clinical phenotype-protein phenotype relationships between novel SLC26A2 variants identified in inherited skeletal dysplasias. *Eur. J. Med. Genet.* **2022**, *65*, 104595. [CrossRef]
11. Spyroglou, A.; Bozoglu, T.; Rawal, R.; De Leonardis, F.; Sterner, C.; Boulkroun, S.; Benecke, A.G.; Monti, L.; Zennaro, M.C.; Petersen, A.K.; et al. Diastrophic dysplasia sulfate transporter (SLC26A2) is expressed in the adrenal cortex and regulates aldosterone secretion. *Hypertension* **2014**, *63*, 1102–1109. [CrossRef] [PubMed]
12. Haila, S.; Saarialho-Kere, U.; Karjalainen-Lindsberg, M.L.; Lohi, H.; Airola, K.; Holmberg, C.; Hastbacka, J.; Kere, J.; Hoglund, P. The congenital chloride diarrhea gene is expressed in seminal vesicle, sweat gland, inflammatory colon epithelium, and in some dysplastic colon cells. *Histochem. Cell. Biol.* **2000**, *113*, 279–286. [CrossRef]
13. Pitule, P.; Vycital, O.; Bruha, J.; Novak, P.; Hosek, P.; Treska, V.; Hlavata, I.; Soucek, P.; Kralickova, M.; Liska, V. Differential expression and prognostic role of selected genes in colorectal cancer patients. *Anticancer. Res.* **2013**, *33*, 4855–4865. [PubMed]
14. Comelli, E.M.; Lariani, S.; Zwahlen, M.C.; Fotopoulos, G.; Holzwarth, J.A.; Cherbut, C.; Dorta, G.; Corthesy-Theulaz, I.; Grigorov, M. Biomarkers of human gastrointestinal tract regions. *Mamm. Genome.* **2009**, *20*, 516–527. [CrossRef] [PubMed]
15. Bjerrum, J.T.; Nyberg, C.; Olsen, J.; Nielsen, O.H. Assessment of the validity of a multigene analysis in the diagnostics of inflammatory bowel disease. *J. Intern. Med.* **2014**, *275*, 484–493. [CrossRef] [PubMed]
16. Zhang, L.; Li, J.; Zhang, Q.; Gao, J.; Zhao, K.; Asai, Y.; Hu, Z.; Gao, H. An Integrative analysis of single-cell RNA-seq, transcriptome and Mendelian randomization for the Identification and validation of NAD(+) Metabolism-Related biomarkers in ulcerative colitis. *Int. Immunopharmacol.* **2025**, *145*, 113765. [CrossRef] [PubMed]
17. Lawrance, I.C.; Fiocchi, C.; Chakravarti, S. Ulcerative colitis and Crohn's disease: Distinctive gene expression profiles and novel susceptibility candidate genes. *Hum. Mol. Genet.* **2001**, *10*, 445–456. [CrossRef]
18. Li, X.L.; Zhou, C.Y.; Sun, Y.; Su, Z.Y.; Wang, X.; Jia, E.N.; Zhang, Q.; Jiang, X.F.; Qi, W.Q.; Xu, Y. Bioinformatic analysis of potential candidates for therapy of inflammatory bowel disease. *Eur. Rev. Med. Pharmacol. Sci.* **2015**, *19*, 4275–4284. [PubMed]
19. Wan, D.; Wang, S.; Xu, Z.; Zan, X.; Liu, F.; Han, Y.; Jiang, M.; Wu, A.; Zhi, Q. PRKAR2A-derived circular RNAs promote the malignant transformation of colitis and distinguish patients with colitis-associated colorectal cancer. *Clin. Transl. Med.* **2022**, *12*, e683. [CrossRef] [PubMed]
20. Fenton, C.G.; Taman, H.; Florholmen, J.; Sorbye, S.W.; Paulssen, R.H. Transcriptional Signatures That Define Ulcerative Colitis in Remission. *Inflamm. Bowel. Dis.* **2021**, *27*, 94–105. [CrossRef]
21. Mitsialis, V.; Wall, S.; Liu, P.; Ordovas-Montanes, J.; Parmet, T.; Vukovic, M.; Spencer, D.; Field, M.; McCourt, C.; Toothaker, J.; et al. Single-Cell Analyses of Colon and Blood Reveal Distinct Immune Cell Signatures of Ulcerative Colitis and Crohn's Disease. *Gastroenterology* **2020**, *159*, 591–608.e10. [CrossRef] [PubMed]
22. Townsend, H.A.; Rosenberger, K.J.; Vanderlinden, L.A.; Inamo, J.; Zhang, F. Evaluating methods for integrating single-cell data and genetics to understand inflammatory disease complexity. *Front. Immunol.* **2024**, *15*, 1454263. [CrossRef] [PubMed]
23. Keever-Keigher, M.R.; Harvey, L.; Williams, V.; Vyhlidal, C.A.; Ahmed, A.A.; Johnston, J.J.; Louiselle, D.A.; Grundberg, E.; Pastinen, T.; Friesen, C.A.; et al. Genomic insights into pediatric intestinal inflammatory and eosinophilic disorders using single-cell RNA-sequencing. *Front. Immunol.* **2024**, *15*, 1420208. [CrossRef] [PubMed]
24. Langfelder, P.; Horvath, S. WGCNA: An R package for weighted correlation network analysis. *BMC Bioinform.* **2008**, *9*, 559. [CrossRef] [PubMed]
25. Subramanian, A.; Tamayo, P.; Mootha, V.K.; Mukherjee, S.; Ebert, B.L.; Gillette, M.A.; Paulovich, A.; Pomeroy, S.L.; Golub, T.R.; Lander, E.S.; et al. Gene set enrichment analysis: A knowledge-based approach for interpreting genome-wide expression profiles. *Proc. Natl. Acad. Sci. USA* **2005**, *102*, 15545–15550. [CrossRef]
26. Korsunsky, I.; Millard, N.; Fan, J.; Slowikowski, K.; Zhang, F.; Wei, K.; Baglaenko, Y.; Brenner, M.; Loh, P.R.; Raychaudhuri, S. Fast, sensitive and accurate integration of single-cell data with Harmony. *Nat. Methods* **2019**, *16*, 1289–1296. [CrossRef] [PubMed]

27. Aran, D.; Looney, A.P.; Liu, L.; Wu, E.; Fong, V.; Hsu, A.; Chak, S.; Naikawadi, R.P.; Wolters, P.J.; Abate, A.R.; et al. Reference-based analysis of lung single-cell sequencing reveals a transitional profibrotic macrophage. *Nat. Immunol.* **2019**, *20*, 163–172. [CrossRef]
28. Jin, S.; Guerrero-Juarez, C.F.; Zhang, L.; Chang, I.; Ramos, R.; Kuan, C.H.; Myung, P.; Plikus, M.V.; Nie, Q. Inference and analysis of cell-cell communication using CellChat. *Nat. Commun.* **2021**, *12*, 1088. [CrossRef] [PubMed]
29. Morabito, S.; Reese, F.; Rahimzadeh, N.; Miyoshi, E.; Swarup, V. hdWGCNA identifies co-expression networks in high-dimensional transcriptomics data. *Cell Rep. Methods* **2023**, *3*, 100498. [CrossRef]
30. Snel, B.; Lehmann, G.; Bork, P.; Huynen, M.A. STRING: A web-server to retrieve and display the repeatedly occurring neighbourhood of a gene. *Nucleic Acids Res.* **2000**, *28*, 3442–3444. [CrossRef]
31. von Mering, C.; Huynen, M.; Jaeggi, D.; Schmidt, S.; Bork, P.; Snel, B. STRING: A database of predicted functional associations between proteins. *Nucleic Acids Res.* **2003**, *31*, 258–261. [CrossRef] [PubMed]
32. Franceschini, A.; Szklarczyk, D.; Frankild, S.; Kuhn, M.; Simonovic, M.; Roth, A.; Lin, J.; Minguez, P.; Bork, P.; von Mering, C.; et al. STRING v9.1 Protein-protein interaction networks, with increased coverage and integration. *Nucleic Acids Res.* **2013**, *41*, D808–D815. [CrossRef] [PubMed]
33. Szklarczyk, D.; Kirsch, R.; Koutrouli, M.; Nastou, K.; Mehryary, F.; Hachilif, R.; Gable, A.L.; Fang, T.; Doncheva, N.T.; Pyysalo, S.; et al. The STRING database in 2023: Protein-protein association networks and functional enrichment analyses for any sequenced genome of interest. *Nucleic Acids Res.* **2023**, *51*, D638–D646. [CrossRef] [PubMed]
34. Shannon, P.; Markiel, A.; Ozier, O.; Baliga, N.S.; Wang, J.T.; Ramage, D.; Amin, N.; Schwikowski, B.; Ideker, T. Cytoscape: A software environment for integrated models of biomolecular interaction networks. *Genome. Res.* **2003**, *13*, 2498–2504. [CrossRef] [PubMed]
35. Chen, E.Y.; Tan, C.M.; Kou, Y.; Duan, Q.; Wang, Z.; Meirelles, G.V.; Clark, N.R.; Ma'ayan, A. Enrichr: Interactive and collaborative HTML5 gene list enrichment analysis tool. *BMC Bioinformatics* **2013**, *14*, 128. [CrossRef]
36. Kuleshov, M.V.; Jones, M.R.; Rouillard, A.D.; Fernandez, N.F.; Duan, Q.; Wang, Z.; Koplev, S.; Jenkins, S.L.; Jagodnik, K.M.; Lachmann, A.; et al. Enrichr: A comprehensive gene set enrichment analysis web server 2016 update. *Nucleic Acids Res.* **2016**, *44*, W90–W97. [CrossRef]
37. Xie, Z.; Bailey, A.; Kuleshov, M.V.; Clarke, D.J.B.; Evangelista, J.E.; Jenkins, S.L.; Lachmann, A.; Wojciechowicz, M.L.; Kropiwnicki, E.; Jagodnik, K.M.; et al. Gene Set Knowledge Discovery with Enrichr. *Curr. Protoc.* **2021**, *1*, e90. [CrossRef]
38. Cooper, H.S.; Murthy, S.; Kido, K.; Yoshitake, H.; Flanigan, A. Dysplasia and cancer in the dextran sulfate sodium mouse colitis model. Relevance to colitis-associated neoplasia in the human: A study of histopathology, B-catenin and p53 expression and the role of inflammation. *Carcinogenesis* **2000**, *21*, 757–768. [CrossRef]
39. Amirmahani, F.; Ebrahimi, N.; Molaei, F.; Faghihkhorasani, F.; Goharrizi, K.J.; Mirtaghi, S.M.; Borjian-Boroujeni, M.; Hamblin, M.R. Approaches for the integration of big data in translational medicine: Single-cell and computational methods. *Ann. N. Y. Acad. Sci.* **2021**, *1493*, 3–28. [CrossRef] [PubMed]
40. Jovic, D.; Liang, X.; Zeng, H.; Lin, L.; Xu, F.; Luo, Y. Single-cell RNA sequencing technologies and applications: A brief overview. *Clin. Transl. Med.* **2022**, *12*, e694. [CrossRef]
41. Liu, S.; Zhao, Y.; Lu, S.; Zhang, T.; Lindenmeyer, M.T.; Nair, V.; Gies, S.E.; Wu, G.; Nelson, R.G.; Czogalla, J.; et al. Single-cell transcriptomics reveals a mechanosensitive injury signaling pathway in early diabetic nephropathy. *Genome. Med.* **2023**, *15*, 2. [CrossRef] [PubMed]
42. Zou, C.; Zan, X.; Jia, Z.; Zheng, L.; Gu, Y.; Liu, F.; Han, Y.; Xu, C.; Wu, A.; Zhi, Q. Crosstalk between alternative splicing and inflammatory bowel disease: Basic mechanisms, biotechnological progresses and future perspectives. *Clin. Transl. Med.* **2023**, *13*, e1479. [CrossRef] [PubMed]
43. Sun, Q.; Han, Y.; He, J.; Wang, J.; Ma, X.; Ning, Q.; Zhao, Q.; Jin, Q.; Yang, L.; Li, S.; et al. Long-read sequencing reveals the landscape of aberrant alternative splicing and novel therapeutic target in colorectal cancer. *Genome. Med.* **2023**, *15*, 76. [CrossRef] [PubMed]
44. Englund, G.; Jacobson, A.; Rorsman, F.; Artursson, P.; Kindmark, A.; Ronnblom, A. Efflux transporters in ulcerative colitis: Decreased expression of BCRP (ABCG2) and Pgp (ABCB1). *Inflamm. Bowel. Dis.* **2007**, *13*, 291–297. [CrossRef] [PubMed]
45. Hennenberg, E.M.; Eyking, A.; Reis, H.; Cario, E. MDR1A deficiency restrains tumor growth in murine colitis-associated carcinogenesis. *PLoS ONE* **2017**, *12*, e0180834. [CrossRef]
46. Min, M.; Peng, L.H.; Sun, G.; Guo, M.Z.; Qiu, Z.W.; Yang, Y.S. Aquaporin 8 expression is reduced and regulated by microRNAs in patients with ulcerative colitis. *Chin. Med. J.* **2013**, *126*, 1532–1537. [CrossRef]
47. Zhao, D.; Qin, D.; Yin, L.; Yang, Q. Integrated Bioinformatics Analysis and Experimental Verification of Immune Cell Infiltration and the Related Core Genes in Ulcerative Colitis. *Pharmgenomics Pers. Med.* **2023**, *16*, 629–643. [CrossRef]
48. Fujino, S.; Andoh, A.; Bamba, S.; Ogawa, A.; Hata, K.; Araki, Y.; Bamba, T.; Fujiyama, Y. Increased expression of interleukin 17 in inflammatory bowel disease. *Gut* **2003**, *52*, 65–70. [CrossRef]
49. Li, J.; Tian, H.; Jiang, H.J.; Han, B. Interleukin-17 SNPs and serum levels increase ulcerative colitis risk: A meta-analysis. *World. J. Gastroenterol.* **2014**, *20*, 15899–15909. [CrossRef]

50. Buran, T.; Batir, M.B.; Cam, F.S.; Kasap, E.; Collu, F.; Celebi, H.B.G.; Sahin, M. Molecular analyses of ADAMTS-1, -4, -5, and IL-17 a cytokine relationship in patients with ulcerative colitis. *BMC Gastroenterol.* **2023**, *23*, 345. [CrossRef]
51. Bunte, K.; Beikler, T. Th17 Cells and the IL-23/IL-17 Axis in the Pathogenesis of Periodontitis and Immune-Mediated Inflammatory Diseases. *Int. J. Mol. Sci.* **2019**, *20*, 3394. [CrossRef] [PubMed]
52. Jiang, P.; Zheng, C.; Xiang, Y.; Malik, S.; Su, D.; Xu, G.; Zhang, M. The involvement of TH17 cells in the pathogenesis of IBD. *Cytokine Growth Factor Rev.* **2023**, *69*, 28–42. [CrossRef] [PubMed]
53. Guo, X.; Rao, J.N.; Liu, L.; Zou, T.T.; Turner, D.J.; Bass, B.L.; Wang, J.Y. Regulation of adherens junctions and epithelial paracellular permeability: A novel function for polyamines. *Am. J. Physiol. Cell. Physiol.* **2003**, *285*, C1174–C1187. [CrossRef] [PubMed]
54. Samak, G.; Chaudhry, K.K.; Gangwar, R.; Narayanan, D.; Jaggar, J.H.; Rao, R. Calcium/Ask1/MKK7/JNK2/c-Src signalling cascade mediates disruption of intestinal epithelial tight junctions by dextran sulfate sodium. *Biochem. J.* **2015**, *465*, 503–515. [CrossRef]
55. Chelakkot, C.; Ghim, J.; Rajasekaran, N.; Choi, J.S.; Kim, J.H.; Jang, M.H.; Shin, Y.K.; Suh, P.G.; Ryu, S.H. Intestinal Epithelial Cell-Specific Deletion of PLD2 Alleviates DSS-Induced Colitis by Regulating Occludin. *Sci. Rep.* **2017**, *7*, 1573. [CrossRef]
56. Xiao, Y.; Lian, H.; Zhong, X.S.; Krishnachaitanya, S.S.; Cong, Y.; Dashwood, R.H.; Savidge, T.C.; Powell, D.W.; Liu, X.; Li, Q. Matrix metalloproteinase 7 contributes to intestinal barrier dysfunction by degrading tight junction protein Claudin-7. *Front. Immunol.* **2022**, *13*, 1020902. [CrossRef]

MDPI AG
Grosspeteranlage 5
4052 Basel
Switzerland
Tel.: +41 61 683 77 34

Biomedicines Editorial Office
E-mail: biomedicines@mdpi.com
www.mdpi.com/journal/biomedicines

www.ingramcontent.com/pod-product-compliance
Lightning Source LLC
Chambersburg PA
CBHW061616220926
51850CB00005B/521
* 9 7 8 3 7 2 5 8 6 3 9 4 5 *